Immunology and Liver

FALK SYMPOSIUM 70

Immunology and Liver

EDITED BY

K.-H. Meyer zum Büschenfelde
I. Medizinische Klinik und
Poliklinik der Universität Mainz
Langenbeckstr. 1
W-6500 Mainz 1
Germany

J.H. Hoofnagle
National Institutes of Health
Department of Health and Human Services
Division of Digestive Diseases and Nutrition
Building 31, Room 9A23
Bethesda
MD 28092
USA

M. Manns
Abteilung für Gastroenterologie und Hepatologie
Zentrum Innere Medizin
Medizinische Hochschule Hannover
Konstanty-Gutschow-Str. 8
W-3000 Hannover 61
Germany

Proceedings of the 70th Falk Symposium held in Basel, Switzerland, October 18–20, 1992

KLUWER ACADEMIC PUBLISHERS
DORDRECHT / BOSTON / LONDON

Distributors

for the United States and Canada: Kluwer Academic Publishers, PO Box 358, Accord Station, Hingham, MA 02018-0358, USA
for all other countries: Kluwer Academic Publishers Group, Distribution Center, PO Box 322, 3300 AH Dordrecht, The Netherlands

A catalogue record for this book is available from the British Library

ISBN 0-7923-8830-5

Library of Congress Cataloging-in-Publication Data

Falk Symposium, 70th (1992 : Basel, Switzerland)
Immunology and liver : proceedings of the 70th Falk Symposium held in Basel, Switzerland, October 18-20, 1992 / Falk Symposium 70 ; edited by K.-H. Meyer zum Büschenfelde, J.H. Hoofnagle, M. Manns.
p. cm.
Includes bibliographical references and index.
ISBN 0-7923-8830-5 (casebound)
1. Liver--Immunology--Congresses. I. Hoofnagle, Jay H. II. Manns, Marianne. III. Title.
[DNLM: 1. Liver--immunology--congresses. 2. Liver Diseases--immunology--congresses. 3. Autoimmune Diseases--immunology. WI 700 F191i 1992]
RC846.9.F35 1992
616.3'62079--dc20
DNLM/DLC
for Library of Congress 93-23189
CIP

Copyright

Published in the United Kingdom by Kluwer Academic Publishers, PO Box 55, Lancaster, UK.

Kluwer Academic Publishers BV incorporates the publishing programmes of D. Reidel, Martinus Nijhoff, Dr W. Junk and MTP Press.

Typeset by Lasertext Ltd, Stretford, Manchester
Printed and bound in Great Britain by Hartnolls Ltd., Bodmin, Cornwall.

Contents

Introduction xi

List of Principal Contributors xiii

SECTION I: BASIC IMMUNOLOGY

1 Production and persistence of antigenic peptide/MHC class II complexes in human antigen-presenting cells
A. Lanzavecchia and C. Watts 3

2 Accessory molecules in T lymphocyte activation by antigens and by superantigens
B. Fleischer 9

SECTION II: IMMUNOLOGY OF HEPATITIS B VIRUS INFECTION

3 The humoral immune response to hepatitis B virus
A. Alberti, D. Cavalletto, L. Chemello, L. Benvegnù, F. Belussi, P. Pontisso and M. Levrero 17

4 Role of immunological tolerance in chronic hepatitis B infection
D. R. Milich and T. Maruyama 26

5 Cellular immune reactions to hepatitis B core antigen
C. Ferrari, F. Fiaccadori and F. V. Chisari 39

6 Cellular immune reactions to hepatitis B envelope antigens
M. Paroli, A. Franco, G. De Petrillo, R. Benevenuto and V. Barnaba 48

7 Immunology of hepadnavirus infection in woodchucks
P. J. Cote 52

8 Genetic variability of hepatitis B virus: potential clinical implications
D. Kremsdorf and C. Brechot 61

SECTION III: IMMUNOLOGY IN HEPATITIS A AND C

9 Immunopathogenesis of hepatitis A virus infection
A. Vallbracht, Y.-D. Stierhof and B. Fleischer 85

10 T-lymphocyte response to hepatitis C virus
S. Abrignani, R. Pileri, D. Unutzmaz, G. Kuo, M. Houghton, M. R. Brunetto, F. Bonino and M. A. Minutello 90

11 Immunopathology of hepatitis C
M. A. Gerber and S. N. Thung 96

12 Immunology and autoimmunity in hepatitis C
F. B. Bianchi, M. Lenzi, F. Cassani, G. Ballardini, F. Giostra, L. Muratori, M. Cataleta, R. Francesconi and D. Zauli 102

13 Clonal analysis of human lymphocyte-B responses to hepatitis C virus structural and non-structural regions
M. U. Mondelli and A. Cerino 105

SECTION IV: CYTOKINES IN THE TREATMENT OF VIRUS-INDUCED LIVER DISEASES

14 Actions of cytokines on immune response and virus replication – an overview
M. Peters 117

15 Innovative therapies for chronic hepatitis B
J. H. Hoofnagle 120

16 The role of interferon-α in virus elimination: viral inhibitors resulting in persistent infection
G. R. Foster and H. C. Thomas 131

SECTION V: MECHANISMS RESPONSIBLE FOR AUTOIMMUNITY

17 Immunoprotection, immunopathology or tolerance – a question of balance
R. M. Zinkernagel 139

18 Autoantibodies as diagnostic markers, probes in cell biology and reporters of cellular activation
E. M. Tan, H. Imai and E. K. L. Chan 145

19 Applications of molecular biology to the analysis of autoantigens
K. F. Sullivan 152

20 Immunological derangements in autoimmunity
N. R. Rose 166

SECTION VI: AUTOIMMUNE CHRONIC ACTIVE HEPATITIS

21 Clinical spectrum and heterogeneity of autoimmune hepatitis: an overview
I. G. McFarlane 179

22 Nuclear antigens in autoimmune hepatitis
M. Nishioka 193

23 Cytoskeleton antibodies in chronic active hepatitis
P. Kurki 206

24 Anti-liver cytosol antibodies in hepatology: autoimmune hepatitis, viral hepatitis C and graft-versus-host disease
N. Abuaf, C. Johanet, E. Soulie, J. Loeper and J.-C. Homberg 215

25 The asialoglycoprotein receptor (ASGPR) as hepatic autoantigen
U. Treichel and T. Poralla 227

26 Autoimmune hepatitis: cellular immune reactions
D. Vergani and G. Mieli-Vergani 233

27 Immunogenetics of autoimmune chronic active hepatitis
E. L. Krawitt and R. J. Albertini 240

28 Therapy of idiopathic autoimmune chronic active hepatitis
B. Combes and W. C. Maddrey 250

SECTION VII: AUTOIMMUNITY AGAINST CYTOCHROME P450 ENZYMES

29 The cytochrome P450 supergene family: a class of autoantigens
E. F. Johnson 259

30 Cytochrome P450 IID6 in autoimmune hepatitis
M. D. Manns 269

31 Mechanisms of adverse drug reactions directed against cytochromes P450
P. Beaune, M. Bourdi, S. Lecoeur, P. Lopez-Garcia, P. Dansette, D. Mansuy, C. Belloc, J.-C. Gautier, D. Larrey, D. Pessayre, R. Catinot and F. Ballet 277

32 Identification and characterization of protein adducts of reactive metabolites by the use of specific antibodies
L. R. Pohl 284

SECTION VIII: PRIMARY SCLEROSING CHOLANGITIS

33 Advances in primary sclerosing cholangitis
R. H. Wiesner 295

34 Immunohistology of primary sclerosing cholangitis
P. Van Eyken and V. J. Desmet 307

35 The immunogenetics of primary sclerosing cholangitis
R. W. Chapman 318

36 Antineutrophil cytoplasmic antibodies in primary sclerosing cholangitis and ulcerative colitis
A. Vidrich and S. R. Targan 324

37 Animal models of sclerosing cholangitis: exploring mechanisms of hepatobiliary inflammation associated with intestinal injury
R. B. Sartor and S. N. Lichtman 330

SECTION IX: PRIMARY BILIARY CIRRHOSIS

38 Primary biliary cirrhosis: definition and epidemiological features
S. Sherlock 341

39 Clinical relevance of different types of mitochondrial antibodies in primary biliary cirrhosis
P. A. Berg and R. Klein 350

40 Molecular basis of mitochondrial autoantigens associated with acyltransferases
M. F. Bassendine, J. M. Palmer, J. Quinn, D. E. J. Jones, A. G. Diamond, O. F. W. James and S. J. Yeaman 361

41 T cell biology and cell surface expression of PDC-E2 in primary biliary cirrhosis
M. E. Gershwin, J. Van de Water, P. S. C. Leung and R. Coppel 373

42 Immunogenetic influences in primary biliary cirrhosis
P. T. Donaldson, D. G. Doherty, J. A. Underhill and R. Williams 383

43 Nuclear autoantibodies in primary biliary cirrhosis
I. R. Mackay, M. J. Rowley and S. F. Whittingham 397

44 Animal models of primary biliary cirrhosis
D. L. Thiele and F. H. Williams 410

45 Disturbed lymphokine production in patients with primary biliary cirrhosis: a functional defect of T lymphocytes?
G. R. Pape, G. Messer, U. Spengler, M.-C. Jung and E. H. Weiss 423

46 Antigen expression and presentation on bile duct epithelium
J. Neuberger, R. Ayres, A. Strain and R. Joplin 435

47 Can enterobacterial antigens induce a primary biliary cirrhosis?
U. Hopf and R. Stemerowicz 447

48 Ursodeoxycholic acid alters hepatocyte membrane structure and function: a therapeutic approach?
U. Leuschner, S. Güldütuna, T. You, S. Bhatti, G. Zimmer and H. P. Dienes 459

49 Therapeutic strategies which interfere with the immune system
R. Poupon, Y. Calmus and R. E. Poupon 462

Index 469

Introduction

The immune system is one of the body's most important organ systems responsible for maintaining the integrity of the organism. This mainly takes place via the immune system's primary function of being able to distinguish between 'self' and 'non-self'. Pathogens that penetrate the organism from outside can thus be identified as foreign and repelled. We are increasingly becoming familiar with the mechanisms by which the immune system functions. This makes it easier for us to understand pathological reactions which, for example in viral infections, mediate the destruction of an organ. In hepatitis infections of the liver, we have had to recognize that it is not the virus itself, but above all the immune reaction to virus-infected cells, that is responsible for the destruction of tissue. On the other hand, autoimmune diseases are occupying an ever greater part of the medical field. Autoimmune diseases are understood to mean pathological processes that are attributable to the immune system identifying parts of its own body as foreign and reacting against them. Autoimmune diseases of the liver are, for one, directed against hepatocytes, i.e. the main cells of the liver. This is the case in so-called autoimmune hepatitis. On the other hand, autoimmunological processes can be directed against the biliary tract, above all against the epithelia of the bile ducts. This can then lead to the development of primary biliary cirrhosis or primary sclerosing cholangitis. There is also a broad range of drugs that cause toxic damage to the liver. Directly hepatotoxic drugs reveal a linearity between the dose taken and the extent of damage to the liver cells. Another aspect is the immune-allergic side-effects caused by drugs. As a general rule, there has usually been prior drug intake, and an allergic predisposition mediates so-called drug-induced hepatitis. After all, the liver itself is not only the target of immunological reactions, but is an essential and integral part of the physiological functions of the immune system. A large number of complement factors are thus produced by the liver. The complement system is a major component of the non-antigen-specific immune system. Kupffer cells in the liver represent a major part of the reticuloendothelial system. Their inability to exercise their pathogenic function in advanced hepatic disease has major consequences for the immune system of the body as a whole.

The Falk Symposium No. 70 directed its focus on current developments in the field of immunological research involving the liver. This concerns the participation of the immune system in acute and chronic viral infections of the liver, but also the diagnosis, pathophysiology and therapy of autoimmune liver diseases. It is becoming increasingly clear that the immunogenetic background is decisive for the manifestation and course of hepatitis. This growing knowledge was also reflected in the symposium. At the end, discussions were held on the current therapeutic principles of the pertinent diseases, principles which increasingly serve as an interface for converting pathophysiological knowledge into therapeutic action, not least by modulation of the immune system. While immunosuppressive therapy represents an *a priori* immunological treatment in autoimmune hepatitis, the action of interferons in chronic viral hepatitis can increasingly be attributed to an interaction with the immune system. Finally, increasing importance is being attached to findings that suggest an influence of ursodeoxycholic acid on the immune system in the treatment of primary biliary cirrhosis or primary sclerosing cholangitis.

We especially wish to thank Dr Herbert Falk for his more than generous support which made it possible to have such an excellent symposium with a wonderful group of outstanding scientists in the field of liver diseases and basic immunology.

List of Principal Contributors

S. ABRIGNANI
Immunobiology Department
Immunobiology Research Institute
Siena (IRIS)
Via Fiorentina 1
I-53100 Siena
Italy

A. ALBERTI
Clinica Medica II
Via Giustiniani, 2
I-35126 Padova
Italy

V. BARNABA
Istituto di Clinica Medica
Via del Policlinico 155
I-00161 Roma
Italy

M. F. BASSENDINE
Medical Molecular Biology Group
Medical School
University of Newcastle upon Tyne
Newcastle upon Tyne NE2 4HH
UK

P. BEAUNE
Laboratoire de Biochimie Metabolique
et Pharmacologique
INSERM U75
CHU Necker
156 Rue de Vaugirard
F-75730 Paris Cedex 15
France

P. A. BERG
Abteilung für Innere Medizin II
Medizinische Universitätsklinik
Otfried-Müller-Str. 10
W-7400 Tübingen 1
Germany

F. B. BIANCHI
Istituto de Clinica Medica Generale e
Terapia Medicale
Policlinico S Orsole
Università di Bologna
Via Massarenti 9
I-40138 Bologna
Italy

C. BRECHOT
Institut Pasteur
28 Rue du Dr Roux
F-75724 Paris Cedex 15
France

R. W. CHAPMAN
Department of Gastroenterology
John Radcliffe Hospital
Headley Way
Headington
Oxford OX3 9DU
UK

B. COMBES
Internal Medicine F4.306
UT Southwestern Medical Center
5323 Harry Hines Blvd
Dallas
TX 75235-8887
USA

P. J. COTE
Georgetown University
Division of Molecular Virology and
Immunology
5640 Fishers Lane
Rockville
MD 20852
USA

V. DESMET
Universitair Ziekenhuisen Leuven
Sint Rafael
Pathol Ontleedkunde B
Minderbroedersstraat 12
B-3000 Leuven
Belgium

P. DONALDSON
Liver Unit
King's College Hospital
Denmark Hill
London SE5 8RX
UK

C. FERRARI
Cattedra Malattie Infective
Università di Parma
Via Gramsci 14
I-43100 Parma
Italy

B. FLEISCHER
Abteilung für Pathophysiologie
I. Medizinische Klinik und Poliklinik der Universität Mainz
Langenbeckstr. 1
W-6500 Mainz 1
Germany

M. A. GERBER
Tulane University Medical Center
Department of Pathology
1430 Tulane Avenue
New Orleans
LA 70112-2699
USA

M. E. GERSHWIN
Division of Rheumatology/Allergy and Clinical Immunology TB 192
University of California at Davis
CA 95616
USA

J.-C. HOMBERG
Laboratoire Central d'Immunologie et d'Hématologie
Hopital Saint-Antoine
184 Rue du Faubourg Saint-Antoine
F-75571 Paris Cedex 12
France

J. H. HOOFNAGLE
National Institutes of Health
Department of Health and Human Services
Division of Digestive Diseases and Nutrition
Building 31, Room 9A23
Bethesda
MD 28092
USA

U. HOPF
Medizinische Klinik und Poliklinik
Universitäts-Klinikum Rudolf Virchow
Standort Charlottenburg
Spandauer Damm 130
W-1000 Berlin 19
Germany

E. F. JOHNSON
Department of Molecular and Experimental Medicine
Division of Biochemistry, NX-4
Scripps Institute
10666 North Torrey Pines Road
La Jolla
CA 90237
USA

E. L. KRAWITT
Department of Medicine
University of Vermont
Given C317
Burlington
VT 05405-0068
USA

P. KURKI
Department of Clinical Research
Sandoz Pharma Ltd
Vattuniemenkatu 8
SF-00210 Helsinki
Finland

A. LANZAVECCHIA
Basel Institute for Immunology
Grenzacher Str. 487
CH-4058 Basel
Switzerland

U. LEUSCHNER
Abteilung für Gastroenterologie
Zentrum der Inneren Medizin
Klinikum der Universität
Theodor-Stern-Kai 7
W-6000 Frankfurt 70
Germany

LIST OF PRINCIPAL CONTRIBUTORS

I. R. MACKAY
Centre for Molecular Biology and Medicine
Monash University
Clayton
Victoria 3168
Australia

M. MANNS
Abteilung für Gastroenterologie und Hepatologie
Zentrum Innere Medizin
Medizinische Hochschule Hannover
Konstanty-Gustschow-Str. 8
W-3000 Hannover 61
Germany

I. G. McFARLANE
Liver Unit
King's College Hospital
Denmark Hill
London
SE5 8RX
UK

K.-H. MEYER ZUM BÜSCHENFELDE
I. Medizinische Klinik und Poliklinik der Universität Mainz
Langenbeckstr. 1
W-6500 Mainz 1
Germany

D. R. MILICH
The Scripps Research Institute
Department of Molecular Biology, GA-1
10666 North Torrey Pines Road
La Jolla
CA 92037
USA

M. U. MONDELLI
Instituto di Malattie Infettive
IRCCS Policlinico S Matteo
viale Taramelli 5
I-27100 Pavia
Italy

J. M. NEUBERGER
Liver Unit
The Queen Elizabeth Hospital
Queen Elizabeth Medical Centre
Edgbaston
Birmingham B15 2TH
UK

M. NISHIOKA
Kagawa Medical School
1750-1, Ikenobe, Mik-cho
Kita-gun 1
Kagawa 761-07
Japan

G. R. PAPE
Medizinische Klinik II
Klinikum Grosshadern
Universität München
Marchioninistr. 15
W-8000 München 70
Germany

M. PETERS
Department of Internal Medicine
Washington University School of Medicine
660 South Euclid Avenue
St Louis
MO 63110
USA

L. R. POHL
Laboratory of Chemical Pharmacology
National Heart, Lung and Blood Institute
Building 10 Room 8N 115
Bethesda MD 20892
USA

R. POUPON
Service d'Hépato-Gastroenterologie
Hopital Saint-Antoine
184 rue du Faubourg Saint-Antoine
F-75571 Paris Cedex 12
France

N. R. ROSE
The John Hopkins University
Department of Immunology and Infectious Diseases
615 N Wolfe Street
Baltimore
MD 21205
USA

R. B. SARTOR
Division of Digestive Diseases
465 Burnett-Womack Building, CB #7080
University of North Carolina at Chapel Hill
Chapel Hill
NC 27599-7080
USA

S. SHERLOCK
Department of Surgery
Royal Free Hospital School of Medicine
Pond St
Hampstead
London NW3 2QG
UK

K. F. SULLIVAN
Department of Cell Biology MB6
Scripps Clinic and Research Foundation
10666 North Torrey Pines Road
La Jolla
CA 92037
USA

E. M. TAN
WM Keck Autoimmune Disease Center
Research Institute of Scripps Clinic, BCR 6
10666 North Torrey Pines Road
La Jolla
CA 92037
USA

S. R. TARGAN
Cedars-Sinai Medical Center
Suite D4063
8700 Beverly Blvd
Los Angeles
CA 90048
USA

D. THIELE
Department of Internal Medicine
UT Southwestern Medical School
5323 Harry Hines Blvd
Dallas
TX 75235
USA

H. C. THOMAS
St Mary's Hospital Medical School
Liver Unit
Praed Street
London W2 8SN
UK

U. TREICHEL
I. Medizinische Klinik und Poliklinik der Universität Mainz
Langenbeckstr. 1
W-6500 Mainz 1
Germany

A. VALLBRACHT
Virologie/FB 2
Universität Bremen
Bibliothekstr. 1
W-2800 Bremen 33
Germany

D. VERGANI
Departments of Immunology and Child Health
King's College School of Medicine and Dentistry
Bessemer Road
London SE5 9PJ
UK

R. H. WIESNER
Gastroenterology Unit
Mayo Clinic and Foundation
200 First Street SW
Rochester
MN 55905
USA

R. M. ZINKERNAGEL
Institute for Experimental Pathology
Department of Pathology
University of Zurich
CH-8091 Zurich
Switzerland

Section I
Basic Immunology

1
Production and persistence of antigenic peptide/MHC class II complexes in human antigen-presenting cells

A. LANZAVECCHIA and C. WATTS

INTRODUCTION

It is well established that, in order to be recognized by helper T cells, soluble antigen has to be captured by antigen-presenting cells (APC) and processed into peptides that bind to MHC class II molecules. Immunoglobulins (Ig) drive efficient antigen capture in antigen-specific B cells and in FcR^+ APC, delivering antigen–antibody complexes as the substrates for proteolytic processing (reviewed in ref. 1). The biosynthetic pathway of class II molecules intersects the endocytic pathway[2,3] and at this level the newly synthesized class II molecules have access to peptides derived from processing of incoming antigens (Fig. 1). This encounter is facilitated by the sorting and protecting action of the Invariant chain[4–6]. Peptide/class II complexes are then transported to the cell surface. Once on the cell surface, class II molecules recycle in peripheral endosomes[7].

One can thus envisage two ways by which peptides can bind to class II molecules in living cells: first they can bind to newly synthesized molecules on their secretory pathway, second they can bind to mature molecules during recycling. Indeed some surface class II molecules are empty and therefore there is some binding capacity[8]; in addition it has been suggested that this capacity may be further increased by a mechanism of peptide exchange[9,10].

While there has been no general consensus on which of these two pathways may be predominant for peptide loading, it is clear that the two mechanisms of loading would lead to very different kinetics of antigen presentation. On the one hand exchange would lead to rapid increase in complex formation by providing a higher capacity but, in the absence of a continuous supply of antigen, would lead to a rapid loss of the antigenic complexes by exchange with self peptides. On the other hand, loading on newly synthesized molecules

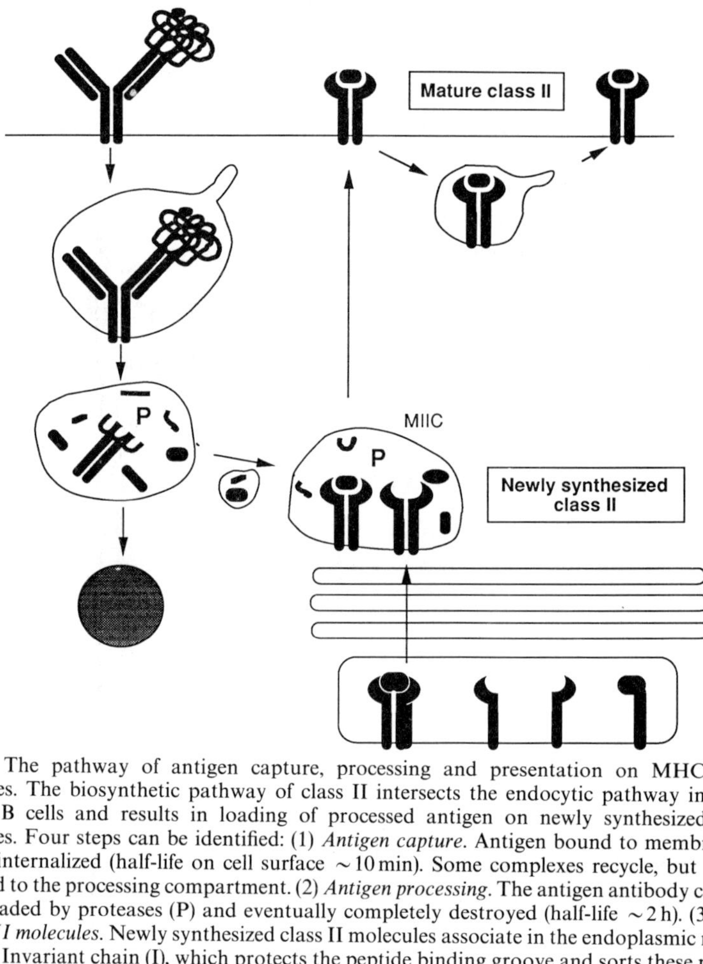

Fig. 1 The pathway of antigen capture, processing and presentation on MHC class II molecules. The biosynthetic pathway of class II intersects the endocytic pathway in antigen-specific B cells and results in loading of processed antigen on newly synthesized class II molecules. Four steps can be identified: (1) *Antigen capture.* Antigen bound to membrane Ig is rapidly internalized (half-life on cell surface ~10 min). Some complexes recycle, but some are delivered to the processing compartment. (2) *Antigen processing.* The antigen antibody complexes are degraded by proteases (P) and eventually completely destroyed (half-life ~2 h). (3) *Binding to class II molecules.* Newly synthesized class II molecules associate in the endoplasmic reticulum with the Invariant chain (I), which protects the peptide binding groove and sorts these molecules in a specialized compartment (MIIC). Here the I chain is removed by proteases and newly synthesized class II molecules with free peptide binding sites come into contact with processed antigen. The mechanism of this intersection has not been yet clarified and may involve specific signals for vesicle fusion. This 'window of opportunity' decides which antigenic peptides can be loaded on class II molecules. (4) *Display of stable complexes.* The newly formed complexes are transported to the cell surface from which they can recycle in the peripheral endosomal compartment. The half-life of the peptide/class II complexes is the same as the half-life of the class II molecules themselves (~30 h). A small fraction (~2%) of surface class II molecules are empty and can bind exogenous peptides, but not processed antigen, since they do not re-enter in the processing compartment

would lead to a more gradual increase in complexes that may be preserved for a longer time.

We have studied in human B cells the loading of MHC class II molecules with antigenic peptides, as well as the stability of peptide/class II complexes, and conclude that in physiological conditions class II molecules bind peptides only once during biosynthesis and these peptides remain bound irreversibly for their lifetime.

PROCESSED ANTIGEN BINDS TO NEWLY SYNTHESIZED CLASS II MOLECULES

When antigen-specific B cells are pulsed with antigen, stimulatory complexes appear only after a lag of approximately 60 min, indicating that antigen processing and class II association requires a much longer time than that taken by class II molecules to recycle in peripheral endosomes[11]. Using the same antigen-specific B cells we developed a biochemical assay that would detect the loading of processed antigen fragments on class II molecules.

When antigen-specific B cells are pulsed in the cold with [^{125}I]antigen and transferred to 37°C, it is possible to follow antigen degradation and the appearance of complexes containing iodinated peptides bound to class II molecules. These peptide/class II complexes appear at approximately 60 min, increase with time and are still present after 40 h (Davidson *et al.*, unpublished), indicating that they are very stable. Using this biochemical readout to measure loading of class II molecules with processed antigen, and lectin chromatography to distinguish newly synthesized from mature class II molecules, we found that iodinated antigen fragments bind only to the newly synthesized class II molecules[12]. In the same experiments exogenously added peptides bound preferentially to surface class II molecules. Thus, while surface class II molecules have some binding capacity for peptides, they cannot bind processed antigen, probably because they cannot re-enter the processing compartment.

IRREVERSIBLE BINDING OF PEPTIDES TO CLASS II MOLECULES IN LIVING CELLS

Our results indicated that peptide exchange on mature class II molecules is not involved in binding processed antigenic peptides, but still did not rule out the possibility that peptide exchange may take place during recycling of mature class II molecules. We reasoned that if there is peptide exchange the half-life of complexes should be much lower than the half-life of class II molecules. If there is no exchange, the half-lives should be the same.

We therefore measured the half-life of peptide class II complexes and related it to the half-lives of the class II molecules themselves[13]. Various APC were pulsed with different concentrations of synthetic peptides corresponding to known T cell epitopes and at different time-points the level of stimulatory complexes was measured in a T cell proliferation assay. Four different epitopes were tested and a similarly long half-life of approximately 25 h was estimated on EBV-B cells, activated T cells and fresh peripheral blood mononuclear cells.

An independent and direct estimate of complex stability was obtained by measuring the half-life of radioiodinated peptide/MHC complexes. The results were in good agreement with those of functional assays, i.e. ~30 h. In addition we showed that preformed peptide class II complexes cannot be displaced in living cells by adding high concentrations of a competing peptide.

Thus, both functional and biochemical assays using different epitopes and different APC indicate that peptide/MHC class II complexes are very stable in living cells with a surprisingly reproducible half-life of ~30 h. This suggested that the dissociation of the complexes might be negligible, and their persistence might be determined essentially by the lifetime of the class II molecules themselves. Indeed we found that the half-life of class II molecules in our EBV-B cells is ~30 h and therefore not significantly different from the half-life of the complexes. We conclude that in living cells antigenic peptides are bound irreversibly to class II molecules, are not displaced under physiological conditions and their turnover reflects the turnover of class II molecules themselves.

A DYNAMIC VIEW OF ANTIGEN UPTAKE PROCESSING AND PRESENTATION

Our results allow assessment of the relative importance of loading during biosynthesis versus peptide exchange on mature molecules. Two experimental findings indicate that in human APC the major pathway is the biosynthetic one. First, processed antigen binds to newly synthesized class II molecules. Second, the half-life of peptide/class II complexes is the same as that of class II molecules themselves, indicating that the molecules are not reused.

An important working principle emerges from these results: an APC is defined not as a cell with high levels of surface class II molecules, but as one that is actually synthesizing these molecules. Class II biosynthesis is tightly regulated in APC such as B cells, macrophages and dendritic cells. Following appropriate stimulation of synthesis by lymphokines increased numbers of MHC molecules will be synthesized and made available for binding incoming antigens. The pre-existing MHC molecules on the cell surface may indeed not only be useless, but may even play a negative role by distracting the CD4 molecules or even the T cell receptor from the productive interaction.

We suggest that the persistence of peptide/MHC complexes is a critical factor for the immune response, since it allows the APC to accumulate processed antigen and keep the memory of antigen encountered over a short time window, allowing presentation at a distant site perhaps several days later. This is illustrated by the behaviour of dendritic cells (reviewed in ref. 14) that pick up and process antigen in non-lymphoid organs (where they have high antigen-capturing capacity and have high class II synthesis) and then move to the T cell areas of secondary lymphoid organs, where they cease class II synthesis, acquire co-stimulatory capacity and wait for antigen-specific T cells. Thus dendritic cells can be viewed as dedicated APC that pick up and process antigen in the periphery and present it at a distance even several days later, a function which is critically dependent on the stability of peptide/class II complexes.

Another example that illustrates the relationship between class II biosynthesis and antigen-presenting function comes from activated T cells. It is known that human activated T cells are class II positive and can present peptide antigens and even protein antigens if these bind to cell surface receptors[15], but have been always considered to be inefficient APC, since long-term T cell lines are unable to present native protein antigens. In the light of these new findings we have now tested the antigen-presenting capacity of T cells and found that recently activated T cells that synthesize class II molecules are indeed capable of presenting soluble antigens (A.L. and C.W., unpublished results). We interpret these findings as an indication that class II biosynthesis is one of the limiting factors in presentation of antigen by activated T cells. Thus, in the case of T cells soon after the activation, presentation of soluble antigen may well play a physiological role in the immune response.

Acknowledgements

We thank Stephane Demotz and Paolo Dellabona for reading the manuscript. The Basel Institute for Immunology was founded and is supported by F. Hoffmann-La Roche Ltd, Basel, Switzerland. This work was partially supported by the Wellcome Trust and the Medical Research Council.

References

1. Lanzavecchia A. Receptor mediated antigen uptake and its effect on antigen presentation to class II restricted T lymphocytes. Annu Rev Immunol. 1990;8:773–93.
2. Cresswell P. Intracellular class II HLA antigens are accessible to transferrin-neuraminidase conjugates internalised by receptor-mediated endocytosis. Proc Natl Acad Sci USA. 1985;82:8188–92.
3. Neefjes JJ, Stollorz V, Peters PJ, Geuze HJ, Ploegh HL. The biosynthetic pathway of MHC class II but not class I molecules intersects the endocytic route. Cell. 1990;61:171–83.
4. Bakke O, Dobberstein B. MHC class II-associated Invariant chain contains a sorting signal for endosomal compartments. Cell. 1990;63:707–13.
5. Lotteau L, Teyton L, Peleraux A, Nilsson T, Karlsson L, Schmid SL, Quaranta V, Peterson PA. Intracellular transport of class II MHC molecules directed by Invariant chain. Nature. 1990;348:600–5.
6. Roche PA, Cresswell P. Invariant chain association with HLA-DR molecules inhibits immunogenic peptide binding. Nature. 1990;345:615–18.
7. Reid PA, Watts C. Cell surface MHC glycoproteins cycle through primaquine sensitive intracellular compartments. Nature. 1990;346:655–7.
8. Shimonkevitz RJ, Kappler J, Marrack P, Grey HM. Antigen recognition by H2-restricted T cells. I. Cell free antigen processing. J. Exp. Med. 1983;158:303–16.
9. Harding CW, Roof RW, Unanue ER. Turnover of Ia-peptide complexes facilitated in viable antigen presenting cells: biosynthetic turnover of Ia versus peptide exchange. Proc Natl Acad Sci USA. 1989;86:4230–4.
10. Adorini L, Appella E, Doria G, Cardinaux F, Nagy ZA. Competition for antigen presentation in living cells involves exchange of peptides bound by class II mHC molecules. Nature. 1989;342:800–3.
11. Roosnek E, Demotz S, Corradin G, Lanzavecchia A. Kinetics of MHC–antigen complex formation on antigen presenting cells. J Immunol. 1988;140:4079–82.
12. Davidson HW, Reid PA, Lanzavecchia A, Watts C. Processed antigen binds to newly synthesized class II molecules in antigen-specific B lymphocytes. Cell. 1991;67:105–16.

13. Lanzavecchia A, Reid P, Watts C. Irreversible association of peptides with class II MHC molecules in living cells. Nature. 1992;357:249–52.
14. Steinman RM. The dendritic cell system and its role in immunogenicity. Annu Rev Immunol. 1991;9:271–96.
15. Lanzavecchia A, Roosnek E, Gregory T, Berman P, Abrignani S. T cells can present antigen such as HIV gp120 targeted to their own surface molecules. Nature. 1988;334:530–2.

2
Accessory molecules in T lymphocyte activation by antigens and by superantigens

B. FLEISCHER

INTRODUCTION

Superantigens are a class of molecules that stimulate T cells by closely mimicking recognition of specific antigen. Prototypes are the enterotoxins produced by *Staphylococcus aureus*. They trigger the T cells by crosslinking variable parts of the T cell receptor with MHC class II molecules on stimulating cells. Although there are many similarities between T lymphocyte activation by antigen recognition and by superantigen binding several fundamental differences exist.

ANTIGEN RECOGNITION BY T LYMPHOCYTES

The physiological ligand for the T cell antigen receptor is a processed peptide presented by MHC molecules. Recently it has been possible to quantitate the number of an antigenic peptide within a cell that can be recognized by its corresponding T cell. A viral peptide in an infected cell is present in approximately 300 copies[1], a self peptide in a tumour cell in approximately 100 copies[2]. Because only a fraction of these peptides will find the appropriate MHC molecule and will be transported to the surface of the cell, it is reasonable to assume that far less than 0.1% of a given MHC molecule will carry the same peptide. Thus the chance of a T cell finding several specific peptides together on an antigen-presenting cell is very low, and one might speculate that very few T receptors, probably much less than 10 molecules, have to be engaged to trigger the T cell.

This surprising sensitivity of the T cell response is due to the requirement for additional so-called co-stimulatory signals derived from the antigen-presenting cells[3–5]. In addition to the antigen-binding T cell receptor and its associated CD3 complex, other cell surface molecules contribute to transmembranes signalling in T cells. The CD4 and CD8 molecules associate with the T cell receptor by binding to non-polymorphic sites of MHC class II and class I proteins respectively, and bring the associated tyrosine $p56^{lck}$ in the vicinity of the T cell receptor. Other co-receptor molecules are the 50 kDa glycoprotein CD2 binding to LFA-3 (CD58) on the antigen-presenting cell, LFA-1 binding to ICAM-1, -2, and -3, and CD28 and CTLA-4 binding to the B7/BB1 antigen. It is remarkable that the expression of LFA-3 and ICAM-1 is up-regulated by activation on several different cell types. This is particularly true for the B7/BB1 antigen, a 46 kDa glycoprotein with very restricted expression. It is not expressed on resting macrophages or B cells but strongly up-regulated after stimulation of these cells. It appears to be present constitutively on dendritic cells. More recent observations show that these co-stimulatory molecules are differentially required for T cell activation. For instance, if naive $CD4^+$ T cells are activated by anti-CD3 antibody, LFA-1-mediated adhesion or signalling appears to be more important than adhesion via CD2 or CD28. In contrast, in preactivated T cells or T cell clones CD2 and CD28 or CTLA-4 appear to be more stringently required[6]. Whether this also holds true for antigen-specific stimulation is still unclear. Furthermore, it has been hypothesized that whereas many of these molecules enhance the delivery of the antigen-specific signal, a few of these molecules provide a distinct additional signal that induces growth and prevents the induction of anergy or tolerance in the responding cell[7]. Of special importance for this latter are the B7 molecules binding to CD28 and CTLA-4[5] and the heat-stable antigen that has been described in the mouse[8].

The hypothesis has been put forward that a major mechanism of tolerance to self tissue may be a general lack of co-stimulatory ligands on tissue cells in contrast to haemopoietic cells[5]. One could therefore speculate that, in turn, the abnormal expression of such molecules could render a tissue cell recognizable for autoreactive T cells.

Blocking studies with monoclonal antibodies have indicated that several of these molecules are mutually required. For instance defects in CD2-mediated adhesion can be compensated by adhesion via LFA-1 and vice-versa[9,10]. Thus the importance of these co-receptors for a T cell response depends on the expression of the respective ligands on the antigen-presenting cell and signals given via one molecule may be replaced by another.

T CELL ACTIVATION BY SUPERANTIGENS

Besides the antigen peptide–MHC molecule complex there is only one other naturally occurring class of ligands for the T cell receptor: the superantigens[11,12]. This is the designation of a group of molecules that have in common an extremely potent activating effect on T lymphocytes of several species. This designation originates from the finding that the mechanism of T lymphocyte stimulation closely mimics the recognition of specific antigen: superantigens crosslink variable parts of the T cell antigen receptor with MHC class II molecules on accessory or target cells. This is true for $CD4^+$, $CD8^+$ and $\gamma\delta^+$ T cells[13]. Toxic shock syndrome toxin-1 of *Staphylococcus aureus* is the prototype superantigen. The superantigens known so far are produced by infectious pathogens, bacteria (*S. aureus* and *S. pyogenes*, both Gram-positive cocci), a mycoplasma (*Mycoplasma arthritidis*) and by murine retroviruses (mouse mammary tumour viruses). It is very surprising that the same molecular mechanism of T cell stimulation has been independently produced three times in evolution by very distinct pathogens. It is thus quite possible that other superantigens will be detected that are not related to these three families of superantigens. In the past few years several other molecules have been reported to have properties characteristic of superantigens. However, in most cases there is only indirect evidence that these molecules are indeed superantigenic; in other cases it is even unlikely. In several cases the superantigenicity comes from contaminations[12]. A major problem with all preparations of staphylococcal or streptococcal proteins is the risk that trace contaminations of extremely potent exotoxins can cause a dramatic mitogenic effect, although they are not detectable by any biochemical assay.

The enormous potency of superantigens is reflected by the biological consequences found when superantigens are introduced into the body. Most prominent are shock-like symptoms caused by an effect of these molecules on T cells, leading to a massive release of lymphokines and monokines. Another important feature of these molecules is the induction of immunosuppression *in vivo*. Although the underlying molecular mechanisms are not completely clear, it is accepted that death of T cells occurs after an initial stimulation *in vivo*[14,15].

As is the case with specific recognition of nominal antigen, the T lymphocyte uses additional adhesion molecules in the response to superantigens. Best studied are T cell responses to the toxins of Gram-positive cocci. Most important appear to be adhesions via CD2 or LFA-1. Monoclonal antibody inhibition studies showed that these adhesions are alternatively required for the stimulation of the T cells if low toxin concentrations are used[10]. This requirement can be completely overcome at high, probably unphysiological, concentrations. Co-stimulatory activity has also been reported for adhesion of VLA-4 to its ligand VCAM-1[16].

Antibodies to CD4 inhibit the response of mouse T cells to staphylococcal enterotoxins and to the retroviral proteins[17]. Nevertheless, $CD4^-$ T cell hybridomas respond to the toxins and the transfection of CD4 into these cells does not enhance the response[18]. Human T cell responses to SE are generally not inhibited by anti-CD4 or anti-CD8 in bulk culture. Only a few human $CD4^+$ T cell clones are weakly inhibitable by anti-CD4. Anti-CD8 never inhibits the response of human or murine $CD8^+$ T cells to the toxins. Furthermore, $CD8^+$ cells easily lyse MHC class I negative cells such as Daudi cells in the presence of the toxins, indicating that CD8 engagement with class I molecules does play a role[19].

Taken together, it is obvious that the requirements for accessory cells to present superantigens at physiological concentrations are similar to those necessary for presentation of peptide antigens. However, it appears that the response to superantigens is less stringently controlled and requires fewer additional signals. We have recently found an example in which antigen-presenting capacity for conventional antigen versus superantigen of an accessory cell can be dissociated. When a known blood-derived antigen-presenting cell, the astrocyte, was used to present a panel of superantigens to unprimed or antigen-specific T cells, we found, surprisingly, that astrocytes could efficiently present peptide antigens but not superantigens to T cells[20]. Although astrocytes can express appropriate levels of MHC class II molecules and adhesion molecules, they turned out to be unable to mediate superantigen-driven T cell activation, even in the presence of rather high concentrations of toxins. In contrast, they could properly present equimolar amounts of nominal antigens to various antigen-specific T cell lines. The inability of astrocytes to support T cell responses to superantigens was not due to a general failure to bind the toxin, and could not be overcome by addition of the cytokines IL-1 or IL-6. The capacity of astrocytes to present superantigens could be reconstituted by the addition of B7-expressing human MHC class II negative cells. A possible explanation may be that the engagement of certain accessory molecules, e.g. CD28, may be more urgently required for superantigen-induced than for antigen-specific stimulation. It appears that astrocytes lack the respective ligands. The response to superantigens may have a stronger requirement for other ligand interaction to replace the missing CD4-derived signal. Apparently this deficiency does not impair the response to a nominal antigen.

This shows that apparently the requirements for co-stimulatory molecules are different, depending on the nature of the antigen or superantigen, of the antigen-presenting cell, and finally also of the responding T lymphocytes.

AUTONOMOUS SIGNALLING VIA A CO-STIMULATORY MOLECULE

Binding of a co-stimulatory molecule to its ligand alone is not sufficient to trigger a T cell. Even cells overexpressing the respective ligands such as LFA-3 or B7 are not able to induce a response in a normal T cell. We have recently found for the first time an exception to this rule[21]. Herpesvirus saimiri (HVS), a T lymphotropic herpesvirus of primates, is able to transform human $CD4^+$ and $CD8^+$ T lymphocytes to continuous growth *in vitro*. These cell lines exhibit the phenotype of activated T cells. They express HLA class II molecules and the IL-2 receptor. We have recently found that the continuous growth of HVS-transformed T cells is due to an activation-dependent production and utilization of IL-2. The cells respond to cell–cell contact with other cells and with each other, with IL-2 production and up-regulation of the IL-2 receptor. The decisive signal given in this interaction is mediated via interaction of CD2 with its ligand CD58 (LFA-3). The evidence for this hypothesis is that monoclonal antibodies to CD2 and CD58, but not to a variety of other cell surface antigens, block proliferation and IL-2 production of HVS-transformed T cells. Furthermore, we could render a non-stimulatory cell stimulatory by transfection with the human CD58 gene. Moreover, sheep erythrocytes are able to activate these transformed cells. Because sheep erythrocytes do not express other surface ligands for human T cells, these experiments show that binding of LFA-3 to CD2 is alone sufficient to activate these transformed cells. It is noteworthy that HVS-transformed T cells can perform all the functions of normal T cells, lymphokine secretion, cytotoxicity and exocytosis of granule esterases. All these activities can be triggered via CD2 by binding to its natural ligand or by anti-CD2 antibodies, but also via the T cell receptor, e.g. by anti-T cell receptor antibodies or by recognition of a bacterial superantigen. Thus HVS-transformed T cells are functionally normal cells that can respond to T cell receptor-mediated signals with the functions of normal T lymphocytes. They are the only transformed human T cells that can be specifically triggered to cytotoxicity and esterase release, and should be a convenient means for the immortalization of functionally normal antigen-specific human T lymphocytes. The only difference compared to normal human T lymphocytes is the response via CD2 to binding of CD58. A possible explanation for this exceptionally strong reactivity to CD2 engagement is that HVS-transformed T cells generally have a lower threshold for stimulation than normal T cells. Thus, transformation by Herpesvirus saimiri apparently brings the T cells in a condition to respond to normally sub-threshold signals with autonomous growth.

CONCLUDING REMARKS

Co-stimulatory signals are essential for T cell immune responses. Their deficiency, imbalance or aberrant utilization can have crucial consequences for T cell-mediated immunopathology and autoreactivity, for immunosuppression or even malignant transformation. It is likely that knowledge of their action will have therapeutic consequences.

References

1. Falk K, Rötzschke O, Deres K, Metzger J, Jung G, Rammensee H-G. Identification of naturally processed viral nonapeptides allows their quantification in infected cells and suggests an allele-specific T cell epitope forecast. J Exp Med. 1991;174:425–34.
2. Wallny H-J, Deres K, Faath S, Jung G, Van Pel A, Boon T, Rammensee H-G. Identification and quantification of a naturally presented peptide as recognized by cytotoxic T lymphocytes specific for an immunogenic tumor variant. Int Immunol. 1992;4:1085–90.
3. Bierer BE, Sleckman BP, Ratnovsky SE, Burakoff SJ. The biologic roles of CD2, CD4 and CD8 in T cell activation. Annu Rev Immunol. 1989;7:579–99.
4. van Seventer GA, Shimizu Y, Shaw S. Roles of multiple accessory molecules in T cell activation. Curr Opin Immunol. 1991;3:294–303.
5. Liu Y, Linsley PS. Costimulation of T cell growth. Curr Opin Immunol. 1992;4:265–70.
6. Damle NK, Klussmann K, Linsley PS, Aruffo A. Differential costimulatory effects of adhesion molecules B7, ICAM-1, LFA-3 and VCAM-1 on resting and antigen-primed CD4+ T lymphocytes. J Immunol. 1992;148:1985–92.
7. Schwartz RM. A cell culture model for T lymphocyte clonal anergy. Science. 1990;248: 1349–55.
8. Liu Y, Jones B, Aruffo A, Sullivan KM, Linsley PS, Janeway CA. The heat stable antigen is a costimulatory molecule for T cell growth. J Exp Med. 1992;175:437–45.
9. Kuijpers KC, Kuijpers TW, Zeijlemaker WP, Lucas CJ, Van Lier RAW, Miedema F. Analysis of the role of leukocyte function antigen-1 in activation of human influenza virus-specific T cell clones. J Immunol. 1990;144:3281–7.

10. Mittrücker HW, Fleischer B. Stimulator cell-dependent requirement for CD2-mediated and LFA-1-mediated adhesions in T-lymphocyte activation by superantigenic toxins. Cell Immunol. 1992;139:108–17.
11. Marrack P, Kappler J. The staphylococcal enterotoxins and their relatives. Science. 1990;248:705–11.
12. Fleischer B, Hartwig U. T-lymphocyte stimulation by microbial superantigens. Chem Immunol. 1992;55:36–64.
13. Fleischer B, Schrezenmeier H. T cell stimulation by staphylococcal enterotoxins. Clonally variable response and requirement for MHC class II molecules on accessory or target cells. J Exp Med. 1988;167:1697–708.
14. Kawabe Y, Ochi A. Programmed cell death and extrathymic reduction of $V\beta 8+$ $CD4+$ T cells in mice tolerant to *Staphylococcus aureus* enterotoxin B. Nature. 1991;349:245–8.
15. MacDonald HR, Baschieri S, Lees RK. Clonal expansion precedes anergy and death of $V\beta 8+$ peripheral T cells responding to staphylococcal enterotoxin B *in vivo*. Eur J Immunol. 1991;21:1963–6.
16. van Seventer GA, Newman W, Shimizu Y, Nutman TB, Tanaka Y, Horgan KJ, Gopal TV, Ennis E, O'Sullivan D, Grey H, Shaw S. Analysis of T cell stimulation by superantigen plus major histocompatibility complex class II molecules or by CD3 monoclonal antibody: costimulation by purified adhesion ligands VCAM-1, ICAM-1 but not ELAM-1. J Exp Med. 1991;174:901–13.
17. Janeway CA, Jr. Selective elements for the $V\beta$ region of the T cell receptor: Mls and the bacterial toxic mitogens. Adv Immunol. 1991;50:1–53.
18. Sekaly RP, Croteau G, Bowman M, Scholl P, Burakoff S, Geha RS. The CD4 molecule is not always required for the T cell response to bacterial enterotoxins. J Exp Med. 1991;173:367–71.
19. Herrmann T, Maryanski JL, Romero P, Fleischer B, MacDonald HR. Activation of MHC class I-restricted $CD8+$ CTL by microbial T cell mitogens. J Immunol. 1990;144:1181–6.
20. Rott O, Tontsch U, Fleischer B. Dissociation of antigen-presenting capacity for peptide antigens versus superantigens of astrocytes. J Immunol. 1993;150:77–85.
21. Mittrücker HW, Müller-Fleckenstein I, Fleckenstein B, Fleischer B. CD2-mediated autocrine growth of Herpesvirus saimiri-transformed human T lymphocytes. J Exp Med. 1992;176: 909–14.

Section II
Immunology of Hepatitis B Virus Infection

3
The humoral immune response to hepatitis B virus

A. ALBERTI, D. CAVALLETTO, L. CHEMELLO, L. BENVEGNÙ, F. BELUSSI, P. PONTISSO and M. LEVRERO

INTRODUCTION

Hepatitis B virus is a double-stranded DNA virus which is responsible in humans for acute and chronic infection, accompanied by a wide spectrum of clinical conditions[1]. The genome of the virus contains at least four different open reading frames (ORF) shown to code for proteins which are expressed in the host during productive infection[2].

These viral proteins, corresponding to the products of the preS/S envelope region, of the pre-C-core nucleocapsid region, of the polymerase gene and of the X gene, are indeed found in serum and/or liver during acute and/or chronic infection, and there is also evidence that they are recognized by the host immune system, with appearance of specific antibodies in serum. Several studies have established that not only the envelope and nucleocapsid structural proteins, but also soluble proteins like the e antigen (HBeAg) and non-structural proteins like the polymerase and X gene products, elicit an antibody response during infection.

Among the different antiviral antibody responses, some have a well-established diagnostic significance and pathogenetic relevance, as the anti-envelope and anti-nucleocapsid antibodies, while the role, if any, of anti-HBpol and of anti-HBx is still unclear.

ANTIBODIES TO HBV DURING ACUTE AND CHRONIC INFECTION

Figure 1 is a simplification of the cascade of the anti-HBV humoral responses occurring during acute infection, as we could derive it from the analysis of serial serum samples of patients with acute hepatitis B.

The anti-HBc, anti-HBe and anti-HBs responses were measured by commercially available ELISA kits (Abbott Laboratories, Chicago, USA),

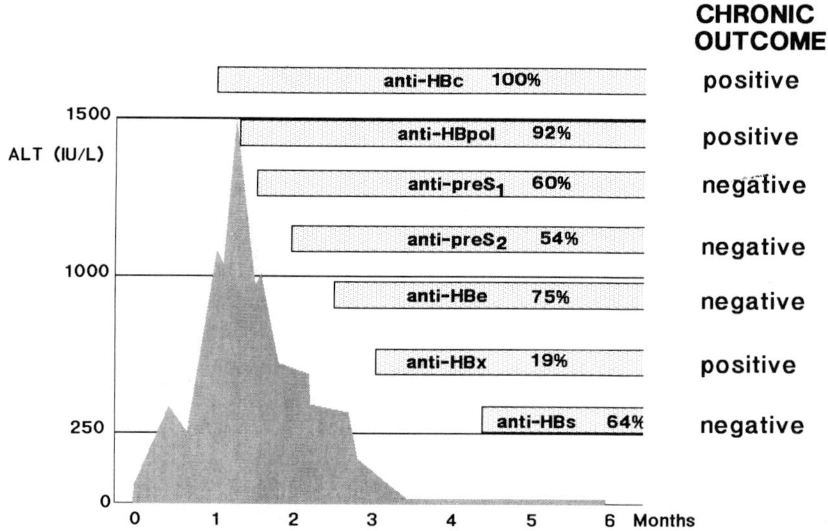

Fig. 1 Schematic representation of the profile of antibodies to HBV during acute hepatitis B in relation to the ALT peak (shaded area). The right-hand side shows the profile seen in patients with chronic evolution

while anti-preS1 and anti-preS2 were determined by solid-phase ELISA using synthetic peptides (see below). Anti-HBx was studied as previously described using fusion proteins expressed in prokaryotic cells[3]. The analysis of anti-HBpol was kindly performed on selected sera by H. Will, using methods previously described[4]. The scheme shown in the figure is representative of the overall results obtained by testing a large series of patients, rather than of the behaviour seen in individual cases. Not all patients with acute hepatitis B were found to develop every antibody reactivity when tested serially during a 12-month follow-up period. The prevalence observed for each antibody is indicated, and ranged from 100% for anti-HBc to 19% for anti-HBx. In patients who recovered from acute hepatitis with transaminases, normalization and HBsAg clearance, anti-HBc usually appeared before the peak in ALT levels, followed by anti-HBpol and by anti-preS1, which was the first anti-envelope reactivity to be detected, usually shortly after the ALT peak. Still later, anti-preS2 and anti-HBe became detectable. Anti-HBx was observed in a few cases, usually at the time of, or shortly after, the normalization of ALT levels, while anti-HBs was a relatively late antibody response. On the right-hand side of Figure 1 we have summarized the profile of anti-HBV antibodies observed in patients with chronic outcome of acute hepatitis B. These patients became anti-HBc, anti-HBpol and anti-HBx-positive, but remained anti-preS1, anti-preS2, anti-HBe and anti-HBs-negative during the follow-up period.

Table 1 Antibodies to preS1 peptides in acute hepatitis

	Antibodies to preS1 sequence		
	No. of cases	*At least one reactivity*	*All three reactivities*
Acute hepatitis B (recovered)			
1–7 days	25	15 (60%)	6 (24%)
1 month	25	6 (64%)	8 (32%)
6–12 months	25	7 (68%)	10 (40%)
5 years	10	5 (50%)	5 (50%)
(Chronic evolution)			
1–7 days	5	0	0
1 month	5	2 (40%)	0
Further follow-up (1–2 years)	5	2 (40%)	0
Acute hepatitis non-B			
1–7 days	10	0	0
1 month	10	0	0

FINE SPECIFICITY OF THE ANTI-PRES1 RESPONSE IN HBV INFECTION

In view of the early appearance of anti-preS1 in acute infection, and its temporal relation with recovery[5], we analysed in more detail the fine specificity of the acute-phase antibodies. Anti-preS1 was investigated by several methods including solid-phase ELISA with synthetic peptides and fusion proteins, competition assays with two monoclonal antibodies reacting with the (27–49) and the (94–117) preS1 sequences, respectively, and a liquid-phase radioimmunoprecipitation assay with radiolabelled preS1-containing particles[6]. This last technique was used to detect antibodies to preS1 conformational epitopes. After preliminary experiments conducted with a series of synthetic peptides covering most of the preS1 sequence, three peptides were selected for further analysis as they were more frequently recognized by human sera. These peptides were derived from the following regions of the preS1 protein: (21–32), (32–47) and (94–117). The (21–32) sequence corresponds, also in our experience[7], to the putative virus binding site for the hepatocyte membrane[8] and antibodies against this epitope may be virus neutralizing[9]. Table 1 summarizes anti-preS1 results obtained with these peptides in 25 patients with self-limited acute hepatitis B, and in five patients who instead had a chronic evolution. All 25 patients who recovered were tested serially during the acute phase, and 10 were tested again 5 years after recovery. More than 50% of patients developed anti-(20–32) and anti-(32–47), and most were positive already during the first few days after onset of clinical symptoms, usually just after the peak in ALT. Both types of antibody remained detectable 5 years after complete recovery.

In sharp contrast with these findings in self-limited hepatitis, anti-(21–32) and anti-(32–47) were never detected in patients with a chronic outcome of hepatitis. A different pattern was observed for anti-(94–117), which was detected with similar prevalences (40–50%) in patients who recovered and in those with chronic outcome. These results were compatible with those

Table 2 Antibodies to preS1 peptides in 66 patients with chronic HBV infection: relation to serological profile and to histological findings

		Antibodies to preS1 sequence		
	n.	*(21–32)*	*(32–47)*	*(94–117)*
Serological profile				
$HBeAg^+/HBV\text{-}DNA^+$	32	0	3 (9%)	9 (28%)
$Anti\text{-}HBe^+/HBV\text{-}DNA^+$	14	0	0	4 (28%)
$Anti\text{-}HBe^+/anti\text{-}HD^+$	10	0	0	0
$Anti\text{-}HBe^+/HBV\text{-}DNA^-$	10	0	2 (20%)	2 (20%)
Histological profile				
CAH/cirrhosis	45	0	3 (7%)	11 (24%)
CPH	11	0	1 (0.9%)	2 (1.8%)
Normal liver or minimal changes	10	0	1 (10%)	2 (20%)

Table 3 Precipitation of the intact HBV particle by anti-(preS1) peptide positive and negative sera

Anti-(21–32) positive (acute phase)	Yes
Anti-(32–47) positive (acute phase)	Yes
Anti-(94–117) positive (chronic phase)	No
Anti-(21–32), Anti-(32–47), Anti-(94–117) negative (acute phase)	Yes

obtained in patients with an established chronic infection. As shown in Table 2, among 66 patients with chronic HBV infection none was positive for anti-(21–32) and few were positive for anti-(32–47), while anti-(94–117) was detectable in about 20% with equal prevalences in the cases with or without HBV-DNA in serum. The presence of anti-(94–117) also did not correlate with histological activity of the underlying liver disease. Sera found positive for anti-(21–32), anti-(32–47) or anti-(94–117) by solid-phase ELISA with synthetic peptides were tested by competition assay against two murine monoclonal antibodies reactive with the (27–49) and (94–117) sequence of preS1, respectively. Using this approach, positivity for anti-preS1 could be confirmed in all but four sera, which were reactive against synthetic peptide (21–32) but were not able to block efficiently the anti-(27–49) monoclonal antibody.

Next we explored whether acute- and chronic-phase sera containing antibodies (IgG) to different preS1 linear epitopes were able to precipitate the intact virion. For this purpose, ^{3}H-labelled HBV particles were used in a solid-phase RIP assay[10]. As shown in Table 3, acute-phase sera positive for anti-(21–32) or for anti-(32–47) were able to precipitate HBV, as was the monoclonal anti-(27–49). On the other hand, anti-(21–32) and anti-(32–47) negative, but anti-(94–117) positive sera from patients with chronic infection failed to precipitate intact virions.

This observation implies that the (94–117) epitope is not exposed on the surface of HBV, a conclusion strengthened by the failure to precipitate HBV

Table 4 Results of inhibition experiments on the precipitation of HBV by acute-phase anti-(preS1) peptide positive and negative sera

Antibody to conformational preS1 epitopes		
	Percentage precipitation of HBV	
Acute-phase serum	*Anti-(32–47) positive*	*Anti-peptide negative*
+ Diluent	98	98
+ {p32–47, p21–32}	19	91
+ preS1 fusion protein	23	92
+ HBs filaments (rich in LHBs)	21	18
+ MHBs particles (CHO)	95	88

by the murine monoclonal antibody specific for the same (94–117) preS1 sequence[11].

EVIDENCE FOR ACUTE-PHASE ANTIBODIES DIRECTED AGAINST CONFORMATIONAL preS1 EPITOPES OF THE HBV SURFACE

When using [^{3}H]HBV particles, acute-phase sera were identified which were able to precipitate the HB virion, but which were negative for antibodies to synthetic peptides as well as to a preS1 fusion protein containing the entire preS1 sequence (Table 3). These sera were anti-preS2 and anti-HBs negative by the most sensitive assays available, and these results were therefore suggestive of the possibility of the presence of anti-preS1 antibodies directed against conformational rather than linear preS epitopes on the virion surface. This interpretation was confirmed by inhibition experiments (Table 4) showing that the ability to precipitate HBV by anti-peptide negative sera was not blocked by an excess of synthetic peptides p(21–32) and p(32–47), or of a preS1 fusion protein, while it was significantly reduced by HBV filamentous particles rich in preS1. The epitope appeared to be preS1 associated, as no inhibition was observed with CHO-derived HBs particles rich in preS2 and S proteins[12]. These findings indicate that patients with acute hepatitis B frequently produce an early antibody response to preS1 which is directed against sequential and conformational epitopes, including the sequence used by the virus to attach to the hepatocyte membrane. These results are in agreement with data from other laboratories[13], and support the hypothesis that such antibody response may be implicated in the mechanism of recovery from the infection.

The data reported on the frequency of antibodies to preS1 in sera of patients with chronic HBV infection have been more controversial than those reported in cases of acute hepatitis B. Several authors have failed to detect anti-preS1 in chronic hepatitis B, while other investigators have described antibodies to preS1 in chronically infected individuals[14]. Such discrepancies could relate to differences in the methods used, and in the patients analysed.

In our own experience, anti-preS1 antibodies were detected in some patients with chronic infection but their specificity often appeared restricted to the C-terminus (94–117) sequence and to an epitope which, apparently, is not expressed on the virion surface. This may explain the coexistence of a large excess of virus particles and of free antibody in serum. The anti-(94–117) response may not play an important pathogenetic role, unlike anti-(21–32) and anti-(32–47) or antibodies to conformational, surface-exposed viral preS1 epitopes detected during acute hepatitis. It remains to be established whether these antibody reactivities are also present in chronic patients, but remain undetectable being continuously adsorbed by circulating virus. Budkowská and her co-workers[15] studied anti-preS1 by inhibition of the binding of a monoclonal antibody to the (28–49) preS1 sequence, and identified a subgroup of patients with chronic hepatitis B who were anti-preS1 positive and eventually normalized aminotransferase levels and cleared serum HBV-DNA during follow-up, events which were not seen in anti-preS1 negative patients. On the basis of these findings the authors concluded that anti-preS1 with specificity for the putative virus binding site for the hepatocyte membrane may play a role in clearance of HBV in chronically infected patients. On the other hand, Petit and colleagues[16], using an immunoblotting assay, did not detect anti-preS1 in any patient with chronic HBV infection, although this study included several cases showing complete and sustained remission of liver disease and termination of virus replication after interferon therapy. We believe that antibodies to preS1 are rarely detectable in chronic HBV infection and those directed against the (21–47) sequence are usually absent, although this does not mean that this defect is central to the mechanism of virus persistence.

The observation that production of anti-preS1 correlates with recovery from HBV infection, and the proposed role of this antibody response in virus neutralization, have stimulated interest for the inclusion of the preS1 proteins in HB vaccines. Recently, recombinant particles containing preS1 have been produced as a new vaccine prototype, but preliminary data indicate poor immunogenicity in humans[17]. HBV recombinant vaccines containing preS2 protein have been developed[12], and we have recently investigated the antibody response obtained in healthy individuals after immunization with such preparations.

ANTI-PRES2 FOLLOWING IMMUNIZATION WITH PRES2 CONTAINING RECOMBINANT PARTICLES

Fifty healthy adult subjects were immunized with Genhevac-B, the Pasteur CHO-derived vaccine which contains preS2 and S protein domains of HBV but lacks preS1. Anti-preS2 was measured in serially collected sera by solid-phase ELISA using a synthetic (120–150) preS2 peptide[18]. The prevalences of anti-preS2 and anti-HBs positivity at different intervals after initiation of the immunization schedule are shown in Fig. 2. Anti-HBs seroconversion occurred in 96% of individuals while anti-preS2 seroconversion was observed in 64%. There was a rather rapid and unexpected decline in anti-preS2

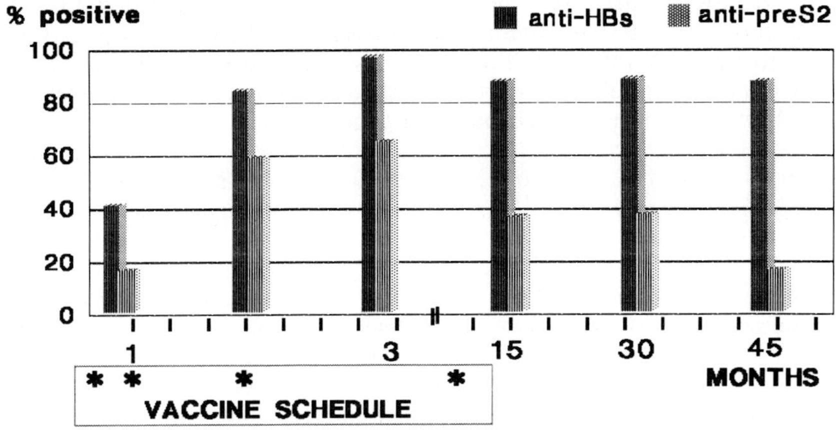

Fig. 2 Rates of positivity for anti-HBs and for anti-preS2 in healthy subjects immunized with a CHO-derived preS2/s vaccine (Genhevac B)

positivity after peak prevalence, which occurred at 3 months. Interestingly, the booster dose given at 12 months was not associated with an enhancement of the anti-preS2 response, which was instead completely lost in several patients during the following months. Forty-five months after the first dose of vaccine, 88% of the subjects were positive for anti-HBs but only 20% retained anti-preS2. These results may be a consequence of the low sensitivity of the method used to detect anti-preS2, or it may reflect a specific suppressor activity generated against the anti-preS2-producing cells[19].

DIAGNOSTIC SIGNIFICANCE OF SEMIQUANTITATIVE ASSESSMENT OF IgM ANTI-HBc IN CHRONIC HBV INFECTION

Another area of interest of recent studies on the humoral immune response to HBV is represented by the significance of IgM anti-HBc in chronic HBV infection. The use of IgM anti-HBc as the most reliable diagnostic marker for acute infection with HBV is well established[20]. It has also been shown that IgM anti-HBc, usually at lower titres compared to those of the acute phase, may persist during chronic infection but their significance, in terms of diagnosis and prognosis, has not been fully elucidated[21,22].

Recently, a semiquantitative microparticle enzyme immunoassay (IMx core-M, Abbott Laboratories, Chicago, USA) has been commercialized and preliminary data would suggest that measurement of IgM anti-HBc with this method may be clinically useful in chronic as well as acute infection. Brunetto and co-workers[23] demonstrated that IgM anti-HBc is detectable in some patients with chronic infection, although antibody titres were significantly lower than those found during acute hepatitis B. Levels of IgM anti-HBc correlated with the degree of activity of liver disease. Furthermore, IgM anti-HBc testing was found particularly useful to predict reactivation of liver disease and to monitor antiviral therapy. In a recent study by

Colloredo-Mels *et al.*[24], IgM anti-HBc testing was confirmed useful for the identification of HBV reactivation in causing flares of hepatitis in patients with chronic HBV infection. These findings will need to be confirmed on a larger number of patients to establish validation of the diagnostic relevance of IgM anti-HBc testing in chronic HBV infection.

ANTIBODIES TO THE PRODUCTS OF THE POLYMERASE AND x GENE OF HBV

Antibodies against the RNAase H domain of the P protein encoded by the polymerase gene of HBV have been detected in patients with acute and chronic infection[25], but it is unclear whether they play any pathogenetic role or may be useful for diagnosis. Using serum samples from experimentally infected chimpanzees and from naturally infected patients, Weiner *et al.*[4] have analysed this antibody response in acute and chronic infection. Anti-HBpol was detected early in the course of acute infection, shortly after anti-HBc. The antibody persisted in most chronic carriers who had evidence of continuing virus replication. However, it declined and eventually disappeared in those who recovered or cleared HBV from serum. These preliminary findings suggest that measurement of anti-HBpol titres during chronic HBV infection may have prognostic value but further data to confirm or disprove such conclusion are clearly needed. With regard to the antibody response against the product of the x gene, there have been conflicting findings as to the correlation of anti-HBx and different phases of HBV infection. There have been reports indicating a close relationship between anti-HBx and HCC in HBsAg-positive patients[26], but this association has not been confirmed in other studies. We have examined anti-HBx in a large collection of patients with different forms of HBV infection and associated liver damage[3]. Although there was a statistically significant association between anti-HBx positivity and markers of ongoing HBV replication, testing for anti-HBx did not appear to add relevant information for the diagnostic and prognostic approach.

References

1. Hoofnagle JH, Sharitz DA, Popper H. Chronic type B hepatitis and the ‘healthy’ HBsAg carrier state. Hepatology. 1987;7:758.
2. Miller RH, Kaneko S, Chung CT, Girones R, Purcell RH. Compact organization of the hepatitis B virus genome. Hepatology. 1989;9:322.
3. Levrero M, Stenler M, Pasquinelli C, Jean-Jean O, Franco A, Balsano C, Diop D, Brechot C, Melegari M, Villa E, Barnaba V, Alberti A, Perricaudet M, Will M. Significance of anti-HBx antibodies in hepatitis B virus infection. Hepatology. 1990;12:485.
4. Weiner T, Schodel F, Jung MC, Pope GR, Alberti A, Fattovich G, Beljoors H, Von Eerd PMC, Will H. Antibodies to the RNAse H domain of hepatitis B virus p protein are associated with ongoing viral replication. J Virol. 1990;64:661.
5. Alberti A, Cavalletto D, Chemello L, Belussi F, Fattovich G, Pontisso P, Ruol A. Fine specificity of human antibody response to preS1 domain of hepatitis B virus. Hepatology. 1990;12:199.

6. Alberti A, Pontisso P, Schiavon E, Realdi G. An antibody which precipitates Done particles in acute hepatitis type B: relation to receptor sites which bind polymerized human serum album or virus particles. Hepatology. 1986;4:220.
7. Pontisso P, Ruvoletto MG, Gerlich WH, Heermann KH, Bardini R, Alberti A. Identification of an attachment site for human plasma liver membranes on hepatitis B virus particles. Virology. 1989;173:522.
8. Neurath A, Kent S, Strick N, Parker K. Identification and chemical synthesis of a host cell receptor binding site on hepatitis B virus. Cell. 1986;46:429.
9. Neurath A, Seto B, Strick N. Antibodies to synthetic peptides from the preS1 region of the hepatitis B virus (HBV) envelope (env) protein are virus-neutralizing and protective. Vaccine. 1989;7:234.
10. Alberti A, Diana S, Scullard G, Eddleston ALNF, Willons R. Detection of a new antibody system reacting with Done particles in hepatitis B virus infection. Br Med J. 1978;2:1056.
11. Takai EA, Machida H, Onhuma H, Miyamoto T, Tanaka K, Baba F, Tsuda S, Ususa T, Nakamura Y, Miyakawa Y, Mayumi M. A solid phase enzyme immunoassay for the determination of IgM and IgG antibodies against translation products of preS1 and preS2 regions of hepatitis B virus. J Immunol Methods. 1986;95:23.
12. Michel ML, Pontisso P, Sobczak E, Malpiece Y, Streeck RE, Tiollais P. Synthesis in animal cells of hepatitis B surface antigen particles carrying a receptor for polymerased human serum albumin. Proc Natl Acad Sci. 1984;81:7708.
13. Theilmann L, Klinkert MQ, Gmelin K, Komerell B, Pfaff E. Detection of antibodies against preS1 protein in sera of patients with hepatitis B virus (HBV) infection. J Hepatol. 1987;4:22.
14. Budkowska A, Dulrenil P, Maillard P, Poynard T, Pillot J. A biphasic pattern of anti-pre responses in acute hepatitis B virus infection. Hepatology. 1990;12:1271.
15. Budkowska A, Dulrenil P, Maillard P, Poynard T, Pillot J, Marcellin P, Loriot MA. Anti-preS responses and viral clearance in chronic hepatitis B virus infection. Hepatology. 1992;15:26.
16. Petit MA, Zoulim F, Berthillar P, Capel F, Li J, Dougnet C, Ferrari C, Trepo C. PreS1 antigen/antibody patterns following interferon therapy in acute and chronic hepatitis B. J Hepatol. 1992:in press.
17. De Wilde M. Future vaccines against hepatitis viruses. Presented at Third International Conference on Current Trends in Chronically Evolving Viral Hepatitis, Pisa, Italy, October 1992.
18. Alberti A, Pontisso P, Tagariello G, Cavalletto D, Chemello L, Belussi F. Antibody response to preS2 and hepatitis B virus induced liver damage. Lancet. 1988;1:1421.
19. Barnaba V, Franco A, Alberti A, Benvenuto R, Balsano F. Selective killing of hepatitis B envelope antigen specific B cells by class-I restricted, exogenous antigen specific T lymphocytes. Nature. 1990;345:258.
20. Lemon SM, Gates NL, Simms TE, Boncroft WH. IgM antibody to hepatitis B core antigen as a diagnostic parameter of acute infection with hepatitis B virus. J Infect Dis. 1981;143:803.
21. Banninger P, Altorfer J, Foresner GG, Pirovino M, Gudat F, Bianchi L, Grob PJ, Schmid M. Prevalence and significance of anti-HBc IgM in acute and chronic hepatitis B and in blood donors. Hepatology. 1983;3:337.
22. Sjogren M, Hoofnagle JH. Immunoglobulin M antibody to hepatitis B core antigen in patients with chronic type B hepatitis. Gastroenterology. 1985;89:252.
23. Brunetto MR, Torrani M, Oliveri F, Piantino P, Rondone A, Calvo PL, Manzini P, Rocca G, Galli C, Bonino F. Monitoring the natural course and response to therapy of chronic hepatitis B with an automated semi-quantitative assay for IgM anti-HBc. J Hepatol. 1992:in press.
24. Colloredo-Mels G, Belloti G, Leandro G, Brunetto M, Scorpiniti A, Fornaciari G, Borzio M, Angeli G, Bonino F, Ideo G. Reactivations of chronic hepatitis B virus infection: patterns of the fluctuations of HBV-DNA ALT and IgM anti-HBc (IMx) during the flare-ups. J Hepatol. 1992;17(Suppl. 1):S14.
25. Weiner T, Weiner K, Tu ZX, Jung MC, Pape GR, Will H. Immunogenicity of human hepatitis B virus P gene derived proteins. J Immunol. 1989;143:3750.
26. Moriarty AM, Alexander H, Lerner RA, Thornton GB. Antibodies to peptides detect new hepatitis B antigen: serological correlations with hepato-cellular carcinoma. Science. 1985;227:429.

4
Role of immunological tolerance in chronic hepatitis B infection

D. R. MILICH and T. MARUYAMA

INTRODUCTION

Hepatitis B virus (HBV) encodes two polypeptides in its core gene. Initiation of translation at the first AUG within the gene results in a 25 kDa precore protein which is secreted as HBeAg after removal of the leader sequence at the amino terminus and 34 carboxyterminal amino acids[1–3]. Initiation at the second AUG (the first AUG on the core mRNA) leads to the synthesis of a 183 amino acid, 21 kDa protein which assembles to form the virion nucleocapsid (HBcAg). HBeAg is collinear with HBcAg in its primary sequence; it has an additional 10 amino acids at the amino terminus and lacks the 34 carboxyterminal amino acids of HBcAg (Fig. 1). Despite this amino acid sequence identity, HBcAg and HBeAg are serologically distinct. However, at the level of T helper (Th) cell recognition HBcAg and HBeAg are highly crossreactive, as shown by murine and human studies[4–7]. Particulate

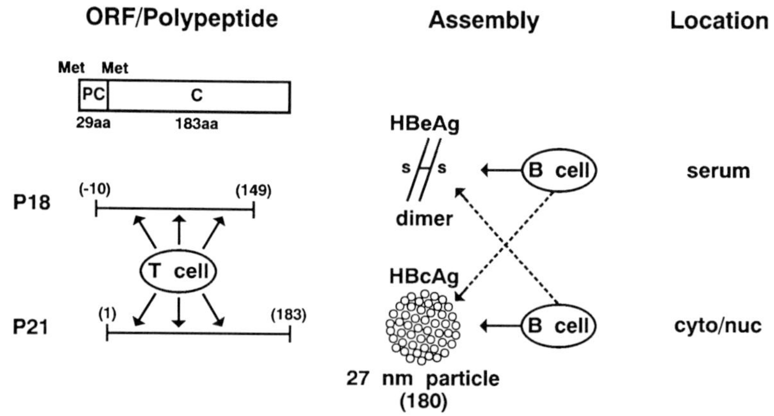

Fig. 1 Comparison of the HBcAg and HBeAg polypeptides, assembly, cellular location, and T and B cell crossreactivity. A broken line depicts lack of crossreactivity

HBcAg is not secreted and serves as the virion nucleocapsid, whereas secreted HBeAg is not a structural component of the virion and is not required for replication or infection[8,9].

Women who are chronic carriers of HBV often infect their infants in the perinatal or postnatal periods, whereas intrauterine infection is much less common[10–13]. The vast majority of untreated infants born to HBeAg-positive mothers become infected, and more than 90% of them become chronic carriers[14]. In contrast, approximately 90% of HBV infections occurring in adults are resolved as acute infections, and only 5–10% result in chronic infections[15]. This dramatic difference in chronicity rates is believed to reflect the immunological status of the host at the time of infection. For example, neonates born to HBV carrier mothers may be immunologically tolerant to viral proteins to which they were exposed *in utero*[16]. The tolerogenic potential of the HBc/HBe antigens is of particular interest because there is evidence that these antigens represent important 'targets' for immune-mediated viral clearance mechanisms[17]. To examine the tolerogenic potential of the nucleocapsid antigens we recently produced inbred HBeAg-expressing transgenic mice (B10.S-Tg31e), and also utilized a neonatal tolerance system in order to investigate the tolerogenic characteristics of the HBeAg[18,19]. Furthermore, we performed an extensive serological analysis of 200 HBeAg-positive chronic hepatitis B (CH-B) carriers in search of evidence of a role for HBeAg-specific tolerance in persistent HBV infection[20].

RESULTS AND DISCUSSION

HBeAg-expressing transgenic mice (B10.S-Tg31e) represent a model system to examine the consequences of *in utero* exposure to HBeAg on HBe/HBcAg-specific immune responses. Characterization of HBe/HBcAg-specific tolerance in B10.S-Tg31e mice and neonatally tolerized mice indicated: (1) T cells but not B cells are tolerized by HBeAg present in the serum at a concentration of 10–100 ng/ml; (2) T cell tolerance elicited by HBeAg also extends to HBcAg-specific T cells; (3) B10.S-Tg31e mice produce anti-HBc but not anti-HBe antibodies upon immunization; (4) the IgG but not the IgM anti-HBc response is diminished in B10.S-Tg31e mice; and (5) the T cell tolerance induced by a single neonatal exposure to HBeAg is reversible and persists for 12–16 weeks[18,19]. It is of interest that many characteristics of immune tolerance demonstrated by B10.S-Tg31e mice parallel the long-term immunological status of neonates born to HBeAg-positive HBV carrier mothers. For example, infants infected perinatally often remain HBeAg-positive, and produce anti-HBc but not anti-HBe antibodies. The correlation of the human serological observations with the murine experimental data suggests the hypothesis that the aberrant immunological responses of neonates born to carrier mothers may also result from *in utero* exposure to HBeAg as occurs in the transgenic model.

Because intrauterine infections are relatively rare, the intact virion does not appear to traverse the placenta, and infection *in utero* most likely results from a defect in the placenta[12,13]. Similarly, it seems unlikely that HBsAg

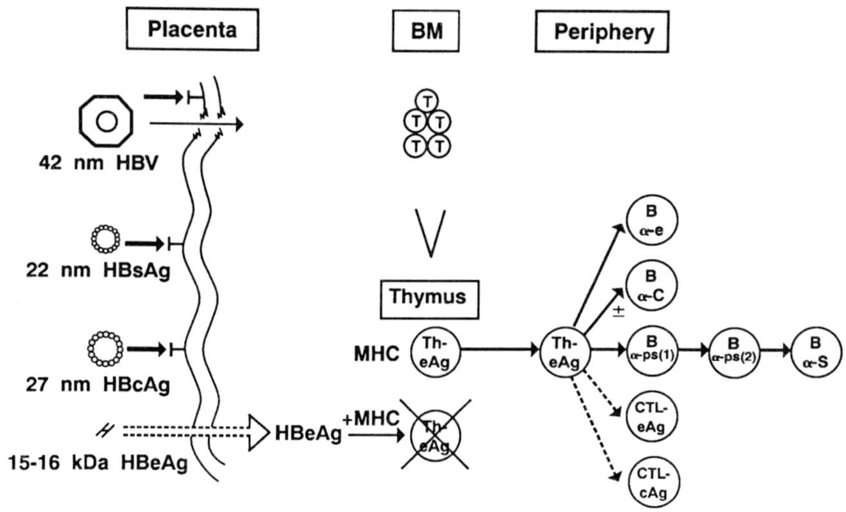

Fig. 2 Schematic of possible mechanism of HBeAg-specific T cell tolerance induction *in utero*. HBV, HBsAg, and HBcAg do not traverse the placenta in the absence of damage, whereas HBeAg may cross the placenta. The encircled T's represent bone marrow-derived prethymocytes. In the thymus the thymocytes undergo positive selection in the absence of HBeAg, and an HBeAg-specific T cell repertoire will emerge and populate the periphery. However, in the presence of HBeAg *in utero* the HBeAg will appear as a self-antigen, and HBeAg-specific T cells will undergo negative selection (that is, clonal deletion or anergy). (From. ref. 53)

crosses the placenta and functions as a tolerogen *in utero* because a high percentage of infants born to HBeAg-positive mothers vaccinated with HBsAg at birth produce anti-HBs antibodies very efficiently[21,22]. Due to its particulate nature, and the fact that HBcAg is not a secreted protein, it is also unlikely that HBcAg can traverse the placenta. However, the small molecular weight HBeAg (15–16 kDa) is secreted into the serum, and may be capable of crossing the placenta (Fig. 2). Placental transit of the intact HBeAg may not be necessary since a peptide fragment of HBeAg (p120–131) injected into neonatal B10.S mice has also been shown to elicit T cell tolerance to the entire HBeAg[19]. In support of the possibility that maternal HBeAg may traverse the placenta are the reports that HBeAg has been detected in neonate cord serum of infants born to HBeAg-positive HBV carrier mothers in the absence of maternally derived HBsAg[23–26].

Because HBeAg is a secreted protein it most likely gains access to the thymus through the circulation. It can be predicted that this mode of antigen presentation within the thymus would lead to the functional deletion of MHC class II-restricted, HBeAg-specific Th cells. For example, HBeAg in the context of MHC would be 'seen' by the immune system as a self antigen (Fig. 2). We suggest that the basic immunological 'defect' in neonates born to HBeAg-positive carrier mothers resides in Th cell tolerance specific for the HBc/HBe antigens[18]. It is important to note that the HBe and HBc antigens are crossreactive at the T cell level. Therefore, HBc/HBe-specific T cell tolerance would preclude Th cell function necessary for anti-HBe and maximal IgG anti-HBc antibody production, and the ability of HBc/HBe-specific Th cells to elicit anti-envelope antibodies[27] would also be impaired. Additionally, HBc/HBe-specific Th cell tolerance may diminish development of a CTL response (CD4 and CD8-mediated), which may be required for the elimination of virus-infected hepatocytes. This central importance of Th cells specific for HBe/HBcAg in terms of the immunoregulation of numerous immune responses during HBV infection is also depicted in Fig. 2. Because of the central regulatory role of HBe/HBc-specific Th cells, the functional absence of this Th cell specificity may impair viral clearance and result in chronic infection.

Although infants born to HBeAg-positive HBV carrier mothers are at high risk for infection and subsequent viral persistence, the infants' age at the time of HBV infection has been shown to be inversely correlated with the rate of chronicity[11]. In the context of an HBc/HBe-specific Th cell tolerance model, this phenomenon can be explained by the reversibility of T cell tolerance apparent for at least 12 weeks of age, but waned thereafter[18]. Therefore, in order for T cell tolerance to the HBc/HBe antigens to be maintained, the tolerogen must be continually present. This suggests that in the absence of the tolerogen, bone marrow (BM)-derived stem cells can migrate to the thymus and give rise to HBc/HBe-specific thymocytes, which can emerge from the thymus, and this 'repertoire renewal process' requires approximately 13–16 weeks in the murine model (Fig. 2). Similarly, in the human system the fetus may be exposed *in utero* to tolerogenic HBeAg but not infected at birth. The longer the elapsed time before HBV infection, the greater the probability of renewing the HBc/HBe-specific T cell repertoire because the neonate would no longer be exposed to the tolerogen (HBeAg)[18].

Cumulatively, the human epidemiological and serological observations, and the murine experimental data, suggest that a function of the HBeAg may be to induce T cell tolerance *in utero*. Indeed, expression of HBeAg may represent a viral strategy to persist in the host subsequent to perinatal infection, which would confer a selective advantage on the conservation of the pre-core domain. This hypothesis of a relationship between HBeAg-specific T cell tolerance and chronic infection also has implications in terms of treatments aimed at interrupting the HBeAg-positive chronic carrier state. Strategies designed to reduce the circulating levels of HBeAg (i.e. the tolerogen) may allow the emergence of HBeAg-specific Th cells. This may be accomplished through anti-viral therapy and/or possibly plasmapheresis. A second and complementary strategy may be to directly up-regulate the Th cell immune response specific for HBeAg. It is interesting to note that interferon-α therapy encompasses both a direct anti-viral activity, and non-specific immune enhancement. Recent studies in the murine HBeAg-transgenic system suggest a more specific immunomodulatory strategy. Although T cell tolerance to HBeAg in the context of B10.S (H-2^s) transgenic mice appears total, T cell tolerance to HBeAg may not be complete in the context of other genetic backgrounds. In fact, (B10.S $\times$ B10)F_1 HBeAg-expressing transgenic mice are significantly less tolerant at the T cell level as compared to B10.S-Tg31e mice[28]. The reduced T cell tolerance of F_1-Tg31e mice is due to the presence of Th cells in the peripheral lymphocytes

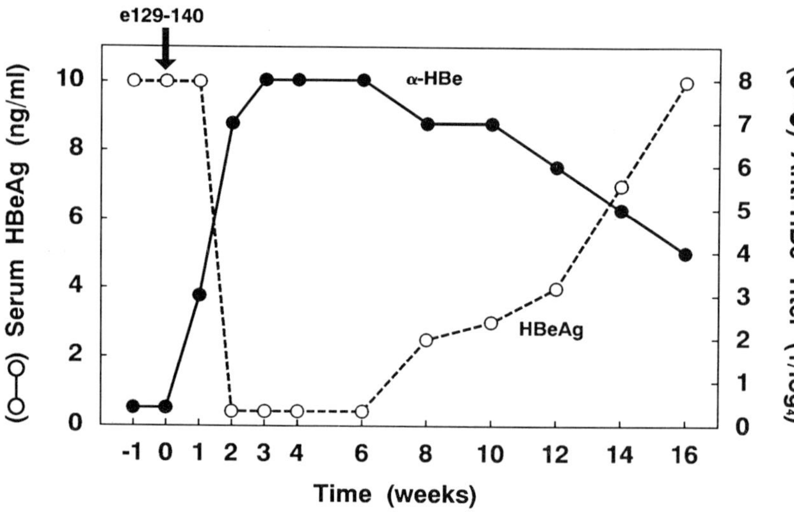

Fig. 3 Induction of seroconversion in HBeAg transgenic mice from HBeAg-positivity to anti-HBe antibody production by the injection of a synthetic T cell site. A group of four (B10.S × B10)F_1-Tg31e mice were injected with the synthetic T cell site representing residues 129–140 of HBeAg, and serum HBeAg concentration and anti-HBe production were measured. (Adapted from ref. 52)

of these mice that are specific for the HBeAg sequence e129–140 and restricted by the I-A^b molecule. Therefore, e129–140-specific Th cells have escaped T cell tolerance induction[28]. Similarly, in the context of HBeAg-positive chronic infection, immunologically silent, HBeAg-specific Th cells may be present and capable of responding to activation. In the murine transgenic model 'quiescent' HBeAg-specific Th cells can be activated by a single injection of the synthetic T cell site e129-140 (Fig. 3). F_1-Tg31e mice secrete HBeAg into the serum at a level of 10 ng/ml and produce no anti-HBe spontaneously; however, an injection with the self T cell peptide e129–140 induces a rapid seroconversion to anti-HBe production with a concomitant neutralization of HBeAg in the serum (Fig. 3). This response is self-limiting but persists for approximately 3 months. The demonstration of residual and functional HBeAg-specific Th cells in the periphery of HBeAg-transgenic mice[28] suggests the possibility that similar HBeAg-specific Th cells can be activated in HBV chronically infected patients. The pattern of HBeAg/anti-HBe seroconversion demonstrated by HBeAg-Tg mice, and illustrated in Fig. 3, has been suggested to be predictive of virus clearance in HBV-infected acute and chronic patients[29,30]. Therefore, at least a portion of CH-B patients may benefit from immune modulation therapy consisting of injection with HBeAg or HBeAg-derived T cell sites[28].

The murine data indicate that the degree of HBeAg-specific T cell tolerance can be variable depending on the MHC of the host, and this may explain the variation in spontaneous HBeAg to anti-HBe seroconversion amongst chronic HBV patients infected at birth. As depicted in Fig. 4, in Tg mice that are H-2^s at the class II MHC locus, HBeAg-specific Th cells that

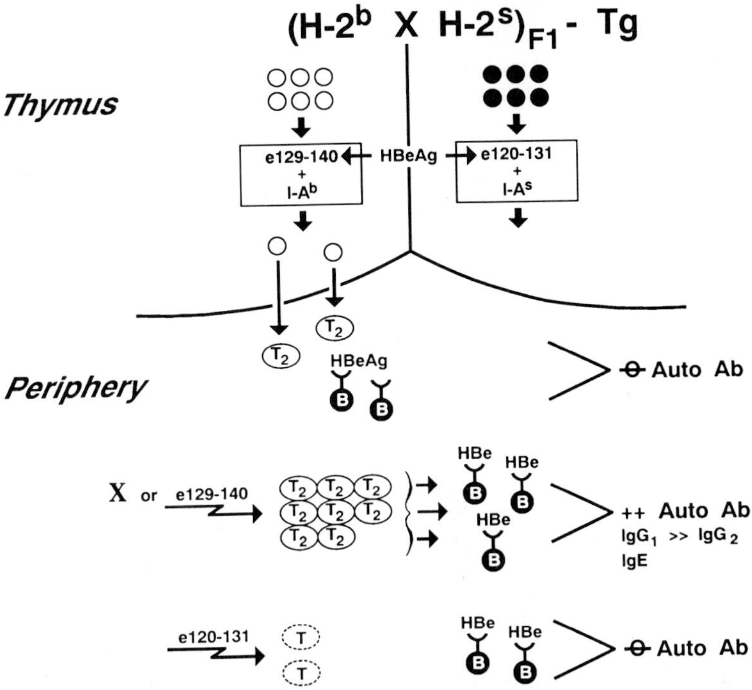

Fig. 4 Schematic of distinct levels of HBeAg-specific T cell tolerance in HBeAg transgenic ($H\text{-}2^b \times H\text{-}2^s)F_1$ mice. See text for details

recognize the e120–131 T cell epitope of endogenous HBeAg are negatively selected (i.e. functionally deleted) in the thymus. However, in Tg mice of the $H\text{-}2^b$ haplotype at least a proportion of Th cells that recognize the e129–140 T cell epitope of HBeAg avoid deletion and migrate to the periphery. Interestingly, these HBeAg-specific Th cells are not activated by the endogenous circulating HBeAg and non-tolerant, HBeAg-specific B cells do not receive T cell helper function and no anti-HBe (autoantibody) is produced. In contrast, the injection of the HBeAg-specific T cell peptide e129–140 into these Tg mice results in activation and expansion of HBeAg-specific Th cells which cooperate with HBeAg-specific B cells to produce anti-HBe autoantibody. Presumably an exogenous, pathogen-derived protein (X) possessing an amino acid sequence homologous to the core of the e129–140 epitope (i.e. e132–138) could also activate the 'quiescent' HBeAg-specific Th cells. The HBeAg-specific Th cells in Fig. 4 have been designated T_2 to represent Th cells of the type 2 phenotype because they proliferate marginally, produce little IL-2, and the autoantibody consists of IgE and IgG predominantly of the IgG_1 isotype. This anti-HBe specific immunoglobulin profile is diagnostic of Th_2 cell function[31,32]. It has yet to be determined whether HBeAg-specific Th cells that evade thymic deletion are primarily of the Th_2 subset or whether Th_2 cells are preferentially activated by B cells presenting endogenous HBeAg. Note that while ($H\text{-}2^b \times H\text{-}2^s)F_1$-Tg mice injected with e129–140 produce anti-HBe autoantibody, F_1-Tg mice injected with e120–131 do not, because Th cells recognizing this epitope restricted by I-A^s have been functionally or physically deleted. Therefore, in this Tg mouse model at least two degrees of HBeAg-specific T cell tolerance can exist depending on MHC genotype.

To examine the relevance of the findings from the Tg murine model in terms of the role of HBeAg-specific tolerance in chronic hepatitis B infection, we have performed an extensive serological analysis of 200 HBeAg-positive CH-B carriers, most of whom were infected perinatally[20]. The hepatitis B virus is not directly cytopathic for the infected hepatocyte, and HBV-induced liver cell injury and subsequent viral clearance is believed to be mediated by 'cellular' immune mechanisms[30]. Despite this fact, historically the serology of CH-B patients has been reported to be remarkably homogeneous regardless of clinical classification (i.e. CAH, CPH, ASC) or degree of liver damage. For example, the sera of CH-B patients contain HBV virions, subviral particles composed of excess envelope proteins (HBsAg and pre-SAg), a secreted form of the nucleoprotein, the hepatitis B e antigen (HBeAg), and antibody to the nucleocapsid (anti-HBc), but remain seronegative for anti-envelope (anti-HBs and anti-pre-S) and anti-HBe antibodies for many years until HBV DNA clearance and loss of serum HBeAg[29,33]. If cellular immune responses are responsible for liver cell injury during chronic active and chronic persistent hepatitis, there should be serological evidence of these underlying cellular processes. However, the presence of HBsAg and HBeAg in the serum may affect the ability to detect circulating antibodies and may obscure the onset of seroconversion. The available commercial assays usually detect anti-HBs and anti-HBe antibodies only after the respective antigens have been cleared from the serum. To address the possibility that antibodies to the structural HBV antigens are produced but not detected in CH-B infection, we have developed sensitive new immunoassays for the detection of anti-HBe and anti-envelope (anti-HBenv) antibodies regardless of the presence of the antigens in serum[34]. We and others[34,35] have utilized a direct binding enzyme immunoassay (EIA) to detect IgG anti-HBe in the sera of HBeAg-positive CH-B patients. This EIA method is more sensitive than the commercial anti-HBe assays which are based on antigen neutralization[34]. To detect anti-envelope antibodies in the presence of a vast excess of the particulate HBsAg, a method of detecting IgG anti-HBenv that is immune complexed (IC) to HBsAg was utilized[34]. The analysis of 200 HBsAg and HBeAg-positive CH-B patients negative for anti-HBs and anti-HBe antibodies by commercial assays revealed: (1) the majority of CH-B patients do indeed demonstrate ongoing humoral immune responses specific for a number of HBV antigens; (2) three representative serological profiles of CH-B infection were identified; (3) these 'silent' immune responses may occur for a number of years prior to liver disease or viral clearance; (4) the quantitative and qualitative characteristics of the immune responses can be correlated with clinical status; and (5) this array of humoral immune responses appears to be mediated exclusively by HBeAg-specific T helper (Th) cells[20].

A summary of the serological profiles exhibited by CH-B patients using novel immunoassays to detect anti-HBe and anti-HBenv antibodies is shown

Table 1 Summary of the serological profiles of CH-B infection and proposed roles of HBeAg-specific Th cells

Clinical diagnosis		*Serological profile*	*n*	*HBeAg-Th*	*Functions*	*Liver disease*	*Tg analogue*
ASC	I	↓α-HBc (G_1) [a]HBV DNA++	20	0	–	0	B10.S
ASC	II	↑α-HBc (G_1) α-HBe (G_1) α-HBenv HBV DNA++	25	Th_2-like	↑*Antibody production*	0	B10
CAH CPH	III	↑↑α-HBc ($G_1 + G_3$) ↑α-HBe ($G_1 + G_3$) ↑α-HBenv HBV DNA + to 0	155	Th_1- like +Th_2-like	↑*Inflammation* ↑MHC ↑CTL ↑DTH ↓HBV α-HBc/HBe → G_3	++ to ±	–

ASC, asymptomatic carrier; CAH, chronic active hepatitis; CPH, chronic persistent hepatitis; *n*, number of patients; G_1 and G_3 refer to IgG subclass; Tg, HBeAg-expressing transgenic mice. (Adapted from ref. 20)

in Table 1. It is notable that virtually all CH-B patients with liver disease (profile III) and 55.6% of ASC patients without disease (profile II) demonstrate ongoing humoral immune responses including anti-HBe and anti-envelope antibody production. Only profile I, representative of 44.4% of ASC patients, is characterized by the absence of anti-HBe and anti-envelope antibody production, although this is the serology which is currently widely believed to characterize all HBeAg-positive CH-B patients. However, another recent study has also indicated a greater incidence of anti-HBe antibody production in HBeAg-positive CH-B patients[35]. Similarly, anti-envelope antibodies may coexist with virions and subviral HBsAg particles for many years prior to viral clearance and loss of HBsAg[20].

The specificity and source of T cell helper function for anti-HBc, anti-HBe, and anti-envelope antibody production in the context of CH-B infection may also be surmised from a complete serological analysis. Because anti-HBc production can occur via a T cell-independent pathway and HBcAg and HBeAg are crossreactive at the Th cell level[36,37], the production of low-titre and predominantly IgG_1 subclass anti-HBc antibodies in the absence of anti-HBe antibody production (profile I) most probably requires little or no HBe/HBcAg-specific Th cell function. Similarly, anti-HBe negative ASC patients produce minimal or no anti-envelope antibodies. We propose that this subset of ASC patients is completely tolerant to HBeAg and lacks sufficient Th cell function to produce antibodies to T cell-dependent HBV antigens. This profile is analogous to HBeAg-expressing Tg mice on a B10.S ($H-2^s$) genetic background (i.e. total tolerance). In contrast, the serological evidence indicates that the anti-HBe positive subset of ASC patients (profile II) possesses adequate HBeAg-specific Th cell function to produce higher-titre anti-HBc as well as anti-HBe antibodies. Additionally, a high proportion of these ASC patients also produce anti-envelope antibody. However, anti-

HBc and anti-HBe antibody titres are significantly higher in CAH patients (profile III) as compared to anti-HBe-positive ASC patients, especially during acute exacerbations of liver injury. A possibly more significant difference can be noted in the IgG subclass distribution of anti-HBc and anti-HBe antibodies produced by ASC versus CAH patients. The ASC patients of both subgroups demonstrate a defect in the production of anti-HBc antibodies of the IgG_3 subclass, and anti-HBe-positive ASC patients also produce low levels of IgG_3 subclass anti-HBe antibodies as compared to CAH patients in which the IgG_3 subclass predominates along with IgG_1. The co-production of IgG_1 and IgG_3 subclass antibodies characterizes the normal human humoral immune response to protein antigens and especially to protein antigens of viral origin including HBV antigens[38–40]. The association of the IgG_3 subclass with viral infection and the identification of interferon (IFN) response elements in the $C\gamma3$ gene[41] suggest that IFN may enhance human IgG_3 subclass antibody production to HBeAg and HBcAg. The ability of Th subsets to influence IgG subclass antibody production via the assortment of lymphokines secreted (i.e. Th_1, IL-2 and IFN-γ; Th_2, IL-4 and IL-5) is well established in the murine system[31] and is also becoming apparent in humans[42]. In the murine system we have observed that certain HBeAg-specific T cell site–MHC combinations preferentially elicit either a Th_1-like (proliferation) or a Th_2-like (antibody) response (unpublished observation). We propose that the production of low-titre and IgG_3 subclass-deficient anti-HBc and anti-HBe responses in ASC versus CAH patients reflects differential engagement of Th subsets amongst these patient groups. The serological profile (II) and absence of cell-mediated liver disease in anti-HBe-positive ASC patients is consistent with an exclusive Th_2-like response. This profile is analogous to the response of HBeAg expressing Tg mice on a B10 (H-2^b) genetic background injected with the e129–140 T cell peptide (i.e. T cell tolerance at the Th_1 subset level, but responsiveness at the Th_2 subset level). In contrast, the serology and evidence of cell-mediated cytotoxic responses in CAH patients (profile III) suggest a Th_1-like or combined Th_1–Th_2-like response. A Th_1-like response is characterized by significant T cell proliferation and by IL-2 production, $CD4^+$ T cell-mediated cytotoxicity (CTL), delayed-typed hypersensitivity (DTH) reactivity, and the varied effects of IFN-γ production (i.e. enhanced MHC expression, direct anti-viral effects, suppression of murine IgE and IgG_1, and enhancement of murine IgG_{2a}[32]).

Both anti-HBe-positive ASC and CAH patients produce anti-envelope antibody. However, anti-envelope antibody production by CH-B-infected patients correlates with anti-HBe production, and does not appear to be mediated by envelope-specific Th cells in as much as the decline in anti-envelope antibody parallels the decline in HBV DNA and HBeAg concentrations at a time when serum envelope antigen concentrations remain elevated. This observation, together with the fact that HBe/HBcAg-specific Th cells have been shown to elicit anti-envelope antibody production[27], suggests that HBeAg-specific Th cells may mediate anti-envelope antibody production in CH-B infection. This hypothesis is consistent with a number of recent reports that have demonstrated HBe/HBcAg-specific T cell proliferative responses but not HBsAg or pre-S-specific T cell proliferation in CH-

B patients[6,7,43,44]. The serological studies also indicate that HBeAg and not the envelope antigens appears to be the focus of Th cell recognition in the context of CH-B infection, and that HBeAg-specific Th cells play a predominant immunoregulatory role in the immune response to multiple HBV antigens. This may, in part, explain the emergence of HBV variants which cannot produce HBeAg (i.e. pre-core mutants) during the course of CH-B infection[45–47]. Such variants may represent escape mutants immunoselected by virtue of greater survival in the milieu of a long-term immune response predominantly regulated by HBeAg-specific Th cells.

The vast majority of the Japanese patients enrolled in this study were infected in the neonatal or perinatal period by HBeAg-positive CH-B-infected mothers, and subsequently became CH-B carriers. Evidence from the HBeAg-expressing transgenic murine model and human epidemiological observations suggest that the HBeAg can traverse the placenta, and *in-utero* exposure to HBeAg may elicit immunological T cell tolerance which may predispose to chronicity[18]. The recent report that neonatal infections with an HBeAg-negative variant of HBV resulted in severe acute rather than chronic infections supports the role of HBeAg-specific tolerance in chronic infection of the neonate[48]. The observation that most CH-B patients possess anti-HBe as well as HBeAg in serum suggests that HBeAg/anti-HBe ICs rather than free HBeAg, may be transported across the placenta. This is consistent with a report that virtually all the HBeAg in the cord blood of infants born to CH-B-infected mothers was immune-complexed[49]. The correlation between anti-HBe production and the degree of liver disease among CH-B patients is consistent with the hypothesis that T cell tolerance to HBeAg leads to chronicity, and suggests that HBeAg-specific T cells emerging from the tolerant state mediate viral clearance and the serological responses described in profiles II and III (Table 1). The HBeAg transgenic murine model provides evidence that the degree of HBeAg-specific Th cell tolerance can be variable, depending on the MHC genotype of the strain (i.e. $H\text{-}2^b$ vs. $H\text{-}2^s$ response)[28]. Furthermore, murine Th_1 and Th_2 subsets appear to differ with respect to tolerance induction[50,51]. Comparable genetic variability among CH-B patients infected at birth may explain the differences in serological profiles and in spontaneous HBV clearance rates.

Acknowledgements

The authors wish to thank Ms René Lang for preparation of the manuscript. This work was supported by National Institutes of Health Grant AI 20720. Toshiyuki Maruyama was supported by a grant from the Japanese government. This is publication no. 7598-MB from the Scripps Research Institute.

References

1. McLachlan A, Milich DR, Raney AK, Riggs MG, Hughes JL, Sorge J, Chisari FV. Expression of hepatitis B virus surface and core antigens: influences of pre-S and precore sequences. J Virol. 1987;61:683–92.

2. Bruss V, Gerlich V. Formation of transmembranous hepatitis B e antigen by cotranslational *in vivo* processing of the viral precore protein. Virology. 1988;163:268–75.
3. Ou J, Laub O, Rutter WJ. Hepatitis B virus gene function: the precore region targets the core antigen to cellular membranes and causes the secretion of the e antigen. Proc Natl Acad Sci USA. 1986;83:1578–82.
4. Milich DR, McLachlan A. The nucleocapsid of the hepatitis B virus is both a T cell dependent and a T cell independent antigen. Science. 1986;234:1398–401.
5. Milich DR, McLachlan A, Moriarty A, Thorton GB. Immune response to hepatitis B virus core antigen (HBcAg): Localization of T cell recognition sites within HBcAg/HBeAg. J Immunol. 1987;139:1223–31.
6. Tsai SL, Chen PJ, Lai MY, Yang PM, Sung JL, Huang JH, Hwang LH, Change TH, Chen DS. Acute exacerbations of chronic type B hepatitis are accompanied by increased T cell responses to hepatitis B core and e antigens. J Clin Invest. 1992;89:87–96.
7. Ferrari C, Penna A, Sansoni P *et al.* Selective sensitization of peripheral blood T lymphocytes to hepatitis B core antigen in patients with chronic active hepatitis type B. Clin Exp Immunol. 1986;67:497–506.
8. Chang C, Enders G, Sprengel R, Peters N, Varmus H, Ganem D. Expression of the precore region of an avian hepatitis B virus is not required for viral replication. J Virol. 1987;61: 3322–5.
9. Schlicht H-J, Salfeld J, Schaller H. The duck hepatitis B virus pre-C region encodes a signal sequence which is essential for synthesis and secretion of processed core proteins but not for virus formation. J Virol. 1987;61:2208–12.
10. Beasley RP, Trepo C, Stevens CE, Szmuness W. The e antigen and vertical transmission of hepatitis B surface antigen. Am J Epidemiol. 1977;105:94–9.
11. Beasley RP, Hwang L. Postnatal infectivity of hepatitic B surface antigen-carrier mothers. J Infect Dis. 1983;147:185–90.
12. Li L, Sheng M-H, Tong S-P *et al.* Transplacental transmission of hepatitis B virus. Lancet. 1989;1:872.
13. Lee S-D, Lo K-J, Tsai Y-T, Wu J-C. Maternal hepatitis B virus DNA in mother–infant transmission. Lancet. 1989;1:719.
14. Stevens CE, Beasley RP, Tsu J, Lee WC. Vertical transmission of hepatitis B antigen in Taiwan. N Engl J Med. 1975;292:771–80.
15. Aldershvile J, Frosner GG, Nielsen JO *et al.* Hepatitis B e antigen and antibody measured by radioimmunoassay in acute hepatitis B surface antigen-positive hepatitis. J Infect Dis. 1980;141:293–308.
16. Thomas HC, Meron J, Water J, Main J. Virus–host interaction in chronic hepatitis B virus infection. Semin Liver Dis. 1988;8:342–9.
17. Mondelli M, Vergani GM, Alberti A *et al.* Specificity of T lymphocyte cytotoxicity to autologous hepatocytes in chronic hepatitis B virus infection: evidence that T cells are directed against HBV core antigen expressed on hepatocytes. J Immunol. 1982;129: 2773–9.
18. Milich DR, Jones JE, Hughes JL *et al.* Is a function of the secreted hepatitis B E antigen to induce immunologic tolerance *in utero.* Proc Natl Acad Sci USA. 1990;87:6599–603.
19. Milich DR, Jones JE, McLachlan A *et al.* Distinction between immunogenicity and tolerogenicity among HBcAg T cell determinants: influence of peptide-MHC interaction. J Immunol. 1989;143:3148–57.
20. Maruyama T, McLachlan A, Iino S, Koike K, Kurokawa K, Milich DR. The serology of chronic hepatitis B infection revisited. J Clin Invest. 1993 (in press).
21. Reichard O, von Sydow M, Dennerstam L *et al.* Prevention by immunisation of hepatitis B in the newborn infant in Stockholm, Sweden. In: Zuckerman AJ, editor. Viral hepatitis and liver disease. New York: Alan R. Liss; 1988:989.
22. Poorvorawan Y, Sanpavat S, Pongpulert W *et al.* Protective efficacy of a recombinant DNA hepatitis B vaccine in neonates of HBe antigen-positive mothers. J Am Med Assoc. 1989;261:3278–81.
23. Arakawa K, Tsuda F, Takahashi K *et al.* Maternofetal transmission of IgG-bound hepatitis B e antigen. Pediatr Res. 1982;16:247–50.
24. Lee S-D, Lo K-J, Wu J-C *et al.* Prevention of maternal-infant hepatitis B virus transmission by immunization: the role of serum hepatitis B virus DNA. Hepatology. 1986;6:369–73.

25. Biswas SC, Gupta I, Ganguly NK *et al.* Prevalence of hepatitis B surface antigen in pregnant mothers and its perinatal transmission. Trans R Soc Trop Med Hyg. 1989;83:698–700.
26. Goudeau A, Lesage G, Denis F *et al.* Lack of anti-HBc IgM in neonates with HBsAg carrier mothers argues against transplacental transmission of hepatitis B virus infection. Lancet. 1983;2:1103–4.
27. Milich DR, McLachlan A, Thornton GB, Hughes JL. Antibody production to the nucleocapsid and envelope of the hepatitis B virus primed by a single synthetic T cell site. Nature. 1987;329:547–9.
28. Milich DR, McLachlan A, Raney AK *et al.* MHC-dependent autoantibody in HBeAg transgenic mice elicited with self T cell peptides and inhibited with non-self peptides. Proc Natl Acad Sci USA. 1991;88:4348–52.
29. Hoofnagle JH, Dusheiko GM, Seeff LB *et al.* Seroconversion from hepatitis B e antigen to antibody in chronic type B hepatitis. Ann Intern Med. 1981;94:744–8.
30. Alberti A, Trevisan A, Fattovich G, Realdi G. The role of hepatitis B virus replication and hepatocyte membrane expression in the pathogenesis of HBV-related hepatic damage. In: Chisari FV, editor. Advances in hepatitis research. New York: Masson; 1984:134–43.
31. Mosmann TR, Coffman RL. Two types of mouse helper T-cell clone. Immunol Today. 1987;8:223–7.
32. Snapper CM, Paul WE. Interferon-γ and B cell stimulation factor 1 reciprocally regulate Ig isotype production. Science. 1987;236:944–7.
33. Realdi G, Alberti A, Rugge M *et al.* Seroconversion from hepatitis B e antigen to anti-HB_e in chronic hepatitis B virus infection. Gastroenterology. 1980;79:195–9.
34. Maruyama T, Thornton GB, Iino S, Kurokawa K, Milich DR. Use of anti-peptide antibodies for the design of antigen-specific immune complex assays. J Immunol Meth. 1992;155:65–75.
35. Sällberg M, Norder H, Lindgh G, Magnius LO. IgG subclasses in circulating immune complexes with hepatitis B e antigen in chronic hepatitis. Clin Exp Immunol. 1991;84: 116–21.
36. Milich DR, McLachlan A, Stahl S *et al.* Comparative immunogenicity of hepatitis B virus core and e antigens. J Immunol. 1988;141:3617–24.
37. Milich DR, McLaclan A. The nucleocapsid of the hepatitis B virus is both a T cell-independent and a T cell-dependent antigen. Science. 1986;234:1398–401.
38. Beck OE. Distribution of virus antibody activity among human IgG subclasses. Clin Exp Immunol. 1981;43:626–32.
39. Sällberg M, Norder H, Linde A, Magnius LO. Subclass pattern of anti-HBc IgG in chronic hepatitis B: relation to HBeAg/anti-HBe and HBV-DNA. In: Zuckerman AJ, editor. Viral hepatitis and liver disease. New York: Alan R. Liss; 1988:244–7.
40. Skvaril F, Joller-Jemelka H. IgG subclasses of anti-HBs antibodies in vaccinated and non-vaccinated individuals and in anti-HBs immunoglobulin preparations. Int Arch Allergy Appl Immunol. 1984;73:330–7.
41. Mills FC, Brooker JS, Camerini-Otero RD. Sequences of human immunoglobulin switch regions: Implication for recombination and transcription. Nucl Acids Res. 1990;18: 7305–16.D.
42. Romagnani S. Human T_H1 and T_H2 subsets: doubt no more. Immunol Today. 1991;12: 256–7.
43. Vento S, Hegarty JE, Alberti A *et al.* T lymphocyte sensitization to HBcAg and T cell-mediated unresponsiveness to HBsAg in hepatitis B virus-related chronic liver disease. Hepatology. 1985;5:192–7.
44. Inoue M, Kakumu S, Yoshioka K *et al.* Hepatitis B core antigen-specific IFN-γ production of peripheral blood mono-nuclear cells in patients with chronic hepatitis B virus infection. J Immunol. 1989;142:4006–11.
45. Brunetto M, Stemler M, Schödel F *et al.* Identification of HBV variants which cannot produce precore derived HBeAg and may be responsible for severe hepatitis. J Gastroenterol. 1989;21:151–4.
46. Carman WF, Jacyna MR, Hadziyannis S *et al.* Mutation preventing formation of hepatitis B e antigen in patients with chronic hepatitis B infection. Lancet. 1989;2:588–90.
47. Okamoto H, Yotsumoto S, Akahane Y *et al.* Hepatitis B viruses with precore region defects prevail in persistently infected hosts along with seroconversion to the antibody against e antigen. J Virol. 1990;64:1298–303.

48. Terazawa S, Kojima M, Yamanaka T *et al.* Hepatitis B virus mutants with precore region defects in two babies with fulminant hepatitis and their mothers positive for antibody to hepatitis B e antigen. Pediatr Res. 1991;29:5–9.
49. Arakawa K, Tsuda F, Takahashi K *et al.* Maternofetal transmission of IgG-bound hepatitis B e antigen. Pediatr Res. 1982;16:247–50.
50. De Wit D, Van Mechelen M, Ryelandt M *et al.* The injection of deaggregated gamma globulins in adult mice induces antigen-specific unresponsiveness of T helper type 1 but not type 2 lymphocytes. J Exp Med. 1992;175:9–15.
51. Burstein H, Shea CA, Abbas AK. Aqueous antigens induce in vivo tolerance selectively in IL-2- and IFN-γ-producing (Th1) cells. J Immunol. 1992;148:3687–91.
52. Milich DR. Immune response to hepatitis B virus proteins: relevance of the murine model. Semin Liver Dis. 1991;11:93–111.

5
Cellular immune reactions to hepatitis B core antigen

C. FERRARI, F. FIACCADORI and F. V. CHISARI

INTRODUCTION

Termination of viral infections is strictly dependent upon a coordinate and efficient development of humoral and cell-mediated immune responses to viral antigens.

While a neutralizing anti-viral antibody response is generally needed for elimination of free circulating viral particles and prevention of virus entry into cells, the HLA class I restricted cytotoxic T lymphocyte (CTL) response against virus-encoded antigens expressed at the membrane of infected cells is believed to play a major role in the clearance of intracellular virus.

Optimal activation of both B cells to produce neutralizing antibodies and CTL to kill infected cells requires the helper effect of HLA class II restricted $CD4^+$ T cells.

CTL RESPONSE AGAINST HBV NUCLEOCAPSID ANTIGENS

Identification by CTL of the infected cells that must be eliminated depends upon the recognition of short peptides associated with HLA class I molecules, derived from the intracellular processing of viral antigens synthesized within the infected cells[1–3].

In several infections the viral nucleoprotein has been shown to serve as a major target for HLA class I restricted CTL[1,4–8]. The potential importance of this antigen for the activation of an anti-viral CTL response in HBV infection was suggested by Mondelli *et al.*[9]. They showed that peripheral blood lymphocytes from patients with acute and chronic hepatitis B may kill autologous hepatocytes *in vitro*. Surprisingly, they reported that this cytotoxicity was specifically inhibited following incubation of the target cells with anti-nucleocapsid but not with anti-envelope antibodies, suggesting that core antigen-specific antibodies and T cells may recognize the same or overlapping epitopes.

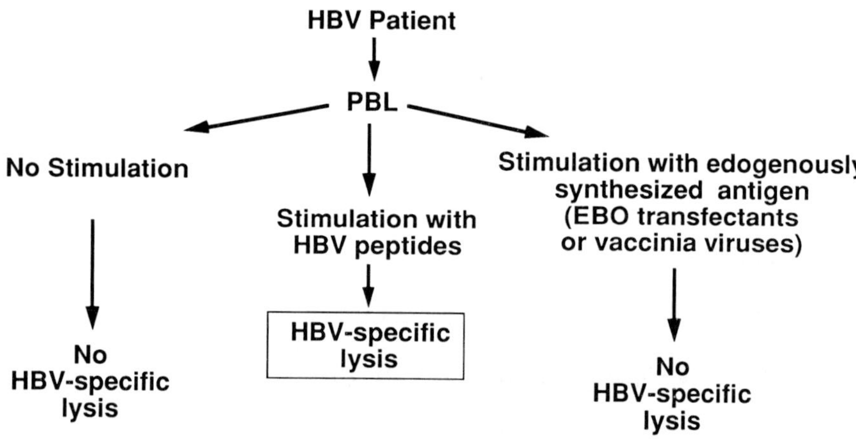

Fig. 1 Experimental strategy for the analysis of HBV-specific cytotoxic activity. PBL isolated from patients with acute and chronic HBV infection were tested for HBV-specific cytolytic activity either (I) immediately after isolation, without prior steps of *in vitro* stimulation, or (II) after 1 or 2 weeks of stimulation with autologous stimulator cells transfected or infected with recombinant HBV core synthetic peptides. Target cells were represented by autologous EBV transformed B-lymphoblastoid cell lines or autologous phytohaemagglutinin-stimulated T cell blasts either infected or transfected with HBV expression vectors, or preincubated with synthetic peptides. Two different eukaryotic expression systems were employed in these studies. The HBV core and precore open reading frames were inserted into the Epstein–Barr virus (EBV)-based plasmid vector EBO-pLPP[28], that is maintained as an episome when transfected into EBV-transformed human B cell lines. The EBO-transfected cells are selected with hygromycin, a selection marker carried by the plasmid. Stable expression of HBV antigens has been obtained following electroporation of EBV-transformed B cells in the presence of each one of the plasmids carrying a specific HBV DNA sequence. The construction and characterization of these vectors have been reported in detail elsewhere[12]. Additionally, recombinant vaccinia viruses that express either the HBV core (V core) or precore (V precore) polypeptides were constructed and used as described[11].

Due to technical limitations inherent in those early studies, however, the reproducibility and specificity of the cytolytic activity, its HLA restriction elements and its cellular phenotype could not be established, and only patients undergoing diagnostic liver biopsies could be studied. Obviously, a different approach was necessary if definitive analysis of the CTL response to HBV encoded antigens was to be achieved.

Since HBV does not efficiently infect human cells *in vitro*, thereby precluding the possibility of producing stimulator/target systems by the conventional approach of human cell infection *in vitro*, we developed an experimental strategy to analyse the HBV-specific CTL response based on the combined use of short synthetic peptides mimicking the processed antigen fragments and of recombinant expression vectors inducing endogenous expression of HBV antigens (Fig. 1). Following this approach a panel of short overlapping synthetic peptides covering the entire amino acid sequence of the HBV core (HBcAg) and e (HBeAg) antigens was synthesized[10]. In addition, two different eukaryotic expression systems were produced: recombinant vaccinia viruses that allow rapid infection of human cell lines

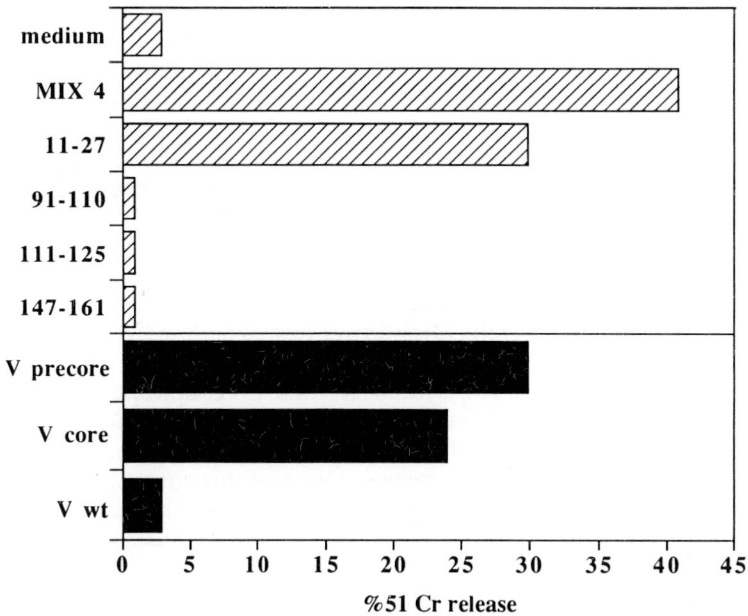

Fig. 2 HBcAg-specific cytotoxic activity in acute hepatitis B. PBL from a patient with acute hepatitis B were initially stimulated with a panel of four pools of overlapping synthetic peptides each one consisting of five or six peptides covering the entire HBV nucleocapsid region. Significant levels of CTL activity were observed only following stimulation with peptide mixture 4 (Mix 4). PBL stimulated *in vitro* with peptide mixture 4 were then tested against autologous target cells prepulsed with the individual peptides included in mixture 4 (11–27, 91–110, 111–125, 147–161, 162–176) and against target cells infected with recombinant vaccinia viruses that express either the HBV core (V core) or precore (V precore) polypeptides or control vaccinia wild-type (V wt). The cytolytic activity is expressed as percentage of ^{51}Cr release by target cells (prelabelled with ^{51}Cr) cocultured with effector CTL[13]

in vitro followed by rapid and efficient, though transient, expression of HBV core and precore polypeptides[11]; and Epstein–Barr virus (EBV)-based plasmid vectors (EBO) that permit stable transfection of EBV-transformed human B cell lines with stable and efficient expression of HBV antigens[12].

HBV-specific CTL were never detected in freshly isolated peripheral blood lymphomononuclear cells (PBL) without prior stimulation *in vitro*, suggesting that HBV-specific CTL are probably present in the peripheral blood compartment at very low frequency (Fig. 1)[13]. In contrast, HBV-specific CTL activity was detectable following PBL stimulation *in vitro* with synthetic peptides[12,13]. This CTL activity was reproducibly induced in HLA-A2 positive patients with acute hepatitis B by a peptide corresponding to HBV core residues 11–27 (Fig. 2). This amino acid sequence is conserved among the major subtypes of HBV and is selectively presented to CTL by HLA-A2, one of the most common HLA class I alleles in the human population.

Importantly, peptide-induced CTL can recognize endogenous HBcAg and HBeAg encoded by recombinant vaccinia and EBO plasmid vectors in autologous HLA class I positive target cells[13]. This finding indicates that the CTL epitope represented by residues 11–27 of HBcAg is actually generated by the intracellular processing of endogenously synthesized core and precore proteins and that, therefore, it is likely available to CTL recognition *in vivo* on the surface of virus-infected liver cells, at the site of antigen synthesis.

The repeated failure to detect a nucleocapsid-specific cytotoxic activity in normal control subjects further confirms that these core-specific CTL must have encountered the antigen *in vivo* and that they have been primed by the natural HBV infection[10–13].

Analysis of the CTL response in patients at different stages of HBV infection shows that the CTL response against HBcAg 11–27 is strong in the peripheral blood of patients who recover from infection (i.e. acute patients) but is absent or very weak in patients who do not succeed in clearing the virus (i.e. chronic patients)[10]. Moreover, this CTL epitope is commonly recognized by HLA-A2 positive patients with acute self-limited hepatitis B (who are primed *in vivo* by the HBV nucleocapsid protein) since virtually all of them develop a vigorous CTL response against this core region peptide[10].

The different responses in patients with acute and chronic evolution of HBV infection finally suggest a pathogenetic role for nucleocapsid-specific CTL in the clearance of HBV infection, raising the possibility that a failure to mount a vigorous CTL response to nucleocapsid antigens may be a factor predisposing to virus persistence and chronic evolution of HBV infection. Further mapping of HBV core sequences recognized by CTL in association with other HLA molecules is now in progress, and results of this analysis will allow us to draw a more complete picture of the CTL response to HBV and its role in virus clearance.

MOLECULAR ANALYSIS OF THE CTL RESPONSE TO HBV NUCLEOCAPSID ANTIGENS

Recent elution studies show that naturally processed peptides present in the groove of the HLA class I molecules are usually 8–10 amino acids long and that allele-specific binding motifs define peptides able to bind distinct HLA molecules[14–17]. For the HLA-A2-restricted T cell epitopes the binding motif is represented by a leucine or isoleucine at position 2 and valine or a residue with aliphatic hydrocarbon side chains at the C-terminus[17,18]. Moreover, the short natural peptides thus far isolated are more efficiently recognized by CTL than the longer synthetic analogues, because of a higher binding affinity to HLA class I molecules[19,20]. This property makes them ideal candidates for the design of synthetic vaccines aimed at inducing a protective CTL response *in vivo*.

To precisely define the optimal amino acid sequences recognized by HBV nucleocapsid-specific CTL we have used a panel of truncated and overlapping synthetic peptides of different length covering the core region 11–27 (Fig. 3) (submitted manuscript).

The HLA-A2 restricted CTL epitope contained within the HBV core sequence 11–27 was mapped at residues 18–27 that define the optimally

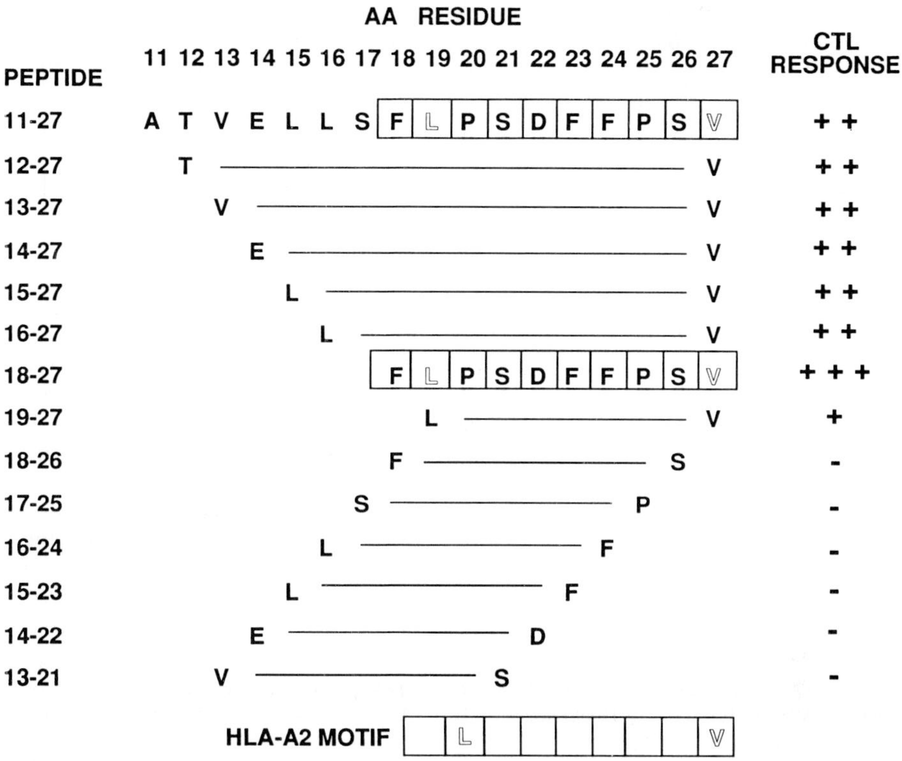

Fig. 3 Peptide 18–27 represents the optimally recognized peptide by HLA-A2-restricted, HBcAg-specific CTL. PBL from a patient with acute hepatitis B were stimulated with peptide 11–27 and then tested against autologous target cells prepulsed with different concentrations of truncated peptides of different length covering the HBcAg 11–27 region. Peptide 18–27 contains the predicted HLA-A2 motif[17,18] with a leucine in position 2 and a valine at the C-terminus. + + +, Significant CTL responses at peptide concentrations equal to or lower than 10 nmol/l; + +, peptide concentrations between 10 and 100 nmol/l; +, peptide concentrations between 1 and 10 μmol/l; –, no CTL response at any of the tested concentrations ranging between 1 nmol/l and 10 μmol/l

recognized peptide (Fig. 3). This 10-mer contains the predicted HLA-A2 binding motif with leucine in position 2 and valine at the C-terminus (submitted manuscript).

In view of the selective association of this nucleocapsid-specific CTL response with the acute stage of self-limited HBV infection and the wide recognition of peptide 18–27 in the HLA-A2 haplotype, this core sequence might represent a potential candidate for a specific immune therapy capable of inducing *in vivo* an efficient anti-HBV specific CTL response in HLA-A2 positive patients.

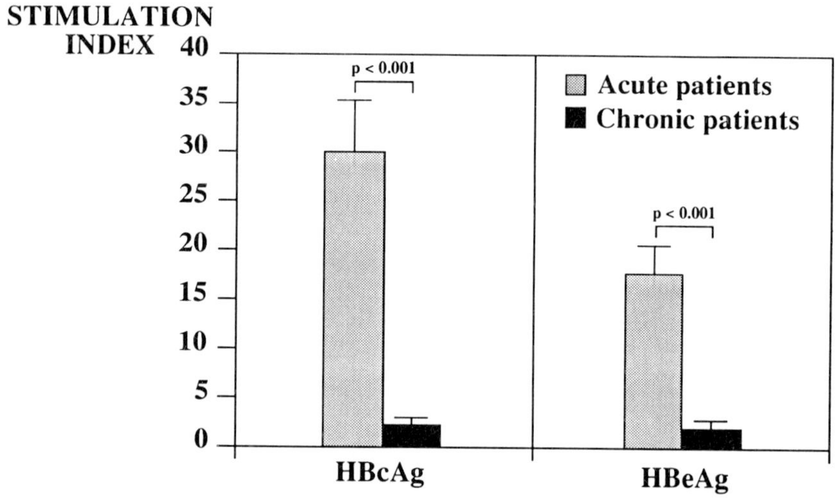

Fig. 4 HLA class II restricted T cell proliferative response to HBcAg and HBeAg in patients with acute (21 cases) and chronic (42 cases) HBV infection. The bars represent the mean values of stimulation index in the two groups of patients. The stimulation index defines the level of T cell proliferative response and is the ratio between the [^{3}H]thymidine incorporated by T cells stimulated with antigen and the [^{3}H]thymidine incorporated by T cells cultured in the absence of antigen

HLA CLASS II RESTRICTED T CELL RESPONSE TO HBV NUCLEOCAPSID ANTIGENS

In contrast to $CD8^+$ CTL that usually recognize viral antigens synthesized within infected cells in association with HLA class I determinants, HLA class II restricted $CD4^+$ T cells generally recognize peptide fragments associated with HLA class II molecules, derived from extracellular antigens which are proteolytically processed in acidified vesicles (endosomes or lysosomes) after endocytosis by specialized antigen-presenting cells[21].

Based on these principles, recombinant and human purified HBV polypeptides have been used as an exogenous source of antigen for *in vitro* stimulation of $CD4^+$ T cells and for analysis of their function in different groups of HBV patients with acute or chronic HBV infection[22]. The results of these studies show that HBV-infected patients who develop a self-limited acute hepatitis express a vigorous HLA class II restricted peripheral blood T cell response to HBcAg and HBeAg[22] (Fig. 4). This response is dramatically lower in patients with chronic HBV infection who do not succeed in clearing the virus[22] (Fig. 4). Whether these defective peripheral blood responses are due to an actual lesion of the immune system in these patients, or are the result of specific viral strategies to evade immune surveillance (such as virus mutations), or reflect a preferential intrahepatic sequestration of virus responsive T cells in the chronic stages of HBV infection, as previously reported[23,24], is under vigorous investigation at this time.

Interestingly, the development of a strong CD4-mediated response to nucleocapsid antigens during acute hepatitis B seems to be temporally associated with the clearance of HBV envelope antigens from the serum[22]. This finding, together with the evidence that this response is defective in the peripheral blood of patients who do not spontaneously clear the virus, suggests that the optimal development of a CD4-mediated response to HBV nucleocapsid antigens following HBV infection may be required for efficient virus elimination. Since the behaviour of this response parallels that of HLA class I restricted CTL, whose activity is similarly vigorous in acute and weak in chronic HBV infection, the apparent involvement of nucleocapsid-specific $CD4^+$ T cells in the pathogenesis of HBV clearance may reflect the helper-dependent activation of nucleocapsid-specific CTL and the elimination of infected cells through their killer function. Alternatively, viral clearance could be facilitated by a direct cooperation between HBcAg-specific helper T cells and HBV envelope-specific B cells, through a mechanism of 'intermolecular' help[25], leading to amplification of the virus-neutralizing anti-envelope antibody response.

FINE SPECIFICITY OF THE CD4-MEDIATED RESPONSE TO HBV NUCLEOPROTEIN

In view of its potential role in HBV clearance the CD4-mediated response to HBcAg could be exploited for the development of anti-HB vaccines with enhanced immunogenic potential. With respect to this possibility it is noteworthy that immunodominant peptides have been identified within the nucleocapsid antigen which are recognized by core-specific $CD4^+$ T cells from patients with acute hepatitis B and different genetic backgrounds[26].

A large panel of short synthetic peptides covering the entire HBV core region were used to study the fine specificity of $CD4^+$ nucleocapsid-specific T cells during HBV infection. Patients with acute hepatitis B were selected for this study since a strong level of T cell response to HBV nucleocapsid antigens is detectable in virtually all of them. Several immunogenic peptides able to induce significant levels of CD4 activation were identified[26]. T cells from individual patients usually recognized more than one peptide fragment. However, a significant proportion of patients were able to recognize three distinct synthetic peptides corresponding to amino acids 1–20, 50–69, and 117–131: in particular, peptide 50–69 was stimulatory for $CD4^+$ T cells from over 90% of acute patients (Fig. 5)[26].

The immunodominance of the T cell epitopes contained within these peptides was demonstrated by their capacity to restimulate *in vitro* the proliferative response of polyclonal HBcAg-specific T cell lines established by PBL stimulation with the whole nucleocapsid protein[26]. In the reciprocal experiments, peptide-induced polyclonal T cell lines established by PBL stimulation with synthetic peptides were able to recognize the native core molecule, demonstrating that the epitopes represented by the stimulatory peptides are actually generated by the intracellular processing of the whole core molecule[26].

Experiments are now in progress to define precisely the HLA restriction elements for these peptides but their 'promiscuous' recognition[27] by T cells

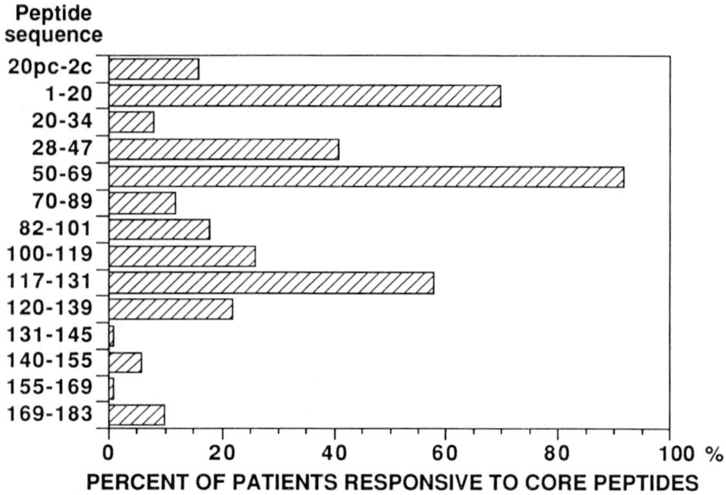

Fig. 5 Fine specificity of the HLA class II restricted T cells response to HBV nucleocapsid antigens. PBL from 27 patients with acute hepatitis B were stimulated with different concentrations of the indicated synthetic peptides and their proliferative response measured after 7 days of culture. Results are expressed as percentage of patients who gave a significant response to the individual core peptides. The T cell response was HLA class II restricted because inhibitable by incubation with anti-HLA class II monoclonal antibodies (not shown)

of different HLA haplotypes is certainly encouraging for their use in a synthetic vaccine that might be effective in a large proportion of the general population.

References

1. Townsend ARM, Rothbard J, Gotch FM, Bahadur G, Wraith D, McMichael AJ. The epitopes of influenza nucleoprotein recognized by cytotoxic T lymphocytes can be defined with short synthetic peptides. Cell. 1986;44:959–68.
2. Gotch FM, Rothbard J, Howland K, Townsend A, McMichael AJ. Cytotoxic T lymphocytes recognize a fragment of influenza virus matrix protein in association with HLA-A2. Nature. 1987;326:881–2.
3. Monaco JJ. A molecular model of MHC class I restricted antigen processing. Immunol Today. 1992;13:173–9.
4. Townsend ARM, Gotch FM, Davey J. Cytotoxic T cells recognize fragments of the influenza nucleoprotein. Cell. 1985;42:457–67.
5. Nixon DF, Townsend ARM, Elvin JG, Rizza CR, Gallway J, McMichael AJ. HIV-1 gag-specific cytotoxic T lymphocytes defined with recombinant vaccinia virus and synthetic peptides. Nature. 1988;336:484–7.
6. Yedwell JW, Bennink JR, Mackett M, Lefrancois L, Lyles DS, Moss B. Recognition of cloned vesicular stomatitis virus internal and external gene products by cytotoxic T lymphocytes. J Exp Med. 1986;163:1529–38.
7. Holt CA, Osorio K, Lilly F. Friend virus-specific cytotoxic T lymphocytes recognized both *gag* and *env* gene-encoded specificities. J Exp Med. 1986;164:211–26.
8. Bangham CRM, Openshaw PJM, Ball LA, King AMQ, Wertz GW, Askonas BA. Human and murine cytotoxic T cells specific to respiratory syncytial virus recognize the viral nucleoprotein (N), but not the major glycoprotein (G) expressed by vaccinia virus recombinants. J Immunol. 1986;137:3973–7.

9. Mondelli M, Mieli-Vergani G, Alberti A, Vergani D, Portman B, Eddleston ALWF, Williams R. Specificity of T lymphocyte cytotoxicity to autologous hepatocytes in chronic hepatitis B virus infection: evidence that T cells are directed against HBV core antigen expressed on hepatocytes. J Immunol. 1982;129:2773–7.
10. Penna A, Chisari FV, Bertoletti A, Missale G, Fowler P, Giuberti T, Fiaccadori F, Ferrari C. Cytotoxic T lymphocytes recognize an HLA-A2-restricted epitope within the hepatitis B virus nucleocapsid antigen. J Exp Med. 1991;174:1565–9.
11. Schlicht HJ, Schaller H. The secretory core protein of human hepatitis B virus is expressed on the cell surface. J Virol. 1989;63:5399–403.
12. Guilhot S, Fowler P, Margolskee R, Ferrari C, Bertoletti A, Chisari FV. Hepatitis B virus (HBV) specific cytolytic T cell response in man: production of target cells by stable expression of HBV encoded proteins in immortalized human B cell lines. J Virol. 1992;66:2670–5.
13. Bertoletti A, Ferrari C, Fiaccadori F, Penna A, Margoleskee R, Schlicht HJ, Fowler P, Guilhot S, Chisari FV. HLA class-I human cytotixic T cells recognize endogenously synthesized hepatitis B virus nucleocapsid antigen. Proc Natl Acad Sci USA. 1991;88: 10445–9.
14. Rotzschke O, Falk K, Deres K, Schild H, Norda M, Metzger J, Jung G, Rammensee HG. Isolation and analysis of naturally processed viral peptides as recognized by cytotoxic T cells. Nature. 1990;348:252–4.
15. Van Bleek GM, Nathenson SG. Isolation of an endogenously processed immunodominant viral peptide from the class I H-$2K^b$ molecule. Nature. 1990;348:213–16.
16. Jardetzky TS, Lane VS, Robinson RA, Madden DR, Wiley DC. Identification of self peptides bound to purified HLA-B27. Nature. 1991;353:326–8.
17. Hunt DF, Henderson RA, Shabanowitz J, Sakaguchi K, Michel H, Sevilir N, Cox AL, Appella E, Engelhard VH. Characterization of peptides bound to the class I MHC molecule HLA-A2.1 by mass spectrometry. Science. 1992;255:1261–3.
18. Falk K, Rotzschke O, Stevanovic S, Jung G, Rammensee H. Allele-specific motifs revealed by sequencing of self-peptides eluted from MHC molecules. Nature. 1991;351:290–6.
19. Cerundolo V, Elliott T, Elvin J, Bastin J, Ramenssee H-G, Townsend A. The binding affinity and dissociation rates of peptides for class I major histocompatibility complex molecules. Eur J Immunol. 1991;21:2069–75.
20. Christinck ER, Luscher MA, Barber BH, Williams DB. Peptide binding to class I MHC on living cells and quantitation of complexes required for CTL lysis. Nature. 1991;352: 67–70.
21. Germain RN. The second class story. Nature. 1991;353:605–6.
22. Ferrari C, Penna A, Bertoletti A, Valli A, Degli Antoni A, Giuberti T, Cavalli A, Petit MA, Fiaccadori F. Cellular immune response to hepatitis B virus-encoded antigens in acute and chronic hepatitis B virus infection. J Immunol. 1990;145:3442–9.
23. Ferrari C, Penna G, Giuberti T, Tong MJ, Ribera E, Fiaccadori F, Chisari FV. Intrahepatic, nucleocapsid antigen-specific T cells in chronic active hepatitis B. J Immunol. 1987;139: 2050–8.
24. Ferrari C, Mondelli MU, Penna A, Fiaccadori F, Chisari FV. Functional characterization of cloned intrahepatic, hepatitis B virus nucleoprotein-specific helper T cell lines. J Immunol. 1987;139:539–44.
25. Milich DR, McLachlan A, Thornton GB, Hughes JL. Antibody production to the nucleocapsid and envelope of the hepatitis B virus primed by a single Synthetic T cell site. Nature. 1987;329:547–9.
26. Ferrari C, Bertoletti A, Penna A, Cavalli A, Valli A, Missale G, Pilli M, Fowler P, Giuberti T, Chisari FV, Fiaccadori F. Identification of immunodominant T cell epitopes of the hepatitis B virus nucleocapsid antigen. J Clin Invest. 1991;88:214–22.
27. Panina P, Tan A, Termijtelen A, Demotz S, Corradin G, Lanzavecchia A. Universally immunogenic T cell epitopes: promiscuous binding to human class II and promiscuous recognition by T cells. Eur J Immunol. 1989;19:2237–42.
28. Canfield V, Emanuel JR, Spickofsky N, Levenson R, Margolskee RF. Ouabain-resistant mutants of the rat Na, K-ATPase alpha2 isoform identified by using an episomal expression vector. Mol Cell Biol. 1990;10:1367–70.

6
Cellular immune reactions to hepatitis B envelope antigens

M. PAROLI, A. FRANCO, G. DE PETRILLO, R. BENVENUTO and V. BARNABA

Hepatitis B virus (HBV) belongs to a strain of viruses that are not cytopathic or are poorly cytopathic in the normal host, but may cause tissue damage by eliciting virus-specific cytotoxic T lymphocyte (CTL) responses essential for the destruction of infected cells and for the consequent limitation of virus replication. Here we consider the immune response by T lymphocytes to the hepatitis B envelope antigen (HBenvAg), a complex molecular structure that constitutes the virus surface and that contains three distinct proteins encoded by the pre-S1, pre-S2, and S regions of the virus genome[1].

Several studies have shown that the humoral and cellular immune response to epitopes of the pre-S1, pre-S2, and S sequences plays an important role in protective immunity against HBV[2–5]. Antibody and cellular responses to HBenvAg have been detected after recovery from acute infection and in HB vaccine recipients, whereas patients with chronic infection may not recognize these antigens, at least at the peripheral B and T cell level[6–9]. Indeed, the recent isolation of both intrahepatic class II ($CD4^+$) and class I ($CD8^+$) major histocompatibility complex (MHC)-restricted pre-S2-specific CTLs in chronic hepatitis B, indicates that HBenvAg may be an important target molecule for killing infected hepatocytes[10]. This is also supported by the observation that in the transgenic (TG) mice model, liver cells expressing HBenvAg are destroyed following the adoptive transfer of class I-restricted HBenvAg-specific CTLs from non-TG syngeneic mice[11].

Since hepatocytes express class II molecules in chronic liver disease[12] and can perform antigen presentation to specific T clones[13], a cytotoxic interaction between hepatic class II-restricted T cells specific for HBenvAg[10] and infected hepatocytes expressing endogenous HBenvAg plus the appropriate class II molecule might participate in the process of lysis of infected cells[14,15]. Furthermore, exogenous HBenvAg has been demonstrated to be presented in association with class I MHC molecules to $CD8^+$ T cells[15,16]. This represents an exception to the rule of class I/class II discrimination. This rule assumes that endogenously synthesized antigens (such as viral proteins) are usually associated with class I molecules in the cytoplasm of infected cells and presented to CD8$^+$ T lymphocytes, while exogenous antigens are taken up by the antigen-presenting cells (APCs) and generally bind to class II molecules in the endosomal compartment, to be thereafter presented to CD4$^+$ T cells[17]. Under these conditions, lysis of uninfected hepatocytes might also occur, because of the capability of exogenous HBenvAg to access not only to class II-, but also to the class I-processing pathway. This would allow the presentation of its peptides to both types of CTLs[10,15,16].

The evidence that HBV infects lymphocytes and macrophages[18–20] suggests that the virus binds to a non-clonally distributed molecule on lymphoid cells and infects them. However, systemic immunosuppression due to direct lymphoid cell lysis is unlikely, since HBV is a non-cytopathic virus. On the other hand, generalized immunosuppression might be a result of a class I-restricted CTL response against HBV-infected lymphocytes, as has been shown for the human immunodeficiency virus (HIV)[21]. In other words, the HBV-specific CTLs, which are essential for limiting virus replication by the destruction of infected cells, could generate a systemic immunosuppression that would also prevent HBV clearance.

In addition soluble HBenvAg may be bound and processed by both T and B uninfected lymphocytes, and presented to class II-restricted HBenvAg-specific CTLs, as well as to class I-restricted CTLs due to its particular tendency to enter the cytoplasmic class I processing pathway[10,15,16].

In this regard we have demonstrated that both CD4$^+$ and CD8$^+$ T clones can efficiently present HBenvAg to class II-restricted CTL[22]. Using this system of T-T presentation, we also showed that transferrin receptor (CD71) was involved in efficient HBenvAg uptake by T cells. Moreover, it can be assumed that antigen-specific CD4$^+$ T clones which kill HBenvAg presenting T cells may participate in generalized immunosuppression by elimination of T lymphocytes. In particular, CD71$^+$ cells expressing class II molecules, as macrophages or activated T cells, could be susceptible to lysis by HBenvAg presentation to class II-restricted CTL, with consequent down-regulating of the T cell response and selective advantage for HBV persistence, further supporting the hypothesis that antigen presentation by T cells may play a role in immunoregulation[23,24].

The role of class II-restricted CTL in immunopathogenesis is further supported by our recent detection of CD4$^+$ T lymphocytes with cytotoxic activity expressing the CD56 molecule among liver-infiltrating T cells of patients with chronic active hepatitis B. Interestingly, these cells were not significantly represented among peripheral lymphocytes from the same patients or from HB vaccine recipients. Furthermore, we generated a large panel of HBenvAg-specific CD4$^+$ T clones from either liver-derived or PBL-derived T lymphocytes, and studied their phenotype and function. All the liver-derived T clones, in contrast with the majority of PBL-derived HBenvAg-specific CD4$^+$ T clones, coexpressed the CD56 surface antigen, and secreted high levels of IFN-γ but not of IL-4, thereby resembling Th1 cells of the mouse. We also found that CD4$^+$ CD56$^+$ clones were highly cytotoxic, and killing was dependent on direct contact between T cells and targets. In another series of experiments we detected the presence of perforin on liver-infiltrating $CD4^+$ $CD56^+$ T cells. The finding that liver-derived but not PBL-derived T cells stained for both CD56 and perforin, suggested a tissue compartmentalization of this CTL subset, that may take part in the amplification of the local immune response and may participate in lysis of virus-infected cells expressing class II molecules, such as the hepatocytes in the course of chronic inflammatory liver diseases[10,12].

Due to their high cytotoxic potential and class II restriction, HBenvAg-specific $CD4^+$ $CD56^+$ T lymphocytes could be involved in the down-regulation of the specific immune responses by elimination of class II-positive APC with impairment of antigen presentation. Selective suppression of antibody responses to HBenvAg due to the killing of antigen-specific B cells has been demonstrated and suggested as a determinant for chronicity of infection[16]. Specific B cells bind very low concentrations of soluble antigens with high affinity via their specific Ig receptors, then internalize and process them through the class II processing pathway, and present their fragments to class II-restricted T cells which have helper activity for the specific B cells. Thus, low concentrations of HBenvAg selectively sensitize antigen-specific B cells for class II-restricted CTLs, which is followed by specific suppression of the antibody response. Moreover, because of the exceptional capability of exogenous HBenvAg to gain access to the class I processing pathway[10,15,16], the specific focusing of HBenvAg by the surface Ig of specific B cells also permits presentation of processed fragments to the conventional class I-restricted CTLs. Thus, both class II- and class I-restricted CTLs, which are abundantly represented in the liver to ensure the killing of infected hepatocytes, can also be responsible for the selective killing of HBenvAg-specific B cells. This leads, on the one hand, to a down-regulation of the specific neutralizing antibody response, and on the other hand, to the establishment of chronic HBV carrier state.

The outcome of HBV infection may be different, including complete recovery from acute disease, establishment of a healthy carrier state or evolution into chronic disease, and is dependent on both viral and host factors. Study of the immune response to HBenvAg may help to understand the complex molecular basis of the interactions between HBV and T cells that ultimately determine the outcome of infection.

References

1. Heermann KH, Goldmann U, Schwartz W, Seyffarth T, Baaumgarten H, Gerlich WH. Large surface protein of hepatitis B virus containing the pre-S sequence. J Virol. 1984;52: 396–402.
2. Alberti A, Pontisso P, Tagariello G, Cavalletto D, Chemello L, Belussi F. Antibody response to pre-S2 and hepatitis B virus induced liver damage. Lancet. 1988;1:1421–4.
3. Klinkert MQ, Theilmann L, Pfaff E, Schaller H. Pre-S1 antigens and antibodies early in the course of acute hepatitis B virus infection. J Virol. 1986;58:522–5.
4. Alberti A, Gerlich WH, Heermann KH, Pontisso P. Nature and display of hepatitis B virus envelope proteins and the humoral immune response. Springer Semin Immunopathol. 1990;12:5–23.
5. Celis E, Kung PC, Chang TW. Hepatitis B virus reactive T lymphocyte clones: antigen specificity and helper function for antibody synthesis. J Immunol. 1984;132:1511–16.

6. Alberti A, Cavalletto D, Chemello L, Belussi F, Fattovich G, Pontisso P, Milanesi G, Ruol A. Fine specificity of human antibody response to the pre-S1 domain of hepatitis B virus. Hepatology. 1990;12:199–203.
7. Barnaba V, Valesini G, Levrero M, Zaccari C, Van Dyke A, Falco M, Musca A, Balsano F. Immunoregulation of the in vitro anti-HBs antibody synthesis in chronic HBsAg carriers and in recently boosted anti-hepatitis B vaccine recipients. Clin Exp Immunol. 1985;60: 209–16.
8. Barnaba V, Levrero M, Ruberti G, Van Dyke A, Perrone A, Musca A, Balsano F. In vitro anti-HBs antibody synthesis from anti-hepatitis B vaccine recipients. Clin Exp Immunol. 1987;70:283–8.
9. Ferrari C, Penna A, Bertoletti A, Cavalli A, Valli A, Schianchi C, Fiaccadori F. The pre-S1 antigen of hepatitis B virus is highly immunogenic at the T cell level in man. J Clin Invest. 1989;84:1314–19.
10. Barnaba V, Franco A, Alberti A, Balsano C, Benvenuto R, Balsano F. Recognition of hepatitis B virus envelope proteins by liver-infiltrating T lymphocytes in chronic HBV infection. J Immunol. 1989;143:2650–5.
11. Moriyama T, Guilhot S, Klopchin K, Moss B, Pinkert CA, Palmiter RD, Brinster RL, Kanagawa O, Chisari FV. Immunobiology and pathogenesis of hepatocellular injury in hepatitis B virus transgenic mice. Science. 1990;248:361–4.
12. Franco A, Barnaba V, Natali PG, Balsano C, Musca A, Balsano F. Expression of class I and class II major histocompatibility complex antigens on human hepatocytes. Hepatology. 1988;8:49–54.
13. Franco A, Barnaba V, Ruberti G, Benvenuto R, Balsano C, Musca A. Liver-derived T cell clones in autoimmune chronic active hepatitis: accessory cell function of hepatocytes expressing class II major histocompatibility complex molecules. Clin Immunol Immunopathol. 1990;54:382–94.
14. Nuchtern JG, Biddison WE, Klausner RD. Class II MHC molecules can use the endogenous pathway of antigen presentation. Nature. 1990;343:74–6.
15. Jin Y, Shih JWK, Berkower I. Human T cell response to the surface antigen of hepatitis B virus (HBsAg). Endosomal and nonendosomal processing pathways are accessible to both endogenous and exogenous antigens. J Exp Med. 1988;168:293–306.
16. Barnaba V, Franco A, Alberti A, Benvenuto R, Balsano F. Selective killing of hepatitis B envelope antigen-specific B cells by class I-restricted, exogenous antigen-specific T lymphocytes. Nature. 1990;345:258–60.
17. Germain RN. The ins and outs of antigen processing and presentation. Nature. 1986;322: 687–9.
18. Romet-Lemonne JJ, McLane MF, Elfassi E, Haseltine WA, Azocar J, Essex M. Hepatitis B virus infects in cultured human lymphoblastoid cells. Science. 1983;221:667–9.
19. Yoffe B, Noonan CA, Melmick JL, Hollinger FB. Hepatitis B virus DNA in mononuclear cells and analysis of cell subsets for the presence of replicative intermediates of viral DNA. J Infect Dis. 1986;153:471–7.
20. Pasquinelli C, Laur F, Chatenouel L, Beaurin G, Gazengel C, Bismuth H, Degos F, Tiollais P, Bach JF, Brechot C. Hepatitis B virus DNA in mononuclear blood cells. A frequent event in HBsAg-positive and -negative patients with acute and chronic liver disease. J Hepatol. 1986;3:95–103.
21. Zinkernagel RM. Virus-triggered AIDS: a T-cell-mediated immunopathology? Immunol Today. 1988;9:370–2.
22. Franco A, Paroli M, Testa U, Benvenuto R, Peschle C, Balsano F, Barnaba V. Transferrin receptor mediates uptake and presentation of hepatitis B envelope antigen by T lymphocytes. J Exp Med. 1992;175:1195–205.
23. Lanzavecchia A. Is suppression a function of class II-restricted cytotoxic T cells? Immunol Today. 1989;10:157–9.
24. Germain RN. Antigen processing and $CD4^+$ T cell depletion in AIDS. Cell. 1988;54: 441–4.

7
Immunology of hepadnavirus infection in woodchucks

P. J. COTE

INTRODUCTION

The eastern woodchuck and the woodchuck hepatitis virus (WHV) are being used to model the immunology of hepadnavirus infection and its applications to hepatitis B virus (HBV) infection and disease of man (reviewed in ref. 1). The woodchuck is uniformly susceptible to WHV infection in the experimental setting when defined virus inocula are used, and acute WHV infections with resolution occur in 80–90% or more of infected yearling and adult woodchucks, while chronic WHV infections occur in 60–70% of infected neonatal woodchucks[2,3]. In chronic WHV infection the woodchuck fails to clear virus and subviral surface antigens (WHsAg) from blood following acute infection of the liver. While cirrhosis is not a common endstage feature of chronic WHV infection, chronic active hepatitis and hepatocellular carcinoma (HCC) invariably develop within 2–4 years[4]. In contrast, successful immune responses to acute infection clear circulating WHV and WHsAg (i.e. induce resolution and recovery), and considerably reduce hepatitis and lower the risk of developing HCC (Table 1). From the fundamental standpoint of virus persistence, however, non-replicating monomeric and multimeric forms of WHV DNA are often detected in the livers of serologically recovered woodchucks, even years after acute infection[5,6]; and when serologically recovered woodchucks develop HCC, WHV DNA is often found in the tumour tissue in integrated form[6]. Thus, resolution of acute WHV infection

Table 1 Neonatal WHV infection: HCC risk

Serological status	*No./total* (%)
(A) Chronic carriers	63/63 (100%)
(B) Recovered	11/63 (17%)
(C) Negative controls	0/108 (0%)

Colony born and held > 3 years
A vs C, B vs C, A vs C; $p < 0.001$

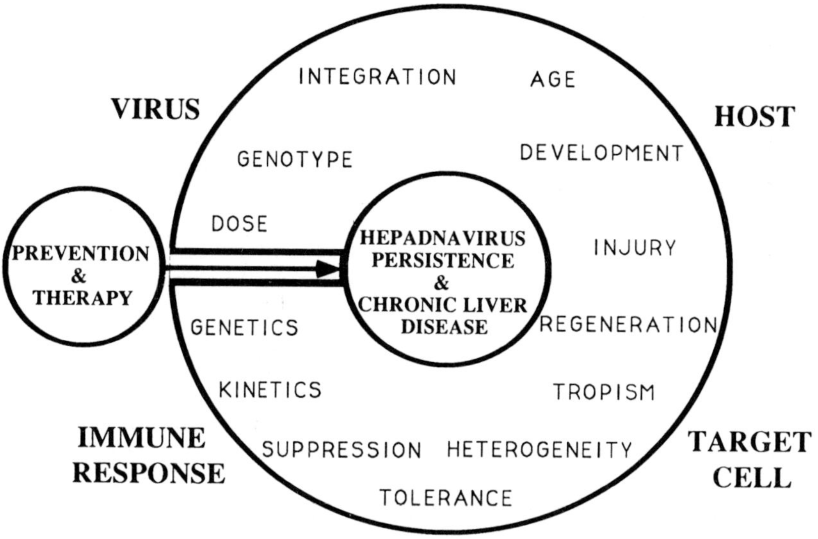

Fig. 1 Variables associated with persistent hepadnavirus infection and chronic liver disease that can be studied in woodchuck/WHV model

does not completely eliminate persistent viral DNA in tissues, or the risk of HCC compared to uninfected animals. However, the immune response to acute infection does eliminate the two major epidemiological risk factors (i.e. surface antigenaemia and viraemia) that are associated with all forms of progressive chronic liver disease in the woodchuck, including HCC.

Many of the HBV model systems that have been described thus far represent powerful tools for answering specific questions and developing hypotheses on the pathogenic mechanisms of hepadnaviruses. The woodchuck model provides a relevant outbred species for controlled testing of such processes as they interact together, naturally with time, or in response to experimental manipulations (Fig. 1). Of all the possible mechanisms involved in such processes the primary goal of this presentation is to examine the role of the immune response to acute infection as the primary determinant in chronicity. In looking more specifically at the immune response to hepadnavirus infection, our laboratory has focused on the T helper/inducer cell. It is the key regulatory cell required for resolution of acute hepadnavirus infection, and should provide a useful target for therapy of chronic hepadnavirus infections. In addition to studies designed to modulate T helper cells *in vivo*, we have also been attempting to characterize their basic immunobiology in the woodchuck. Our overall goal here is to eventually develop the woodchuck as a predictive model for the cellular, molecular, and immunogenetic processes that function during the immune response to hepadnavirus infection. Such information will allow us to develop and test novel preventive and therapeutic strategies for WHV and HBV infection.

IMMUNOBIOLOGY OF THE WOODCHUCK

The woodchuck is a relatively new and important model species for the study of hepadnavirus infection, immune response, and disease pathogenesis. Little is known about its immunobiology, and there are no available reagents, analogous to human and murine immune systems. Our laboratory is currently active in cross-screening antibody, cytokine, and genetic reagents for application to the model, and in the development of woodchuck-specific reagents to permit more definitive studies in the future. Thus far we have found that peripheral blood mononuclear cells (PBMC) of the woodchuck undergo DNA synthesis and cell division *in vitro* in response to mitogens such as LPS and concanavalin A (ConA), and while they readily incorporate radiolabelled uridine and adenine into cellular nucleic acids, they fail to incorporate significant amounts of labelled thymidine (and thymidine analogues) into cellular DNA[1,7]; therefore, measurement of *in vitro* proliferation by this method is not applicable in the woodchuck model, and other methods have been developed. For example, *in vitro* assays for two important T cell cytokines have been developed recently: one for woodchuck interleukin-2 (IL-2) and another for woodchuck interferon-γ (IFN-γ) (P. Cote, B. Fernie, and J. L. Gerin, manuscripts in preparation). We hope to further apply these assays to substantiate the mechanisms proposed from *in vivo* studies (see below).

IMMUNOMODULATION OF WHV INFECTION

Our laboratory has tested several immunological hypotheses in the woodchuck model by using outcome of infection and disease as the primary endpoints. Needless to say, these studies are of the type that cannot be performed in humans, or readily in any of the other HBV model systems. We have focused on the modulation of T helper cells in the *in vivo* setting, primarily early during infection. One of the rationales for acute-phase studies is to define early events in the cascade leading to chronicity or resolution, which should then permit the development of more rational therapies for chronic infections based on cause–effect relationships.

Chronicity and tolerance to e-antigen

The e-antigen tolerance hypothesis was proposed by Dr Milich from his studies in murine model systems[8]. It is not known in humans when and whether tolerance to e-antigen occurs as proposed, or if it causes or is involved in maintenance of chronic HBV infection. While there is yet no documented proof for the existence of a native e-antigen/antibody system in the woodchuck, we have attempted to examine the e-tolerance hypothesis in woodchucks using both virological and immunological approaches.

Using a virological approach we showed that infection of neonates with 5×10^6 genomic equivalents of cloned wild-type WHV8 inoculum resulted in a 70% rate of chronicity; a site-directed pre-core mutant of this clone (i.e.

Table 2 Outcome of infection in woodchucks given rWHeAg at birth and challenged with WHV at 8 weeks of age

Group	No. infected	Acute (%)		Outcome (%)	
		WHV	*WHsAg*	*Chronic*	*anti-WHs*
WHeAg−	12	8 (67)	8 (67)	4 (33)	3 (25)
WHeAg+	15	9 (60)	8 (53)	3 (20)	10 (67)*

Data are numbers of animals and percentages
*$p < 0.05$

a model e-minus mutant) produced no carriers among five neonates in a high-dose pilot study (~ 3–5×10^8 genomic equivalents)[9]. In a more recent and larger study at 5×10^6 genomic equivalents, the pre-core mutant has thus far (i.e. as of 5 months post-infection) produced only seven potential carriers out of 23 neonatal infections (30%; $p < 0.02$ vs control). While these results may suggest that e-antigen is a correlate of chronicity in WHV infection, they are preliminary pending; (a) follow-up of the animals; (b) titration of virus to endpoint to show equal ratios of physical to infectious particles; and (c) demonstration in WHV infection of native e-antigen and its associated antibodies and tolerogenic epitopes.

To examine the possible tolerogenicity of an e-like antigen in the woodchuck, we used a recombinant WHeAg developed by Dr Florian Schoedel of the Max Planck Institute and designed an antigen administration–WHV challenge study in woodchucks analogous to the rHBeAg tolerization–priming experiments in mice[8]. In our study (Table 2), we administered 30 μg of recombinant WHeAg in incomplete Freund's adjuvant at birth to neonatal woodchucks, and challenged them with WHV at 8 weeks of age (i.e. when the normal frequency of developing chronic infections is lower than at birth). There was no evidence that any of the e-treated animals were protected from infection. Administration of WHeAg at birth did not influence acute WHV infection when animals were challenged at 8 weeks of age, nor was the outcome of infection in terms of chronicity different from controls as of 9 months post-infection. However, the frequency of anti-WHs responses following acute-phase infection was higher in the e-treated animals, suggesting that e-antigen could provide help for anti-WHs responses.

Thus: (a) neonatal woodchucks were primed by rWHeAg rather than tolerized; (b) priming with rWHeAg enhanced anti-WHs responses to WHV challenge; and (c) there was no effect of subtle modulatory responses caused by priming on acute WHV infection or its outcome. These results question whether the tolerance hypothesis is relevant for outbred species (e.g. woodchucks), and, by inference, humans. However, in defence of further testing of tolerance mechanisms in woodchucks, we would need to establish conditions, if they exist, under which tolerance can be induced experimentally in neonatal woodchucks, including *in utero* methods.

Chronicity and post-exposure priming with WHsAg

This approach bears more directly on T helper cell expansion and its role in the outcome of WHV infection and disease. In this case we used priming doses of WHsAg vaccine in a post-exposure setting following high-dose challenge of neonates[1]. Placebo-controlled data showed that two priming doses of vaccine, which failed to induce early anti-WHs, did not prevent infection by high-dose virus challenge, but did decrease the rate of chronicity as of 1 year and the rate of HCC as of 3 years following acute infection. This study implies that vaccine induced expansion of WHsAg-specific T helper cells early during infection protected against chronicity and HCC as outcomes of acute infection. The precise timing of the post-exposure vaccination window to achieve such an effect has not been established, but it should be noted from other studies in our laboratory[1] that a single vaccination with surface antigen in combination with ara-AMP and IL-2 at 5 months post-infection (i.e. when 30–35% of infected woodchucks normally begin to resolve the neonatal infection) did not increase the frequency of resolved infections relative to controls. This indicated that chronicity in neonatally infected woodchucks is established by 5 months of age, which corresponds to the late acute phase of infection.

Chronicity and post-exposure immunosuppression with CsA

If early T helper cell expansion to surface antigen alone can protect against chronicity, we asked whether immunosuppression of all T helper responses would increase the rate of chronicity. In these experiments[10,11], we applied the adult model of WHV infection and used the T helper cell immunosuppressive agent, cyclosporin A (CsA), to ask whether and when it would affect the outcome of infection. In these experiments[10,11], non-immunosuppressed, adult control animals showed a 0% rate of chronicity, as expected, whether left untreated or given an oil vehicle. When animals were immunosuppressed throughout the incubation and acute phase of infection, there was an overall rate of chronicity at 1 year of 92%. There was no increase in chronicity, or reactivation of infections, when animals were treated for 10 weeks beginning at or near the end of the acute phase (i.e. from 8 to 18 weeks post-inoculation). However, the rate of chronicity was increased to 55% when animals were treated for 10 weeks during the acute phase, and there was a remarkable 50% rate of chronicity when animals were treated for only the first 4 weeks post-inoculation, which involved mainly the incubation phase[11]. In summary, immunosuppression of T helper responses for even short intervals during the incubation was sufficient to increase the risk of chronicity. Based on the mechanism of action of CsA, the results suggested that IL-2-dependent T helper cell expansion occurs early in the response to WHV infection and is required to interdict chronic infection. The results also have important clinical implications when organ and liver transplantations are complicated by HBV infection.

To further substantiate immunological mechanisms operating in the woodchuck, we applied our newly developed *in vitro* assay for woodchuck IL-2. In a representative control experiment using a murine IL-2-dependent NK cell line (Table 3), CsA had no effect on the direct assay of standard recombinant human IL-2. In the experiment with woodchuck peripheral

Table 3 CsA inhibits IL-2 production by ConA-stimulated woodchuck PBMC: assay of supernate IL-2 activity on murine NKA cells

Woodchuck PMBC supernate		*NKA assay*		
ConA (*μg/ml*)	*CsA* (*ng/ml*)	*CsA* (*ng/ml*)	*hrIL-2* (*IU/ml*)	*c.p.m.*
		0	0	2468
		0	18	97903
		1000	18	89450
0	0			2601
80	0			115216
80	1000			6178
80	250			8591
80	50			18613

Fifty microlitres of woodchuck PBMC supernate was assayed on NKA cells (1:4 final dilution); hrIL-2 is human recombinant IL-2 (Cetus); c.p.m. is the average count for NKA assays performed in duplicate

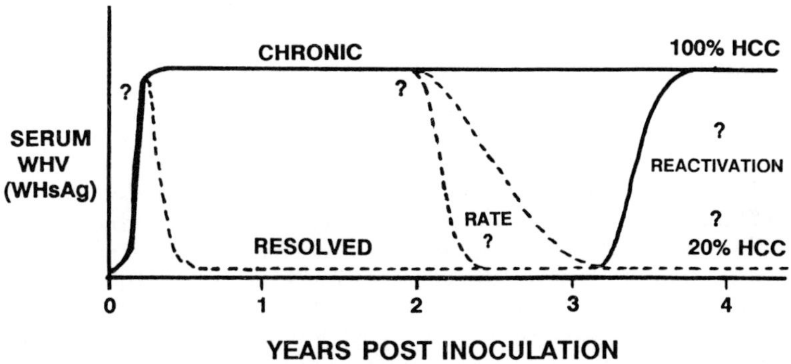

Fig. 2 Serological response patterns of virus and surface antigen during WHV infection

blood mononuclear cells (PBMC) (Table 3), supernatants from unstimulated woodchuck PBMC had no effect on the uptake of thymidine by the IL-2-dependent cells, while those from ConA-stimulated PBMC contained assayable IL-2, except when CsA was added to the cultures at the time of stimulation. The activity in the ConA supernates from woodchuck PBMC was specifically due to IL-2 alone, because it was inhibited completely by an excess of crossreactive rabbit antibody to human IL-2 (P. Cote *et al.*, manuscript in preparation). Studies are in progress using the IL-2 and IFN-γ assays to study antigen-specific responses of PBMC during WHV infection.

Late-stage modulation of chronic WHV infections

In a follow-up of natural and CsA-induced chronic WHV infections we have observed several serological profiles which have bearing on the long-term outcome and prognosis for treatment of chronic hepadnavirus infections (Fig. 2). The course of naturally resolved infections is associated with a 20%

Table 4 Potential applications of models for hepadnavirus chronicity in the woodchuck

WHV chronicity	*Model*		*Mechanism(s) Same: yes/no*
	Neonate	*Adult*	
Early cause	Yes	Yes	?
Maintenance	Yes	Yes	?
Response/therapy	Yes	Yes	?
Resolve late			
spontaneous	No	Yes	No
experimental	?	?	?
Reactivation			
spontaneous	Yes	No	No
experimental	?	?	?
Chronic hepatitis	Yes	Yes	?
HCC	Yes	Yes	Yes

Neonatal = experimentally infected at birth; adult = experimentally infected and CsA-treated

rate of HCC, compared to chronic carriers which always develop HCC. While neonatal chronic infections can be modulated with antiviral nucleotide analogues and immune modulators, neither has been able thus far to effect a permanent cure. One additional point is that 1–2% of neonatal infections appear to resolve for up to 1 or 2 years, but then reactivate into the chronic pattern with HCC (Fig. 2). It may be possible to model this further experimentally in animals with resolved infections using steroids.

In CsA-induced chronic infections we observed two patterns of response in six of the initial carriers followed now for 3 years[10,11]. In three animals there was natural maintenance of the chronic infection (i.e. WHV and WHsAg positive in blood) and development of HCC, as expected. Unlike natural chronic infections in neonates, the pattern in the other three adult carriers involved spontaneous resolution with loss of both serum WHV and WHsAg, generally occurring between $1\frac{1}{2}$ and 2 years post-infection (e.g. Fig. 2). No HCC has been detected in these animals thus far. If these patterns of resolution are permanent, then the results suggest further possibilities for immunological therapies to eliminate circulating WHV and WHsAg in natural chronic infections. The question then becomes whether such late-stage clearance, including its timing relative to the acute phase, and its rate of occurrence (Fig. 2), will have an impact on decreasing all of the progressive manifestations of chronic liver disease, including HCC.

SUMMARY AND FUTURE DIRECTIONS

In summary (Table 4), CsA-induced chronicity in adults and experimental chronicity in the neonate can both be used to model early events that cause chronicity in the different settings, and both can be used to identify factors associated with the long-term maintenance of chronicity and development of hepatitis and HCC in active chronic infections. CsA can perhaps be used to help model adult chronicity for antivirals and immunotherapeutics,

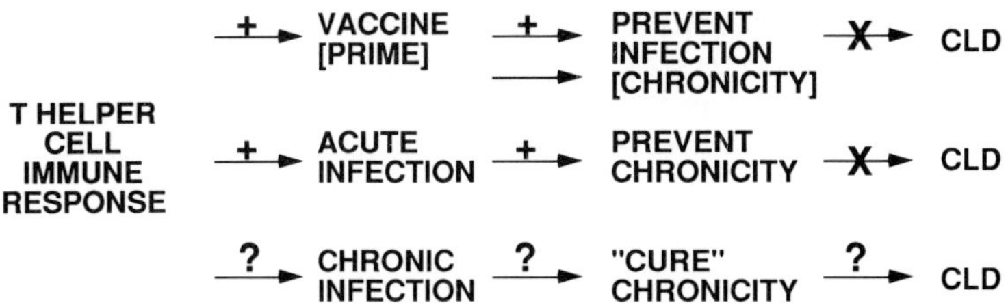

Fig. 3 Role of T helper cell immune response in WHV infection and disease. CLD = chronic liver diseases, including hepatocellular carcinoma; + = positive stimulation or effect; X = reduction in effect; ? = potential effect

provided a control carrier group is used to monitor spontaneous resolution. Reactivation is rare in either setting, but may be able to be modulated experimentally in either system. Natural resolution of long-term chronic infections seems more frequent in the CsA model. This might represent a failure to establish T helper cell tolerance during the response to CsA, or represent the emergence of T helper cells from an anergic state. The serological pattern may be analogous to natural seroconversions that sometimes occur in chronic HBV carriers (e.g. HBeAg/anti-HBe; HBsAg/anti-HBs). An understanding of such mechanisms should lead to more improved therapeutic modalities for adult and neonatal chronic HBV infection.

The above studies also raise further questions. For example, although an adequate IL-2-dependent T helper response appears to function in resolution of acute infection, why do IL-2 and other cytokines, such as interferons, fail to consistently induce recovery in chronic carriers? What are the other defects downstream in the immunological cascade that promote chronicity? And what defects, if any, represent 'lock-out' mechanisms that could set in, once chronicity is established, and frustrate direct immunological intervention (e.g. T suppression or peripheral anergy of T helper cells). The immune responses to vaccine and acute infection are the only proven means of prevention and 'natural therapy' for protecting the host against chronic hepadnavirus infection and chronic liver disease (Fig. 3). In the future we hope to identify cause–effect immunological mechanisms, and characterize their timing, response rates, and defects, by using *in vivo* studies in the woodchuck with supporting *in vitro* immunological modelling. Then it should be possible to test rationally developed immunological strategies aimed at the T helper cell for their efficacy in eliminating chronic hepadnavirus infection and decreasing the progression of chronic liver disease leading to HCC (Fig. 3).

Acknowledgements

The author would like to thank the organizing committee for the invitation to present this work on behalf of the Woodchuck Hepatitis Virus Program and its investigators, Drs J. L. Gerin, B. C. Tennant, B. E. Korba, B. Fernie, B. Baldwin, W. Hornbuckle, R. Miller, and R. H. Purcell. Dr L. Johnson is the NIAID Project Officer for the WHV programme. The author also acknowledges the contributions to this presentation involving WHeAg by Drs F. Schoedel, D. Peterson, and D. R. Milich. This work was supported by contracts AI-72623 and AI-52585 between the National Institutes of Health and the Georgetown and Cornell Universities, respectively.

References

1. Cote PJ, Korba BE, Tennant BC, Gerin JL. Immunopathogenesis and immunomodulation of WHV infection. In: Hollinger FB, Lemon SM, Margolis H, editors. Viral hepatitis and liver disease. Baltimore: Williams & Wilkins; 1991:244–51.
2. Tennant BC, Hornbuckle WE, Baldwin BH, King JM, Cote P, Popper H, Purcell RH, Gerin JL. Influence of age on the response to experimental woodchuck hepatitis virus infection. In: Zuckerman AJ, editor. Viral hepatitis and liver disease. New York: Alan R. Liss; 1988:462–4.
3. Gerin JL, Cote PJ, Korba BE, Tennant BC. Hepadnavirus-induced liver cancer in woodchucks. Cancer Detect Prevent. 1989;14:227–9.
4. Popper H, Roth L, Purcell RH, Tennant BC, Gerin JL. Hepatocarcinogenicity of the woodchuck hepatitis virus. Proc Natl Acad Sci USA. 1987;84:866–70.
5. Korba BE, Cote PJ, Wells FV, Baldwin B, Popper H, Purcell RH, Tennant BC, Gerin JL. Natural history of WHV infections during the course of experimental viral infection: molecular virologic features of the liver and lymphoid tissues. J Virol. 1989;63:1360–70.
6. Korba BE, Wells FV, Baldwin B, Cote PJ, Tennant BC, Popper H, Gerin JL. Hepatocellular carcinoma in woodchuck hepatitis virus-infected woodchucks: presence of viral DNA in tumor tissue from chronic carriers and animals serologically recovered from acute infections. Hepatology. 1989;9:461–70.
7. Korba BK, Cote PJ, Gerin JL. Mitogen-induced replication of woodchuck hepatitis virus in cultured peripheral blood lymphocytes. Science. 1988;241:1213–16.
8. Milich DR, Jones JE, Hughes JL, Price J, Raney AK, McLachlan A. Is a function of the secreted hepatitis B e antigen to induce immunologic tolerance *in utero*? Proc Natl Acad Sci USA. 1990;87:6599–603.
9. Chen H-S, Kew M, Hornbuckle WE, Tennant BC, Cote PJ, Gerin JL, Purcell RH, Miller RH. The precore gene of the woodchuck hepatitis virus genome is not essential for viral replication in the natural host. J Virol. 1992;66:5682–4.
10. Cote PJ, Korba BE, Steinberg H, Ramirez-Maija C, Baldwin B, Hornbuckle WE, Tennant BC, Gerin JL. Cyclosporine A modulates the course of woodchuck hepatitis virus infection and induces chronicity. J Immunol. 1991;146:3138–44.
11. Cote PJ, Korba BE, Baldwin B, Hornbuckle WE, Tennant BC, Gerin JL. Immunosuppression with cyclosporine A during the incubation period of experimental woodchuck hepatitis virus infection increases the frequency of chronic infection in adult woodchucks. J Infect Dis. 1992;166:628–31.

8
Genetic variability of hepatitis B virus: potential clinical implications

D. KREMSDORF and C. BRECHOT

INTRODUCTION

Acute infection by hepatitis B virus (HBV) leads to chronic carriage in about 5% of adults and 40 to 80% of babies born to infected mothers[1]. During the natural course of chronic HBV infection there is a progressive decline in viral replication, as shown by low levels of serum HBV DNA and HBeAg (which become undetectable in routine assays) and by seroconversion to anti-HBe. Reactivation of viral replication is marked by the reappearance of serum HBV DNA; HBeAg is usually also present, but anti-HBe can persist (Fig. 1)[2–6].

The mechanisms involved in the development of chronic carriage are still poorly understood, although it is clear that persistent viral replication is a major risk factor for chronic active hepatitis (CAH). As with other viral infections, the outcome of HBV infection reflects a balance between the host immune response and the ability of the virus to escape it[2,3,7–10]. The HBV genome is a 3.2 kb DNA (Fig. 2)[6–11]. Like other members of the hepadnavirus family, its replication involves reverse transcription of an RNA pregenome, which occurs after packaging of the RNA pregenome; this latter process requires the polymerase protein acting in cis[6,11–13]. The reverse transcription step probably accounts for the greater genetic variability of the HBV genome than that of other 'classical' DNA viruses. The first evidence of this genetic variability was the serological heterogeneity of HBsAg: all known HBV subtypes share a common 'a' determinant, together with one of the mutually exclusive d/y and w/r epitopes; additional specificities have since been identified in the ayw and adw serotypes. A 'q' determinant, initially found in the adw4 subtype, might in fact be expressed by all HBsAg serotypes[14,15]. Nucleotide sequence analysis now suggests that a single mutation in the S gene may account for a change from one subtype to another, or for the loss of a determinant[14–18]. On the basis of comparative sequence analysis of HBV DNA isolated at different times from a single chronic HBV carrier, it has been estimated that the rate of substitution in the HBV core gene is

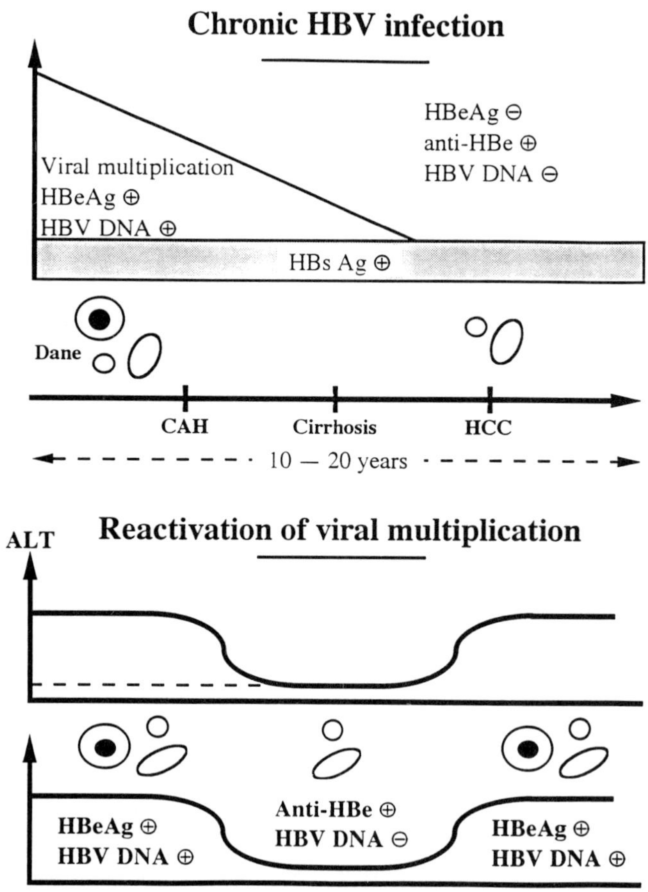

Fig. 1 Level of serum HBV DNA and viral proteins during the natural course of chronic HBV infection (upper panel) and in reactivation of viral multiplication (lower panel).

about 2.2×10^{-5} per nucleotide per year[19], a figure about 100-fold higher than for herpes virus and 10-fold lower than for retroviruses (Table 1). Nucleotide sequence analysis of 32 HBV strains showed a higher-than-expected divergence between genotypes and serotypes; the rate of synonymous substitution in the polymerase gene was about 4.57×10^{-5} per site per year[20]. Since these figures are about 100 times lower than those observed for retroviruses, it has been postulated that HBV replication may not depend exclusively on reverse transcription[15,20].

The development of the polymerase chain reaction (PCR) has now provided rapid access to partial nucleotide sequences of a number of HBV DNA molecules isolated from HBV-infected individuals with various clinical manifestations. The aim of this review is to examine the potential implications of the mutant forms of HBV DNA that have now been identified by means of PCR.

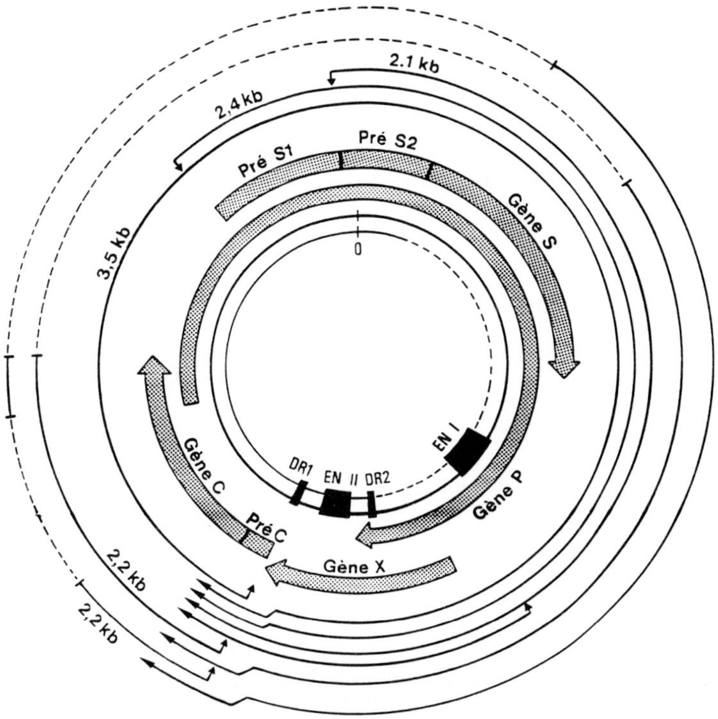

Fig. 2 Genetic organization of HBV genome. The broad arrows surrounding the genome represent the four large open reading frames encoding for envelope (PreS1, PreS2 and S), capsid (PreC and C), polymerase (P) and X proteins. The thin arrows represent the HBV mRNAs (dotted lines represent deleted regions in the singly and doubly spliced HBV mRNAs). Direct repeats (DR1 and DR2) cis-acting elements involved in replication and gene regulation elements (enhancer I and II) are indicated on the map.

Table 1 HBV genetic variability

Viruses or animals	*ORF*	*Number of codons*	*Synonymous substitutes per site per year*	*Non-synonymous substitutes per site per year*
HBV	P	843	4.57×10^{-5}	1.45×10^{-5}
	PreS	163	7.62×610^{-5}	2.57×10^{-5}
	S	259	5.75×10^{-5}	0
	C	212	5.54×10^{-5}	1.75×10^{-5}
	X	154	7.90×10^{-5}	5.45×10^{-5}
MMLV	Gag	537	1.16×10^{-3}	0.54×10^{-3}
Mammals	α-Globin	141	3.94×10^{-9}	0.56×10^{-9}

Orito et al., Proc Natl Acad Sci, 1989;86:7059
Okamoto et al., Jpn J Exp Med, 1987;57:231

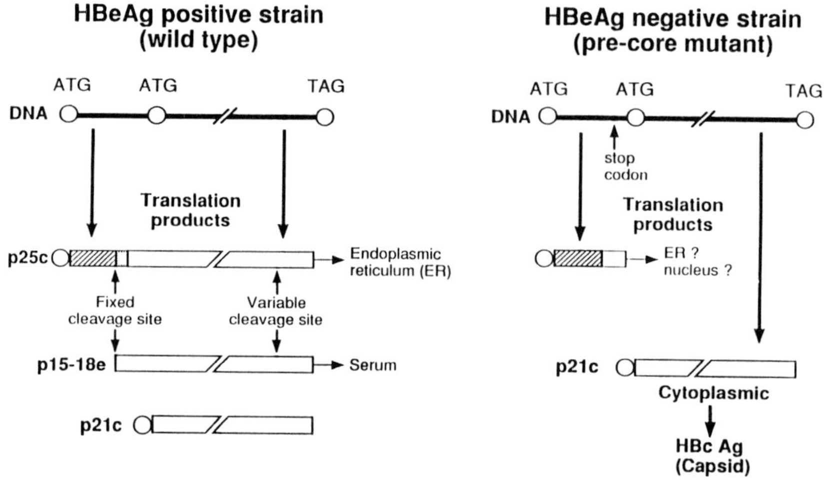

Fig. 3 Translational products from the PreC/C genes of normal and mutant strains of HBV (from Carman et al.[51]).

THE HBV GENOME AND PROTEINS

Four open reading frames (ORF) have been identified; they encode the PreS1/PreS2/S, PreC/C, polymerase and X proteins, respectively[6,21,22] (Fig. 2). The large, middle and small PreS/S proteins are major constituents of the viral envelope and the hepatitis B surface antigen (HBsAg), while the hepatitis B core antigen (HBcAg) is carried by the viral capsid. The polymerase shows both reverse transcriptase and DNA polymerase activities and includes distinct domains encoding for a terminal protein, and a RNase H activity. A 'spacer' region within these functional domains overlaps with the PreS ORF and is not essential for the polymerase function; the latter can thus tolerate the higher variability generally observed in the PreS sequence[11].

The PreC sequence encodes a 29-amino-acid hydrophobic peptide which engages the PreC/C 25 kd protein into the endoplasmic reticulum when translation of the PreC mRNA is initiated at the PreC ATG[21,22]. The secretory HBeAg is generated, after cleavage of the 19 *N*-terminal PreC residues, and by processing of its C-terminal part, giving rise to a 16–18 kd molecule (Fig. 3). Initiation of translation at the core ATG leads to the synthesis of a 21 kd cytoplasmic peptide bearing the HBcAg determinants, which form the viral capsid (Fig. 3). A sequence referred to as the 'e' signal is essential for packaging of RNA pregenome and polymerase, and overlaps with the 3′ PreC and 5′ core sequences[23].

During infection, the virus binds to the hepatocyte via the PreS/S proteins to an unidentified 'receptor'; a peptide (21–47) on the *N*-terminal portion of PreS1 is critical for this process, but other domains on the PreS2 and S proteins are also probably involved[22,24]. Penetration of HBV DNA into the nucleus is followed by its transition from a circular 'relaxed' form to a supercoiled (CCC DNA) form. This CCC DNA is the template for viral

Table 2 Prevalence of PreC stop codon in chronic hepatitis

	HBeAg+	*anti-HBe+*	*Reference*
CH/CAH[a]	10/42	61/64	Brunetto et al.[27]
	1/5	8/8	Carman et al.[28]
	0/3	3/3	Takeda et al.[30]
		41/42	Santantonio et al.[43]
		26/29	Naoumov et al.[36]
	0/1	6/6	Okamoto et al.[37]
		14/19	Minami et al.[31]
		7/7	Brunetto et al.[26]
		11/11	Fioradalisi et al.[29]
		7/7	Tur-Kaspa et al.[53]
AC[b]		5/5	Carman et al.[28]
	0/5	11/12	Okamoto et al.[37]
		1/1	Minami et al.[31]
		5/5	Tur-Kaspa et al.[53]

[a]CH = chronic hepatitis; CAH = chronic active hepatitis.
[b]AC = asymptomatic carrier.

messenger RNAs and for the pregenomic RNA; its amount in the nucleus is tightly regulated by the PreS sequences[13].

HBV MUTANTS IN HBsAg-POSITIVE PATIENTS

Mutations in the PreC sequence

A G-to-A mutation at nucleotide 1896 of the preC region, which generates a stop codon (TAG), is very frequent[25–44]. Because it interrupts the PreC/C open reading frame at amino acid 28, this stop codon prohibits the synthesis of HBeAg (Fig. 3). The mutation was initially described in Italy and Greece, and recent studies have shown it to be present in most Italian anti-HBe-positive chronic carriers with chronic active hepatitis (Table 2). For example, PreC-mutant HBV DNA was detected in 61/64 and 41/42 Italian subjects with CAH[27,43]. This mutation has now also been detected in various geographical areas, including France, Germany, Bulgaria, Japan and Israel[30–33,36,37,40,41], although it was not found in a recent South African study[45].

Most of these patients in fact have a mixture of wild-type and mutant HBV DNA, at a ratio which varies both from subject to subject and during the course of the infection in a given patient[4,33,40]. It is important to realize that different procedures do not provide exactly the same information: direct sequencing, hybridization of amplified products to specific oligonucleotide probes and amplification with primers specific for the mutation permit rapid identification of the major viral DNA molecules but will not identify minor forms. In contrast, sequencing of a number of clones derived from the amplified products provides a more comprehensive evaluation of the various minor viral DNA molecules but is time-consuming. This 'mixed bag' of molecules accounts for the detection of the PreC mutant in a significant proportion of HBeAg-positive subjects. For example, both wild-type and

Table 3 Prevalence of PreC stop codon in acute hepatitis

Acute benign hepatitis	
0/10	Omata et al.[38]
0/8	Kosaka et al.[34]
0/7	Okamoto et al.[37]
8/8	Carman et al.[50]
Fulminant hepatitis	
7/7	Omata et al.[38]
8/15	Carman et al.[51]
3/3	Yotsumoto et al.[42]
9/10	Kosaka et al.[34]
5/5	Liang et al.[35]

mutant HBV DNA were found in 10/42 HBeAg-positive and 19/64 anti-HBe-positive Italian patients and in 15/29 anti-HBe-positive Bulgarian patients[27,36]. However, it remains to be explained why some patients are anti-HBe-positive despite the absence of detectable wild-type HBV DNA. Possible explanations are past infection by a wild-type HBV DNA and cross-reactivity to a modified core gene product.

Another striking feature in the original description of these mutants was their apparent association with severe liver disease. They were first identified in studies of Italian and Greek chronic HBV carriers who were anti-HBe-positive and who had severe chronic active hepatitis with ongoing HBV replication despite a negative serological test for HBeAg[28,44,46]. Subsequent reports confirmed the association of these mutants with chronic active hepatitis, elevated transaminase levels and high serum levels of HBV DNA[26,27,36,37]. In Bulgaria, patients who were predominantly infected by a PreC mutant had higher levels of ALT and HBV DNA than those infected principally by a major wild-type virus[36]. This difference apparently bore no relationship to the duration of the liver disease or the patients' age. In Italy, severe liver disease refractory to interferon treatment has been reported in anti-HBe-positive patients with ongoing HBV replication, and most were subsequently shown to be infected by a PreC mutant[47]. In follow-up studies, a decrease in PreC-mutant DNA associated with the emergence of detectable wild-type DNA corresponded to a fall in serum ALT and HBV DNA levels[27]. Conversely, reactivation of HBV DNA replication can be associated with an acute exacerbation of the liver disease: patients with CAH and predominantly mutant HBV DNA often show a 'flare up' pattern of liver cell necrosis intersected with a course of an asymptomatic carrier state[27]. The duration of the chronic carrier state is another important parameter. The PreC mutant prevails during long-term HBV infection and after both spontaneous and therapeutically induced seroconversion to anti-HBe[48,49]. With regard to treatment by interferon alpha, it is important to note that, despite evidence for the selection of PreC mutants, the detection of mutant HBV DNA before treatment does not appear to have prognostic value[33,47].

PreC mutants were not detected in patients with acute, self-resolving hepatitis in Japan, despite the analysis of serial samples (and several clones for each sample in some studies) during clearance of the viral DNA (Table 3)[34,37,38]. In contrast, the preC mutation was detected, in one study, in all

Greek patients with acute hepatitis[50]. Finally, the stop codon at nucleotide 1896 was detected in three independent studies of Japanese, Greek and Israeli patients with acute fulminant hepatitis B due to nosocomial, transfusional, sexual or intrafamilial transmission (Table 3)[34,35,38,42,51]. In Israel, 5 of 5 subjects contaminated from a single HBsAg-positive, anti-HBe-positive donor had a PreC mutant[35]. As direct sequencing was used, the presence of an associated wild-type HBV DNA could not be ruled out but the mutant was clearly the major form. The same PreC mutant was also the major form in the donor, and the partial HBV DNA sequence was identical, clearly supporting the presumed sources of transmission[35]. In Japan, three studies gave similar results: 7/7, 3/3 and 9/10 subjects with fulminant hepatitis B had the PreC mutation. Interestingly, 5 cases were due to sexual or grandmother-to-child transmission: all the contaminants were anti-HBe-positive, and the analysis of several HBV DNA clones from the patients and the contaminants failed to detect wild-type HBV but yielded the same HBV sequence[34,38,42]. None of these investigations gave evidence for coinfection by hepatitis delta or C viruses. These thought-provoking results should be interpreted in the light of clinical reports of hepatitis B after mother-to-child transmission and sexual contamination by anti-HBe-positive individuals[52].

While all these data strongly argue for a link between infection by PreC mutants and severe liver disease, recent reports from Italy, Israel, and Japan indicate that PreC mutants also occur in asymptomatic chronic carriers (Table 2)[28,31,37,53]. This was well illustrated in a recent survey of chronic HBV carriers in Italy: repeat liver biopsies over a 10-year period showed a normal histology, despite the presence of a PreC mutant[39]. For our part, we recently failed to detect the PreC mutation in a series of French patients with fulminant hepatitis[54]. Similarly, a report from the USA also indicates a low incidence of PreC mutants in fulminant hepatitis[55]. Finally, some evidence suggests intrafamilial transmission of HBV PreC mutants without the occurrence of severe hepatitis[56].

There is probably an intricate interplay of epidemiological and virological factors in the course of infection by these HBV mutants that complicates the interpretation of the results. It is also important to bear in mind that a viral phenotype probably depends on a combination of mutations at various sites of the genome, as clearly shown for HIV and SIV. It is thus interesting that an additional mutation has been detected on the PreC sequence at codon 29 (replacing a glycine by an aspartic acid) in some patients with chronic or fulminant hepatitis[26,28,29,36,38,42,43], and that an increase in the proportion of molecules with the double mutation was shown at the time of contamination of the sexual partner[42]. It has also recently been suggested that a mutation at codon 12 of the core (replacing a threonine by a serine) may be associated with CAH and fulminant hepatitis in anti-HBe-positive carriers, and might be selectively present on HBV DNA molecules with the PreC 1896 stop codon[57].

Other mutations since identified include one at the second nucleotide of the PreC translation initiation codon and the appearance of stop codons at positions 1817-1819 and 1874-1876; all three mutations prevent HBeAg synthesis[33]. A recent interesting study of HBV DNA from patients with

HBsAg-positive, anti-HBe-positive hepatocellular carcinoma (HCC) showed the absence of the PreC 1896 stop codon in 9/9 tumour samples, while it was shown in 4/6 adjacent non-tumorous samples, and 8/9 liver samples from tumour-free subjects with CAH[58]. In addition, a mutation at codon 24 of the PreC sequence was detected in the tumour specimens; it eliminates the cystein at this position and might therefore modify the conformation of the protein[58]. The implications of these results are unclear but, if confirmed, would suggest that integration of the viral DNA (which occurs early in the chronic stage) might prevent subsequent mutations in the absence of replication.

MUTATIONS OF THE CORE GENE

HBV DNA with mutations on the core sequence have also been reported by several investigators[19,40,41,59,60]. We have identified an in-frame 36 bp insertion located 6 bp after the core ATG, together with a 6 bp deletion (2257 to 2262) in an HBsAg-positive, HBeAg-positive subject with CAH[40]. These mutations were associated with genetic rearrangements on the PreS/S gene and were selected during the course of the infection[40]. Interestingly, the first 26 bp of the insert turned out to be identical to the last 26 bp of an insert found in an independent isolate, but the origin (cellular?) of these sequences has not been determined[60].

HBV DNA molecules with core mutations were recently described in 15/20 and 7/11 Japanese patients with HBsAg-positive CAH (16/20 and 11/11 were also HBeAg-positive)[41,59]. The mutations were located between nucleotides 2150 and 2254, and 2062 and 2192, respectively. Deletions and missense mutations were detected mostly in codons 84 to 101. PreC mutations were associated with the C mutations in 1/16 and 3/4 of these HBe-positive, anti-HBe-positive patients, respectively[59]. In contrast, there were no mutations in the 20 asymptomatic (HBs-positive, HBeAg-positive) carriers enrolled in the two studies, but a follow-up study of some of them showed that the emergence of the C mutants coincided with an elevation of ALT activity and the development of CAH[41,59]. Deletions in the core gene had also been described in four Japanese asymptomatic HBV carriers (repeat liver tests were not available); they ranged from 13 to 1071 bp, and overlap the core, Pol or X open reading frames[19].

It is still not known if there are specific links between mutations on the PreC and C sequences, although some recent evidence suggests an association between the PreC 1896 mutation and a mutation at codon 12 of HBcAg (discussed in the previous section).

MUTATIONS ON THE PreS/S GENES

Various forms of rearrangement in the PreS/S ORFs have been identified. An early description came from Japan, where a 143 bp deletion was detected by cloning (without prior amplification) in the PreS region (nt 2831–2975) in an asymptomatic HBV carrier[19].

We recently analysed defective HBV strains with rearrangements in the PreS/S region in two HBsAg-positive patients with CAH, one of whom also had HCC[9,40]. In the first case, 9/12 clones showed a 183-bp in-frame deletion (nt 2995–3177) in the PreS1 region; additional rearrangements were shown in the 5′ part of PreS2 in 3 of the 9 clones, while the remaining 3 (with no 183 bp deletion) had small insertions and deletions in the 5′ part of PreS1. The defective HBV DNA was first detected in circulating viral particles. In peripheral blood mononuclear cells only defective HBV DNA was detected, which contrasted with a mixture of different molecules in the liver and serum. Epitope mapping confirmed the integrity of the 21–47 PreS1 amino acid sequence (which probably mediates binding of HBV to the hepatocyte) and the loss of epitopes encoded by the *C*- and *N*-terminal parts of PreS1 and PreS2, respectively. In the second patient, we detected the emergence of and takeover by the mutant in serial serum samples obtained over a 6-year period[40]. In the same individual, we identified an HBV DNA molecule with extensive rearrangements in the PreS1 region (numerous mutations and a stop codon at position 3028–3030) and point mutations in the 5′ part of the PreS2 and S ORFs[40]. They were associated with modifications of the core sequence (described in the previous section) and with a frameshift in the polymerase sequence which prohibited synthesis of a full-length polymerase product. Electron microscopy showed abnormal circulating HBV particles containing the mutant HBV DNA. Sequencing of several clones at different times of the chronic infection showed a very significant increase in the mutant HBV, which was the only form detectable at the end of the follow-up period. This clearly suggests a selective advantage on the part of the mutant.

Recent evidence from other investigators suggests that such rearrangements in the PreS gene are frequent events[61]. Indeed, 7/22 isolates from Italian chronic HBV carriers showed deletions, mostly in the 5′ part of PreS2, together with mutations in the PreS1 region of 6/7 mutants which gave rise to truncated products; five of the mutants lacked the PreS2 translation initiation codon; furthermore, there was again evidence for the selection of PreS2 mutant HBV DNA in some subjects treated with interferon alpha[61].

Another indicator of the potential importance of mutations in the viral envelope genes is the recent description of so-called ‘escape mutants’ in Italy, Gambia, and Japan during the follow-up of childhood immunization programmes[62,63]. Some children, despite apparently effective vaccination, were subsequently serum HBsAg-positive or anti-HBc-positive. Sequencing of the S ORF showed a single mutation at amino acid 145 (located in a highly antigenic domain for the ‘a’ determinant), replacing the glycine with an arginine[62,63] (Fig. 4). A study of Japanese babies infected at birth (despite vaccination and immunization with hepatitis B immune globulin) showed an additional mutation, at amino acid 126, associated with the change at amino acid 145[64] (Fig. 4). The same amino acid substitution was detected during treatment with a monoclonal anti-HBs antibody after liver transplantation to prevent reinfection of the graft[65]. The serum showed reduced binding to monoclonal antibodies specifically recognizing this loop of the ‘a’ determinant.

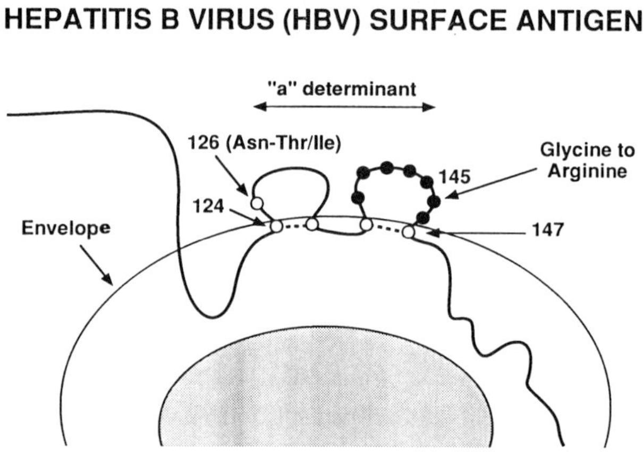

Fig. 4 Localization of the mutant amino acids in the common 'a' determinant domain on HBsAg (from Carman et al.[62]).

The number of cases so far reported is limited. These findings do, however, strongly support the selection of these HBV DNA molecules through immune pressure and might therefore have important implications for strategies to prevent HBV infection.

GENERATION OF DEFECTIVE HBV PARTICLES FROM SPLICED HBV RNA

We have recently shown that spliced HBV RNA is packaged following reverse transcription *in vivo* (Fig. 5)[66]. Defective particles (with no PreS or 5′ part of S ORFs) are thus generated and detectable in serum together with complete virions; a similar finding has now been made in woodchucks[67]. Studies *in vitro* have shown that the removal of large sections of the HBV genome does not prevent the synthesis of albeit defective viruses that are helper-dependent for their replication. Cotransfection of subgenomic and full-length HBV DNAs leads to a reduction in wild-type virus production. It is thus plausible that the secreted defective HBV particles generated by the encapsidation of subgenomic HBV genomes synthesized from the spliced HBV RNA act as defective interfering particles: indeed, synthesis of defective interfering particles is a feature shared by several viruses and might lead to persistent infection[68]. It is also interesting that a delegated integrated HBV DNA sequence identified in the hepatocellular carcinoma-derived cell line PLC/PRF/5 is in fact generated by integration of a cDNA resulting from reverse transcription of a spliced HBV RNA[69]. Synthesis of defective HBV particles from these spliced HBV RNAs and integration of the cDNAs into the host genome might therefore contribute to the persistence of HBV infection and, possibly, to liver cell transformation.

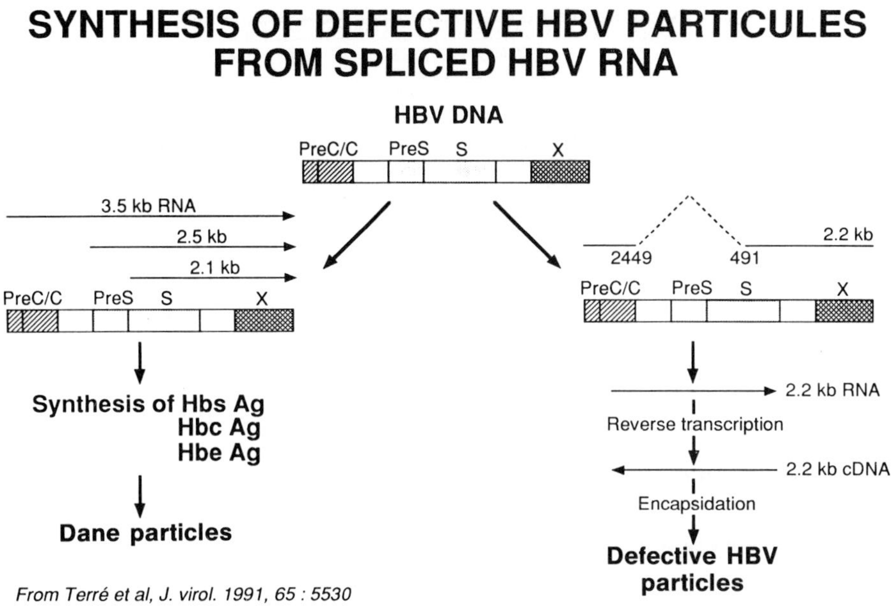

Fig. 5 Representation of the processing for the generation of defective HBV particles from the singly spliced HBV mRNA.

HBV MUTANTS IN HBsAg-NEGATIVE PATIENTS

Several authors have identified HBV DNA sequences in the serum, liver and circulating mononuclear cells of patients with acute and chronic hepatitis, as well as those with primary liver cancer, who lack standard serological markers of HBV infection[7,49,70–106] (Table 4). It has been shown that 50 to 60% of HBsAg-negative patients with anti-HBsAg and anti-HBcAg and chronic liver disease have HBV sequences in their serum[79,98]. HBsAg determinants have been detected in the serum of some of these patients by means of a radioimmunoassay with anti-HBs monoclonal antibodies[71,75,85,88].

Transmission experiments with chimpanzees showed that the viral DNA sequences were contained in infectious particles[71,75,86,88]. The two serological profiles in infected animals provided clues as to the nature of the HBV genomes[71,75,88]. In some animals, serum HBsAg became clearly detectable with regular assays during acute hepatitis, thus demonstrating that a small amount of circulating HBV DNA was present in the patient whose serum was used for injection. This resembled the situation in infections by so-called 'HBV-2'[107,108], in which the unusual serological pattern (anti-HBc negativity) mostly reflects an abnormal host immune response. In addition, the core sequence of HBV DNA from HBsAg-positive, anti-HBc-negative subjects was identical to that of wild-type HBV[108]. In contrast, other animals with acute hepatitis did not develop the usual HBV serological markers, and some were infected despite the presence of anti-HBs before inoculation. The

Table 4 HBV DNA in serum HBsAg negative patients. Detection by PCR

	HBV DNA (PCR)	*Geographical*	*References*
Chronic hepatitis	3/11[a]	Japan	Kaneko et al
	2/13	France	Loriot et al
	4/9	Senegal	Coursaget et al
	2/36	France	Porchon et al
	3/26	France	Barlet et al
	0/11	Japan	Yokosoka et al
	4/8	Japan	Kaneko et al
	21/67[c]	Israel	Liang et al
	39/217		
Primary liver	2/3 HCC	Italy	Pontisso et al
(Hepatocarcinoma = HCC)	0/6 Hepatoblastomas		
	18/31 HCC	Senegal	Coursaget et al
	10.19 HCC[d]	France/Italy	Paterlini
	6/8 HCC	South Africa	
	36/61		
Asymptomatic carriers	9[b]/206	Taiwan	Wang et al
	7/42	Senegal	Coursaget et al
	8/107	Taiwan	Shih et al
Acute post-transfusional	1/19	France	Thiers et al
fulminant	1/9	Taiwan	Wang et al
	6/12 (Liver)	France, USA	Wright et al

[a]Patients HBsAg+ with subsequent negativation of serum HBsAg during follow-up.
[b]2/9 without any HBV serological marker.
[c]11/21 without any HBV serological marker.
[d]6/13 without any HBV serological marker.

level of viral replication in these patients and in inoculated chimpanzees was consistently low. Transmission experiments have shown that a mutant HBV can persist in a non-replicating episomal form in the hepatocyte nucleus[86]. In the case of another HBV isolate, it was found that seronegativity was due to a defect blocking viral DNA synthesis. This defect was associated with a point mutation in the 5′ part of the polymerase gene, resulting in an inability to package pregenomic RNA in core particles[95]. It is thus plausible that genetic variability is involved, at least in part, in the establishment of viral latency. However, additional factors are probably involved in these unusual patterns, e.g. changes in the host immune response.

We have inoculated three distinct HBsAg-negative, HBV DNA-positive sera into chimpanzees which then developed acute hepatitis[75,87,88]. HBV DNA-related sequences were detected in the animals' serum and/or liver by spot test, Southern blot or PCR techniques. To investigate the integrity of the HBV DNA Sequences, the full HBV genomes were amplified using sets of primers located throughout the HBV genome. Amplified products of the expected size were obtained with all the sets of primers tested. This indicated that no major deletion or insertion had occurred in the viral genomes. To determine the complete nucleotide sequence of these HBV isolates, the PCR products were cloned and sequenced. Extensive sequence homology with subtype ayw was found (less than 1% divergence), a result in agreement with studies of two other HBV isolates from patients lacking serological markers[86,97]. The point mutations were located throughout the genomes and no clusters were observed. Most of the mutations failed to induce amino acid changes[87]. Significantly, however, amino acid changes did occur in the antigenic determinants of the viral envelope and capsid and thus might have been involved in the negative serological results[87,88]. None of the point mutations were located in the enhancer elements or viral gene promoters, except in one case[87]. In this latter isolate, four mutations were located in a region (nucleotides 2900 to 3137) which contains the regulatory elements of the surface antigen promoter 109, while two (positions 3104 and 3117) were located in specific sequence sites for DNA binding proteins. These mutations could also be involved in the lack of serological markers. To study the expression of envelope proteins, the PreS2/S-encoding sequences of two of these HBV isolates were inserted in a eucaryotic expression vector[87]. The constructs were then transfected into mouse L fibroblast cells and the secretion of HBV surface antigens was tested for by means of a standard RIA for HBsAg or an RIA based on monoclonal antibodies directed against preS2 (F124) and S (F39.20) viral epitopes. PreS2 and S viral epitopes were detected with both constructs, with both polyclonal and monoclonal antibodies. Interestingly, reactivity with the monoclonal antibody F124 was observed with one isolate despite amino acid changes in the domain recognized by this antibody[87]. Thus, the HBsAg seronegativity of the patients and chimpanzees could not only be due to these genetic variations modifying the structure of PreS2 and HBsAg. Taken together, the results clearly indicate that the genetic modifications we detected in the HBV DNA of seronegative individuals could not alone explain the apparent absence of HBsAg from the serum.

Other explanations relate to the importance of the immune response to the virus. Indeed, circulation of HBsAg in immune complexes has been demonstrated in the serum of HBsAg-negative individuals[110] and a minor or absent immune response to HBsAg has been documented after vaccination, something that could also occur with HBsAg[111]. Taken together, these different observations suggest that a combination of viral and/or host factors result in the unusual serological profiles.

Finally, the detection of HBV DNA in HBsAg-negative alcoholics points to a further possibility. Alcohol has been shown to modify the exportation of several proteins by the liver and it is tempting to speculate that this might be the case for HBsAg. Recent experiments performed on HBsAg-producing transgenic mice indeed indicate that alcohol can reduce the secretion of HBsAg into the serum[112,113].

POTENTIAL EFFECTS OF THESE MUTATIONS

Several issues are raised by the identification of such HBV mutants *in vivo*. First, their structure might point to previously unrecognized antigenic epitopes and regulatory pathways for HBV DNA replication and HBV gene expression. Most studies have been based on the mouse model, *in-vitro* analysis of stimulated T and B lymphocytes, and transfection of various cell lines with complete or deleted Hepadna virus genomes. Therefore, the appearance of some of these mutations during the course of HBV infection may reflect their selection under immune pressure. On the other hand, these mutations might, at least in part, be 'random' events occurring during viral DNA replication and generating defective viruses, and have no implications for the course of the infection. Various mechanisms (that are probably inter-related) may well determine the immunopathological effects of such mutations:

(1) Modification, elimination or creation of epitopes engendering the immune response to the virus

PreS/S-encoded proteins play a major role in the generation of neutralizing antibodies[3]. Several of the mutations reported in both HBsAg-negative and HBsAg-positive individuals modify B and T cell epitopes, particularly those affecting the *C*-terminal and *N*-terminal parts of PreS1 and PreS2, respectively, and those in the S gene[9,40,87,88]. In 'escape mutants', the amino acid substitution in the S protein lies in one of the two loops forming the 'a' antigenic determinant[62–64]. Mutations in the core gene might have profound effects on the synthesis of epitopes recognized by CTL; the cluster of mutations in the 84–101 amino acid domain of HBc might point to the importance of this region[59].

Mutations in the PreC sequence abolish HBeAg synthesis and may be viewed in several ways: like HBcAg, HBeAg has been considered a target for both CTL and ADCC[8,114,115], abrogation of its synthesis might thus diminish the immune response to HBV and thereby account for its 'escape' during the course of chronic infection or its rapid selection in fulminant hepatitis. On the other hand, since HBeAg is thought to mediate tolerance to HBV in the newborn infants of infected mothers[52], possibly by transplacental passage, the absence of HBeAg might rather enhance the immune response. Furthermore, a truncated PreC peptide created by the stop codon at position 1896 might form a new endogenous peptide target for CTL; indeed, synthesis of such a peptide has recently been demonstrated in the liver of patients infected by a PreC mutant[116].

It is possible that mutations located in the vicinity of known epitopes affect their conformation, meaning that it is in fact a combination of several mutations that confers a selective advantage of the mutant. For example, creation of a PreC mutation *in vitro* can lead to an accumulation of HBcAg similar to that observed in cases of fulminant and chronic hepatitis. However, a recent transfection study with a full-length cloned PreC mutant isolated *in vivo* did not lead to such accumulation[117].

(2) Direct effects of viral proteins on infected cells

Although HBV is not considered cytopathic, accumulation of the large envelope protein in transgenic mice and HBcAg in cultured cells are both cytotoxic[118,119]. These are clearly experimental data, but they might provide information on a more generalized phenomenon. Truncated PreS2/S proteins can also have a transactivating effect on cellular genes (e.g. myc and fos) and it is thus conceivable that some abnormal HBV proteins generated by mutations affect the cell machinery[120]. It will be particularly interesting to investigate whether or not they modify the response of cellular genes to interferon, as is the case for the terminal polymerase protein and HBcAg[121,122]. As stated above, it will be important to determine whether or not HBcAg accumulates in hepatocytes.

(3) Modifications of HBV gene expression, HBV DNA replication, and the assembly and secretion of viral proteins

The mutation at position 1896 affects the replication of HBV DNA *in vitro*, a finding in keeping with *in-vivo* observations[117]. In fact there are several potential stop codons which can be generated in the PreC sequence and it has been suggested that only some of these are viable, accounting in part for the selection of the stop codon at codon 28[117]. Mutations in a given region of HBV DNA can have several concomitant effects, due to the superposition of different regulatory elements in this small DNA molecule. For example, mutations in the 3′ and 5′ parts of the PreC and C genes can modify the encapsidation and assembly of core particles[23]. This might be important in understanding the accumulation of free replicating HBV DNA molecules in tumour cell cytoplasm without the synthesis of HBcAg.

Mutations in the PreS genes may lead to an accumulation of the supercoiled form (CCC DNA) of HBV DNA which is involved in the persistence of HBV infection, a prediction based on experiments with deleted duck hepatitis virus (DHBV). Accumulation of CCC DNA might also be toxic for the cell. Part of the PreS sequence could be involved in regulating the synthesis of the relaxed circular form of HBV DNA during replication. The PreS1-encoded large protein is one of the molecules involved in the penetration of the virus into the hepatocyte and is also involved in the assembly of the virus. Finally, the different mutations described in the polymerase gene of some mutants might explain the low replication levels in some patients.

It is thus clear that the various mutations described can potentially interfere with the expression of HBV and its infectivity.

IMPLICATIONS AND FUTURE PERSPECTIVES

On the basis of the published data, it is difficult to determine the implications of these mutants, but it is likely that a mixture of random events and mutations provide the virus with a selective advantage vis-à-vis the immune response.

In HBsAg-positive patients there is fairly good evidence that HBV DNA molecules with the 1896 PreC mutation are generally selected, possibly under immune pressure, during the course of chronic HBV infection. Mutations in

PreS1 and PreS2 also probably arise from the immune response to the virus. Some studies have shown a selective increase in mutant forms during the natural course of HBV infection and during interferon therapy, results consistent with these mutations being located in important epitopes or regulatory elements.

The link between certain mutations and the severity of the liver disease is far less clear. In fact, the discrepancies between different studies reflect epidemiological variations and the fact that several mutations at different regions of the HBV genome generate a given phenotype. This has been established in other viral infections such as HIV and SIV and it is therefore important to emphasize that most studies so far reported have focused on very limited parts of the viral genome. Another difficulty arises from the 'mixed bag' of viral DNA; the proteins detected can thus be synthesized by the wild-type virus, the mutant or both. In addition, transregulatory effects can modify viral gene expression.

It will be of major importance to clone complete mutant genomes and to analyse their intrinsic properties *in vitro*; it will also be necessary to design *in-vivo* approaches to investigate their interplay with the host immune system, thus performing *in vivo* mapping of the HBV epitopes.

In HBsAg-negative subjects such investigations have confirmed the concept of persistent HBV infection in individuals who, on the basis of serological criteria, should have cleared the virus or lack markers of HBV infection. While the importance of persistent HBV infection in the pathogenesis of chronic hepatitis is not clear, particularly with regard to the role of HCV in non-A, non-B infections, it might be a risk factor for liver cancer. Finally, the recent description of 'escape mutants' with point mutations in the S gene provides a link between observations made in HBsAg-positive and HBsAg-negative individuals suggesting that infection can occasionally occur despite apparently effective immunization.

References

1. Stevens CE, Beasley RP, Tsui J, Lee WC. Vertical transmission of hepatitis B antigen in Taiwan. N Engl J Med. 1975;292:771.
2. Baker, BL, Di Bisceglie M, Kaneko S, Miller R, Feinstone SM, Waggoner JG, Hoffnagle JH. Determination of hepatitis B virus DNA in serum using the polymerase chain reaction: clinical significance and correlation with serological and biochemical markers. Hepatology. 1991;13:632–6.
3. Eddleston ALWF. Overview of HBV pathogenesis. In: Viral hepatitis and liver disease. Baltimore: Williams and Wilkins; 1991:234–7.
4. Fattovich G, Brollo L, Alberti A, Pontisso P, Giustina G, Realdi G. Long term follow-up of anti-HBe positive chronic active hepatitis B. Hepatology. 1988;8:1651–4.
5. Housset C, Pol S, Carnot F, Dubois F, Nalpas B, Housset B, Berthelot P, Bréchot C. Interactions between human immunodeficiency virus-1, hepatitis delta virus and hepatitis B virus infections in 260 chronic carriers of hepatitis B virus. Hepatology. 1992;15:578–83.
6. Tiollais P, Pourcel C, Dejean A. The hepatitis B virus. Nature. 1985;317:489–95.
7. Bréchot C. Hepatitis B virus (HBV) and hepatocellular carcinoma. HBV DNA status and its implications. J. Hepatol. 1987;4:269–79.
8. Ferrari C, Penna A, Cavalli A, Bertoletti A, Valli A, Missale G, Pilli M, Giuberti T, Fiaccamori F. Human cellular immune response to hepatitis B virus (HBV) envelope and

nucleocapsid antigen. In: Viral hepatitis and liver disease. Baltimore: Williams and Wilkins; 1991:238–243.
9. Gerken G, Kremsdorf D, Capel F, Petit, M-A, Dauguet C, Manns MP, Myer Zum Buschenfelde KH, Bréchot C. Hepatitis B defective virus with rearrangements in the PreS gene during chronic HBV infection. Virology. 1991;183:555–65.
10. Guilhot S, Fowler P, Portillo G, Margolskee RF, Ferrari C, Bertoletti A, Chisari FV. Hepatitis B virus (HBV) specific cytotoxic T-cell responses in humans: production of target cells by stable expression of HBV-encoded proteins in immortalized human B-cell lines. J. Virol. 1992;66:2670–8.
11. Miller RH, Kaneko S, Chung CT, Girones R, Purcell RH. Compact organization of the hepatitis B virus genome. Hepatology. 1989;9:322–7.
12. Bartenschlager R, Schaller H. Hepadnaviral assembly is initiated by polymerase binding to the encapsidation signal in the viral RNA genome. EMBO J. 1992;9:3413–20.
13. Wu TT, Coudreay LD, Liuc W, Mason W, Jilbert A. Hepadna virus synthesis. In: Viral hepatitis and liver diseases. Baltimore: Williams and Wilkins; 1991:114–121.
14. Norder H, Hammas B, Löfdahl S, Courroucé AM, Magnius LO. Comparison of amino acid sequences of nine different serotypes of hepatitis B surface antigen and genomic classification of the corresponding hepatitis B virus strains. J Gen Virol. 1992;73:1201–8.
15. Okamoto H, Tsuda F, Sakugawa H, Sastroewigugo RI, Imai M, Miyakawa Y, Mayumi M. Typing hepatitis B virus by homology in nucleotide sequence: comparison of surface antigen subtypes. J Gen Virol. 1988;69:2575–83.
16. Okamoto H, Omi S, Wang Y, Itoh Y, Tsuda F, Tanaka T, Akahane Y, Miyakawa Y, Mayumi M. The loss of subtypic determinants in alleles, d/y or w/r, on hepatitis B surface antigen. Mol Immunol. 1989;26:197–205.
17. Gerin JL, Alexander H, Shih JWK, Purcell RH, Dapolito G, Engle R, Green N, Sutcliffe JG, Shinnick TM, Lerner RA. Chemically synthesized peptides of hepatitis B surface antigen duplicate the d/y specificities and induce subtype-specific antibodies in chimpanzees. Proc Natl Acad Sci. 1983;80:2365–9.
18. Okamoto H, Imai M, Tsuda F, Tanaka T, Miyakawa Y, Mayumi M. Point mutation in the S gene of hepatitis B virus for a d/y or w/r subtypic change in two blood donors carrying a surface antigen of compound subtype adyr or adwr. J Virol. 1987;3030–4.
19. Okamoto H, Imai M, Kametani M, Nakamura T, Mayumi M. Genomic heterogeneity of hepatitis B virus in a 54-year-old woman who contracted the infection through materno-fetal transmission. Jpn J Exp Med. 1987;57:231–6.
20. Orito E, Mizokami M, Ina Y, Moriyama EN, Kameshima N, Yamamoto M, Gojobori T. Host-independent evolution and a genetic classification of the hepadnavirus family based on nucleotide sequence. Proc Natl Acad Sci. 1989;86:7059–62.
21. Ganem D, Varmus HE. The molecular biology of the hepatitis B viruses. Annu Rev Biochem. 1987;56:651–93.
22. Gerlich WH, Heerman KH. Hepatitis B virus proteins and virus assembly. In: Viral hepatitis and liver disease. Baltimore: Williams and Wilkins; 1991:121.
23. Junker-Niepman M, Bartenschlager R, Schaller H. A short cis-acting sequence is required for hepatitis B virus pregenome encapsidation and sufficient for packaging of foreign RNA. EMBO J. 1990;9:3389–96.
24. Dash S, Rao KVS, Panda SK. Receptor for Pre-S1 (21–47) component of hepatitis B virus on the liver cell: role in virus cell interaction. J Med Virol. 1992;37:116–21.
25. Brown JL, William F, Carman F, Thomas HC. The clinical significance of molecular variation within the hepatitis B virus genome. Hepatology. 1992;15:144–8.
26. Brunetto MR, Stemler M, Bonino F, Schodel F, Oliveri F, Rizetto M, Verme G, Will H. A new hepatitis B virus strain in patients with severe anti-HBe positive chronic hepatitis. Br J Hepatol. 1990;10:258–61.
27. Brunetto MR, Giarin MM, Oliveri F, Chiaberge E, Baldi M, Alfarano A, Serra A, Saracco G, Verme G, Will H, Bonino F. Wild-type and e antigen-minus hepatitis B viruses and course of chronic hepatitis. Proc Natl Acad Fr. 1990;88:4186–90.
28. Carman WF, Hadziyannis S, McGarvey MJ, Jacyna MR, Karayiannis P, Makris A, Thomas HC. Mutation preventing formation of hepatitis B e antigen in patients with chronic hepatitis B infection. Lancet. 1989; 588–90.
29. Fiordalisi G, Cariani E, Mantero G, Zanetti A, Tanzi E, Chiaramonte M, Primi D. High

genomic variability in the Pre C region of hepatitis B virus in anti-HBe, HBV-DNA position chronic hepatitis. J Med Virol. 1990;31:297–300.
30. Takeda K, Akahane Y, Suzuki H, Okamoto H, Tsuda F, Miyakawa Y, Mayumi M. Defects in the precore region of the HBV genome in patients with chronic hepatitis B after sustained seroconversion from HBeAg to anti-HBe induced spontaneously or with interferon therapy. Hepatology. 1990;12:1284.
31. Minami M. Point mutations in the hepatitis B virus precore region in Japanese patients with chronic HBV infection. J Kyoto Pref Univ Med. 1992;101:235–43.
32. Gerken G, Goergen B, Teuber G, Meyer Zum Buschenfelde KH. High prevalence of HBe-minus variants in anti-HBe positive chronic carriers in central Europe. J Hepatol. 1992;16:P1–24.
33. Günther S, Meisel H, Reip A, Miska S, Krüger DH, Will H. Frequent and rapid emergence of mutated Pre-C sequences in HBV from e-antigen positive carriers who seroconvert to anti-HBe during interferon treatment. Virology. 1992;187:271–9.
34. Kosaka Y, Takase K, Kojima M, Shimizu M, Inoue K, Yoshiba M, Tanaka S, Akahane Y, Okamoto H, Tsuda F, Miyakawa Y, Mayumi M. Fulminant hepatitis B: induction by hepatitis B virus mutants defective in the precore region and incapable of encoding e antigen. Gastroenterology. 1991;100:1087–94.
35. Liang TJ, Hasegawa K, Rimon N, Wands JR and Ben-Porath E. A hepatitis B virus mutant associated with an epidemic of fulminant hepatitis. N Engl J Med. 1991;324:1705–9.
36. Naoumov NV, Schneider R, Grötzinger T, Jung MC, Miska S, Pape GR, Will H. Precore mutant hepatitis B virus infection and liver disease. Gastroenterology. 1992;102:538–43.
37. Okamoto H, Yotsumoto S, Akahane Y, Yamanaka T, Miyazaki Y, Sugai Y, Tsuda F, Tanaka T, Miyakawa Y, Mayumi M. Hepatitis B viruses with precore region defects prevail in persistently infected hosts along with seroconversion to the antibody against e antigen. J Virol. 1990;64:1298–303.
38. Omata M, Ehata T, Yokosuka O, Hosoda K, Ohto M. Mutations in the precore region of hepatitis B virus DNA in patients with fulminant and severe hepatitis. N Engl J. 1991;324:1699–704.
39. Raimondo G, Meucci G, Rodino G, Sardo MA. Detection of wild-type and 'E minus' HBV populations in liver tissue of chronic healthy HBsAg carriers. J Hepatol. 1992;16:P1–23.
40. Tran A, Kremsdorf D, Capel F, Housset C, Dauguet C, Petit MA, Bréchot C. Emergence of and takeover by hepatitis B virus (HBV) with rearrangements in the Pre-S/S and Pre-C/C genes during chronic HBV infection. J Virol. 1991;65:3566–74.
41. Wakita T, Kakumu S, Shibata M, Yoshioka K, Ito F, Shinagawa T, Ishikawa T. Detection of Pre-C and core region mutants of hepatitis B virus in chronic hepatitis B virus carriers. J Clin Invest. 1991;88:1793–801.
42. Yotsumoto S, Kojima M, Shoji I, Yamamoto K, Okamoto H, Mishiro S. Fulminant hepatitis related to transmission of hepatitis B variants with precore mutations between spouses. Hepatology. 1992;16:31–5.
43. Santantonio T, Jung MC, Miska S, Pastore G, Pape GR, Will H. Prevalence and type of Pre-C HBV mutants in anti-HBe positive carriers with chronic liver disease in a highly endemic area. Virology. 1991;183:840–4.
44. Brunetto MR, Stemler M, Schödel F, Will H, Ottobrelli A, Rizzetto M, Verme G, Bonino F. Identification of HBV variants which cannot produce precore derived HBeAg and may be responsible for severe hepatitis. Gastroenterology. 1989;21:151–4.
45. Xu J, Brown D, Harrisson T, Lin Y, Dusheiko G. Absence of hepatitis B virus precore mutants in patients with chronic hepatitis B responding to interferon alpha. Hepatology. 1992;15:1002–6.
46. Bonino F, Rosina F, Rizzeto M, Rizzi R, Chiaberge E, Tardanico R, Callea F, Verme G. Chronic hepatitis in HBsAg carriers with serum HBV-DNA and anti-HBe. Gastroenterology. 1986;90:1268–73.
47. Santantonio T, Jung MC, Schneider R, Pastore G, Pape GR, Will H. Selection for a pre-C stop codon mutation in hepatitis B virus variant with a pre-C initiation codon mutation during interferon treatment. J Hepatol. 1991;13:368–71.
48. Carman WF, Dourakis S, Karayiannis P, Crossey M, Drobner R, Thomas HC. Incidence of hepatitis B viraemia, detected using the polymerase chain reaction, after successful therapy of hepatitis B virus carriers with interferon alpha. J Med Virol. 1991;34:114–18.

49. Loriot MA, Marcellin P, Bismuth E, Martinot-Peignoux M, Boyer N, Degott C, Erlinger S, Benhamou P. Demonstration of hepatitis B virus DNA by polymerase chain reaction in the serum and the liver after spontaneous or therapeutically induced HBeAg to anti-HBe or HBsAg to anti-HBs seroconversion in patients with chronic hepatitis B. Hepatology. 1991;15:32–6.
50. Carman WF, Hadziyannis S, Karayiannis P, Fagan EA, Tassopoulos NC, William R, Thomas HC. Association of the precore variant of HBV with acute and fulminant hepatitis B infection. In: Viral hepatitis and liver disease. Baltimore: Williams and Wilkins; 1991:216–19.
51. Carman WF, Fagan EA, Hadziyannis S, Karayiannis K, Tassopoulos N, William R, Thomas H. Association of a precore genomic variant of hepatitis B virus with fulminant hepatitis. Hepatology. 1991;14:219–22.
52. Shiraki K, Yoshihara N, Sakurai M, Eto T, Kawana T. Acute hepatitis B in infants born to carrier mothers with the antibody to hepatitis B e antigen. J Pediatr. 1980;97:768.
53. Tur-Kaspa R, Klein A, Aharonson S. Hepatitis B virus precore mutants are identical in carriers from various ethnic origins and are associated with a range of liver disease severity. Hepatology. 1992;16:1338–42.
54. Féray C, Gigou M, Samuel D, Bernuau J, Bismuth H, Bréchot C. Low pevalence of precore mutations in hepatitis B virus (HBV) DNA in fulminant hepatitis type B in France. J. Hepatol. (in press).
55. Liang TJ, Hasegawa K, Feng CY. Hepatitis B virus precore mutants and fulminant hepatitis B in USA. Molecular Biology of Hepatitis B viruses. La Jolla, California. 1992:113.
56. Barlet V, Zarski JP, Petit MA, Bichard P, Seigneurin JM. Transmission familiale du mutant Pre-C du virus de l'hépatie B. AFEF. Paris. 1992:55.
57. Carman WF, McIntyre G, Hadziyannis S, Fattovich G, Alberti A. Mutation of HBcAg after loss of HBeAg and association with progressive disease. J Hepatol. 1992;16:P1–26.
58. Manzin A, Menzo S, Bagnarelli P, Varaldo PE, Bearzi I, Carloni G, Galibert F, Clementi M. Sequence analysis of the hepatitis B virus Pre-C region in hepatocellular carcinoma HCC and non tumoral liver tissues from HCC patients. Virology. 1992;188:890–5.
59. Ehata T, Omata M, Yokosuka O, Hosoda K, Ohto M. Variations in codons 84–101 in the core nucleotide sequence correlate with hepatocellular injury in chronic hepatitis B virus infection. J Clin Invest. 1992;89:332–8.
60. Bhat RA, Ulrich PP, Vyas GN. Molecular characterization of a new variant of hepatitis B virus in a persistently infected homosexual man. Hepatology. 1990;11:271–6.
61. Santantonio T, Jung MC, Schneider R, Fernholz D, Milella M, Monno L, Pastore G, Pape GR, Will H. Hepatitis B virus genomes that cannot synthesize Pre-S2 proteins occur frequently and as dominant virus populations in chronic carriers in Italy. Virology. 1992;188:948–52.
62. Carman WF, Zanetti AR, Karayiannis P, Waters J, Manzillo G, Tanzi E, Zuckerman AJ, Thomas HC. Vaccine-induced escape mutant of hepatitis B virus. Lancet. 1990;336:325–9.
63. Harrison TJ, Hopes EA, Oon CJ, Zanetti AR, Zuckerman AJ. Independent emergence of a vaccine-induced escape mutant of hepatitis B virus. J Hepatol. 1991;13:S105–7.
64. Okamoto H, Yano K, Nozaki Y, Matsui A, Miyazaki H, Yamamoto K, Tsuda F, Machida A, Mishoro S. Mutations within the S gene of hepatitis B virus transmitted from mothers to babies immunized with hepatitis B immune globulin and vaccine. Pediatr Res. 1992;32:3–9.
65. McLahon G, McCarthy LA, Dottavio D, Ostberg L. Surface antigen and polymerase gene variations in hepatitis B virus isolates from a monoclonal antibody-treated liver transplant patient. In: Viral hepatitis and liver disease. Baltimore: Williams and Wilkins; 1991:219–221.
66. Terre S, Petit MA, Bréchot S. Defective hepatitis B virus particles are generated by packaging and reverse transcription of spliced viral RNAs in vivo. J Virol. 1991;65: 5539–43.
67. Hantz O, Baginski I, Fourel I, Chemin I, Trepo C. Viral spliced RNA are produced, encapsidated and reverse transcribed during in vivo woodchuck hepatitis virus infection. Virology. 1992;190:193–200.
68. Holland J. Defective viral genomes. Fields Virol. 1990;1:151.
69. Ziemer M, Garcia P, Shaul Y, Rutter WJ. Sequence of hepatitis B virus DNA incorporated into the genome of a human hepatoma cell line. J Virol. 1985;53:885–92.

70. Wands JR, Lieberman HM, Muchmore E, Isselbacher K, Shafritz DA. Detection and transmission of hepatitis B virus-related agents formerly designated 'non-A', 'non-B'. Proc Natl Acad Sci. 1982;79:7552–6.
71. Wands JR, Fujita YK, Isselbacher KJ, Schellekens H, Dazza M-C, Thiers V, Tiollais P, Bréchot C. Identification and transmission of a hepatitis B virus-related variant. Proc Natl Acad Sci. 1986;83:6608–12.
72. Wang JT, Wang TH, Sheu JC. Detection of hepatitis B virus DNA by polymerase chain reaction in plasma of volunteer blood donors negative for hepatitis B surface antigen. J Infect Dis. 1991;163:397–9.
73. Wright TL, Hsu H, Donegon E. Hepatitis C virus not found in fulminant non-A, non-B hepatitis. Ann Intern Med. 1991;115:111–12.
74. Thiers V, Fujita Y, Takahashi H, Schellekens H, De Reus A, Driss F, Degott C, Isselbacher K, Tiollais P, Wands J, Bréchot C. Hepatitis B virus DNA sequences in the serum of HBsAg-negative patients with chronic liver disease. In: Viral hepatitis and liver disease. New York: Liss; 1988:553–7.
75. Thiers V, Nakajima E, Kremsdorf D, Mack D, Schellekens H, Driss F, Goudeau A, Wands J, Sninsky J, Tiolais P, Bréchot C. Transmission of hepatitis from hepatitis-B-seronegative subjects. Lancet. 1988;1273–6.
76. Tanaka Y, Esumi M, Shikata T. Persistence of hepatitis B virus DNA after serological clearance of hepatitis B virus. Liver. 1990;10:6–10.
77. Shafritz DA, Lieberman HM, Isselbacher KJ, Wands JR. Monoclonal radioimmunoassay for hepatitis B surface antigen: demonstration of hepatitis B virus DNA or related sequences in serum and viral epitopes in immune complexes. Proc Natl Acad Sci. 1982;79:5675.
78. Rumi MG, Colombo M, Romeo R, Colucci G, Gringeri A, Mannucci PM. Serum hepatitis B virus DNA detects cryptic hepatitis B virus infection in multitransfused hemophilic patients. Blood. 1990;75:1654–9.
79. Repp R, Mance A, Bertram U, Nieman H, Gerlich WH, Lampert F. Persistent hepatitis B virus replication in mononuclear blood cells as a source of reinfection of liver transplants. Transplantation. 1991;52:5.
80. Pol S, Thiers V, Nalpas B, Gazengel C, Carnot F, Tiollais P, Wands JR, Berthelot P, Bréchot C. Monoclonal anti-HBs antibodies radioimmunoassay and serum HBV-DNA hybridization as diagnostic tools of HBV infection: relative prevalence among HBsAg-negative alcoholics, patients with chronic hepatitis or hepatocellular carcinomas and blood donors. Eur J Clin Invest. 1987;17:515–21.
81. Paterlini P, Driss F, Nalpas B, Pisi E, Franco D, Berthelot P, Bréchot C. Persistence of hepatitis B and hepatitis C viral genomes in primary liver cancers from HBsAg negative patients: a study of low endemic area. Hepatology. 1992;17:20–9.
82. Paterlini P, Gerken G, Nakajima E, Terre S, D'Errico A, Grigioni W, Nalpas B, Franco D, Wands J, Kew M, Pisi E, Tiollais P, Bréchot C. Polymerase chain reaction to detect hepatitis B virus DNA and RNA sequences in primary liver cancers from patients negative for hepatitis B surface antigen. N Engl J Med. 1990;323:80–5.
83. Pontisso P, Morsica G, Ruvoletto MG, Barzon M, Perilongo G, Basso G, Ceccheto G, Chemello T, Alberti A. Latent hepatitis B virus infection in childhood hepatocellular carcinoma. Cancer. 1992;69:2731–5.
84. Marcellin P, Martinot-Peignoux M, Loriot MA, Giostra E, Boyer N, Thiers V, Benhamou JP. Persistence of hepatitis B virus DNA demonstrated by polymerase chain reaction in serum and liver after loss of HBsAg induced by antiviral therapy. Ann Intern Med. 1990;2:112–3.
85. Liang TJ, Baruch Y, Ben-Porath E, Enat R, Bassan L, Brown NV, Rimon N, Blum HE, Wands JR. Hepatitis B virus infection in patients with idiopathic liver disease. Hepatology. 1991;13:1044–51.
86. Liang TJ, Blum HE, Wands JR. Characterization and biological properties of a hepatitis B virus isolated from a patient without hepatitis B virus serologic markers. Hepatology. 1990;12:204–12.
87. Kremsdorf D, Garreau F, Duclos H, Thiers V, Schellekens H, Petit MA, Bréchot C. Complete nucleotide sequence and viral envelope protein expression of a hepatitis B virus DNA derived from a hepatitis B surface antigen seronegative patient. J Hepatol. 1993; in press

88. Kremsdorf D, Thiers V, Garreau F, Nakajima E, Chappey C, Shellekens H, Wands JR, Sninsky J, Tiollais P, Bréchot C. Nucleotide sequence analysis of hepatitis B virus genomes isolated from serologically negative patients. In: Viral hepatitis and liver disease. Baltimore: Williams and Wilkins; 1991:222–6.
89. Hadchouel M, Pasquinelli C, Fournier JG, Hugon RN, Scotto J, Bernard O, Bréchot C. Detection of mononuclear cells expressing hepatitis B virus in peripheral blood from HBsAg positive and negative patients by in situ hybridization. J Med Virol. 1988;24:27–32.
90. Figus A, Blum HE, Vyas GN, De Vergilis S, Cao A, Lippi M, Lai E. Hepatitis B viral nucleotide sequences in non-A, non-B or hepatitis B virus-related chronic liver disease. Hepatology. 1984;4:364–8.
91. Fagan EA, Davidson FD, Trowbridge R, Carman WF, Smith HM, Tedder R, Williams R. Detection of hepatitis B virus DNA sequences in liver in HBsAg seronegative patients with liver disease with and without anti-HBe antibodies. Q J Med. 1991;78:123–34.
92. Bréchot C, Degos F, Lugassy C, Thiers V, Zafrani S, Franco D, Bismuth G. Hepatitis B virus DNA in patients with chronic liver disease and negative tests for hepatitis B surface antigen. N Engl J Med. 1985;312:270–6.
93. Bréchot C, Scotto J, Charnay P, Hadchouel M, Degos F, Trepo C. Detection of hepatitis B virus DNA in liver and serum: a direct appraisal of the chronic carrier state. Lancet. 1981:765–67.
94. Bréchot C, Hadchouel M, Scotto J, Fonck M, Potet F, Vyas GN, Tiollais P. State of hepatitis B virus DNA in hepatocytes of patients with hepatitis B surface antigen-positive and negative liver disease. Proc Natl Acad Sci USA. 1981;78:3906–10.
95. Blum HE, Galun E, Liang J-T, Von Weizseker F, Wands JR. Naturally occurring missense mutation in the polymerase gene terminating hepatitis B virus replication. J Virol. 1991;65:1836–52.
96. Blum HE, Offensperger W-B, Walter E, Offensperger S, Gerok W. Latent hepatitis B virus infection in a patient serologically immune to hepatitis B virus infection. Liver. 1988;8:307–16.
97. Blum HE, Liang J-T, Galun E, Wands JR. Persistence of hepatitis B viral DNA after serological recovery from hepatitis B virus infection. Hepatology. 1991;14:56–63.
98. Kaneko S, Miller RH, Feinstone SM, Unoura M, Kobayashi K, Hattori S, Purcell RH. Detection of serum hepatitis B virus DNA in patients with chronic hepatitis using the polymerase chain reaction. Proc Natl Acad Sci. 1989;86:312–16.
99. Barlet V, Zarski JP, Thelu MA, Seigneurin JM. Advantage of PCR for detecting low amounts of HBV DNA in patients' sera. Res. Virol. 1991;142:373–9.
100. Kaneko S, Feinstone SM, Miller RH. Characterization of primers for optimal amplification of hepatitis B virus DNA using the polymerase chain reaction assay. J Virol Meth. 1990;29:225–9.
101. Coursaget P, Le cann P, Leboulleux D, Diop MT, Bao O, Coll AM. Detection of hepatitis B virus DNA by polymerase chain reaction in HBsAg negative Senegalese patients suffering from cirrhosis or primary liver cancer. FEMS Lett. 1991;35–8.
102. Porchon C, Kremsdorf D, Pol S, Lunel-Fabiani F, Driss F, Opolon P, Berthelot P, Bréchot C. Serum hepatitis C virus RNA and hepatitis B virus DNA in non-a and non-B post transfusional and sporadic chronic hepatitis. J Hepatol. 1992;16:184–9.
103. Shih YS, Shim KS, Lampertico P. Detection of hepatitis C virus sequences in liver tissues by the polymerase chain reaction. Lab Invest. 1991;65:408–11.
104. Yokosuka O, Omata M, Hosoda K. Detection and direct sequencing of hepatitis B virus genome by DNA amplification method. Gastroenterology. 1991;10075–81.
105. Wright TL, Mamish D, Combs C, Kim M, Donegan E, Ferrel L, Lake J, Roberts J, Ascher N. Hepatitis B virus and apparent fulminant non-A non-B hepatitis. Lancet. 1992;339: 952–5.
106. Thiers V, Lunel-Fabiani F, Valla D, Opolon P, Bréchot C. Post transfusional anti-HCV negative non-A non-B hepatitis: serological and polymerase chain reaction analysis for hepatitis C and hepatitis B viruses. J Hepatol. 1993: in press.
107. Coursaget P, Bourdil C, Adamowicz P, Chotard J, Diop Mar I, Yvonnet B, Mevelec MN, Barrès JL, N'Doye R, Chiron JP. HBsAg positive reactivity in man not due to hepatitis B virus. Lancet. 1987;12:1354–7.
108. Gallagher M, Fields H, De La Torre N, Ebert J, Krawczyuski K. Characterization of HBV2 by experimental infection of primates. In: Viral hepatitis and liver disease. Baltimore:

Williams & Wilkins; 1991:227–8.
109. Raney AK, Milich DR, McLachlan A. Complex regulation of transcription from the hepatitis B virus major surface antigen promoter in human hepatoma cell lines. J Virol. 1991;65:4805–11.
110. Ackerman Z, Gazitt LY, Wands JR, Bréchot C, Kew M, Shouval D. Unmasking of circulating hepatitis B surface antigen (HBsAg) following removal of immune complexes from serum of HBsAg-negative patients with chronic liver disease and hepatocellular carcinoma. In: Viral hepatitis and liver disease. New York: Liss; 1988;783–5.
111. Maynard JE, Kane MA, Alter MJ, Hadler SC. Control of hepatitis B by immunization: global perspectives. In: Viral hepatitis and liver disease. New York: Liss; 1988: 967–8.
112. Nalpas B, Pourcel C, Felman G, Housset C, Tiollais P, Bréchot C, Berthelot P, Farza H. Chronic alcohol intoxication decreases the serum level of hepatitis B surface antigen in transgenic mice. J Hepatol. 1992;15:118–24.
113. Nalpas B, Driss F, Pol S, Hamelin B, Housset C, Bréchot C, Berthelot P. Association between HCV and HBV infection in hepatocellular carcinoma and alcoholic liver disease. J Hepatol. 1991;12:70–4.
114. Oldstone MBA. Viral persistence. Cell. 1989;56:517–20.
115. Schlicht HJ, Schaller H. The secretory core protein of human hepatitis B virus is expressed on the cell surface. J Virol. 1989;63:5399–404.
116. Dienes HP, Gerken G, Goergen B, Autschbach F, Gerlich W, Heermann F, Meyer Zum Büschenfelde K-H. Histopathology and hepatitis B virus associated antigens in liver tissue of patients with severe anti-HBe-positive chronic hepatitis. J Hepatol. 1992;16:P1–15.
117. Tong S, Diot C, Gripon P, Vitvistski L, Trepo C, Guguen Guillouzou C. In vitro replication competence of a cloned hepatitis B virus variants with non sense mutations in the distal Pre C region. Virology. 1990;181:733–7.
118. Chisari FV, Filippi P, McLachlan A, Milich DR, Riggs M, Sun S, Palmiter RD, Pinkert CA, Brinster RL. Expression of hepatitis B virus large envelope polypeptide inhibits hepatitis B virus surface antigen secretion in transgenic mice. J Virol. 1986;60:880–7.
119. Roingeard P, Romet-Lemonne JL, Leturcq D, Goudeau A, Essex M. Hepatitis B virus core antigen (HBcAg) accumulation in an HBV nonproducer clone of HepG2-transfected cells is associated with cytopathic effect. Virology. 1990;179:113–20.
120. Kekulé AS, Lauer U, Meyer M, Caselman WH, Hofschneider PH, Koshy R. The preS2/2 region of integrated hepatitis B virus DNA encodes a transcriptional transactivator. Nature. 1990;343:457–61.
121. Foster GR, Acrkrill AM, Goldin RD, Kerr IM, Thomas HC, Stark GR. Expression of the terminal protein region of hepatitis B virus inhibits cellular responses to interferons and double-stranded RNA. Proc Natl Acad Sci. 1991;88:2888–92.
122. Whitten TM, Quets AT, Schloemer RH. Identification of the hepatitis B virus factor that inhibits expression of the beta interferon gene. J Virol. 1991;65:4699–704.

Section III
Immunology in Hepatitis A and C

9
Immunopathogenesis of hepatitis A virus infection

A. VALLBRACHT, Y.-D. STIERHOF and B. FLEISCHER

Hepatitis A virus (HAV) was first identified by electron microscopy in 1973 by Feinstone *et al.*[1]. Due to its biochemical and biophysical characteristics, this virus was classified in the enterovirus genus of the picornavirus family (enterovirus type 72). However, recent studies at the cellular and molecular level support the view that HAV should be classified in a distinct genus of the picornaviruses[2].

Besides demonstrating unique properties in its capsid as well as in the 5′ non-translated region of its genome, HAV also differs considerably from the enterovirus genus in its biological behaviour. Cell culture studies have shown that HAV regularly leads to a persistent infection, in the course of which little or no cytolytic mechanisms are seen. Immunofluorescence microscopy investigations have shown that 100% of cells are infected after the HAV infection is established, with large amounts of infectious particles being released in the supernatant[3]. The proliferation rate of cells with persistent HAV infection is essentially the same as uninfected cells[3].

Electron microscopic studies show HAV particles accumulating in vesicles in these carrier cells (Fig. 1). All relevant studies suggest that virus particles are released from the intact cell in numerous small vacuoles or vesicles. Although the persistence of HAV *in vitro* differs from the course of an HAV infection *in vitro*, there are a number of apparent similarities in the type of HAV antigens and HAV-infected vesicles and vacuoles in hepatocytes, macrophages and Kupffer cells. The vesicles shown here were from HAV-infected liver tissue of experimentally infected marmosets and chimpanzees, but are also found in human biopsies[4–6].

These studies *in vitro* suggest a mechanism for viral persistence and prolonged release in liver cells. However, the absence of well-documented cases of chronicity of HAV infection in humans indicates that there are efficient recognition and elimination mechanisms of the host immune system, where cellular immune responses play a central role.

The histological picture of acute HAV infection is characterized by the infiltration of the hepatic tissue by mononuclear cells of which $CD8^+$ T cells

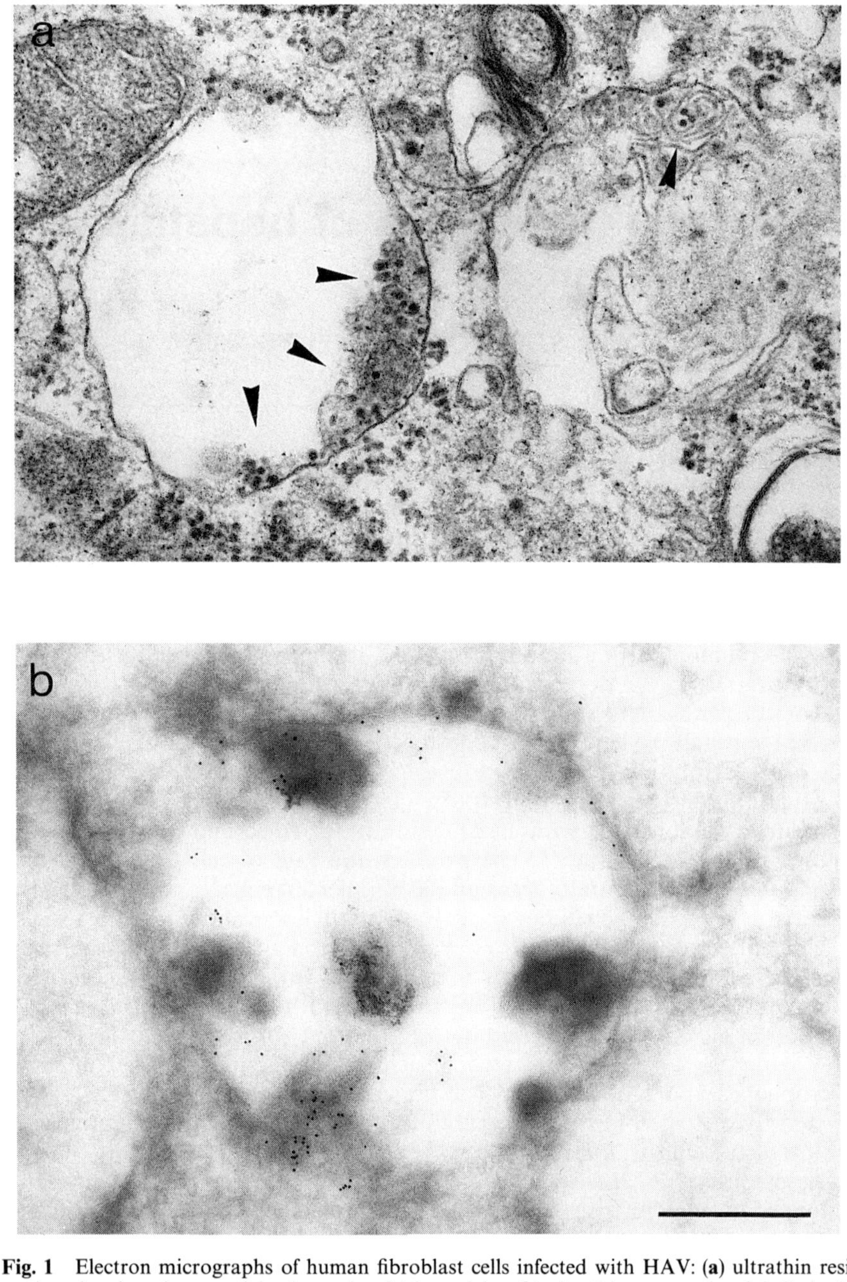

Fig. 1 Electron micrographs of human fibroblast cells infected with HAV: (**a**) ultrathin resin section showing virus particles (arrowheads) in vesicles; (**b**) ultrathin cryosection labelled with human anti HAV IgG and protein A–9 nm gold. Gold particles are detectable in vesicles. Bar = 0.5 μm

Table 1 Incidence of HAV-specific cytolytic $CD8^+$ T lymphocytes in liver and peripheral blood during acute HAV infection

T-lymphocyte clones derived from patient	*Days after onset of jaundice*	*Number of isolated clones*		*HAV-specific cytoxicity of $CD8^+$ clones*	
		$CD4^+$	*$CD8^+$*	*No. positive/ no. tested*	*Percentage*
Patient 1					
Liver	12	21	72	15/28	53.5
Peripheral blood	12	—	26	0/26	0.0
Patient 2					
Liver	38	42	35	11/26	42.3
Peripheral blood	30	—	120	3/114	2.6

Table 2 HAV-specific cytotoxicity and IFN-γ production by liver-derived $CD8^+$ clones from a patient with acute HAV infection

	Specific lysis of autologous targets (%)		*IFN-γ production (IU/ml)*	
Clone no.	*HAV-infected*	*Uninfected*	*HAV-infected*	*Uninfected*
1	71	5	64	<16
2	73	3	60	<16
3	76	3	70	<16
4	5	4	40	<16
5	4	5	<16	<16
6	9	3	<16	<16
7	92	8	280	<16
8	3	4	<16	<16
9	5	2	<16	<16
10	3	4	<16	<16
11	81	4	130	<16
12	4	4	64	<16

are the most common cell type. The establishment of an HLA congruent system, in which HAV-infected autologous skin fibroblasts serve as target cells, enabled us to determine the functional capacity of these $CD8^+$ cells in infiltrating HAV-infected liver tissue[7–9]. T-cell clones were isolated from liver biopsy and from the peripheral blood of patients with acute HAV infection, with subsequent analysis of the $CD8^+$ clones regarding their HLA-restricted, HAV-specific cytolytic activity. Table 1 shows the accumulation of these HAV-specific, $CD8^+$ cytolytic cells at the liver infection site.

Preliminary investigations using vaccinia constructs suggest that cytotoxic T cells in the infected cells recognize the structural proteins of the P1 region of the HAV genome (J. Stapleton, unpublished results).

While these cytolytic effector cells interact with the persistently HAV-infected target cells, interferon-γ (1FN-γ), an effective mediator in HLA expression, is produced (Table 2). Although few or no HLA class I antigens are expressed on hepatocytes, we have shown that this effect can be heightened considerably in the course of an HAV infection[10]. Thus, IFN-γ induction probably plays a central role in the efficiency of HAV elimination.

Our *in-vitro* results of recent years suggest that although HAV infection at the cellular level represents a persistent infection, a highly effective mechanism of recognizing HAV antigens together with histocompatibility antigens is apparently quite capable of eliminating this persistent infection in the hepatocytes.

Faecal shedding of HAV significantly precedes elevation of serum enzyme levels, although an enteric site of replication has yet to be demonstrated for HAV[11,12]. Most if not all faecally shed HAV appears to be replicated in the liver, reaching the intestinal tract by excretion in bile. This stage of HAV infection in the hepatocytes might be considered a persistent phase lasting < 2 weeks, in which host-cell metabolism and viral replication are kept in equilibrium. This persistent phase is comparable to the behaviour of HAV in cell cultures. Later, this balance seems to be upset *in vivo* by cell-mediated immunological mechanisms, which in turn lead to hepatocellular necrosis and elevation of serum transaminase levels[8,13].

The anicteric course of HAV infection cannot therefore be attributed solely to replication in the oropharynx and gastrointestinal tract, as is the case with polio infection. Infection of the liver, with a proliferation of the virus in a limited number of hepatocytes and the elimination of these infected cells by immunopathogenetic responses must be assumed to be the basis of inapparent HAV infection.

Clinically, this immunologically mediated cell destruction of acute HAV infection is normally characterized by a brief, self-limiting phase. However, the clinical manifestations of acute HAV infection range from asymptomatic to prolonged or relapsing cases, fulminant hepatitis and death[14–17].

HAV-specific cytotoxic T cells also seem to play an essential role in the protracted and relapsing form of HAV infection, in which elevated aminotransferases persist for several months. In these cases the highest cytolytic activity against HAV is observed in peripheral blood lymphocytes obtained 8–12 weeks after the onset of symptoms[7]. The recent description of HAV infection at an intensive-care unit for premature infants with virus excretion periods of up to 7 months[18] is most probably due to the immature cellular immune system of these children.

Further studies are needed to confirm the hypothesis that highly effective cell-mediated immune mechanisms lead to liver cell destruction and elimination of the virus in HAV infection. However, clinical findings seem to support *in-vitro* findings.

References

1. Feinstone SM, Kapikian AZ, Purcell RH. Hepatitis A: detection by immune electron microscopy of a virus-like antigen associated with acute illness. Science. 1973;182:1026–8.
2. Wimmer E, Murdin AD. Hepatitis A virus and the molecular biology of picornaviruses: a case for a new genus of the family picornaviridae. In: Hollinger FB, Lemon SM, Margolis HS, editors. Viral hepatitis and liver disease. Baltimore: Williams & Wilkins; 1990:31–41.
3. Vallbracht A, Hofmann L, Wurster KG, Flehmig B. Persistent infection of human fibroblasts by hepatitis A virus. J Gen Virol. 1984;65:609–15.
4. Shimizu YK, Shikata T, Beninger PR, Sata M, Setoyama H, Abett, Tanikawa K. Detection of hepatitis A antigen in human liver. Infect Immun. 1982;36:320–4.

5. Shimizu YK, Mathiesen LR, Lorenz D, Drucker J, Feinstone SM, Wagner JA, Purcell RH. Localization of hepatitis A antigen in liver tissue by peroxidase-conjugated antibody method: light and electron microscopic studies. J Immunol. 1978;121:1671–9.
6. Huang SN, Lorenz D, Gerety RJ. Electron and immunoelectron microscopic study on liver tissues of marmosets infected with hepatitis A virus. Lab Invest. 1979;41:63–71.
7. Vallbracht A, Gabriel P, Maier K, Hartmann F, Steinhardt HJ, Müller C, Wolf A, Mannck KH, Flehmig B. Cell-mediated cytotoxicity in hepatitis A virus infection. Hepatology. 1986;6:1308–14.
8. Vallbracht A, Maier K, Stierhof YD, Wiedmann KH, Flehmig B, Fleischer B. Liver-derived cytotoxic T cells in hepatitis A virus infection. J Infect Dis. 1989;160:209–17.
9. Fleischer B, Fleischer S, Maier K, Wiedmann KH, Sacher M, Thaler H, Vallbracht A. Clonal analysis of infiltrating T lymphocytes in liver tissue in viral hepatitis A. Immunology. 1990;69:14–19.
10. Maier K, Gabriel P, Koscielniak E, Stierhof YD, Wiedmann KH, Flehmig B, Vallbracht A. Human gamma interferon production by cytotoxic T lymphocytes sensitized during hepatitis A virus infection. J Virol. 1988;62:3756–63.
11. Stapleton JT, Lange DK, Le Duc JW, Binn LN, Jansen RW, Lemon SM. The role of secretory immunity in hepatitis A virus infection. J Infect Dis. 1991;163:7–11.
12. Scholz E, Heinricy U, Flehmig B. Acid stability of hepatitis A virus. J Gen Virol. 1989;70:2481–5.
13. Gabriel P, Vallbracht A, Flehmig B. Lack of complement-dependent cytolytic antibodies in hepatitis A virus infection. J Med Virol. 1984;20:23–31.
14. Glikson M, Galun E, Oren R, Tur-Kaspa R, Shouval D. Relapsing hepatitis A. Review of 14 cases and literature survey. Medicine. 1992;71:14–23.
15. Vallbracht A, Gabriel P, Zahn J, Flehmig B. Hepatitis A virus infection and the interferon system. J Infect Dis. 1985;152:211–13.
16. Fagan E, Yousef G, Brahm J, Garelick H, Mann G, Wolstenholme A, Portmann B, Harrison T, Mowbray JF, Mowat A, Zuckerman A, Williams R. Persistence of hepatitis A virus in fulminant hepatitis and after liver transplantation. J Med Virol. 1990;30:131–6.
17. McDonald GSA, Courtney MG, Shattock AG, Weir DG. Prolonged IgM antibodies and histopathological evidence of chronicity in hepatitis A. Liver. 1989;9:223–8.
18. Rosenblum LS, Villarino ME, Nainan OV, Melish ME, Hadler SC, Pinsky PP, Jarnis WR, Ott LE, Margolis HS. Hepatitis A outbreak in a neonatal intensive care unit: Risk factors for transmission and evidence of prolonged viral excretion among preterm infants. J Infect Dis. 1991;164:476–82.

10
T-lymphocyte response to hepatitis C virus

S. ABRIGNANI, P. PILERI, D. UNUTZMAZ, G. KUO, M. HOUGHTON, M. R. BRUNETTO, F. BONINO and M. A. MINUTELLO

Hepatitis C virus (HCV) is an RNA virus responsible for the majority of blood-borne non-A–non-B hepatitis[1]. Chronic hepatitis develops in at least half of infected patients, and progresses to liver cirrhosis in 20% of the chronic cases[2]. Although the HCV genome has been completely sequenced[3], the viral particles have not yet been isolated. A first step in designing an HCV vaccine is the identification of the components involved in protective immunity. At present it is not known what role the immune response plays in the course of HCV infection, since the study of the antibody response to HCV, although critical for developing means of diagnosis, cannot address this matter directly.

T lymphocyte responses to viruses may have two opposing effects: on the one hand they may be critical for protection, either directly through $CD8^+$ T killer cells[4], or indirectly through $CD4^+$ T cells which help B lymphocytes to produce neutralizing antibodies[5]; on the other hand, T cells may be harmful, mainly through $CD8^+$ T cells which damage infected tissues in the process of clearing the virus[6–8].

$CD4^+$ and $CD8^+$ T cells recognize antigens as peptides bound to major histocompatibility complex (MHC) class II and class I molecules, respectively, on the surface of an antigen-presenting cell (APC)[9]. Generally, peptides generated by proteolytic degradation of antigens such as viral particles or viral proteins internalized by APCs, bind to MHC class II, whereas peptides generated by proteolytic degradation of antigens which are synthesized *de novo* within APCs, as is the case in virus-infected cells, can bind both to MHC class I and to MHC class II.

The $CD4^+$ T cell response to viral proteins is usually essential for protection, since these cells are needed to help antibody production by B cells, and possibly to support priming of $CD8^+$ T cells specific for virus-infected cells[10].

At present, all information on the immune response to HCV comes from serological studies. To assess the role played by the cellular immune response

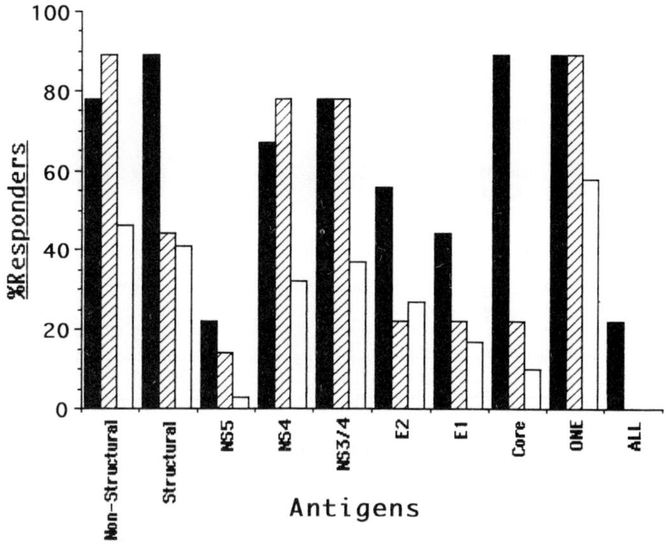

Fig. 1 T cell response to core correlated with benign course of HCV infection. Summary of 7-day proliferation assays for PBMC from 41 chronic hepatitis C patients (open bars), 11 individuals in remission (hatched bars) and 11 healthy seropositives (solid bars). Data are listed as percentage of responders (SI $\geqslant 4$) to at least one HCV protein (One), all HCV proteins (All), structural (core, E1 and E2), non-structural (NS3, NS4 and NS5), or the individual HCV proteins. The prevalence of proliferative responses either to core in the healthy seropositive group was significantly higher than in the other two groups ($p < 0.001$). Differences in the proliferative responses to the other antigens were not significantly different in the three groups ($p > 0.05$)

in the outcome of HCV infection we studied the $CD4^+$ T lymphocyte response to viral antigens in infected individuals with different clinical courses. Using six recombinant proteins corresponding to the putative core, envelope-1, envelope-2, non-structural proteins NS3, NS4 and NS5 of HCV, we assessed the specificity of liver-infiltrating T cells and the T lymphocyte proliferative responses of peripheral blood mononuclear cells from 63 HCV-seropositive individuals: 41 patients with chronic hepatitis C, 11 patients whose chronic hepatitis C was successfully treated with interferon-α (IFN-α), and 11 healthy individuals seropositive for anti-HCV.

To assess the priming of T cells by HCV infection *in vivo* we first selected HCV-seropositive individuals with different clinical outcomes of infection and measured the proliferative response of their peripheral blood mononuclear cells (PBMCs) to six different HCV proteins *in vitro*. Figure 1 shows that: (a) regardless of the course of infection, NS3 and NS4 were the most immunogenic proteins of HCV for peripheral blood $CD4^+$ T cells; (b) differences in the PBMC responses between chronic patients who were in remission and those with ongoing chronic hepatitis, were quantitative more than qualitative; (c) healthy seropositives were the only individuals whose PBMCs responded, in some cases, to all HCV proteins; (d) there was a significant correlation between presence of PBMC response to core and a

Table 1 CD4$^+$ T cell clones specific for HCV antigens

Patient no.	*Cell source*	*Core*	*E1*	*NS1*	*NS3*	*NS4*	*NS5*
1	Blood				2	6	3
13	Liver					12	
13	Blood					10	
14	Liver					4	
15	Blood	5				11	
25	Blood	2					
31	Blood	1					
50	Blood		2	2			
71	Liver					27	
71	Blood					22	
110	Blood		3				
		8	5	2	2	92	3

benign course of infection ($p < 0.001$), whereas responses to all the other proteins did not show any significant correlation with the course of infection ($p > 0.05$).

Although the study of the T cell responses in the peripheral blood is critical to the understanding of both the immunogenicity of the virus and the immune status of the individual, it does not necessarily reflect the pattern of T cell responses present at the site of the disease. Since information on the local immune response may be relevant to the understanding of the pathogenesis of hepatitis, we assessed the specificity of liver-infiltrating T lymphocytes from liver biopsies. We obtained antigen-specific T cell lines only from three biopsies cultured with NS4, whereas with all the other proteins we failed to obtain antigen-specific T cell lines from 19 liver samples. The absence of antigen-specific responses in most of the biopsies was not related to the inability of these cells to respond to activation stimuli *in vitro*, since we obtained T cell lines stimulated with the mitogen phytohaemagglutinin (PHA) from all the liver samples.

Finally, we have established HCV-specific CD4$^+$ T cell clones from cell lines isolated from both PBMCs and liver biopsies. Table 1 shows that (a) it was possible to isolate CD4$^+$ MHC-class II restricted T cell clones specific for any HCV antigen from the blood of infected individuals, (b) NS4 specific T cell clones were the only HCV specific T cells we could isolate from liver biopsies. Studies are in progress to investigate structural and functional differences between NS4 specific T cell clones obtained from blood and liver of the same individuals.

DISCUSSION

All the putative HCV proteins, except NS2 which was not available in purified recombinant form, were expressed intracellularly in yeast as SOD fusion proteins, and purified after denaturation with SDS. The use of denatured proteins may result in an underestimation of the B cell response, because of the presence of antibodies directed to conformational epitopes of the proteins. In contrast, T cell responses generally are not influenced by protein conformation, in that they recognize short peptides generated by proteolytic degradation of the antigen[9]. Therefore, T cell responses assessed with denatured antigens should give the same spectrum of response to the viral proteins which occurs *in vivo*.

The CD4$^+$ T cell response was studied in three groups of HCV seropositive individuals (total of 63 patients), who differed with regard to the clinical outcome of infection: 41 patients with chronic hepatitis, 11 patients whose chronic hepatitis went into remission after IFN treatment, and 11 healthy seropositives.

Altogether, our data show that, regardless of the clinical course of HCV infection, NS3 and NS4 were the most immunogenic proteins for CD4$^+$ T cells. The high immunogenicity of NS4 was further proven by the finding that the only HCV-specific T cell lines obtained from liver biopsies were specific for NS4.

Since NS4 is a putative non-structural protein of HCV[3], it should not be present in the virion particles. Therefore, the high frequency of MHC class II restricted CD4$^+$ T cells specific for NS4, may imply a high-affinity binding to MHC class II of peptides derived from endogenously synthesized NS4 in infected cells. Alternatively, it is possible that this protein is shed by infected cells, captured by macrophages or specific B cells, and presented to CD4$^+$ T cells. The last hypothesis could also explain the serology data demonstrating that NS4 (C100-3) is a highly immunogenic protein for antibody responses[1]. Indeed, NS4 can be considered as an immunodominant region of HCV, both for humoral and MHC class II restricted CD4$^+$ T cell responses.

The absence of detectable PBMC proliferation to any HCV protein in 35% (22/63) of the individuals is intriguing, since they had HCV-specific antibodies, the production of which usually requires CD4$^+$ T cell help[10]. Proliferation experiments performed in the absence of CD8$^+$ T cells allow us to exclude that this was due to a suppressor effect of CD8$^+$ T cells (data not shown). Although we could not rule out the possibility that these PBMCs recognize the protein NS2, which was not available to us, it is possible that HCV-specific T cells help B cells, though they were present at a frequency which is below the sensitivity of our assay. Alterntively, since proteins, such as E1 and E2, show considerable sequence heterogeneity among HCV isolates[11], one could speculate that, in these individuals, CD4$^+$ T cells were present but recognized variable regions of HCV proteins. Such T cells would not be detected in proliferation assays performed with recombinant proteins from HCV isolates different from the patients' isolates.

The relationship between the immune response to the various proteins of a virus and the course of infection is critical to vaccine development. When T cell proliferation is correlated with the clinical phase of infection, there was a clear trend indicating that healthy seropositives responded to HCV proteins better than patients from the other two groups. Most important, there was a significant correlation between presence of T cell response to core and the healthy-seropositive status ($p < 0.001$). It is interesting to note that we detected by PCR the presence of HCV RNA in the sera of six of nine healthy seropositives, and all these viraemic individuals responded to core. This shows that the majority of these individuals are in fact healthy carriers of HCV, and indicates that the T cell response to core, although associated with a benign course of the infection, does not coincide with elimination of the virus.

Although it is well established that almost all patients with chronic hepatitis C have serum antibodies to core (c22), it is not surprising that only a few of these patients have a detectable T cell proliferative response to core. It is indeed well known that antibody responses to a given viral protein can occur in the absence of a T cell response to the same protein, provided that there are T cell responses to other proteins of the same virus. This so-called intermolecular help[12] could account for the dissociation between T and B cell responses to core in chronic patients.

We cannot exclude the possibility that a strong T cell response to core occurs as a consequence of a favourable course of the infection, but it may well be that $CD4^+$ T cell responses to core epitopes are critical to keep HCV infection under control by the immune system. With the hepatitis B virus, $CD4^+$ T cells specific for the core (HBcAg) have been shown to help production of anti-envelope antibodies[12], which are virus-neutralizing. It is noteworthy, in this context, that the HCV-core gene is highly conserved among different virus isolates, whereas the putative envelope genes E1 and E2 exhibit considerable sequence variability[11]. Therefore, T cell responses to core should be unaffected by the occurrence of viral mutants that might arise in infected individuals[13,14]. It is tempting to speculate that $CD4^+$ T cell response to core could provide continuous help for B cells and $CD8^+$ T cells specific for new variable regions of HCV mutants, both of which may be required to maintain humoral and cellular responses protective against the disease.

References

1. Kuo G, Choo Q-L, Alter HJ *et al.* An assay for circulating antibodies to a major etiologic virus of human non-A, non-B hepatitis. Science. 1989;4:362–4.
2. Dienstag JL. Hepatitis non-A, non-B: C at last. Gastroenterology. 1990;99:1177–80.
3. Choo Q-L, Richman KH, Han JH *et al.* Genetic organization and diversity of the hepatitis C virus. Proc Natl Acad Sci USA. 1991;88:2451–5.
4. Byrne JA, Oldstone MBA. Biology of cloned cytotoxic T lymphocytes specific for lymphocytic choriomeningitis virus: clearance of virus in vivo. J Virol. 1984;51:682–6.
5. Raff MC. Role of thymus-derived lymphocytes in the secondary humoral immune response in mice. Nature. 1970;226:1257–9.
6. Zinkernagel RM, Haenseler E, Leist TP, Cerny A, Hengartner H, Althage A. T cell mediated hepatitis in mice infected with lymphocytic choriomeningitis virus. J Exp Med. 1986;164:1075–92.
7. Barnaba V, Franco A, Alberti A, Benvenuto R, Balsano F. Selective killing of hepatitis B envelope antigen-specific B cells by class I-restricted, exogenous antigen-specific T lymphocytes. Nature. 1990;345:258–60.
8. Moriyama T, Guilhot S, Klopchin K *et al.* Immunobiology and pathogenesis of hepatocellular injury in hepatitis B virus transgenic mice. Science. 1990;248:361–4.
9. Morrison LA, Lukacher A, Braciale VL, Fan DP, Braciale TJ. Differences in antigen presentation to MHC class I and class II-restricted influenza virus-specific cytolytic T lymphocyte clones. J Exp Med. 1986;163:903–21.

10. Sprent J, Webb SR. Function and specificity of T cell subsets in the mouse. Adv Immunol. 1987;41:39–133.
11. Weiner AJ, Brauer MJ, Rosenblatt J *et al.* Variable and hypervariable domains are found in the regions of HCV corresponding to the flavivirus envelope and NS1 proteins and the pestivirus envelope glycoproteins. Virology. 1991;180:842–8.
12. Milich DR, McLachlan A, Thornton GB, Hughes JL. Antibody production to the nucleocapsid and envelope of the hepatitis B virus primed by a single synthetic T cell site. Nature. 1987;329:547–9.
13. Pircher H, Moskophidis D, Rohrer U, Bürki K, Hengartner H, Zinkernagel RM. Viral escape by selection of cytotoxic T cell-resistant virus variants *in vivo.* Nature. 1990;346: 629–32.
14. Phillips RE, Rowland-Jones S, Nixon DF *et al.* Human immunodeficiency virus genetic variation that can escape cytotoxic T cell recognition. Nature. 1991;354:453–9.

11
Immunopathology of hepatitis C

M. A. GERBER and S. N. THUNG

INTRODUCTION

Hepatitis C virus (HCV) is the predominant aetiological agent of non-A–non-B hepatitis around the world[1–3]. It frequently leads to chronic hepatitis which may progress to cirrhosis and hepatocellular carcinoma[4–7]. The histological types of hepatitis associated with HCV infection range from acute hepatitis to massive hepatic necrosis, and from chronic persistent hepatitis to chronic active hepatitis with or without cirrhosis[8–13]. At present the pathogenesis of liver injury in hepatitis C is unknown. Two major mechanisms of liver damage in HCV infection are proposed: (1) direct cytopathic effect of HCV, and (2) immune-mediated cell injury induced by HCV. In an attempt to elucidate the pathogenesis of hepatitis C, we studied a series of liver biopsy specimens of chronic hepatitis C by immunopathological and molecular techniques.

MATERIALS AND METHODS

Liver biopsy specimens from 13 patients with anti-HCV-positive chronic hepatitis and four HCV-negative control patients were studied. Nucleic acids were extracted by the guanidinium method from formalin-fixed, paraffin-embedded tissue sections[14]. Non-translated (NT) sequences of HCV RNA were detected by reverse double polymerase chain reaction (PCR)[15]. Genomic and replicative strands of HCV were distinguished by strand-specific PCR[16]. Inflammatory cell infiltrates in the liver biopsy specimens were phenotyped by immunohistochemical staining with a panel of monoclonal antibodies to B lymphocytes, T lymphocytes, activated T and B lymphocytes, dendritic histiocytes, macrophages, granulocytes, and HLA antigens using the avidin biotin peroxidase complex method[17].

RESULTS

Histologically, HCV-infected patients showed chronic persistent hepatitis or chronic active hepatitis with or without cirrhosis. The majority of the biopsy

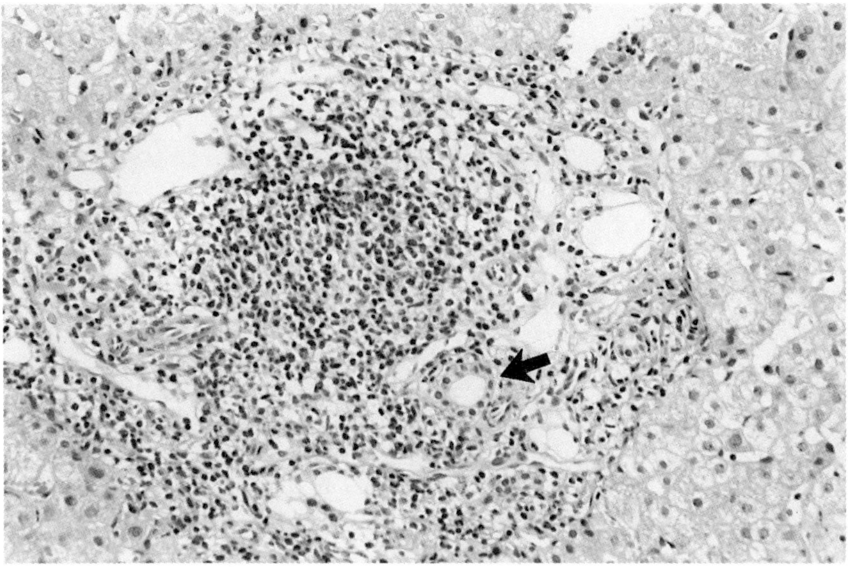

Fig. 1 Dense lymphoid aggregate in a portal tract of a patient with chronic hepatitis C. The bile duct (arrow) is slightly distorted (H&E × 210)

specimens revealed characteristic changes of chronic hepatitis C, i.e. macro- or microvesicular steatosis, lymphoid aggregates in portal tracts (Fig. 1), and bile duct damage (Fig. 2). Lymphoid aggregates in portal tracts contained predominantly T cells, as well as B cells, and dendritic histiocytes. The bile ducts showed epithelial degeneration and lymphocyte infiltration. There was no detectable expression of HLA class II antigens in bile duct epithelial cells. Liver tissue of all anti-HCV-positive patients except for two contained the plus (genomic) strand of HCV RNA as demonstrated by reverse double PCR. In eight of these 11 patients, minus (replicative) strands of HCV RNA were also detected. Both plus and minus strands of HCV RNA correlated with anti-HCV reactivity in serum at significance levels of $p < 0.005$ and $p < 0.05$, respectively. There was, however, no statistically significant correlation of any of the histological parameters or the histological activity index (Knodell)[18] and the presence or absence of genomic or replicative HCV RNA sequences.

DISCUSSION

In contrast to hepatitis B virus (HBV) infection, little is known about the mechanism of hepatocyte injury in chronic HCV infection. There is evidence in support of either a direct cytopathic effect of HCV or immune-mediated cell injury induced by HCV[19]. This virus belongs to the family of flaviviridae, members of which are often directly cytopathic, i.e. yellow fever virus[20,21]. In some cases of HCV infection, hepatocytes show cytopathic changes

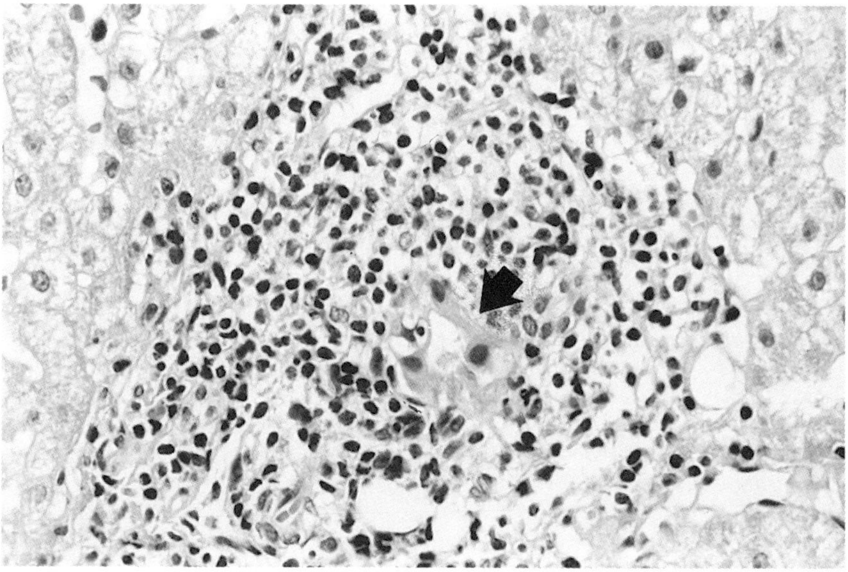

Fig. 2 A damaged bile duct (arrow) in the centre of a lymphoid aggregate in a different portal tract of the same patient as in Fig. 1 (H&E × 340)

without significant inflammatory infiltration of the liver parenchyma[19]. A recent immunohistochemical study of the expression of HCV antigens in liver biopsy specimens demonstrated that HCV-positive livers exhibited higher aminotransferase levels and more intralobular inflammation and fibrosis than HCV-negative livers[22,23]. These findings support the theory that HCV is directly cytopathic.

On the other hand, the immune hypothesis of liver injury in hepatitis C is also supported by several lines of evidence:

1. HCV infection is often associated with a variety of autoimmune manifestations[24], particularly Sjögren's syndrome[25], mixed cryoglobulinaemia[26–29], vasculitis[30], and skin diseases such as erythema nodosum and urticaria[31]. A number of autoantibodies have been demonstrated in the serum of anti-HCV-positive patients, including anti-liver/kidney microsomal antibody type 1, and anti-GOR antibody[32,33]. Both autoantibodies may be related to molecular mimicry based on sequence homology between the HCV polyprotein and P450 IID6 or nuclear antigen (GOR) respectively[34].
2. A number of viruses, including HBV, may infect lymphocytes and alter the immune response of the patient. Recently, HCV RNA sequences were demonstrated in the lymphocytes of patients with chronic hepatitis C[35].
3. Over half of liver specimens of chronic hepatitis C show dense lymphoid aggregates in portal tracts, often in association with damaged bile ducts. Some of these lymphoid aggregates contain germinal centres with

dendritic cells and B lymphocytes surrounded by T lymphocytes. These lymphoid aggregates, as well as the lymphoid infiltrates in the hepatic parenchyma, may mediate an immune response of the host to the HCV-infected hepatocytes. In over half of liver specimens with hepatitis C, the bile duct epithelium is infiltrated by lymphocytes, but there is no aberrant expression of HLA class II antigens in bile duct epithelial cells as seen in primary biliary cirrhosis, hepatic allograft rejection, and graft-versus-host disease[17].

4. Our studies did not demonstrate a correlation between the histological activity of hepatitis C and the presence or absence of HCV RNA sequences, either genomic or replicative, in liver tissues.

These findings support the hypothesis that HCV is not directly cytopathic and that immune mechanisms mediate hepatocyte injury in chronic hepatitis C. Finally, about half of chronic hepatitis C patients initially respond to the antiviral agent interferon-α, but many responders relapse after cessation of therapy[36,37].

In conclusion, current evidence supports both mechanisms of hepatocyte injury in chronic hepatitis C, i.e. a direct cytopathic effect of HCV as well as immune-mediated damage perhaps triggered by HCV. An animal model of HCV infection and further detailed studies of infected patients are needed to define the exact mechanism of hepatocyte and bile duct injury in hepatitis C and to develop an effective therapeutic strategy.

Acknowledgement

This work was supported by NIH grant RO1CA54576.

References

1. Kuo G, Choo Q-L, Alter HJ, Gitnick GL, Redeker AG, Purcell RH, Miyamura T, Dienstag J, Alter MJ, Stevens CE, Tegtmeier GE, Bonino F, Colombo M, Lee WS, Kuo C, Berger K, Shuster JR, Overby LR, Bradley DW, Houghton M. An assay for circulating antibodies to a major etiologic virus of human non-A, non-B hepatitis. Science. 1989;244:362–4.
2. Weiner AJ, Kuo G, Bradley DW, Bonino F, Saracco G, Lee C, Rosenblatt J, Choo Q-L, Houghton M. Detection of hepatitis C viral sequences in non-A, non-B hepatitis. Lancet. 1990;335:1–3.
3. Alter HJ, Purcell RH, Shih JW, Melpolder JC, Houghton M, Choo Q-L, Kuo G. Detection of antibody to hepatitis C virus in prospectively followed transfusion recipients with acute and chronic non-A, non-B hepatitis. N Engl J Med. 1989;321:1494–500.
4. Kiyosawa K, Akahane Y, Nagata A, Furata S. Hepatocellular carcinoma after non-A, non-B post-transfusion hepatitis. Am J Gastroenterol. 1984;79:777–81.
5. Oka H, Kurioka N, Kim K, Kanno T, Kuroki T, Mizoguchi K, Kobayashi K. Prospective study of early detection of hepatocellular carcinoma in patients with cirrhosis. Hepatology. 1990;12:680–7.
6. Okuda K. Hepatitis C virus and hepatocellular carcinoma. In: Tabor E, DiBisceglie AM, Purcell RH, editors. Etiology, pathology, and treatment of hepatocellular carcinoma in North America. Houston: Gulf; 1991;119–26.
7. DiBisceglie AM. Chronic viral hepatitis and hepatocellular carcinoma in the United States. In: Tabor E, DiBisceglie AM, Purcell RH, editors. Etiology, pathology, and treatment of hepatocellular carcinoma in North America. Houston: Gulf; 1991:127–36.

8. Gerber MA, Thung SN. Viral hepatitis: Pathology. In: Berk JE, Haubrich WS, Kalser MH, Roth JLA, Schaffner F, editors. Bockus Gastroenterology, Vol. V. Philadelphia: W.B. Saunders; 1985:2825–55.
9. Bach N, Thung SN, Schaffner F. The histological features of chronic hepatitis C and autoimmune chronic active hepatitis: a comparative analysis. Hepatology. 1992;15:572–7.
10. Scheuer PJ, Ashrafzadeh P, Sherlock S, Brown D, Dusheiko GM. The pathology of hepatitis C. Hepatology. 1992;15:567–71.
11. Gerber MA. Chronic hepatitis C: the beginning of the end of a time-honored nomenclature? Hepatology. 1992;15:733–4.
12. Thung SN, Gerber MA, Popper H. Basic morphologic patterns of viral hepatitis A, B, non-A, non-B, and delta agent in animal and man. In: Chisari FV, editor. Advances in hepatitis research. New York: Masson; 1983:293–302.
13. Gerber MA, Krawczynski K, Alter MJ, Sampliner RE, Margolis HS, Sentinel Counties Chronic non-A, non-B Hepatitis Study Team. Histopathology of community acquired chronic hepatitis C. Mod Pathol. 1992;5:483–6.
14. Akyol G, Dash S, Shieh CY-S, Malter JS, Gerber MA. Detection of hepatitis C virus sequences by polymerase chain reaction in fixed liver tissue. Mod Pathol. 1992;5:501–4.
15. Shieh YS-C, Shim K-S, Lampertico P, Balart LA, Jeffers LJ, Thung SN, Regenstein R, Reddy KR, Farr G, Schiff E, Gerber MA. Detection of hepatitis C virus sequences in liver tissue by polymerase chain reaction. Lab Invest. 1991;65:408–11.
16. Gerber MA, Shieh YS-C, Shim K-S, Thung SN, Demetris AJ, Schwartz M, Akyol G, Dash S. Detection of replicating hepatitis C virus sequences in hepatocellular carcinoma. Am J Pathol. 1992;141:1271–7.
17. Danque POV, Bach N, Schaffner F, Gerber MA, Thung SN. Bile duct injury in chronic hepatitis C. Mod Path. 1993;(in press).
18. Knodell RH, Ishak KG, Black WC, Chen TS, Craig R, Kaplowitz N, Kiernan TW, Wollman J. Formulation and application of a numerical scoring system for assessing histological activity in asymptomatic chronic active hepatitis. Hepatology. 1981;1:431–5.
19. Dienes HP, Popper H, Arnold W, Lobeck H. Histologic observations in human hepatitis non-A, non-B. Hepatology. 1982;2:562–71.
20. Miller RH, Purcell Rh. Hepatitis C virus shares aminoacid sequence similarity with pestiviruses and flaviviruses as well as members of two plant virus supergroups. Proc Natl Acad Sci USA. 1990;87:2057–61.
21. Feinstone SM. The virology of hepatitis C. Gastroenterology. 1991;1:26–8.
22. Hiramatsu N, Hayashi N, Haruna Y, Kasahara A, Fusamoto H, Mori C, Fuke I, Okayama H, Kamada T. Immunohistochemical detection of hepatitis C virus-infected hepatocytes in chronic liver disease with monoclonal antibodies to core, envelope and NS3 regions of the hepatitis C virus genome. Hepatology. 1992;16:306–11.
23. Krawzynski K, Beach M, Bradley D, Kuo G, DiBisceglie A, Houghton. Hepatitis C virus antigen in hepatocytes: immunomorphologic detection and identification. Gastroenterology. 1992;03:622–9.
24. McFarlane IG. Autoimmunity and hepatotropic viruses. Semin Liver Dis. 1991;11:223–33.
25. Haddad J, Deny P, Munz-Gotheil C, Ambrossine J-C, Trinchet J-C, Pateron D, Mal F, Callard P, Beaugrand M. Lymphocytic sialadenitis of Sjogren's syndrome associated with chronic hepatitis C virus liver disease. Lancet. 1992;339:321–3.
26. Pascual M, Perrin L, Giostra E, Schifer JA. Hepatitis C virus in patients with cryoglobulinemia type I. J Infect Dis. 1990;162:569–70.
27. Ferri C, Greco F, Longombardo G, Palla P, Moretti A, Marzo E, Fosella PV, Pasero G, Bombardieri S. Hepatitis C virus antibodies in mixed cryoglobulinemia patients. Arthritis Rheum. 1991;34:1606–10.
28. Ferri C, Greco F, Longombardo G, Palla P, Moretti A, Marzo E, Mazzone A. Association between hepatitis C virus and mixed cryoglobulinemia. Clin Exp Rheumatol. 1991;9:621–4.
29. Casato M, Pucillo LP, Lagana B, Taliani G, Goffredo F, Bonomo L. Cryoglobulinemia and hepatitis C virus. Lancet. 1991;337:1047–8.
30. Hearth-Holmes M, Zahradka SL, Baethge BA, Wolf RE. Leukocytoclastic vasculitis associated with hepatitis C. Am J Med. 1991;90:765–6.
31. Domingo P, Ris J, Martines E, Casas F. Erythema nodosum and hepatitis C. Lancet. 1990;336:1377.

32. Lumel F, Abuaf N, Frangeul L, Grippon P, Perrin M, LeCos Y, Valla D, Borotto E, Yamamoto A-M, Huraux J-M, Opolon P, Homberg JC. Liver/kidney microsome antibody type 1 and hepatitis C virus infection. Hepatology. 1992;16:630–6.
33. Michel G, Ritter A, Gerken G, Meyer Zum Buschenfelde KH, Decker R, Manns MP. Anti-GOR and hepatitis C virus in autoimmune liver diseases. Lancet. 1992;339:267–9.
34. Hosein B, Fang X, Wang CY, Lenzi M, Cassani F, Ballardini G, Bianchi FB, Mishiro S, Unoura M, Kaneko S, Kobayashi K. Anti-HCV, anti-GOR, and autoimmunity. Lancet. 1992;339: 871–2.
35. Zignego AL, Macchia D, Monti M, Thiers V, Mazzetti M, Foschi M, Maggi F. Infection of peripheral mononuclear blood cells by hepatitis C virus. J Hepatol. 1992: in press.
36. DiBisceglie AM, Martin P, Kassianides C, Lisker-Melman M, Murray L, Waggoner J, Goodman Z, Banks SM, Hoofnagle JH. Recombinant interferon alpha therapy for chronic hepatitis C. A randomized, double-blind placebo-controlled trial. N Engl J Med. 1989;321:1506–10.
37. Davis GL, Balart LA, Schiff ER, Linday K, Bodenheimer HC Jr, Perrillo RP, Carey W, Jacobson IM, Payne J, Dienstag JL, VanThiel DH, Tamburro C, Lefkowitch J, Albrecht J, Meschievitz, Ortego TJ, Gibas A, the Hepatitis Interventional Therapy Group. Treatment of chronic hepatitis C with recombinant interferon alpha. A multicenter randomized, controlled trial. N Engl J Med. 1989;321:1501–6.

12
Immunology and autoimmunity in hepatitis C

F. B. BIANCHI, M. LENZI, F. CASSANI, G. BALLARDINI, F. GIOSTRA, L. MURATORI, M. CATALETA, R. FRANCESCONI and D. ZAULI

Concepts regarding autoimmune hepatitis (AIH) are at present being extensively revised: this is largely due to the availability of tests to detect antibodies to HCV peptides and HCV-RNA in serum and liver. In particular, an intriguing relationship between HCV infection and cryptogenic hepatitis with markers of autoimmunity has been consistently detected in countries of the Mediterranean area and Japan, although not in the United States or Britain[1]. This has stimulated a redefinition of diagnostic criteria (biochemical and immunological parameters) and response to corticosteroid treatment by an International Autoimmune Hepatitis Group, whose proposals will soon be available for discussion.

At the moment the identification of AIH relies on three major criteria: (1) the cryptogenic nature of the liver disease; (2) the demonstration of serum autoantibodies (in particular antinuclear and anti-smooth muscle antibodies, which identify type 1 AIH, anti-liver and kidney microsomes (LKM1) which identify type 2 AIH); (3) an '*ex juvantibus*' criterion, the rapid and complete response of liver tests (transaminases, bilirubin, γ-globulin) to corticosteroid therapy.

In 1990–1 we presented evidence that the vast majority of *AIH type* 2 (*LKM1-positive*) *adult cases* were also anti-HCV positive. This conclusion was first reached using first- and second-generation ELISAs with recombinant and synthetic HCV peptides, and the results validated by second-generation RIBA[2,3]. When tested for serum HCV-RNA by a 'nested' PCR (with primers from the 5′ NC region) 17 of the 18 anti-HCV positive sera tested were found to be positive[4]. The group of Homberg in Paris added the important observation that, differently from adults, paediatric anti-LKM1-positive AIH cases did not have anti-HCV[5]. This was confirmed in our series. From the experimental work of Manns *et al.* we know that anti-LKM1 recognizes a sequence of cytochrome P450 IID6 molecule, which shares a short amino acid sequence homology with peptides encoded by HCV and herpes simplex virus[6]. When tested by counterimmunoelectrophoresis or immuno-'western' blotting with rat liver microsomes as source of antigen, both anti-HCV-positive and -negative anti-LKM1 sera display a common pattern of reactivity. In contrast, when recombinant P450 IID6 is used as antigen in an immunoblot assay the number of positive reactions with anti-LKM1/anti-HCV sera is significantly lower, despite similar LKM1 titres of anti-LKM1. Moving from the observation that an anti-HCV and serum HCV-RNA-positive patient, who developed anti-LKM1 after an ALT peak during interferon treatment, was positive for HLA-DR3 (known to be associated with a variety of autoimmune disorders with serum autoantibodies, including AIH type 1)[8], we assayed anti-LKM1-positive cases for the presence of HLA-DR3 phenotype. In the 24 cases studied (20 anti-HCV-positive, four anti-HCV-negative) a significant association was found, which was even higher when only anti-LKM1/anti-HCV-positive cases were considered.

In our series of *AIH type 1 (ANA and/or SMA positive)* anti-HCV (second-generation tests) was present in 46% of cases[9]. We found that the small group of AIH type 1 patients with both ANA and SMA were consistently anti-HCV negative which was significantly different from what was found in cases with only one reactivity[10]. There was no obvious explanation for this result. We have tested 12 AIH type 1 patients (six anti-HCV-positive, six negative) for serum HCV-RNA, selected on the basis of the availability of a suitable sample for PCR analysis. A complete concordance was found between anti-HCV and HCV-RNA in these 12 specimens which confirmed previous Italian findings[11]. Interestingly, HLA-DR3 phenotype was found in four of the five anti-HCV/HCV-RNA-negative as well as three of the four anti-HCV/HCV-RNA-positive patients.

In our experience, anti-GOR testing added little. This antibody is elicited by HCV infection through a molecular mimicry mechanism between a HCV peptide and a nuclear autoantigen. Anti-GOR antibodies were confined to a proportion of patients with both AIH types 1 and 2 who were positive for anti-HCV. Anti-GOH was never detected in anti-HCV-negative patients with AIH[12].

Our working hypothesis is that, along with a true 'primary' AIH, HCV is able to trigger a form of chronic hepatitis with autoimmune markers in genetically predisposed persons. This HCV-related AIH is indistinguishable from the 'primary' form. This hypothesis can and must be tested in order to select a rational therapeutic option.

References

1. Lenzi M, Johnson PJ, McFarlane IG, Ballardini G, Smith HM, McFarlane BM, Bridger C, Vergani D, Bianchi FB, Williams R. Antibodies to hepatitis C virus in autoimmune liver disease: evidence for geographical heterogenicity. Lancet. 1991;338:277–80.
2. Lenzi M, Ballardini G, Fusconi M, Cassani F, Selleri L, Volta U, Zauli D, Bianchi FB. Type 2 autoimmune hepatitis and hepatitis C virus infection. Lancet. 1990;335:258–9.
3. Fusconi M, Lenzi M, Ballardini G, Miniero R, Cassani F, Zauli D, Bianchi FB. Anti-HCV testing in autoimmune hepatitis and primary biliary cirrhosis. Lancet. 1990;336:823.
4. Garson JA, Lenzi M, Ring C, Cassani F, Ballardini G, Briggs M, Tedder RS, Bianchi FB. Hepatitis C viraemia in adults with type 2 autoimmune hepatitis. J Med Virol. 1991;34:223–6.

5. Lunel F, Homberg JC, Grippon P, Perrin M, Blanc C, Bernared B, Cadranel JF, Abuaf N, Valla D, Opolon P, Huraux JM. Type 2 autoimmune hepatitis and hepatitis C virus: a study group of 83 patients. J Hepatol. 1991;13(Suppl. 2):S47.
6. Manns PM, Griffin KJ, Sullivan KF, Johnson EF. LKM-1 autoantibodies recognize a short linear sequence in P450IID6, a cytochrome P-450 monooxygenase. J Clin Invest. 1991;88:1370–8.
7. Mackay IR, Morris P. Association of autoimmune chronic active hepatitis with HLA-A1. Lancet. 1972;2:793–5.
8. Muratori L, Zauli D, Giostra F, Ballardini G, Lenzi M, Cassani F, Bianchi FB. LKM_1 appearance in a HLA-DR3+ patient with chronic hepatitis C during Interferon treatment. J Hepatol. 1992:in press.
9. Cassani F, Ballardini G, Fusconi M, Lenzi M, Volta U, Zauli D, Bianchi FB. Anti-HCV antibodies detected by ELISA in autoimmune and cryptogenic chronic liver diseases. J Hepatol. 1991;12:269–70.
10. Cassani F, Muratori L, Manotti P, Lenzi M, Fusconi M, Ballardini G, Selleri L, Volta U, Zauli D, Miniero R, Bianchi FB. Serum autoantibodies and the diagnosis of type-1 autoimmune hepatitis in Italy: a reappraisal in the light of hepatitis C virus infection. Gut. 1992;33:1260–3.
11. Magrin S, Craxì A, Fabiano C, Almasio P, Palazzo U, Pinzello GB, Provenzano G, Pagliaro L, Choo QL, Kuo G, Polito A, Han J, Houghton M. Hepatitis C virus replication in 'autoimmune' chronic hepatitis. J Hepatol. 1991;13:364–7.
12. Lenzi M, Cassani F, Ballardini G, Bianchi FB, Mishiro S, Unoura M, Kaneko S, Kobayashi K. Anti-HCV, anti-GOR, and autoimmunity. Lancet. 1992;339:872–3.

13
Clonal analysis of human lymphocyte-B responses to hepatitis C virus structural and non-structural regions

M. U. MONDELLI and A. CERINO

GENETIC ORGANIZATION OF HEPATITIS C VIRUS

Hepatitis C virus (HCV) is a 9.4 kb, single-stranded, polyadenylated, positive sense RNA virus which causes acute and chronic liver disease and hepatocellular carcinoma[1-6]. The viral genome encodes for a polyprotein of 3010–3011 amino acids which undergoes extensive post-translational processing[1,7,8]. The 5′ untranslated region (UTR) is highly conserved and contains efficient *cis*-acting elements which repress or enhance translation at its 5′ terminus and near its 3′ terminus, respectively[9]. Additional small open reading frames (ORF), upstream from the enhancer element, may also down-regulate translation[9].

Evidence based on hydrophobicity plots and sequence homologies suggests that HCV may be distantly related to pestiviruses and flaviviruses[10]; however, the assignment of definite function to putative polypeptide domains is still under investigation. The structural region is located upstream from the non-structural region and comprises a conserved nucleocapsid protein of 19–22 kDa[7,8,11], and two extensively glycosylated envelope polypeptides, E1 (gp33–35) and E2/NS1 (gp70–72), which, similarly to the core protein, are not secreted as they are tightly bound to the endoplasmic reticulum. Recent studies suggest that the processing of structural polypeptides from the polyprotein precursor requires host signal peptidases[12]. Evidence indicates that substantial sequence heterogeneity exists among virtually all HCV isolates in the aminoterminal region of E2/NS1, suggesting that this subregion of the envelope may be under strong immune selection[13]. The non-structural region includes four proteins with poorly defined functions. NS2 is probably a membrane-anchored protein. The NS3 polypeptide contains a serine protease domain responsible for cleavage of non-structural proteins from the polyprotein precursor[14], similar to the NS3 protein of yellow-fever virus[15]. The function of the NS4 protein is also poorly understood, but it encompasses the subregion originally identified as containing immunodominant antibody-binding sites[2]. Finally, by analogy with Flaviviridae, NS5 is thought to contain the viral replicase[10].

ANTIBODY RESPONSE TO HCV POLYPEPTIDES

Evidence from prospective studies of post-transfusion hepatitis indicates that antibodies to the c100-3 fusion protein, derived from the NS4 region, appear several weeks to months after acute onset[2,4,16] and persist through chronicity, probably reflecting viral replication[17]. Fine specificity studies on anti-NS4 antibodies using synthetic oligopeptides showed the presence of several sequential immunodominant epitopes within 5-1-1, a 42-amino acid fragment of c100-3, and near the C-terminus of c100-3[2,18].

Antibodies to NS3 and nucleocapsid (core) proteins appear significantly earlier than anti-NS4 and have been clearly shown to be useful diagnostic markers of acute HCV infection[19–21]. Moreover, antibodies to the highly conserved core protein may be the only serological marker of exposure to HCV and may persist for several years after recovery[21]. The fine specificity of antinucleoprotein antibodies has been studied in some detail. The available evidence suggests the existence of at least two major epitopes at the aminoterminal end of the nucleoprotein region at positions 5-23 and 39-74[22–24] and probably a minor epitope closer to the C-terminus[23]. Interestingly, weak but significant sequence homology and immunological crossreaction have been found with residues 4–20 of the HCV core protein and residues 15–29 of a host-derived peptide, designated GOR[25,26] providing additional support for the concept that HCV may induce autoimmunity[27].

Unpublished data indicate that, unlike most HCV polypeptides, the fine specificity of the antibody response to the NS3 region cannot be defined with synthetic peptides, suggesting that lymphocyte-B responses to this region are probably directed at conformational epitopes; however, the coordinates of such epitopes are largely unknown.

The NS5 region, which includes the putative viral polymerase, has recently received attention since it may identify some uniquely reactive sera that do not recognize other HCV polypeptides. Indeed, analyses of serial samples from patients with acute hepatitis demonstrated early seroconversion to NS5 region antigens in the absence of other serological markers[28]. In a preliminary survey, antibodies to NS5 were found in 79% of patients with chronic HCV infection compared with 83% of sera reactive with c100-3 (NS4), 90% with c22-3 (core), and 88% with c33c (NS3)[28]. Epitope mapping studies, using molecularly cloned sequences encoding the putative RNA polymerase gene, indicated the existence of major antibody-binding sites in a region 3′, and contiguous with, c100-3 (a.a. 1872-1989) and further downstream in a region thought to be the 5′ portion of the NS5 gene product (a.a. 2097-2428)[29].

Little is known on the significance and specificity of antibodies to the envelope glycoproteins. Preliminary evidence would suggest that both sequential and conformational epitopes are present on the HCV envelope; however, native conformational epitopes, obtained by expressing E1 and E2/NS1 in recombinant vaccinia virus vectors, are more immunogenic than linear epitopes and have been shown to be responsible for early seroconversion during the course of infection[30]. Furthermore, immunization with native envelope glycoproteins was associated with eradication of HCV infection in a chimpanzee, and it has been suggested that anti-E1 may be involved in virus neutralization[31].

The biological significance of antibodies to the various HCV polypeptides, as well as their fine specificities, are largely unknown. In this chapter we describe the isolation and fine characterization of stable EBV-transformed human lymphocyte-B clones which secrete abundant quantities of immunoglobulin specific for the HCV structural and non-structural regions.

PRODUCTION OF HUMAN MONOCLONAL ANTIBODIES TO HCV

Human monoclonal antibodies (hmAb) provide novel ways to probe the lymphocyte B repertoire in health and disease. However, the development of hmAb technology has met with several difficulties due to the instability of the cell lines, the low level of specific antibody secretion, and the poor cloning efficiency, particularly when using lymphoblastoid cells[32,33]. In order to overcome these problems, some investigators have fused human lymphocytes B with human/mouse myeloma heterohybrids; however, in such systems human chromosomes are unstable and may occasionally be deleted. Despite the potential emergence of technical pitfalls, lymphocyte B immortalization with EBV has been extensively used for hmAb production, because of its simplicity and because EBV can bind to and penetrate virtually all lymphocytes B, theoretically allowing exploration of the whole lymphocyte B repertoire.

Over the past few years we have used the traditional EBV transformation technique to generate HCV-specific lymphocyte B clones[34,35]. In an effort to maximize lymphocyte B growth at low cell density, we have employed supplements which significantly improve cell cloning efficiency[34]. Moreover, lymphocyte B clones were shown to be remarkably stable without significant loss of specific antibody secretion after over 2 years in continuous culture.

Peripheral blood mononuclear cells, depleted of lymphocytes T, are usually obtained from patients with histologically documented chronic hepatitis and circulating antibodies to HCV. Following infection with EBV, cells are plated at low cell density in microtitre wells. After several weeks in culture, each well is tested for the presence of specific antibody, and positive microcultures are then repeatedly cloned until stable antigen-specific cell lines are identified. The following criteria are considered as indicative of monoclonality: (1) secretion of only one immunoglobulin H and L chain; (2) stability of antibody secretion as a function of time in culture; (3) typically restricted banding pattern on isoelectrofocusing (Fig. 1); (4) 100% of wells secreting specific antibody following at least two subcloning cycles.

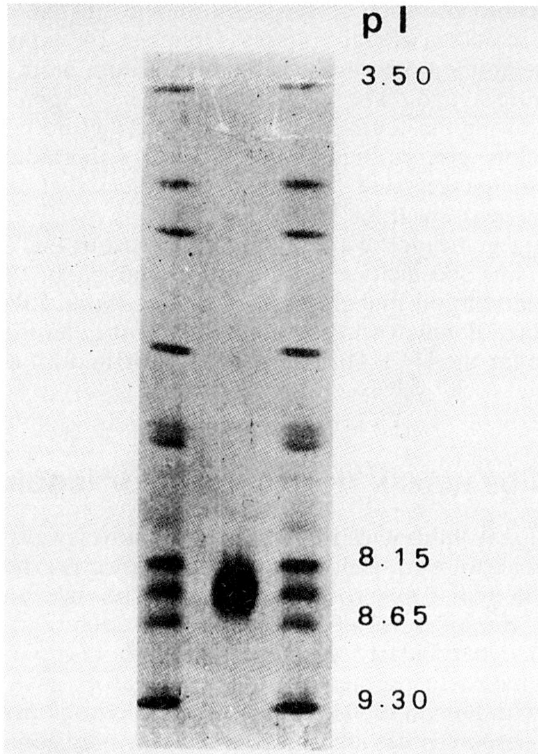

Fig. 1 Isoelectrofocusing of mAb D10 shown in the central lane. Side lanes indicate pI standards

HUMAN MONOCLONAL ANTIBODIES TO HCV NON-STRUCTURAL PROTEINS

We initially concentrated on the HCV NS4 region. Four lymphocyte B lines, from a total of 1152 cultures, secreted significant levels of 5-1-1/c100-3 specific antibodies, as assessed by ELISA and recombinant immunoblot assay, and were stable for a time sufficient to allow further characterization. Two of these lines generated several stable lymphocyte B clones that fulfilled the criteria established for monoclonality, and that still secrete abundant quantities of NS4-specific immunoglobulin after 30 months of continuous culture. Analysis of the IgG H and L chains secreted by such clones revealed the presence of IgG1(κ) only.

The fine specificity of the NS4-specific hmAb was determined using five synthetic oligopeptides (20-mers) overlapping by 14 amino acid residues and covering virtually all the 5-1-1 fragment of the c100-3 protein. Peptide coordinates, determined according to the HCV prototype sequence[7], were as follows: peptide 1: 1688–1707; peptide 2: 1694–1713; peptide 3: 1700–1719; peptide 4: 1706–1725; peptide 5: 1712–1731. To confirm the results obtained in the direct binding assay, we performed competitive inhibition

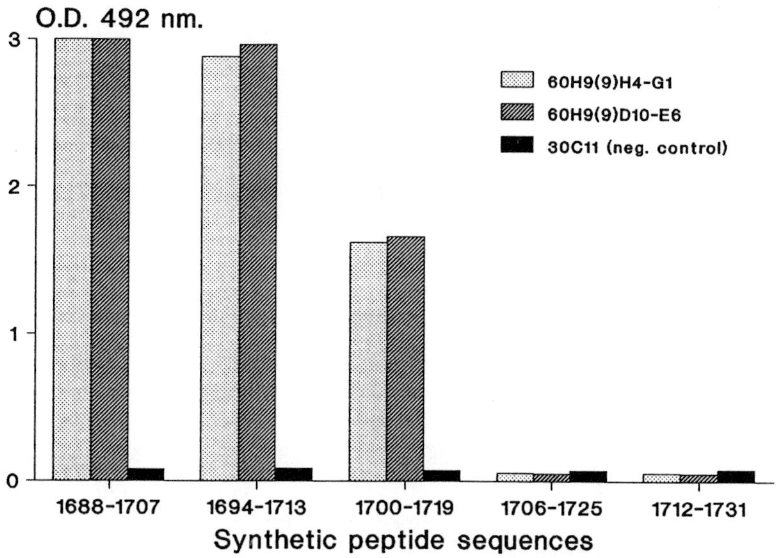

Fig. 2 Fine specificity of IgG secreted by lymphocyte B clones D10 and H4. Five overlapping peptides covering the 5-1-1 region were utilized in an ELISA as described in Materials and Methods. 30C11 is a supernatant from an irrelevant EBV-transformed B cell line non-secreting anti-NS4 antibodies

studies in which increasing concentrations of the same soluble peptides employed for epitope mapping were incubated in solution with constant concentration of human mAb anti-NS4 prior to transfer to ELISA plates coated with the recombinant fusion protein c100-3[35]. hmAb D10 and H4 displayed high-affinity binding to peptides 1 and 2 and, to a lesser extent, peptide 3, whereas no significant binding to peptides 4 and 5 was documented (Fig. 2). These results indicate that antibodies secreted by the NS4-specific lymphocyte-B cloned lines recognize a sequential epitope located at the aminoterminal end of the 5-1-1 fragment. The minimal sequence is conceivably comprised within residues 1700–1705 (VLYREF) of the HCV prototype-deduced amino acid sequence shared by peptides 1, 2 and 3. These findings are further supported by experiments showing complete inhibition of binding of human mAb anti-NS4 to solid-phase c100-3 by soluble peptides 1 and 2, partial inhibition by peptide 3 at over 200-fold molar excess, and no effect of peptides 4 and 5 (data not shown). The dissociation constant (K_d) for peptide 1, calculated according to a modified Friguet's technique[19], was found to be 3.3×10^{-8} mol/l, consistent with that of an IgG. Recently we were able to confirm the fine specificity data reported above by pepscan analysis using pin-bound 12-mers overlapping by 11 amino acid residues. As shown in Fig. 3, significantly raised absorbance values were noted when mAb D10 was allowed to bind to peptides 128–132 which contain the minimal hexamer VLYREF recognized by our mAb, further confirming the sequential nature of the epitope. Comparative experiments indicated that the recognition pattern of the majority of patients' sera was indeed remarkably

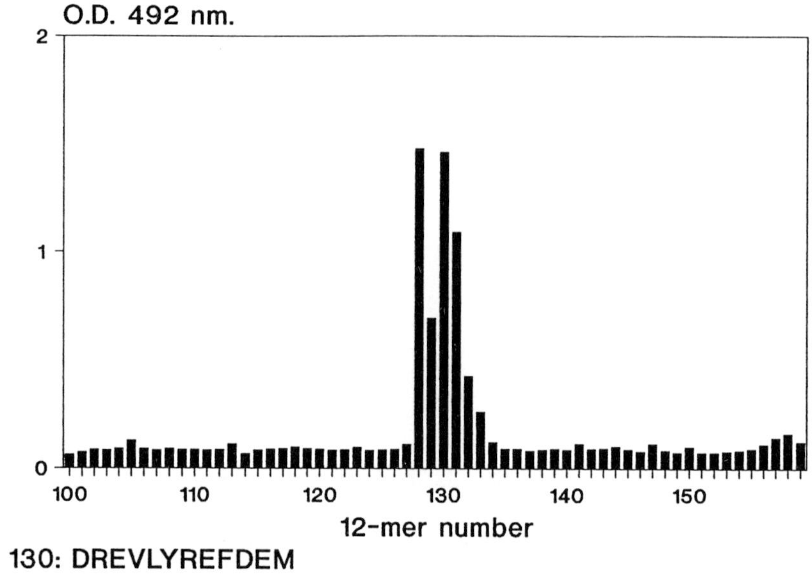

Fig. 3 Fine specificity of human mAb D10 determined by pepscan analysis. The mAb was tested on pin-bound 12-mers, scaled by one amino acid residue, covering the entire NS4 region sequence. Shown here is the critical region recognized by the mAb. 12-mer 130, DREVLYREFDEM, contains the minimal epitope defined by initial experiments using 20-mers

similar to that of human mAb D10 and H4, suggesting that the N-terminal sequence of 5-1-1 is immunodominant with respect to the NS4 region of HCV. Analysis of the hydrophilicity plot of that region revealed an extensive hydrophilic domain spanning from residues 1699 to 1714. These findings, indicating hydrophilic residues within 5-1-1 that are likely to be exposed on a helix, are consistent with our data showing a major sequential lymphocyte B epitope at the aminoterminus of 5-1-1.

Recently we were able to generate another IgG1(κ) hmAb specific for the NS3 non-structural protein; however, its fine specificity is presently under investigation (data not shown).

A HUMAN MONOCLONAL ANTIBODY SPECIFIC FOR THE HCV NUCLEOPROTEIN

In a further set of experiments we elected to analyse the human antibody response to the HCV nucleoprotein at the clonal level. Following transformation of patients' mononuclear cells with EBV, several oligoclonal lymphocyte B lines were obtained which secreted antibodies reactive in commercial HCV II generation assays. However, of the initial 23 short-term lines, only two were stable enough to allow further characterization, and one was found to meet the stringent criteria for monoclonality. The clone, designated B12.F8, secreted abundant quantities of IgG1(κ) which, in addition to second-generation antigens, recognized a highly purified recombinant core protein

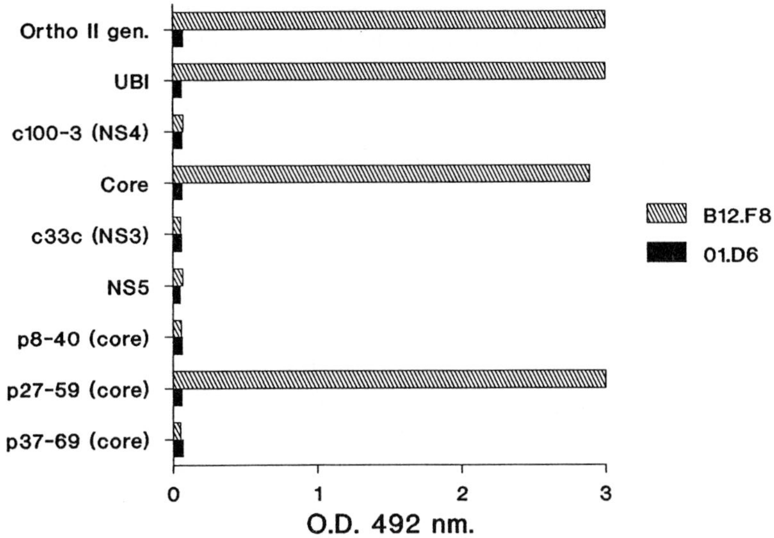

Fig. 4 Broad and fine antigen specificity of hmAb B12.F8. In addition to the various recombinant proteins listed in the graph, binding to synthetic core oligopeptides was also tested to determine the specific epitope recognized by the hmAb. 0.1D6 is an irrelevant EBV-transformed B-cell line

preparation (c22-3), but failed to recognize recombinant c33c (NS3), c100-3 (NS4) and part of NS5 (Fig. 4). Several attempts were made to determine the fine specificity of hmAb B12.F8. Initially, pepscan analysis using pin-bound 12-mers covering the entire HCV nucleoprotein region revealed weakly increased optical density values above background around a.a. 33–35 (not shown). The most reproducible results, however, were obtained with relatively long overlapping synthetic 33-mers, covering the immunoreactive region of the HCV nucleoprotein (residues 8–69 of the HCV prototype sequence). As shown in Fig. 4, hmAb B12.F8 displayed high-affinity binding (K_d: 4.5×10^{-7} mol/l) to the sequence 27–59. Moreover, the same peptide exerted a highly significant dose-dependent inhibition of hmAb B12.F8 binding to recombinant core protein bound to the solid phase, attesting to the specificity of the reaction (data not shown).

We next determined whether sera from patients with HCV infection containing antibodies to the core protein also recognized the synthetic 33-mers employed to analyse the fine specificity of hmAb B12.F8. All sera examined showed significant binding to peptides 8–40 and 27–59, whereas only about two-thirds of the sera showed low-titre binding to 37–69. These findings suggest that hmAb B12.F8 recognizes a major epitope within the aminoterminal region of the HCV nucleoprotein, which may have important biological implications.

CONCLUSIONS AND OUTLOOK

Applications of hmAb technology in the diagnosis and treatment of infectious diseases, such as hepatitis C, are manifold, particularly since the epitopes recognized by human lymphocytes B may be different from those recognized by murine cells. Thus, hmAb can be used to purify biologically important native polypeptides for use as immunogens, or for passive immunotherapy or enhancement of the response to vaccines using preformed Ag/mAb complexes. Other uses include the delivery of antiviral drugs as conjugates to selected cells expressing defined ligands for the antibody and the production of antiidiotypes which could be used either as antigens in diagnostic assays or as alternative vaccines. It is also anticipated that the use of HCV-specific hmAb will help to elucidate the biology and function of the different HCV proteins in the virus life cycle, as well as their possible role in the pathogenesis of HCV-induced hepatocellular injury.

Acknowledgements

We thank Dr W. Habets, Organon Teknika, Boxtel, The Netherlands, for performing pepscan analysis of human monoclonal antibodies, and Drs C. Rosa and F. Bonelli, Sorin Biomedica, Saluggia, Italy, for providing synthetic peptides derived from the NS4 and core regions.

References

1. Choo Q-L, Kuo G, Weiner AJ *et al.* Isolation of a cDNA clone derived from a blood-borne non-A, non-B hepatitis genome. Science. 1989;244:359–62.
2. Kuo G, Choo Q-L, Alter HJ *et al.* An assay for circulating antibodies to a major etiologic virus of human non-A, non-B hepatitis. Science. 1989;244:362–4.
3. Kubo Y, Takeuchi K, Boonmar S *et al.* A cDNA fragment of hepatitis C virus isolated from an implicated donor of posttransfusion non-A, non-B hepatitis in Japan. Nucl Acids Res. 1989;17:10367–72.
4. Alter HJ, Purcell RH, Shih JH *et al.* Detection of antibodies to hepatitis C virus in prospectively followed transfusion recipients with acute and chronic non-A, non-B hepatitis. N Engl J Med. 1989;321:1494–500.
5. Colombo M, Choo Q-L, Del Ninno E *et al.* Prevalence of antibodies to hepatitis C virus in Italian patients with hepatocellular carcinoma. Lancet. 1989;2:1006–8.
6. Mondelli MU, Colombo M. The emerging picture of hepatitis C. Dig Dis. 1991;9:245–52.
7. Houghton M, Choo Q-L, Kuo G. Eur Patent Appl. 88,310,922.5 and Publ. no. 318,216.
8. Takamizawa A, Mori C, Fuke I *et al.* Structure and organization of the hepatitis C virus genome isolated from human carriers. J Virol. 1991;65:1105–13.
9. Yoo BJ, Shyamala V, Spaete RR *et al.* Regulation of gene expression by the 5′ end and 3′ regions of hepatitis C viral RNA. Abstract presented at the 1st annual meeting on Hepatitis C Virus and Related Viruses, Molecular Virology and Pathogenesis. Venice, July 1992. Proceedings, p. 26.
10. Miller RH, Purcell RH. Hepatitis C virus shares amino acids sequence similarity with pestiviruses and flaviviruses as well as members of plant virus supergroups. Proc Natl Acad Sci USA. 1990;87:2057–61.
11. Takeuchi K, Kubo Y, Boonmar S *et al.* The putative nucleocapsid and envelope protein genes of hepatitis C virus determined by comparison of the nucleotide sequences of two isolates derived from an experimentally infected chimpanzee and healthy human carriers. J Gen Virol. 1990;71:3027–33.

12. Hijikata M, Kato N, Ootsuyama Y *et al.* Gene mapping of the putative structural region of the hepatitis C virus genome by *in vitro* processing analysis. Proc Natl Acad Sci USA. 1991;88:5547–51.
13. Weiner AJ, Brauer MJ, Rosenblatt J *et al.* Variable and hypervariable domains are found in the regions of HCV corresponding to the Flavivirus envelope and NS1 proteins and the Pestivirus envelope glycoproteins. Virology. 1991;180:842–8.
14. Choo Q-L, Lee C, Eckart M *et al.* The NS3 domain of HCV encodes a serine protease responsible for cleavage of nonstructural proteins from the polyprotein precursor. Abstract presented at the 1st annual meeting on Hepatitis C Virus and Related Viruses, Molecular Virology and Pathogenesis. Venice, July 1992. Proceedings, p. 25.
15. Chambers TJ, Weir RC, Grakoui A *et al.* Evidence that the N-terminal domain of nonstructural protein NS3 from yellow fever virus is a serine protease responsible for site-specific cleavages in the viral polyprotein. Proc Natl Acad Sci USA. 1990;87:8898–902.
16. Esteban JI, Gonzalez A, Hernadez JM *et al.* Evaluation of antibodies to hepatitis C virus in a study of transfusion-associated hepatitis. N Engl J Med. 1990;323:1107–12.
17. Weiner AJ, Kuo G, Bradley DW *et al.* Detection of hepatitis C viral sequences in non-A, non-B hepatitis. Lancet. 1990;335:1–3.
18. Dreesman GR, Frenzel GD, Burk KH *et al.* Identification of an immunodominant HCV epitope and its application for immunoassays. Abstract presented at the 1st annual meeting on Hepatitis C Virus and Related Viruses, Molecular Virology and Pathogenesis. Venice, July 1992. Proceedings, p. 78.
19. Hosein B, Fang CT, Popowsky MA *et al.* Improved serodiagnosis of hepatitis C virus infection with synthetic peptide antigen from capsid protein. Proc Natl Acad Sci USA. 1991;88:3647–51.
20. Harada S, Watanabe Y, Takeuchi K *et al.* Expression of processed core protein of hepatitis C virus in mammalian cells. J Virol. 1991;65:3015–21.
21. van der Poel CL, Cuypers HTM, Reesink HW *et al.* Confirmation of hepatitis C virus infection by new four-antigen recombinant immunoblot assay. Lancet. 1991;337:317–19.
22. Okamoto H, Munekata E, Tsuda F *et al.* Enzyme-linked immunosorbent assay for antibodies against the capsid protein of hepatitis C virus with a synthetic oligopeptide. Jpn J Exp Med. 1990;60:223–33.
23. Nasoff MS, Zebedee SL, Inchauspe G *et al.* Identification of an immunodominant epitope within the capsid protein of hepatitis C virus. Proc Natl Acad Sci USA. 1991;88:5462–6.
24. Okamoto H, Tsuda F, Machida A *et al.* Antibodies against synthetic oligopeptides deduced from the putative core gene for the diagnosis of hepatitis C virus infection. Hepatology. 1992;15:180–6.
25. Mishiro S, Hoshi Y, Takeda K *et al.* Non-A, non-B hepatitis specific antibodies directed at host-derived epitope: implication for an autoimmune process. Lancet. 1990;336:1400–3.
26. Mishiro S, Takeda K, Hoshi Y *et al.* An autoantibody cross-reactive to hepatitis C virus core and a host nuclear antigen. Autoimmunity. 1991;10:269–73.
27. Hosein B, Fang X, Wang C-Y. Anti-HCV, anti-GOR, and autoimmunity. Lancet. 1992;339:871.
28. Lesniewski RR, Desai SM, Johnson RG *et al.* Enhanced detection of hepatitis C virus (HCV) infection using antigens from the putative polymerase (NS5) gene product. Abstract presented at the 1st annual meeting on Hepatitis C Virus and Related Viruses, Molecular Virology and Pathogenesis. Venice, July 1992. Proceedings, p. 76.
29. Desai SM, Dailey SH, Casey JM *et al.* Antigenic epitopes within NS5 region of HCV. Abstract presented at the 1st annual meeting on Hepatitis C Virus and Related Viruses, Molecular Virology and Pathogenesis. Venice, July 1992. Proceedings, p. 77.
30. Chien DY, Choo Q-L, Spaete D *et al.* Diagnosis of hepatitis C virus (HCV) infection using the native structure antigens from viral envelope regions. Abstract presented at the 1st annual meeting on Hepatitis C Virus and Related Viruses, Molecular Virology and Pathogenesis. Venice, July 1992. Proceedings, p. 75.
31. Houghton M, Choo Q-L, Weiner AJ *et al.* Vaccine approaches to HCV. Abstract presented at the 1st annual meeting on Hepatitis C Virus and Related Viruses, Molecular Virology and Pathogenesis. Venice, July 1992. Proceedings, p. 144.
32. James K, Bell GT. Human monoclonal antibody production. Current status and future prospects. J Immunol Methods. 1987;100:5–40.

33. Pistillo MP, Mazzoleni O, Tanigaki N *et al.* Human anti-HLA monoclonal antibodies: production, characterization and applications. Hum Immunol. 1988;21:265–78.
34. Cerino A, Mondelli MU. Identification of an immunodominant B cell epitope on the hepatitis C virus nonstructural region defined by human monoclonal antibodies. J Immunol. 1991;147:2692–6.
35. de Lalla C, Cerino A, Rosa C *et al.* Physicochemical properties of a human monoclonal antibody specific for the NS4 region of hepatitis C virus. J Hepatol. 1993: in press.

Section IV
Cytokines in the Treatment of Virus-induced Liver Diseases

14
Actions of cytokines on immune response and virus replication – an overview

M. PETERS

Cytokines are small proteins which act locally at the site of inflammation or immune responses. Interferons (IFN) are small pleiotropic molecules which have antiproliferative, antiviral and immunomodulatory actions[1]. IFN comprises three types: α, β and γ. While all IFNs have similar actions the relative importance of each differs in that IFN-γ is predominantly immunomodulatory and IFN-α/β predominantly antiviral and antiproliferative.

IFN-α is a group of proteins encoded on the short arm of chromosome 9. There are at least 23 IFN-α genes, six of which are pseudogenes. The remainder have active protein products, some of which may differ in their relative level of effects e.g. IFN-α-J has no natural killer (NK) activity but normal antiproliferative activity. Presently available recombinant IFNs are the products of one gene or a consensus sequence. It may be that different genes do have subtle but distinct effects that impact on response to therapy. IFN-γ is the product of a single gene on the long arm of chromosome 12.

IFN-α and IFN-β share the same single-chain receptor encoded on chromosome 21[2]. IFN-γ receptor is encoded on chromosome 6 and requires an accessory molecule encoded on chromosome 21. It may be that IFN-α and IFN-β receptors also have accessory molecules which increase affinity and explain the observed differences between receptor binding of IFN-α and IFN-β.

Once IFN-α/β is bound to its receptor a series of novel events occur which lead to transcription of IFN-responsive genes (IRG) as early as 15 min[3]. Recent data have shown that IFN signalling occurs through phosphorylation and subsequent binding of three cytoplasmic proteins (ISGF3α) which translocate to the nucleus and when associated with another DNA binding protein (ISGFγ) bind to the interferon-stimulated response element (ISRE). These proteins are called IFN-stimulated gene factors (ISGFs)[3]. ISGF1 is constitutively expressed. ISGF2 is induced by IFN-α and IFN-γ 90 min after receptor–ligand interaction, and depends on protein synthesis. ISGF3 is induced by IFN-α and IFN-β after 5 min and is independent of protein synthesis. ISGF3 contains three ISGFα proteins, 113, 91, and 84 kDa, all of which have been cloned[3]. These proteins contain SH2 (src-like) domains which often are associated with tyrosine kinases. Studies of mutant cell lines that are unresponsive to IFN[5] revealed that these lines lacked a tyrosine kinase, tyk2. Cell fractionation studies suggested that the kinase was associated with the membrane fraction, presumably interacting with the receptor[6]. Studies of IFN-γ revealed that receptor–ligand interaction leads to phosphorylation of the 91 kDa ISGF3α, suggesting that IFN-γ signalling uses a similar but not identical mechanism[3,4].

IFN-stimulated response elements (ISRE) are consensus sequences located in the 5′ regulatory regions of IFN-responsive genes[7]. ISGF3 binds to this region via the 40 kDa ISGFγ DNA binding protein. Transcription of certain genes occurs within 15 min of receptor–ligand binding and peaks at 2 h. IFN-γ has a closely associated ISRE sequence at an overlapping but distinct site to which IFN-γ-associated transcriptional factor (GAF) binds[3]. The roles of ISGF1 and ISGF2 are less clear. Many genes are transcriptionally activated by IFNs including 2′5′oligoA synthetase (2′5′OAS), major histocompatibility gene class I and II (the latter by IFN-γ only); β_2-microglobulin and protein kinases. IFN induces a dsRNA-phosphokinase (PK), which is a serine/threonine specific PK. This PK phosphorylates the α-subunit of eIF-2, a eukaryotic translation initiation factor. This phosphorylation blocks further translation, thereby blocking viral replication. PK mutants have been created which show malignant transformation, suggesting that dsRNA PK is critical for both antiviral and antiproliferative effects of IFN[8].

IFN cannot be discussed in isolation without consideration of other cytokines. Cell–cell interaction may be cognate with contact or may be cytokine-mediated. The role of cytokines includes assisting cell–cell communication, response amplification and response regulation[9]. Cytokines are small polypeptides which are transiently produced and have a relatively short duration of action at local sites. There is great overlap between different cytokines in terms of effects and interplay between cytokines, which are both positive and negative[9]. While many cytokines are produced by many cells, lymphocytes and monocytes predominate. T lymphocytes produce many of the cytokines and can be separated into TH1 and TH2 cell types which drive the immune response differently. TH1 cells secrete IL-2, IFN-γ and TNF, and are involved in macrophage activation and delayed-type hypersensitivity. TH2 cells secrete IL-4, IL-5, IL-6 and IL-10, and predominate in IgE and IgA responses. The main T cell growth factor is IL-2, although other cytokines can promote T cell growth. The cytokine cascade involves macrophage activation with subsequent immune stimulation followed by regulation (depending on the relative proportion of cytokines produced) and induction of inflammation by proinflammatory cytokines, IL-1, IL-6 and TNF. Many of these cytokines interact with IFNs. TNF induces or enhances production of IL-1, IL-6, GM-CSF and IL-2 receptor expression. TNF has both inflammatory and acute-phase reactant responses.

Viral interaction with cytokines can aid or inhibit host defences[10]. Some viruses produce proteins which can (1) mimic cytokines, such as viral IL-10, a product of Epstein–Barr virus or (2) mimic cytokine receptors, such as Shope fibroma virus which encodes a soluble form of TNF receptor. Other viruses can inhibit transcriptional activation. Examples include the adenovirus type 5 E1A oncogene, which decreases the level of ISGFs and the terminal protein of the hepatitis B virus polymerase gene which inhibit the response to IFN by lack of transcriptional activation. HSV and SV40 make non-functional 2′5′OAS, thus evading IFN effects. Adenovirus inhibits protein kinase activity.

Cellular and viral responses to IFNs need to be assessed in the light of signalling mechanisms and interactions between various cytokines induced both in the primary response in host defence and then during antigen-specific responses. Viruses have adapted mechanisms for evasion of the host's immune system by mimicking host proteins or altering them. Synergism between cytokines may prove of value in recovering an antiviral effect.

References

1. Peters M. Mechanisms of action of interferons. Semin Liver Dis. 1989;9:235–9.
2. Sen GC, Lengyel P. The interferon system: a bird's eye view of its biochemistry. J Biol Chem. 1992;267:5017–20.
3. Schindler C, Shuai K, Prezioso VR, Darnell JE, Jr. Interferon-dependent tyrosine phosphorylation of a latent cytoplasmic transcription factor. Science. 1992;257:809–12.
4. Lew DJ, Decker T, Darnell JE Jr. Alpha interferon and gamma interferon stimulate transcription of a single gene through different signal transduction pathways. Mol Cell Biol. 1989;9:5404–11.
5. Velazquez L, Fellous M, Stark GR, Pellgrini S. A protein tyrosine kinase in the interferon alpha/beta signalling pathway. Cell. 1992;70:313–22.
6. David M, Larner AC. Activation of transcription factors by interferon-alpha in a cell-free system. Science. 1992;257:813–15.
7. Williams BRG. Transcriptional regulation of interferon-stimulated genes. Biochemistry. 1991;200:1–11.
8. Koromilas AE, Roy S, Barber GN, Katze MG, Sonenberg N. Malignant transformation by a mutant of the IFN-inducible dsRNA-dependent protein kinase. Science. 1992;257: 1685–9.
9. Screiber RD. Cytokines: structure, function and their role in immune response amplification. In: Schwartz B, ed. Immunology. Kalamazoo, MI: The Upjohn Co. 1991;84–97.
10. Taylor JL, Grossberg SE. Recent progress in interferon research: molecular mechanisms of regulation, action, and virus circumvention. Virus Res. 1990;15:1–26.

15
Innovative therapies for chronic hepatitis B

J. H. HOOFNAGLE

INTRODUCTION

Hepatitis B is an important cause of morbidity and mortality of acute and chronic liver disease and is ranked as the ninth most common cause of death worldwide[1]. In the United States, chronic hepatitis B virus (HBV) infection affects approximately 1 million persons and accounts for approximately 10% of cases of chronic liver disease and cirrhosis. Of the more than 2500 liver transplants performed yearly in the United States, about 6% are done on patients with end-stage liver disease due to hepatitis B[2].

Until recently there have been no specific therapies of proven benefit for chronic hepatitis B. In the past few years a series of randomized controlled trials have demonstrated that interferon-α (IFN-α) is effective in inducing remissions in disease activity in 25–40% of patients with chronic hepatitis B[3–6]. These remissions are characterized by a loss of hepatitis B virus (HBV) DNA and hepatitis B e antigen from serum, followed by a fall of serum aminotransferases into the normal range and improvement in liver biopsy histology. Remissions in disease induced by interferon have been found to be sustained and often accompanied, many years later, by a loss of hepatitis B surface antigen (HBsAg) from serum and development of antibody (anti-HBs)[7]. Thus, IFN-α therapy in doses of 5–10 million units given three times weekly for 4–6 months is now the standard, accepted treatment for chronic hepatitis B.

IFN-α, however, is far from being a completely satisfactory therapy for chronic hepatitis B. Less than 50% of patients respond to a course of therapy, and many subjects are not eligible for treatment, such as those on immunosuppressive therapy, who have decompensated cirrhosis or who are inactive carriers of HBsAg. Furthermore, IFN-α has to be given parenterally for up to 6 months and has many side-effects, some of which are severe and even life-threatening[8]. Finally, therapy with interferon is expensive. Obviously, more effective, better tolerated and less expensive therapies are needed for this important and serious form of liver disease.

INNOVATIVE THERAPIES FOR CHRONIC HEPATITIS B

New approaches to therapy of chronic hepatitis B fall into two categories: antiviral and immunomodulatory agents. This duality of approach reflects the duality of the pathogenesis of chronic hepatitis B[9]. Thus, HBV is a hepatotrophic virus, but most evidence indicates that HBV is not directly cytopathic. Instead, the hepatocellular injury in hepatitis B appears to be due to the host immune response to the virus or viral products.

NEW ANTIVIRAL AGENTS FOR CHRONIC HEPATITIS B

Two recent factors have greatly stimulated research into antiviral therapy of chronic hepatitis B. First has been the world-wide search for anti-retroviral agents that might have activity against HIV, a virus similar to HBV[10]. Second has been the development of cell culture systems (such as primary hepatocytes and 2.2.15 cells)[11–17] as well as animal models of HBV replication (such as woodchuck and duck hepatitis B virus)[18–25]. These model systems have allowed for efficient screening of antiviral compounds for activity against HBV. As a result a great number of antiviral agents have been identified that show promise and deserve evaluation as therapy of chronic hepatitis B (Table 1). Several of these agents deserve discussion.

Table 1 Antiviral agents in chronic hepatitis B

Adenine arabinoside (Ara-A)
Adenine arabinoside monophosphate (Ara-AMP)
Acyclovir
Deoxyacyclovir
Ganciclovir
Suramin
Foscarnet
Dideoxynucleosides (DDI, DDA, DDC, DDG)
Ribavirin
Fluoro-iodo-arabinofurasyl uracil (FIAU)
3-Thiacytidine (3TC)
Anti-sense oligonucleotides
Ribozymes

Adenine arabinoside (Ara-A) and *adenine arabinoside monophosphate* (Ara-AMP) are nucleoside (adenine) derivatives with potent activity against HBV and HBV-like agents *in vitro* and *in vivo*[16,17,20,24,25]. In pilot studies in humans, Ara-A was found to lead to a rapid, marked decrease in HBV levels in serum and liver[26]. Subsequently, a phosphorylated derivative Ara-AMP was developed that had the advantage that it was more soluble and could be given by intramuscular injection twice a day rather than requiring continuous intravenous infusion. The promise of Ara-AMP as a definitive therapy led to several randomized controlled trials in humans. In three studies from the United States, Ara-AMP did not lead to an increased rate of HBV DNA clearance or disease remission when given for up to 4 weeks[27–29]. Furthermore, the duration of treatment was limited because of the frequency of neuromuscular toxicity that arose after 3–4 weeks of treatment. In contrast, three studies from Europe suggested that Ara-AMP led to remissions in disease in 25–50% of patients and was reasonably well tolerated[30–32]. These discrepancies remain unexplained. Thus, Ara-AMP had marked inhibitory activity against HBV and some evidence of long-term benefit in chronic hepatitis B; however, toxicity limits the duration of therapy with Ara-AMP and short courses do not appear to be adequate for an acceptable rate of long-term responses.

Recently, derivatives of Ara-AMP that are rapidly taken up by the liver (lactosaminated albumin conjugated Ara-AMP) have been developed and shown to retain the potency of the original drug in animal model systems[33]. These liver-targeted nucleoside analogues have the potential of being more potent and less toxic than the native compounds. Preliminary studies suggest that these derivatives are active against HBV in humans[34]. Further, controlled trials of these agents are needed.

Acyclovir, *deoxyacyclovir* and *ganciclovir* are nucleoside analogues with potent activity against several herpesviruses; all three agents have also demonstrated some activity against HBV-like agents in cell culture or animal model systems[14,15,24,25,35]. Unfortunately, acyclovir and ganciclovir require parenteral (intravenous) administration to achieve the serum concentrations needed to inhibit HBV. The need for intravenous infusion has limited the duration of treatment with these agents[36–38]. Deoxyacyclovir has better oral absorption than acyclovir, but absorption is not entirely reliable. In clinical studies, neither short courses of intravenous acyclovir nor longer courses of oral formulations have been effective in lowering HBV DNA levels or inducing long-term responses in chronic hepatitis B[36,38].

Suramin is a novel antiviral agent that has been extensively evaluated in HIV infection. In an animal model, suramin appeared to have marked activity against HBV replication[18,21]. However, in small clinical trials, suramin was found to be too toxic and to have little effect on human HBV[39]. The discrepancy between results obtained in animal models and in human disease is a factor that has to be weighed in all studies of new agents.

Foscarnet (phosphonoformate) is a antiviral agent that inhibits HBV DNA polymerase activity *in vitro*[40], but that was found to be only poorly effective in inhibiting HBV DNA levels in animal model systems[19,41]. In a small trial in humans, foscarnet given intravenously for 7–14 days led to only a modest, transient decrease in serum HBV DNA levels; long-term responses did not occur with the short courses of treatment[42]. The need to administer foscarnet by intravenous infusion and its modest effects on HBV DNA limit its usefulness for treatment of chronic hepatitis B.

The *dideoxynucleosides* are antiviral agents that have been extensively evaluated against HIV[10]. In animal models, dideoxyadenine (DDA), dideoxycytodine (DDC), dideoxyguanosine (DDG) and dideoxyinosine (DDI) all had potent inhibitory activity against HBV-like viruses[22,23]. The activity against HBV replication was less impressive and less reliable in cell culture systems[13,15,17]. However, the oral availability of these compounds and their relative lack of toxicity which were documented in studies of patients with AIDS encouraged trials in chronic hepatitis B. In a pilot, dose-escalating study, however, DDI demonstrated no appreciable inhibitory activity against serum HBV DNA levels in humans, and prolonged therapy did not induce long-term responses[43]. The discrepancies between the results obtained in the duck hepatitis B virus model and in humans suggest that there are important species differences in these related viruses. Other dideoxynucleosides with greater activity against the human HBV *in vitro* have been identified, such as DDG[17], the carbocyclic analogue of deoxyguanosine (2′CDG)[13], and 2′,6′-diamino-purine-2′,3′-dideoxyriboside (DDDAPR)[15]; these compounds deserve further evaluation.

Ribavirin is a purine nucleoside analogue that has been shown to be effective in treating respiratory syncytial virus infections in children. The relative safety of ribavirin and its excellent oral absorption prompted a pilot study of three different doses of ribavirin given for 6 months in 18 patients with chronic hepatitis B[44]. During treatment, serum levels of HBV DNA decreased slightly (20–25%) and serum aminotransferase activities improved. However, no patients cleared HBV DNA and there were no obvious long-term beneficial effects of treatment. These results indicate that ribavirin is not effective in chronic hepatitis B as a single agent, but may play a role in combination with other agents.

Fluoro-iodo-arabinofurasyl-uracil (*FIAU*) is one of a family of fluorinated nucleoside analogues developed originally for their activity against herpesviruses which were subsequently shown to have activity against woodchuck hepatitis B virus[25,34] and against human HBV in cell culture systems[17]. Concerns over toxicity have limited human trials of these agents. Among these fluorinated nucleoside analogues, FIAU was found to be relatively non-toxic and well absorbed orally, thus deserving further evaluation in humans. In a pilot study among patients with HIV infection who were coinfected with HBV, FIAU led to a rapid, marked inhibition of HBV DNA and to clearance of virus in some patients despite therapy for only 10 days[45]. Subsequently, a dose-finding study was carried out in patients with chronic hepatitis B who were not infected with HIV[46]. Again, FIAU led to rapid, marked decreases in serum HBV DNA levels in all patients at doses that were well tolerated. Treatment for 1 month led to clearance of HBV in a proportion of patients. Further studies with more prolonged therapy with FIAU are now under way.

3-*Thiacytidine* (3TC) is another nucleoside analogue that was first evaluated extensively in patients with HIV infection. Studies of 3TC among patients with HIV infection demonstrated that the drug was well absorbed orally and was well tolerated even when given for a prolonged period. In cell culture systems, 3TC was found to have a marked inhibitory effect on replication of HBV[47]. Analysis of preliminary results of trials of 3TC in patients with HIV infection identified a few patients who were also infected with HBV. In these patients, 3TC therapy led to a marked decrease in serum HBV DNA levels. These results have led to a pilot study of several doses of 3TC in patients with chronic hepatitis B without HIV infection, which is currently under way in Europe and North America.

Molecular techniques offer more innovative approaches to antiviral therapy of chronic hepatitis B, especially the techniques of gene transfer and modification of RNA processing to inhibit HBV replication. Thus, cell culture systems have been used to demonstrate that *antisense oligonucleotides* delivered into hepatocytes harbouring HBV DNA can inhibit viral replication[48]. Furthermore, *in vitro* systems have shown that *ribozymes* can be designed to target sites within HBV RNA which cleave the pregenome of the virus and inhibit replication[49]. These new techniques are not immediately practical to treat humans, but they do provide a direction for future work in designing safe and effective treatments for this disease.

Thus, many antiviral agents have shown promise in cell culture or animal model systems. In several situations, however, the activity detected *in vitro* was not detectable *in vivo*; in other situations the activity detected against HBV-like agents in animal models was not detected against the human HBV or *in vivo* in human trials. In addition, some agents that appeared promising in model systems have been found to be too toxic or too difficult to administer to humans for the prolonged period necessary to treat hepatitis B. However, the continued search for safe and effective agents has provided some promise that an agent will be identified that has marked inhibitory activity against human HBV, and can be administered easily and safely for a prolonged period. Ultimately, these agents may be used alone or in combination with IFN-α.

IMMUNOLOGICAL THERAPY OF CHRONIC HEPATITIS B

Several immunostimulatory or immunomodulatory substances have been evaluated as therapies for chronic hepatitis B (Table 2). The major impedance to these studies are the lack of understanding of the immunological response to hepatitis B and the paucity of agents that effectively stimulate immunological responses.

Table 2 Immunomodulatory agents in chronic hepatitis B

Levamisole
Phyllanthus amarus
IFN-α and IFN-β
IFN-γ
Interleukin-2
Thymosin
Granulocyte–macrophage colony stimulating factor
Short course of corticosteroids
Specific immunotherapies (anti-HBs, bone marrow transplantation)

Levamisole is a widely used anti-parasitic agent that has been shown to augment immune responses in animals and humans. Preliminary studies demonstrated promising activity of prolonged therapy with levamisole in inducing long-term remissions in chronic hepatitis[50]. However, when subjected to a randomized, double-blind controlled trial, levamisole therapy was not associated with a higher rate of remission in chronic hepatitis B than occurred spontaneously. Furthermore, there was little information on whether levamisole improved immune responsiveness of HBV or viral antigens.

Plant extracts of *Phyllanthus amarus* were reported to inhibit viral replication in the woodchuck HBV model, and to be very effective in inducing clearance of HBV and hepatitis B surface antigen in humans[51]. This plant extract, which had been used as a herbal medicine in India, was given orally, and evidently had no appreciable side-effects. Its mechanism of action was unclear. In subsequent studies from other investigators, however, extracts of *Phyllanthus amarus* did not demonstrate any activity against HBV *in vitro* or *in vivo*[23]. Furthermore, other controlled trials failed to reproduce the clinical benefits of therapy with this substance[52,53].

The success of *IFN-α* in treating chronic hepatitis B[3–6] led to the evaluation of other cytokines and lymphokines in this disease. The rationale for using various cytokines in treating chronic hepatitis B has been not only their antiviral effects, but perhaps more importantly their immunostimulating or immunomodulating activities. Cytokines that have been evaluated in man include IFN-α, IFN-β and IFN-γ, interleukin 2, thymosin and granulocyte-macrophage colony-stimulating factor (GM-CSF).

IFN-β is similar to IFN-α, sharing 70% homology and a common cell surface receptor. All available evidence suggests that IFN-α and IFN-β have similar antiviral activities against hepatitis B and similar toxicities[54]. It is possible that IFN-α and IFN-β can be used interchangeably. IFN-β may play some role in treatment of patients who become resistant to IFN-α because of the development of neutralizing antibodies.

IFN-γ is both structurally and antigenically quite different from IFN-α and IFN-β, having no nucleotide homology and a separate cell surface receptor. IFN-γ has antiviral activity against HBV; however, it appears to be less potent and more toxic than IFN-α or IFN-β[54]. In prospective studies, IFN-γ treatment led to little inhibition in HBV DNA levels and virtually no long-term responses[55–57]. Furthermore, IFN-α and IFN-γ did not appear to be synergistic in their antiviral activities against HBV[55].

Interleukin-2 (IL-2) has major effects on T cell growth and differentiation, and might be expected to have beneficial activity in patients with chronic hepatitis B. While preliminary trials of IL-2 therapy were promising[58], subsequent studies have not supported any evidence that IL-2 has antiviral activity against HBV or leads to remissions in disease[59]. Furthermore, in cell culture systems, IL-2 has little effect on HBV replication[60]. Furthermore, IL-2 itself has hepatotoxic effects[61].

Thymosin is a general term used for lymphopoietic factors produced by the thymus which modulate immune responses. Several thymic factors including thymosin α_1 have been cloned, sequenced, expressed as peptides in eukaryotic vectors and purified for use in humans[62]. Studies in the chimpanzee model of hepatitis B suggested that thymosin had little effect on hepatitis B[63]. Nevertheless, in the woodchuck hepatitis B virus model, prolonged treatment with thymosin led to a gradual decrease in levels of virus in the serum and liver[25]. In a prospective controlled trial in 12 patients with chronic hepatitis B, thymosin was associated with a high rate of clearance of HBV DNA and remission in disease activity[64]. The mechanism of action of thymosin was unclear; it did not appear to inhibit viral replication directly but may have augmented T cell responses leading to immunological clearance of HBV. These promising results have led to a multicentre, randomized controlled trial of thymosin that is under way in the United States.

Granulocyte–macrophage colony stimulating factor (GM-CSF) and other haematopoietic growth and differentiation factors have been used to stimulate depressed bone marrow responses in patients receiving chemotherapy. Some of these factors have been found to have antiviral effects. Consequently, pilot studies of therapy of chronic hepatitis B were initiated to evaluate the effects of GM-CSF on levels of HBV DNA and disease activity. In preliminary studies some degree of viral inhibition was noted, but there was little long-term effect[65]. Larger controlled trials of more prolonged courses of GM-CSF, perhaps in combination with other agents, are warranted.

Another approach to increasing immunological responsiveness in chronic hepatitis B is to administer a *short course of corticosteroids*[66]. The subsequent withdrawal of corticosteroids typically induces an acute exacerbation of the underlying hepatitis and a decrease in HBV DNA levels[67]. During this exacerbation there seems to be a heightened rebound in the immune response which may make the patient more likely to respond to a subsequent course of IFN-α[66] or Ara-AMP[28]. However, prospective studies have failed to show any benefit of pretreatment with prednisone over and above treatment with IFN-α alone[5]. Furthermore, prednisone treatment can induce severe and even life-threatening exacerbations of disease in chronic hepatitis B.

Specific immunomodulatory therapy, directed at the specific immunological defect that underlies the viral persistence, has great appeal as an approach to therapy of chronic hepatitis B[9]. Despite its appeal, however, this approach is very problematical, largely because the actual immune defect that is responsible for chronic HBV infection is not known. It is not clear what immunocyte (B, CD4, CD8, NK or other cell) is defective in patients with chronic hepatitis B, or what antigenic target (HBsAg, HBcAg, HBeAg) is important in the immune response that accounts for clearance of virus. Recent studies on immunological models of chronic HBV infection suggest that the disease is due to a deficiency in the T cell responses to either HBsAg or the nucleocapsid gene product HBcAg[9]. This concept requires confirmation in humans. Interestingly, therapy with specific immunological factors or cells may be the most reliable means of proving the importance of the immune system in sustaining chronic infection with HBV.

Trials of specific immunotherapy of chronic hepatitis B have not been done. However, there have been intriguing reports of dramatic improvements in chronic hepatitis B which in retrospect can be interpreted as resulting from specific immunotherapy. Thus, case reports of recovery from chronic hepatitis B after immunotherapy with monoclonal antibodies to HBsAg suggest that active production of anti-HBs might help clear chronic HBV infection[68]. This antibody therapy has been carried out largely in patients with hypogammaglobulinaemia. Whether this therapy is applicable to patients with chronic hepatitis B with normal immunoglobulin levels has not been shown, and awaits the large-scale production of human monoclonal antibodies.

Another form of possible immunotherapy has been shown by several recent reports of recovery from chronic hepatitis B after bone marrow transplantation. Several independent groups have reported that a percentage of patients with chronic hepatitis B who undergo bone marrow transplantation for malignant disease (leukaemia or lymphoma) have been found to clear HBsAg and resolve the chronic liver disease after successful engraftment[69–72]. Retrospective analyses demonstrated that, in every case of clearance of HBsAg after bone marrow transplantation, the donor of the marrow has had anti-HBs *and* anti-HBc. Thus, it is likely that B cells that produce antibodies to hepatitis B or alternatively T cells that react with HBV antigens are transferred during engraftment, and that these reconstituted cells account for the clearance of the chronic viral infection. These reports are extremely provocative and lead one to suggest that a modification of bone marrow transplantation might be used to treat patients with chronic hepatitis B. If further analyses of marrow transplantations can dissect out which cell type and which antigenic target is important, rational specific immunotherapies could be designed. Thus, one might isolate antigen-specific cytolytic T cells that react with HBsAg or HBcAg from a patient with chronic hepatitis B, stimulate the cells in culture to proliferate, and then reinfuse the activated T cells. Alternatively, gene transfer techniques might be used to inser the relevant T cell receptor or immunoglobulin gene into cells which can be reinfused. These forms of specific immunotherapy are not practical at present, but represent approaches to therapy of chronic hepatitis B that may be useful in the future.

Thus, at present, therapy for chronic hepatitis B remains problematical. A 4–6-month course of moderately high doses of IFN-α induces a remission in disease in 25–40% of patients, but this therapy is difficult and expensive. New therapies are needed for chronic hepatitis B and can be classified into antiviral therapies and immunomodulatory therapies. The most promising antiviral agents for chronic hepatitis B are some of the newer nucleoside analogues which are well absorbed orally, and appear to be safe enough to allow therapy for a prolonged period (which seems to be necessary in this chronic viral infection). However, immunomodulatory therapies may eventually play a key role in treating this disease, as they are directed against the underlying defect that sustains the chronic infection. Advances in knowledge about immunology and the liver will help in eventually developing a rational, safe and effective therapy for this important liver disease.

References

1. Everhart JE, Hoofnagle JH. Chronic end-stage liver disease. Gastroenterology. 1992;103: in press.
2. Annual Report of the US Scientific Registry for Organ Transplantation and the Organ Procurement and Transplantation Network. UNOS, Richmond, VA, and the Division of Organ Transplantation, Health Resources and Services Administration, Bethesda, MD, 1990.
3. Alexander GJM, Brahm J, Fagan EA *et al.* Loss of HBsAg with interferon therapy in chronic hepatitis B virus infection. Lancet. 1987;1:66–8.
4. Hoofnagle JH, Peters MG, Mullen KD *et al.* Randomized controlled trial of a four-month course of recombinant human alpha interferon in chronic type B hepatitis. Gastroenterology. 1988;95:1318–25.
5. Thomas HC, Duscheiko GM, Lok ASF *et al.* Comparative study of three doses of interferon alpha-2a in chronic active hepatitis B. In: Hollinger FB, Lemon SM, Margolis HS, editors. Viral hepatitis and liver disease. Baltimore: Williams & Wilkins; 1991:641–2.

6. Perrillo RP, Schiff ER, Davis GL *et al.* A randomized controlled trial of interferon alfa-2b alone and after prednisone withdrawal for the treatment of chronic hepatitis B. N Engl J Med. 1990;323:295–301.
7. Korenman J, Baker B, Waggoner J *et al.* Long-term remission in chronic hepatitis B after alpha-interferon therapy. Ann Intern Med. 1991;114:629–34.
8. Renault PF, Hoofnagle JH. Side effects of alpha interferon. Semin Liver Dis. 1989;9: 273–8.
9. Peters M, Vierling J, Gershwin ME *et al.* Immunology and the liver. Hepatology. 1991;13:977–94.
10. Mitsuya H, Broder S. Strategies for antiviral therapy in AIDS. Nature. 1987;325:773–8.
11. Tuttleman JS, Pugh JC, Summers J. *In vitro* experimental infection of primary duck hepatocyte cultures with duck hepatitis B virus. J Virol. 1986;58:17–25.
12. Sells MA, Zelent AZ, Shvartsman M, Acs G. Replicative intermediates of hepatitis B virus in Hep-G2 cells that produce infectious virions. J Virol. 1987;84:1005–9.
13. Price PM, Banergee R, Acs G. Inhibition of the replication of hepatitis B virus by the carbocyclic analogue of 2′deoxyguanosine. Proc Natl Acad Sci USA. 1989;86:8541–4.
14. Ueda K, Tsurimoto T, Nagahata T, Chisaka O, Matsubara K. An *in vitro* system for screening anti-hepatitis B virus drugs. Virology. 1989;169:213–16.
15. Lee B, Luo W, Suzuki S, Robbins MJK, Tyrell DLJ. *In vitro* and *in vivo* comparison of the abilities of purine and pyrmidine 2′3′-dideoxynucleosides to inhibit duck hepadnavirus. Antimicrob Agents Chemother. 1989;33:336–9.
16. Fourel I, Gripon P, Hantz O *et al.* Prolonged duck hepatitis B virus replication in epithelial cells: a useful system for antiviral testing. Hepatology. 1989;10:186–91.
17. Korba BE, Gerin JL. Use of a standardized cell culture assay to assess activities of nucleoside analogs against hepatitis B replication. Antiviral Res. 1992;17:1–16.
18. Tsiquaye KN, Collins P, Zuckerman AJ. Screening of antiviral drugs for treatment of hepatitis B. J Hepatol. 1986;2:S45–8.
19. Sherker AH, Hirota F, Omata M, Okuda K. Foscarnet decreases serum and liver duck hepatitis B virus DNA in chronically infected ducks. Gastroenterology. 1986;91:818–24.
20. Hirota K, Sherker AH, Omata M *et al.* Effects of adenine arabinoside on serum and intrahepatic replicative forms of duck hepatitis B virus in chronic infection. Hepatology. 1987;7:24–8.
21. Petcu DJ, Aldrich CE, Coates L *et al.* Suramin inhibits *in vitro* infection by duck hepatitis B virus, Rous sarcoma virus, and hepatitis delta virus. Virology. 1988;167:385–92.
22. Kassianides C, Hoofnagle JH, Miller RH *et al.* Inhibition of duck hepatitis B virus replication by 2′,3′-dideoxycytidine. Gastroenterology. 1989;97:1275–80.
23. Martin P, Kassianides C, Korenman J *et al.* 2′d′-dideoxyinosine (DDI) and dideoxyguanosine (DDG) are potent inhibitors of hepadnaviruses in vivo. Gastroenterology. 1989;96:628 (abstract).
24. Bishop N, Civitico G, Wang Y *et al.* Antiviral strategies in chronic HBV infection: I. Establishment of a suitable in vitro system using the duck hepatitis B virus model. J Med Virol. 1990;31:82–9.
25. Korba BE, Cote PJ, Tennant BC, Gerin JL. Woodchuck hepatitis virus infection as a model for the development of antiviral therapies against HBV. In: Hollinger FB, Lemon SM, Margolis HS, editors. Viral hepatitis and liver disease. Baltimore: Williams & Wilkins; 1991;641–2.
26. Pollard RB, Smith JL, Beal A *et al.* Effect of vidarabine on chronic hepatitis B infection. J Am Med Assoc. 1978;239:1648–50.
27. Hoofnagle JH, Hanson RG, Minuk GY *et al.* Randomized controlled trial of adenine arabinoside monophosphate for chronic type B hepatitis. Gastroenterology. 1984;86: 150–7.
28. Perrillo RP, Regenstein GF, Bodicky CJ *et al.* Comparative efficacy of adenine arabinoside 5′ monophosphate and prednisone withdrawal followed by adenine arabinosine 5′ monophosphate in the treatment of chronic active hepatitis B. Gastroenterology. 1985;88: 780–6.
29. Garcia G, Smith CI, Weissberg JI *et al.* Adenine arabinoside monophosphate in combination with human leukocyte interferon in the treatment of chronic hepatitis B. A randomized, double-blind, placebo-controlled trial. Ann Intern Med. 1987;107:278–85.

30. Weller IVD, Lok ASF, Mindel A *et al.* Randomized controlled trial of adenine arabinoside 5′ monophosphate (ara-AMP) in chronic hepatitis B virus infection. Gut. 1985;26:745–51.
31. Ouzan D, Chevallier M, Laffranchi B *et al.* Therapeutic efficacy of ara-AMP in symptomatic HBeAg positive CAH. A randomized placebo control study in heterosexuals. Hepatology. 1986;6:1151 (abstract).
32. Marcellin P, Ouzan D, Degos F *et al.* Randomized controlled trial of adenine arabinoside 5′ monophosphate (ara-AMP) in chronic active hepatitis B: comparison of the efficacy in heterosexual and homosexual patients. Hepatology. 1989;10:328–31.
33. Ponzetto A, Forzani B, Busi C *et al.* Adenine arabinoside monophosphate and acyclovir monophosphate coupled to lactosaminated albumin inhibit woodchuck hepatitis virus replication at low doses. Hepatology. 1991;14:16–23.
34. Fiume L, Torrani-Cerenzia MR, Bonino F *et al.* Inhibition of hepatitis B virus replication by vidarabine monophosphate conjugated with lactosaminated serum albumin. Lancet. 1988;2:13–15.
35. Hantz O, Allaudeen HS, Ooka T *et al.* Inhibition of human and woodchuck hepatitis virus DNA polymerase by the triphosphates of acyclovir, 1-(2′deoxy-2′-fluoro-beta-D-arabinofuranosyl)-5-iodo-cytosine and E-5-(2-bromovinyl)-2′-deoxyuridine. Antiviral Res. 1984;4:187–99.
36. Alexander GJM, Fagan EA, Hegarty JE *et al.* Controlled clinical trial of acyclovir in chronic hepatitis B virus infection. J Med Virol. 1987;21:81–7.
37. Locarnini SA, Guo K, Lucas CR, Gust ID. Inhibition of HBV DNA replication by ganciclovir in patients with AIDS. Lancet. 1989;2:1225–6.
38. Berk L, Schalm SW, de Man RA *et al.* Failure of acyclovir to enhance the antiviral effect of alpha lymphoblastoid interferon on HBe seroconversion in chronic hepatitis B. A multicentre randomized controlled trial. J. Hepatol. 1992;14:305–9.
39. Loke RHT, Anderson MG, Coleman JC *et al.* Suramin treatment for chronic active hepatitis B-toxic and ineffective. J Med Virol. 1987;21:97–9.
40. Nordenfelt E, Helgstrand E, Oberg B. Trisodium phosphonoformate inhibits hepatitis B Dane particle DNA polymerase. Acta Path Microbiol Scand, Sect B. 1979;87:75–6.
41. Nordenfelt E, Widell A, Hansson BG *et al.* No *in vivo* effect of trisodium phosphonoformate on woodchuck hepatitis virus production. Acta Path Microbiol Immunol Scand. 1982;90:449–51.
42. Bain VG, Daniels HM, Chanas A *et al.* Foscarnet therapy in chronic hepatitis B virus e antigen carriers. J Med Virol. 1989;29:152–5.
43. Fried MW, Korenman, Hoofnagle JH *et al.* A pilot study of 2′,3′dideoxyinosine (DDI) in chronic hepatitis B. Gastroenterology. 1991;100:A741 (abstract).
44. Fried M, Fong T-L, Swain MG *et al.* Hepatitis B virus DNA suppression during long-term therapy with ribavirin. Gastroenterology. 1992;102:A808 (abstract).
45. Paar DP, Hooton TM, Smiles KA *et al.* The effect of FIAU on chronic hepatitis B virus (HBV) infection in HIV-infected subjects. Fed Proc. 1992:in press.
46. Fried MW, Di Bisceglie AM, Straus SE *et al.* FIAU, a new oral anti-viral agent, profoundly inhibits HBV DNA in patients with chronic hepatitis B. Hepatology. 1992;16:127A (abstract).
47. Doong SL, Tsai CH, Schinazi RF *et al.* Inhibition of the replication of hepatitis B virus in vitro by 2′,3′-dideoxy-3′-thiapyrimidine and related analogues. Proc Natl Acad Sci USA. 1991;88:8495–9.
48. Wu GY, Wu CH. Specific inhibition of hepatitis B viral gene expression in vitro by targeted antisense oligonucleotides. J Biol Chem. 1992;267:12436–9.
49. Weizsaecker FV, Blum HE, Wands JG. Ribozyme mediated cleavage of hepatitis B and duck hepatitis B virus RNA. Hepatology. 1992;16:88A (abstract).
50. Fattovich G, Brollo L, Pontisso P *et al.* Levaminsole therapy in chronic type B hepatitis. Results of a double-blind randomized trial. Gastroenterology. 1986;91:692–6.
51. Thyagarajan SP, Subramanian S, Thirunalasundar T *et al.* Effect of *Phyllanthus amarus* on chronic carriers of hepatitis B virus. Lancet. 1988;2:764–6.
52. Leelarasamee A, Trakulsomboon S, Maunwongyathi P *et al.* Failure of *Phyllanthus amarus* to eradicate hepatitis B surface antigen from symptomless carriers. Lancet. 1990;335: 1600–1 (letter).
53. Berk L, de Man RA, Schalm SW *et al.* Beneficial effects of *Phyllanthus amarus* for chronic hepatitis B, not confirmed. J Hepatol. 1991;12:405–6 (letter).

54. Bisset J, Eisenberg M, Gregory P *et al.* Recombinant fibroblast interferon and immune interferon for treating chronic hepatitis B virus infection. Patients' tolerance and the effect on viral markers. J Infect Dis. 1988;157:1076–80.
55. Di Bisceglie AM, Rustgi VK, Kassianides C *et al.* Therapy of chronic hepatitis B with recombinant alpha and gamma interferon. Hepatology. 1990;11:266–70.
56. Lau JYN, Lai CL, Wu PC *et al.* A randomised controlled trial of recombinant interferon-gamma in Chinese patients with chronic hepatitis B virus infection. J Med Virol. 1991;34: 184–7.
57. Marcellin P, Loriot MA, Boyer N *et al.* Recombinant human gamma-interferon in patients with chronic active hepatitis B: pharmacokinetics, tolerance and biological effects. Hepatology. 1990;12:155–8.
58. Nishioka M, Kagawa H, Shirai M *et al.* Effects of human recombinant interleukin 2 in patients with chronic hepatitis B: a preliminary report. Am J Gastroenterol. 1987;82: 438–42.
59. Zeniya M, Takahashi H, Sata H *et al.* The effects of recombinant interleukin 2 on HBe antigen positive chronic hepatitis B. Jpn J Med. 1991;30:292–8.
60. Muller C, Bergmann KF, Gerin JL, Korba BE. Production of hepatitis B virus by stably transfected monocytic cell line, U937: a model for extrahepatic hepatitis B virus replication. J Infect Dis. 1992;165:929–33.
61. Fisher B, Keenan AM, Garra BS *et al.* Interleukin-2 induces profound reversible cholestasis: a detailed analysis in treated cancer patients. J Clin Oncol. 1989;7:1852–62.
62. Goldstein AL, Low TLK, Thurman GB *et al.* Current status of thymosin and other hormones of the thymus gland. Recent Prog Hormone Res. 1981;37:369–415.
63. Eichberg JW, Seeff LB, Lawlor DL *et al.* Effect of thymosin immunostimulation with and without corticosteroid immunosuppression on chimpanzee hepatitis B carriers. J Med Virol. 1987;21:25–37.
64. Mutchnick MG, Appelman HD, Chung HT *et al.* Thymosin treatment of chronic hepatitis B. A placebo controlled pilot trial. Hepatology. 1991;14:409–15.
65. Martin J, Bosch O, Quiroga JA *et al.* Recombinant human granulocyte–macrophage colony stimulating factor (rhGM-CSF) in the treatment of chronic hepatitis B. Hepatology. 1992;16:67A (abstract).
66. Perrillo RP, Regenstein FG, Eters MG *et al.* Prednisone withdrawal followed by recombinant alpha interferon in the treatment of chronic hepatitis B. A randomized controlled trial. Ann Intern Med. 1988;109:95–100.
67. Hanson RF, Peters MG, Hoofnagle JH. Effects of immunosuppressive therapy with prenisolone on B and T lymphocyte function in patients with chronic type B hepatitis. Hepatology. 1986;6:173–9.
68. Lever AML, Waters J, Brook MG *et al.* Monoclonal antibody to HBsAg for chronic hepatitis B virus infection with hypogammaglobulinaemia. Lancet. 1990;335:1529 (letter).
69. Chen P-M, Fan S, Liu C-J *et al.* Changing of hepatitis B virus markers in patients with bone marrow transplantation. Transplantation. 1990;49:708–16.
70. Reed EC, Myerson D, Corey L, Meyers JD, Allogeneic marrow transplantation in patients positive for hepatitis B surface antigen. Blood. 1991;77:195–200.
71. Lok ASF, Liang RHS, Chung H-T. Recovery from chronic hepatitis B. Ann Intern Med. 1982;116:957 (letter).
72. Shouval D, Ilan Y, Nagler A *et al.* Ablation of persistent hepatitis B virus infection through adoptive transfer of immunity following bone marrow transplantation from an HBV immune donor. J Hepatol. 1992;16:S12 (abstract).

16
The role of interferon-α in virus elimination: viral inhibitors resulting in persistent infection

G. R. FOSTER and H. C. THOMAS

Interferons (IFN) are a group of related cytokines first identified by their ability to inhibit the replication of influenza virus[1]. IFNs are divided into two types: type I IFNs comprise some 22 different IFN-α subtypes as well as a single IFN-β subtype. Type II IFNs comprise a single subtype: IFN-γ. Type I IFNs are induced by many viruses and they act as inhibitors of viral replication. Type II IFNs are produced by activated T lymphocytes and function as immunomodulatory cytokines. Over the past few years considerable progress has been made in determining how type I IFNs exert their antiviral effects, and it has recently become clear that many viruses can inhibit the antiviral properties of type I IFNs assisting in the development of chronic viral infections.

Type I IFNs exert their effects by activating a set of cellular genes[2]. Once activated these genes allow the production of a wide range of proteins, some of which are able to inhibit viral replication. Activation of IFN-inducible genes occurs via a protein synthesis independent cellular transduction pathway (Fig. 1). IFN-α binds to a cellular receptor[3] that then activates a protein complex known as Eα[4] (E is a cellular factor that is also known as ISGF3[5]). The activation of Eα is believed to be due to phosphorylation of one or more of the components of Eα (C. Schindler and J. Darnell, personal communication). Eα contains at least three different protein subunits[5] and once activated by receptor-bound IFN Eα binds to another protein (Eγ) to form a complex–active E[5]. Active E then migrates to the cell nucleus where it binds to a DNA sequence (the ISRE[6]) that is found in the promoter region of all IFN-inducible genes. Binding of E to the ISRE activates gene transcription and results in the synthesis of a large number of proteins. The cellular transduction pathway used by IFN-γ is not yet fully understood.

The functions of many IFN-inducible genes are still unknown; however, some have been well characterized and have specific antiviral properties. 2′-5′A oligoadenylate synthetase (2-5A) is an IFN-inducible enzyme that is

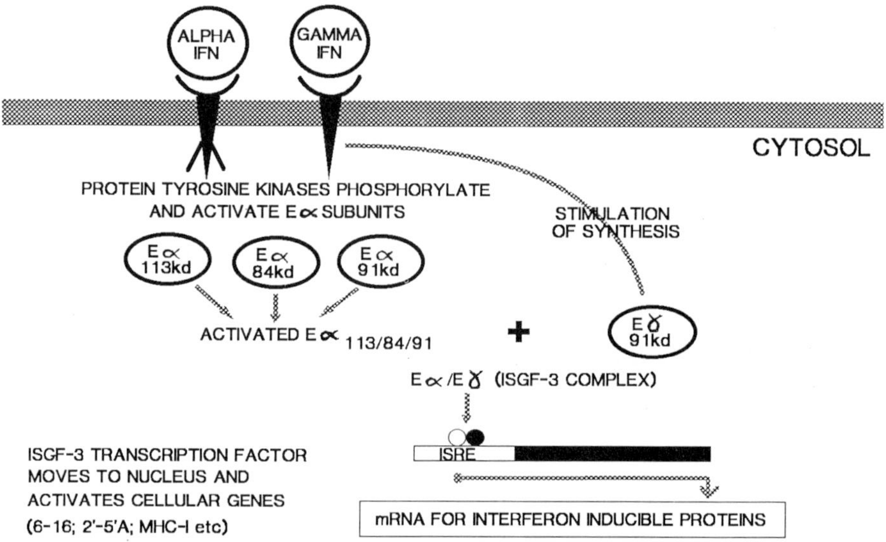

Fig. 1 Activation of interferon inducible genes. IFN-α binds to a cellular receptor and activates one or more of the Eα protein subunits. The active Eα protein complex then binds to another protein (Eγ) to form active E (also known as ISGF3). The active protein complex then migrates to the nucleus where it activates gene transcription by binding to an element (the ISRE) that is found in the promoter of all interferon-inducible genes. The transactivation pathway used by IFN-γ is poorly understood, but IFN-γ can interact with the IFN-α pathway by increasing the synthesis of the Eγ subunit of E

activated by double-stranded RNA (dsRNA)[7]. Once activated 2-5A catalyses the synthesis of a family of 2′-5′-linked oligonucleotides that activate a ribonuclease (RNAaseL). This ribonuclease is then able to destroy dsRNA. Since dsRNA is normally found only in cells that contain replicating RNA viruses 2-5A is activated only in infected cells; hence uninfected cells are spared the deleterious effects of an active ribonuclease. p68 protein kinase is another IFN-inducible protein that is activated by dsRNA[8]. Once activated this kinase phosphorylates the protein synthesis initiation factor eIF-2, and inhibits protein synthesis by preventing the initiation of translation. Hence 2-5A and p68 kinase are IFN-inducible proteins capable of inhibiting the replication of viruses containing dsRNA. Other IFN-inducible proteins have more specific antiviral activities. For example the Mx protein specifically inhibits the replication of the influenza virus[9].

In addition to activating the synthesis of specific antiviral proteins, IFNs (both types I and II) also act as immunomodulators. To be recognized by immunocytes antigenic viral proteins must first be presented to the immune system in association with MHC antigens. Viral antigens that are recognized by cytotoxic T cells are first degraded in the cytoplasm by a complex of enzymes known as the proteasome[10]. The peptide fragments are then transported into the endoplasmic reticulum by transporter enzymes[11] where they associate with the MHC class I proteins. The antigen–MHC complex is then expressed on the cell surface where it can be recognized by

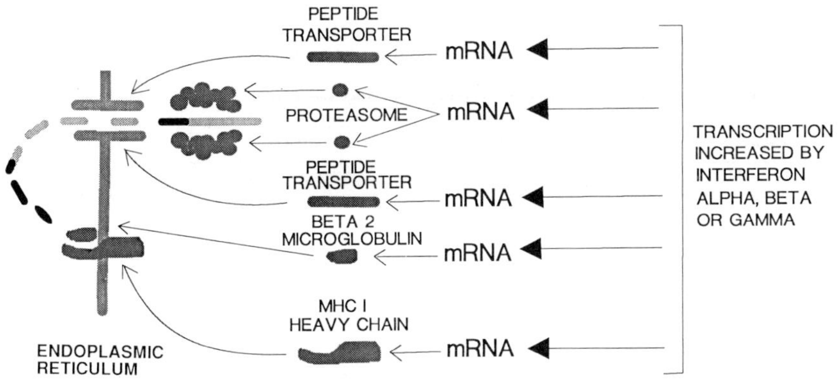

Fig. 2 Interferon induction of antigen processing and presentation of proteins to the immune system. Interferon increases the transcription of a number of genes that are involved in the processing of viral antigens. The proteasome proteins form a complex that degrades viral proteins and presents them to the transporter protein. This protein carries the peptide fragments into the endoplasmic reticulum where they combine with β microglobulin and the MHC proteins. The resulting complex is then expressed on the cell surface where it can act as an immunological target

immunocytes (Fig. 2). It has long been known that IFNs can increase the synthesis of MHC proteins, and recent work has shown that IFNs can also increase cellular synthesis of both the proteasome and transporter proteins (J. Trowsdale, ICRF, London, personal communication). Hence IFNs can amplify the antigen presentation pathway by increasing the presentation of viral proteins, thus allowing cytotoxic T cells to recognize and eliminate infected cells.

IFNs, particularly IFN-γ, also assist in the development of an antiviral immunological response by directly activating immunocytes. IFN-γ is released by activated lymphocytes, whereupon it activates a number of other cells directly (such as macrophages) and indirectly, by stimulating the release of other cytokines[12]. IFNs thus play a central role in the development of an antiviral immunological response – they increase expression of viral antigens on the cell surface and they activate the cells of the immune system.

IFNs are very potent antiviral agents. It is therefore not surprising to find that a number of viruses have developed strategies for avoiding the antiviral effects of IFN (summarized in Fig. 3). The p68 kinase and 2-5A synthetase enzymes are both activated by dsRNA. This form of RNA is produced by many viruses and thus the virus contains the seeds of its own destruction. The reovirus, serotype 1, produces a protein, sigma 3, which is able to sequester dsRNA and thereby prevent activation of the dsRNA-activated antiviral proteins[13]. This mechanism may be used by other viruses – recent work suggests that the delta antigen produced by the hepatitis delta virus may also sequester viral RNA and thus prevent activation of the antiviral enzymes (A. McNair and I. M. Kerr, HCT, unpublished data). Other viruses inactivate the dsRNA-activated enzymes by interacting directly with them. A number of adenoviral strains produce RNAs (the VA RNAs) that bind to

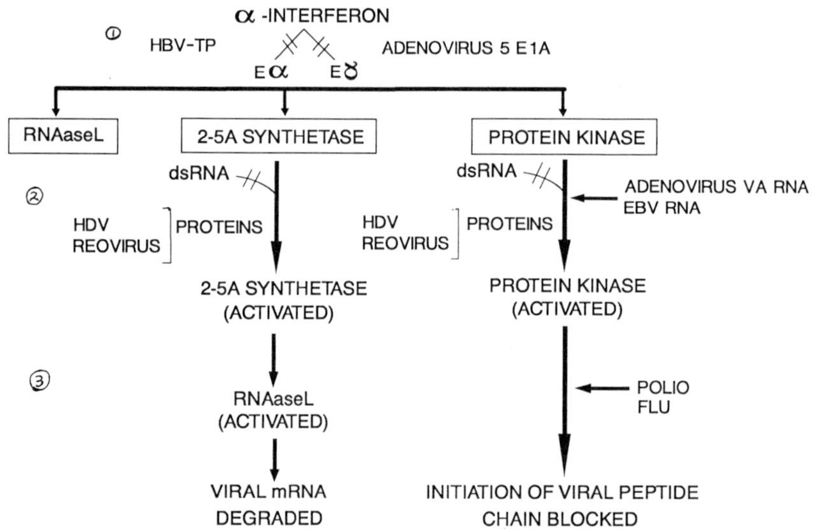

Fig. 3 Virus inhibition of the antiviral effects of interferon. Some viruses (e.g. hepatitis B and certain adenoviral strains) inactivate the signal transduction pathway by inhibiting the formation of the transactivating factor E (1). Other viruses, e.g. reoviruses and adenoviruses, allow interferon-inducible proteins to form but inhibit their activation by double-stranded RNA (2). A third group of viruses (e.g. polio) may inhibit the action of antiviral proteins by enhancing their degradation (3). HBV-TP = hepatitis B virus terminal protein, HDV = hepatitis delta virus, EBV = Epstein–Barr virus

the p68 kinase and inactivate it[14] and the Epstein–Barr virus may produce RNAs that act in a similar fashion. The poliovirus may inactivate the kinase by inducing proteolytic cleavage of the enzyme[15] and there is some evidence to suggest that the influenza virus may inactivate the kinase using a similar method. Other viruses (e.g. HIV) do not inactivate the kinase but they produce proteins (TAT in the case of HIV) that prevent kinase production[16]. Hence some viruses have developed mechanisms to inactivate specific IFN-inducible antiviral proteins.

Inactivation of the cellular inhibitors of viral replication is clearly of great advantage to a virus. However, IFNs can also inhibit viral replication by activating the immune system. Some viruses have evolved strategies that allow them to overcome this effect of IFN. The BCRF1 protein of Epstein–Barr virus is homologous to, and capable of mimicking the activity of, interleukin-10[17]. Interleukin-10 inhibits the production of IFN-γ in activated T cells and hence the Epstein–Barr virus can inhibit the IFN-induced activation of the immune system.

A number of viruses have developed mechanisms that allow them to overcome some of IFN's antiviral effects. Clearly a virus that could completely inhibit all of IFN's effects would have a significant survival advantage and it is not surprising to find that some viruses have evolved such mechanisms. The E1A protein of the oncogenic adenoviruses completely inhibits the cellular response to IFN by preventing the activation of the transactivating factor E[18]. Similarly, a fragment of the hepatitis B viral polymerase protein (terminal protein) can inhibit the effects of IFN by preventing the formation of active Eα[19]. It is not yet clear what role these IFN inhibitors play in the pathogenesis of human chronic viral infections but recent work has shown that for the hepatitis B virus patients who overproduce the IFN inhibitor, terminal protein, have a poor response to therapeutic IFN (G. R. Foster, R. D. Goldin and M. J. McGarvey, HCT, unpublished data), suggesting that this natural IFN inhibitor may play a significant role in viral pathogenesis.

IFN is a major component of the host response to viral infections. It antagonizes viral replication directly and enhances the immunological eradication of infected cells. It is not surprising to find that some viruses that cause chronic infections have become resistant to the effects of IFN. Viral resistance may be conferred by viral inhibition of a single component of the IFN-induced antiviral response, or it may involve complete inhibition of the cellular response to IFN. A complete understanding of the mechanisms of viral resistance will no doubt lead to the development of therapies that can overcome them and restore the potent antiviral properties of these natural antiviral compounds.

References

1. Isaacs A, Lindenmann J. Virus interference 1. The interferon. Proc Roy Soc Lond B. 1957;147:258–67.
2. Taylor J. Inhibition of interferon activity by actinomycin. Biochem Biophys Res Commun. 1964;14:447–51.
3. Uze G, Lutfalla G, Gresser I. Genetic transfer of a functional human interferon a receptor into mouse cells: cloning and expression of its cDNA. Cell. 1990;60:225–34.
4. Dale TC, Rosen JM, Guille MJ *et al.* Overlapping sites for constitutive and induced DNA binding factors involved in interferon-stimulated transcription. EMBO J. 1989;8:831–9.
5. Kessler DS, Veals SA, Fu XY, Levy DE. IFNa regulates nuclear translocation and DNA-binding affinity of ISGF3, a multimeric transcriptional transactivator. Genes Devel. 1991;4:1753–65.
6. Levy D, Larner A, Chaudhuri A *et al.* Interferon-stimulated transcription: isolation of an inducible gene and identification of its regulatory region. Proc Natl Acad Sci USA. 1986;83:8929–33.
7. Williams and Silverman (eds). The 2-5A system. New York: Liss; 1984.
8. Samuel CE. Mechanism of interferon action. Phosphorylation of protein synthesis initiation factor eIF-2 in interferon treated cells by a ribosome associated kinase processing site specificity similar to hemin-regulated rabbit reticulocyte kinase. Proc Natl Acad Sci USA. 1979;76:600–4.
9. Staeheli P, Haller O, Boll W *et al.* Mx protein: constitutive expression in 3T3 cells transformed with cloned Mx DNA confers selective resistance to influenza virus. Cell. 1986;44:147–58.
10. Kelly A, Powis SH, Glynne R *et al.* Second proteosome related gene in the human class II region. Nature. 1991;353:667–8.
11. Trowsdale J, Hanson, Mockridge I *et al.* Sequences encoded in the class II region of the MHC related to the ABC superfamily of transporters. Nature. 1990;349:7412–14.
12. Trinchieri G, Perussia B. Immune interferon: a pleiotropic lymphokine with multiple effects. Immunol Today. 1985;6:131–6.
13. Imani F, Jacobs BL. Inhibitory activity for the interferon-induced protein kinase is associated with the reovirus serotype 1 o3 protein. Proc Natl Acad Sci USA. 1988;85: 7887–91.
14. Kitajewski J, Schneider RJ, Safer B *et al.* Adenovirus VAI RNA antagonises the antiviral

action of interferon by preventing activation of the interferon-induced eIF-2a kinase. Cell. 1986;45:195–200.

15. Black T, Safer B, Hovanessian A, Katze MG. The cellular 68,000 Mr protein kinase is highly autophosphorylated and activated yet significantly degraded during poliovirus infection: implications for translation regulation. J Virol. 1989;63:2244–51.
16. Roy S, Katze MG, Parkin NT *et al.* Control of the interferon induced 68 kilodalton protein kinase by the HIV-1 TAT gene product. Science. 1990;247:1216–19.
17. Hsu DH, de Waal MR, Fiorentino DF *et al.* Expression of interleukin-10 activity by Epstein–Barr virus protein BCRF1. Science. 1990;250:830–2.
18. Ackrill AM, Foster GR, Laxton CD *et al.* Inhibition of the cellular response to interferons by products of the adenovirus type 5 E1A oncogene. Nucl Acid Res. 1991;19:4387–93.
19. Foster GR, Ackrill AM, Goldin RD *et al.* Expression of the terminal protein region of hepatitis B virus inhibits cellular responses to interferons a and g and double stranded RNA. Proc Natl Acad Sci USA. 1991;88:2888–92.

Section V
Mechanisms responsible for Autoimmunity

17
Immunoprotection, immunopathology or tolerance – a question of balance

R. M. ZINKERNAGEL

INTRODUCTION

The desirable part of immune protection is the elimination of infectious agents. Cytopathic viruses must be stopped before too many host cells are destroyed by the virus, therefore quick and efficient cell-mediated immunoprotection by cytotoxic T cells (CTL) is essential for the survival of the host. Since CTLs destroy virus-infected cells to stop and eliminate virus, immunoprotection is mediated by immunopathology. The latter aspect may become more obvious in diseases caused by non-cytopathic viruses, since only CTLs but not the virus itself cause pathology. Because non-cytopathic viruses do not kill the host directly, they have been able to develop varying balanced states with the immune system; they may even be able to escape immune surveillance without harming the host. Hepatitis B virus infection in humans[1–3] and lymphocytic choriomeningitis virus infection in mice[4–7] may serve as classical examples.

T CELL-MEDIATED HEPATITIS

Lymphocytic choriomeningitis disease in mice develops after intracerebral injection of LCMV only in immunocompetent mice[4–6]. Mice lacking T cells, or those immunosuppressed by irradiation or cytostatic drugs, do not develop inflammatory reactions and thus no LCM disease, but they fail to eliminate virus and as a result become LCMV carriers. LCM disease has been carefully analysed and has been clearly shown to be T cell-mediated[8]. Lethal LCM disease apparently depends upon effector T cells being preferentially recruited to the acutely infected leptomeninges.

Alternatively viscerotropic LCMV infecting liver cells may recruit cytotoxic T cells to the liver, and these cause liver cell destruction[7]. The resulting LCMV-induced hepatitis in mice has been monitored histologically and by the determination of changes in serum levels of aminotransferases and alkaline phosphatase. The kinetics of histological disease manifestations, increases of liver enzyme levels in the serum, and cytotoxic T cell activities in livers and spleens all correlated, and were found to be dependent upon several parameters such as the LCMV-isolate, the virus dose and route of infection, and the general genetic background of the murine host. The degree of immunocompetence of the murine host is important since T cell-deficient nu/nu mice never developed hepatitis, whereas nu/+ or +/+ mice always did. Thus LCMV-induced hepatitis in mice is an immunopathologically mediated disease caused by T cell-mediated destruction of infected liver cells. Overall, this disease parallels many aspects of acute viral hepatitis in humans, which is caused by hepatitis B virus.

MHC–DISEASE ASSOCIATION

In both LCMV hepatitis and hepatitis B, disease depends upon the balance between the rate of virus spread and the immune response. An efficient T cell-mediated immune response leads to rapid elimination of the virus, limited cell and tissue damage and therefore limited disease. Absence of an immune response results in unchecked growth of virus and in a virus-carrier state. Slow and low immune responsiveness allows extensive spread of virus with chronic T-cell mediated tissue destruction. Since major transplantation antigens bind foreign antigen fragments more or less well, and thus determine whether a T cell response is efficiently induced, they may drastically influence the balance between virus and immune-mediated tissue damage. Amongst many other variables characteristic for the virus or the host, severity of disease has also been shown to be determined by major transplantation antigens in both hepatitis B virus infections in humans[3,9] and in LCMV infections in mice[10].

The influence of major transplantation antigens on susceptibility to T cell-mediated disease caused by infection with the non-cytopathic virus lymphocytic choriomeningitis virus (LCMV) was evaluated in B10 H-2-congenic mice. Susceptibility to early T cell-mediated liver cell destruction (day 7–9) and early mortality (> day 12) was H-2D^q linked and correlated directly with early (~day 6–8) and high cytotoxic T cell activity. In contrast, susceptibility to become an LCMV-carrier, inability to rapidly clear virus or the tendency to develop late hepatitis (day 14–17) was linked to D^k and correlated with absence of early cytotoxic T cell activity. Thus H-2D-regulated T cell immune responses controlling both virus spread and immunopathology may directly determine the type and severity of disease. The results illustrate that susceptibility to disease caused by one virus may be linked to distinct MHC alleles dependent upon the disease parameter studied.

VIRAL ESCAPE BY SELECTION OF CYTOTOXIC T CELL-RESISTANT VIRUS VARIANTS *IN VIVO*

The equilibrium between virus and immune system may also be modulated if the virus mutates the epitopes recognized by cytotoxic T cells[11]. Examples of such T cell epitope mutants have recently been found for LCMV and HIV[12]. Mice expressing a transgenic T cell receptor specific for LCMV-GP aa32-42 and D^b (see ref. 13) can eliminate 10^2–10^4 plaque-forming units (pfu) of LCMV (pfu) very efficiently. If 10^6 pfu LCMV are injected, virus is apparently not cleared by transgenic mice. Analysis of surviving virus in these transgenic hosts revealed that it expressed a mutation in the glycoprotein GPaa32–42, and therefore were no longer recognized by the transgenic effector T cells. Thus cytotoxic T cell responses are able, during a primary infection *in vivo*, to rapidly select mutant virus that escapes the dominant T cell recognition and as a consequence is no longer efficiently eliminated in these transgenic mice. Such variants were readily detected in TCR transgenic mice because T cell recognition is mainly directed against one viral epitope with high frequency; therefore potentially protective T cell responses against other LCMV epitopes are either not generated at all or appear relatively late in the TCR transgenic mice. These experiments document that, like antibody-driven selection, cytotoxic T cell responses may also efficiently select virus mutants in a given individual. Antibody-driven selection of mutant virus has been demonstrated *in vitro* with single neutralizing antibodies. Selection cannot be induced with two or more distinct monoclonal antibodies at the same time, only if they are used in sequence. Similar stepwise selection may be postulated for T cell-escape without avoiding several distinct T cell responses. Although theoretically possible, it is probably rare that as a result of such a multistep selection, virus may spread through a species population. In most instances, cytotoxic T cell-dependent selection is relevant to the individual only. Because cytotoxic T cells recognize virus as peptide fragments of various viral gene products in a strictly class 1 MHC-dependent fashion, virus can survive immune selection only in this individual (or individuals with the same major transplantation antigens).

VIRUS-TRIGGERED ACQUIRED IMMUNOSUPPRESSION

It has been known for some time that LCMV causes immunosuppression in mice. When re-evaluating this in various mouse strains using different LCMV isolates, we found that an LCMV infection of mice suppressed their capacity to mount an IgM or IgG response to vesicular stomatitis virus (VSV)[14]. Mice preinfected with LCMV were considerably more susceptible to disease caused by VSV, which is usually non-pathogenic for mice if injected subcutaneously or intravenously.

The extent of immune suppression by LCMV depended upon the following parameters: different LCMV virus isolates influenced immune reactivity differently. LCMV-WE and some other LCMV isolates such as LCMV-AGG or LCMV-DOC caused immunosuppression, whereas LCMV-ARM did so only rarely. Mouse strains differed considerably with respect to susceptibility to this immunosuppression; the MHC played some yet poorly defined role, but non-MHC genes also had a major influence. The kinetics of induction of the described impairment of mice to respond with T cell-dependent IgM and/or a strictly T cell-dependent IgG response to a subsequent virus infection paralleled that usually characteristic for the induction of an anti-LCMV T cell response starting on day 6 after LCMV infection and reaching maximum levels around day 8–10. The following experimental results[15] suggested that, similar to LCMV-hepatitis[7], the antiviral T cell response was responsible for immunosuppression. When neonatally infected LCMV-carrier mice were evaluated with respect to their immune responsiveness they were found to mount anti-VSV, IgM and IgG responses comparable to normal control mice. T cell-deprived nude mice infected with LCMV also made normal IgM responses. This indicated that LCMV alone is not immunosuppressive, and that the observed immune suppression is not caused by the action of interferons on VSV. In contrast, LCMV-infected nude mice that received LCMV immune cytotoxic T cells exhibited suppressed antibody responses[15]. Also, while LCMV-infected mice failed to mount an antibody response, similarly infected mice that were treated with anti-CD8 antisera some days before they received the VSV infection mounted normal IgM and IgG responses. These results are compatible with the view that antiviral cytotoxic T cells are responsible for immune suppression in this model infection.

This immune suppression has been analysed further by monitoring lymphocyte subset composition in spleens of mice acutely infected with LCMV by using FACS analysis. We found no drastic reduction in the absolute numbers of T helper cells or B cells, but an increase in the number of cytotoxic T cells. Studies of the lymph follicles and germinal centres in spleens of T cell competent ICR mice showed the following characteristic changes during an acute LCMV infection: by day 3–4 most of the typical distributions of cells expressing CD4, CD8, IgM or macrophage markers were comparable to that in controls. However, in immunocompetent mice the follicular structure was massively destroyed between day 6 and 14 after LCMV infection[16]. The usual architecture of germinal centres in spleens reappeared slowly after day 12. Thus the orderly structure of germinal centres is drastically altered, and this may be responsible for the failure of LCMV-infected mice to mount an IgM and IgG response.

These findings may be relevant to our understanding of acquired immunodeficiency which is caused by the human immunodeficiency viruses (HIV)[17]. As in LCMV infections, recent evidence suggests that cytotoxic T cells may actually be instrumental in controlling HIV replication, but may also be responsible for destroying lymphocytes and macrophages and thus causing immune suppression. The example of HIV infections in humans may therefore in a way represent the ultimate perversity in the balance between host immune system and infectious agent: non-cytopathic viruses infect lymphocytes and macrophages, the essential partners of an immune response, which are then destroyed by the immune response; i.e. the virus infection misleads the immune system to partially destroy itself; thereby virus may be able to persist.

T CELL TOLERANCE AND RESPONSES TO VIRAL ANTIGENS IN TRANSGENIC MICE: IMPLICATIONS FOR THE PATHOGENESIS FOR IMMUNOPATHOLOGICAL DISEASE

Conventional immunological tolerance to virus by negative selection of reactive T cells in the infected thymus due to transplacental transmission of virus, from carrier mother to offspring permits the non-cytopathic virus to persist in the host without causing disease[4–6,13].

Yet another mechanism by which virus may escape immune surveillance may be by hiding in immunologically privileged sites, where viruses may be ignored by the immune system. To analyse this possibility transgenic mice were generated that express a T cell receptor specific for a viral peptide (aa 32–42 of the lymphocytic choriomeningitis virus glycoprotein LCMV-GP) presented by the class I transplantation antigen H-2D^b (see ref. 13). Other mice express the viral glycoprotein (LCMV-GP) exclusively (as far as tested) in pancreatic islet cells[18]. Both mice were used to study cytotoxic T cell reactivity and tolerance to a peripheral antigen in GP-single and TCR/GP-double transgenic mice. These experiments reveal that self-epitopes that are genetically self and presented by class I antigens may not be considered immunologically self if expressed solely extrathymically, despite the fact that they are antigenic and can be recognized by induced effector T cells. Thus, a 'self-antigen' that is presented on cells which can induce neither tolerance nor an immune response is immunologically ignored. If the same antigen is expressed immunogenically on proper antigen-presenting cells in these mice after infection with LCMV, then a T cell response is induced promptly, causing immunopathology. This experiment may illustrate the possibility that non-cytopathic virus may hide from immune surveillance in non-lymphohaemopoietic cells without causing disease[19].

CONCLUSION

Several examples of distinct balances between non-cytopathic viruses and CD8$^+$ T cell-mediated immunity have been summarized. They reach from tolerance and virus carrier state, to immunopathology, to acute protective immunity. Both viral and host parameters influence the balance, and modulation of either side may modify immunopathological consequences of infection and disease.

References

1. Bianchi L. The immunopathology of acute type B hepatitis. Springer Semin Immunopathol. 1981;3:421–38.
2. Mondelli M, Eddleston ALWF. Mechanisms of liver cell injury in acute and chronic hepatitis B. Semin Liver Dis. 1984;4:47–58.
3. Peters M, Vierling J, Gershwin ME, Milich D, Chisari FV, Hoofnagle JH. Immunology and the liver. Hepatology. 1991;13:977–94.
4. Buchmeier MJ, Welsh RM, Dutko FJ, Oldstone MBA. The virology and immunobiology of lymphocytic choriomeningitis virus infection. Adv. Immunol. 1980;30:275–312.
5. Hotchin J. The biology of lymphocytic choriomeningitis infection: virus induced immune

disease. Cold Spring Harbor Symp Quant Biol. 1962;27:479–99.
6. Lehmann-Grube F. Lymphocytic choriomeningitis virus. Virol Monogr. 1971;10:1–173.
7. Zinkernagel RM, Haenseler E, Leist TP, Cerny A, Hengartner H, Althage A. T cell mediated hepatitis in mice infected with lymphocytic choriomeningitis virus. J Exp Med. 1986;164:1075–92.
8. Cole GA, Nathanson N, Prendergast RA. Requirement for theta-bearing cells in lymphocytic choriomeningitis virus-induced central nervous system disease. Nature. 1972;238:335–7.
9. Eddleston ALWF, Williams R. HLA and liver disease. Br Med Bull. 1978;34:295–300.
10. Leist TP, Althage A, Haenseler E, Hengartner H, Zinkernagel RM. MHC-linked susceptibility or resistance to disease caused by a noncytopathic virus varies with the disease parameter evaluated. J Exp Med. 1989;170:269–77.
11. Pircher HP, Moskophidis D, Rohrer U, Bürki K, Hengartner H, Zinkernagel RM. Viral escape by selection of cytotoxic T cell-resistant virus variants in vivo. Nature. 1990;346: 629–33.
12. Philips RE, Rowland-Jones S, Nixon DF, Gotch FM, Edwards JP, Ogunlesi AO, Elvin JG, Rothbard JA, Bangham CR, Rizza CR, McMichael AJ. Human immunodeficiency virus genetic variation that can escape cytotoxic T cell recognition. Nature. 1991;354:453–9.
13. Pircher HP, Bürki K, Lang R, Hengartner H, Zinkernagel R. Tolerance induction in double specific T-cell receptor transgenic mice varies with antigen. Nature. 1989;342:559–61.
14. Roost P, Charan S, Gobet R, Rüedi E, Hengartner H, Althage A, Zinkernagel M. An acquired immunodeficiency in mice caused by infection with lymphocytic choriomeningitis virus. Eur J Immunol. 1988;18:511–18.
15. Leist TP, Rüedi E, Zinkernagel RM. Virus-triggered immune suppression in mice caused by virus-specific cytotoxic T cells. J Exp Med. 1988;167:1749–54.
16. Odermatt B, Eppler M, Leist TP, Hengartner H, Zinkernagel RM. Virus-triggered acquired immunodeficiency by cytotoxic T-cell dependent destruction of antigen-presenting cells and lymph follicle structure. Proc Natl Acad Sci USA. 1991;88:8252–6.
17. Rosenberg ZF, Fauci AS. The immunopathogenesis of HIV infection. Adv Immunol. 1989;47:377–431.
18. Ohashi PS, Oehen S, Bürki K, Pircher HP, Ohashi CT, Odermatt B, Malissen B, Zinkernagel R, Hengartner H. Ablation of 'tolerance' and induction of diabetes by virus infection in viral antigen transgenic mice. Cell. 1991;65:305–17.
19. Zinkernagel RM, Pircher HP, Ohashi PS, Oehen S, Odermatt B, Mak TW, Arnheiter H, Bürki K, Hengartner H. T and B cell tolerance and responses to viral antigens in transgenic mice: implications for the pathogenesis of autoimmune versus immunopathological disease. Immunol Rev. 1991;122:133–71.

18
Autoantibodies as diagnostic markers, probes in cell biology and reporters of cellular activation

E. M. TAN, H. IMAI and E. K. L. CHAN

INTRODUCTION

A common feature of many systemic autoimmune diseases is a humoral immune response manifested by the production of autoantibodies targeted against intracellular proteins and nucleic acids (for review see ref. 1). The autoimmune diseases include systemic lupus erythematosus, scleroderma, Sjögren's syndrome, mixed connective tissue disease, dermatomyositis and polymyositis. In these systemic autoimmune diseases, autoantibodies are present in high titre and in the majority of patients with each categorical disease. Each disease is characterized by a rather distinctive profile of antibodies reacting with a restricted number of intracellular antigens. Thus, definitions of the specificities of the autoantibodies have been useful adjuncts in the diagnosis of several autoimmune diseases. As discussed previously, many of these autoantibodies are not likely to be involved in the pathogenesis of tissue lesions[1,2]. Since most of the autoantigens in this group of diseases are intracellular in location, autoantibodies would have to penetrate cell membranes in order to gain access to their cognate antigens. In the living cell membrane these autoantibodies, which are normal immunoglobulins in structure and function, would not be expected to penetrate cell membranes. So far as is known, only a few intracellular antigens such as DNA and histones have been detected in extracellular fluids, and in such situations pre-existing autoantibodies in the circulation could react with their cognate antigens to form antigen–antibody immune complexes and initiate a cascade of inflammation by the activation of complement and other inflammatory mediators.

ASSOCIATION OF AUTOANTIGENS WITH SUBCELLULAR PARTICLES

Autoantibodies have been used as effective reagents to screen cDNA libraries in order to isolate DNA encoding autoantigens. In other instances autoantibodies have been used to isolate purified antigens and amino acid sequencing of these isolated antigens has enabled construction of oligonucleotide probes for the screening of cDNA or genomic libraries. This has resulted in the elucidation of the molecular structure of the majority of autoantigens and, in many cases, the function of these autoantigens has been deduced by the presence of characteristic motifs. In other cases cloned antigens and the respective autoantibodies have been used as reagents to define function in various experimental systems. These studies have shown an interesting feature of intracellular autoantigens in that they are frequently associated with, or components of, subcellular particles. Some of this information is shown in Table 1. Autoantibodies to DNA and histones which are integral components of the nucleosome are present in systemic lupus erythematosus. Autoantibodies to an antigen called Sm were first defined by immunodiffusion analysis as a precipitin reaction. The Sm antigen has been shown to be a family of several proteins which are components of small nuclear ribonucleoprotein particles engaged in the splicing of precursor-mRNA. PCNA (proliferating cell nuclear antigen), another target antigen of lupus autoantibodies, is an auxiliary protein of DNA polymerase delta-regulated DNA replication. So far, most of the antigens known to react with lupus autoantibodies reside in the nucleoplasm. Of interest are antigens which are targeted by autoantibodies in scleroderma. Most of these are resident in the nucleolus, including fibrillarin, a component of the U3-ribonucleoprotein particle involved in preribosomal RNA processing[3] and a protein doublet called nucleolus organizer region-90 (NOR-90) proteins, which have been shown to be RNA polymerase I transcription factors[4,5].

Table 1 Association of autoantigens with subcellular particles

Subcellular particles	*Function*	*Antigenic components*
Nucleosome	Genome repository	DNA, Histones
Small nuclear ribonucleoprotein particles	Splicing of pre-mRNA	Sm proteins, U1-RNP proteins, U-RNAs
DNA replication particles	DNA polymerase delta-regulated DNA replication	PCNA (proliferating cell nuclear antigen)
Centromere/kinetochore	Mitosis	Centromere proteins 19, 80 and 140 kDa
Nucleolus organizer region (NOR)	RNA polymerase I transcription factor	NOR protein doublet of 93 and 89 kDa
U3 ribonucleoprotein particle	RNA polymerase I transcription termination	Fibrillarin (34 kDa protein)
Ribosomes	mRNA translation	Ribosomal P proteins tRNA synthetases, $tRNA^{His,Thr,Ala}$

Centromere proteins of 19, 80 and 140 kDa are associated with the centromeric regions and kinetochore plates of condensed chromosomes in mitosis. It has been shown recently that these centromere proteins can be localized by immunoelectron microscopy in the nucleolus[6].

AUTOANTIBODIES INHIBIT FUNCTION OF SUBCELLULAR PARTICLES

In many cases where the function of the antigen is known and where there are experimental systems for studying such functions, it has been shown that human autoantibodies have the special property of inhibiting function. This is shown in Table 2. Human autoantibody to PCNA from patients with lupus has been used to inhibit DNA polymerase delta-regulated DNA replication and in helping to elucidate the finding that DNA polymerase delta is involved with leading strand DNA synthesis[7]. Similarly, lupus autoantibodies have been used effectively in showing the involvement of a number of small nuclear ribonucleoproteins (snRNPs) in the ordered assembly of these ribonucleoproteins on precursor-mRNA and elucidating sequential steps in the splicing process[8]. Antibodies to tRNA synthetases which are present in patients with dermatomyositis and polymyositis have been detected on the basis of their abilities to inhibit the charging of transfer RNAs with their respective amino acids and similarly, antibodies to DNA topoisomerase I and RNA polymerase I (from scleroderma patients) and to pyruvate dehydrogenase E2 (from patients with primary biliary cirrhosis) have been used to demonstrate inhibition of the functions shown in Table 2[9–11]. This property of autoantibodies should be distinguished from antibodies derived experimentally by immunization with purified antigens. Many experimentally induced antibodies to these antigens are reactive with epitopes revealed only on denatured proteins, and are incapable of inhibiting function[12]. On the other hand, autoantibodies obtained from patients are often incapable of reacting with denatured antigens but react primarily with antigens in native form, suggesting that the epitopes recognized by many autoantibodies are conformation-dependent. These and other features have suggested that autoantibodies are reacting with epitopes which are the active sites or

Table 2 Autoantibodies inhibiting function of subcellular particles

Autoantibody to	*Function inhibited*
PCNA (proliferating cell nuclear antigen)	DNA polymerase delta-regulated DNA replication
Sm/U1 ribonucleoproteins	Splicing of pre-mRNA
Ribosomal P0, P1 and P2 proteins	mRNA translation
tRNA synthetases (Jo-1, PL7, PL-12)	Charging of tRNAs with His, Thr and Ala
DNA topoisomerase I	Changing DNA topology or relaxing supercoil
RNA polymerase I	28S and 18S rRNA synthesis
Pyruvate dehydrogenase E2	Binding of lipoic acid to mitochondrial enzymes

functional domains of antigens and that the immunogen driving the autoimmune response may be an activated form of the subcellular particle[13].

AUTOIMMUNE PHENOMENA IN HEPATOCELLULAR CARCINOMA AND OTHER MALIGNANCIES

Recently, we have been interested in antinuclear antibodies (ANAs) which have been found in patients with hepatocellular carcinoma (HCC) and other malignancies. HCC is a well-studied form of liver cancer and arises primarily in patients with chronic liver disease such as chronic hepatitis or liver cirrhosis[14]. By immunofluorescence microscopy it was shown that patients with HCC and other malignancies display a variety of ANAs which react with components in the nucleoplasm and nucleolus. The initial studies focused on defining the molecular identity of nucleolar antigens recognized by ANAs in cancer patients[15]. A spectrum of nucleolar fluorescence was identified which demonstrated characteristics previously described for certain nucleolar antigens associated with autoimmune diseases (Fig. 1). In frame A, patient W.K. had an antibody which reacted in a distinctive fashion with condensed chromosomes in a metaphase cell. In frame B, patient I.I. had antibodies which reacted with the nucleolus organizer region in a mitotic cell, and in frame C the anti-nucleolar antibody reacted only with interphase nucleoli in a homogeneous morphological pattern. The sera were further analysed in Western blot immunoassays as well as other studies, and were shown to be autoantibodies which reacted with fibrillarin (a 34 kDa component of U3-RNP), NOR-90 protein (doublets of 93 and 89 kDa) and nucleophosmin, also known as protein B23, a 37 kDa protein localized to the granular regions of the nucleolus (Fig. 2). We have now defined the reactivities of anti-nucleolar antibodies from five patients – three with HCC, one with adenocarcinoma of the lung and one with dysgerminoma. The results are depicted in Table 3.

It can be seen by referring to Table 1 that the antigens fibrillarin and NOR-90 had been previously described in patients with the autoimmune disease scleroderma. These patients with HCC were not known clinically to have any features of scleroderma.

These studies have shown that autoimmune phenomena manifested by the production of autoantibodies to intracellular components can be demonstrated in certain other diseases such as in some patients with cancer. These and other studies show that the stimulus which drives the autoimmune response is not disease-specific, although it might be observed predominantly in one disease and only occasionally in others. Many of these observations further support the notion that autoantibody responses are antigen-driven and that the immunogen is a subcellular particle. As discussed earlier, these subcellular particles are engaged in important cellular functions associated with cell activation, proliferation or mitosis. In addition to the functions of U3-RNP particles and the nucleolus organizer region described in Table 1, nucleophosmin or protein B23 has been implicated in mitogenic functions associated with the nucleolus.

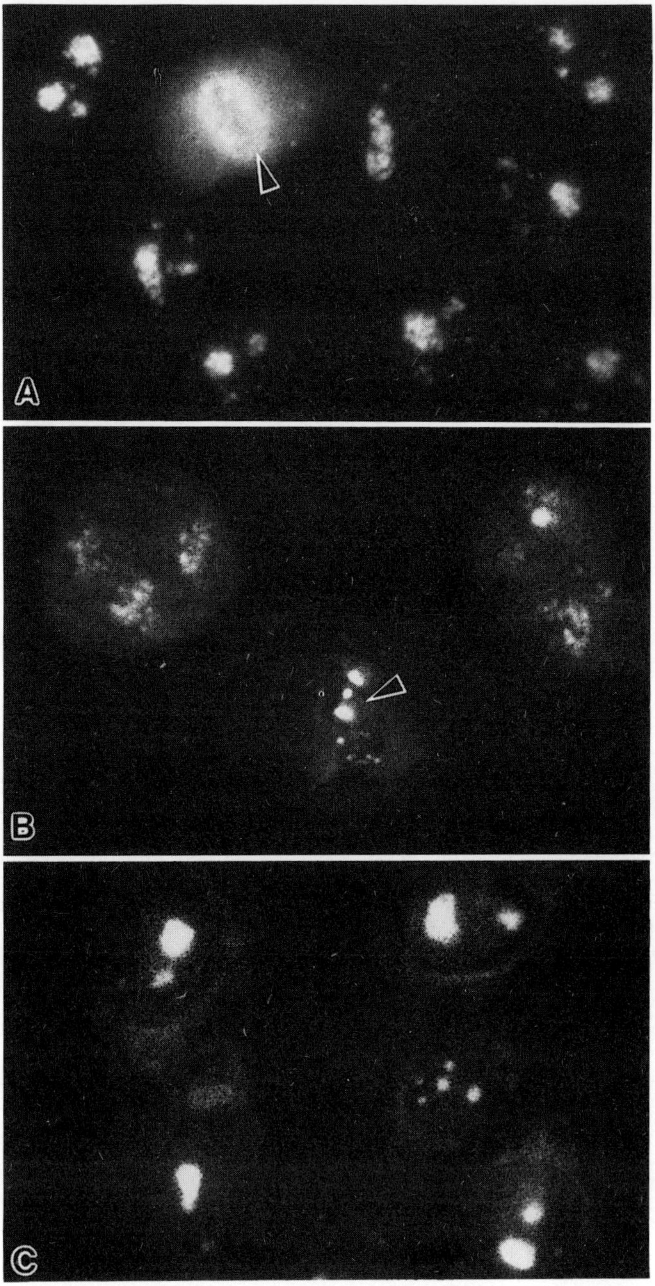

Fig. 1 Indirect immunofluorescence microscopy on HEp-2 cells was used to demonstrate anti-nucleolar antibodies in three patients with hepatocellular carcinoma. **A**: Patient W.K. with autoantibody to fibrillarin showed a clumpy nucleolar pattern with staining around condensed chromosomes in a metaphase cell (arrowhead). **B**: Patient I.I. with autoantibody to NOR-90 showed speckled nucleolar staining with smaller condensed dots depicting staining of NORs in a metaphase cell (arrowhead). **C**: Homogeneous nucleolar staining demonstrated by patient W.S., with autoantibody to protein B23. Weaker staining of the nuclear membrane and cytoplasm may be related to other autoantibodies present in this serum. (× 800)

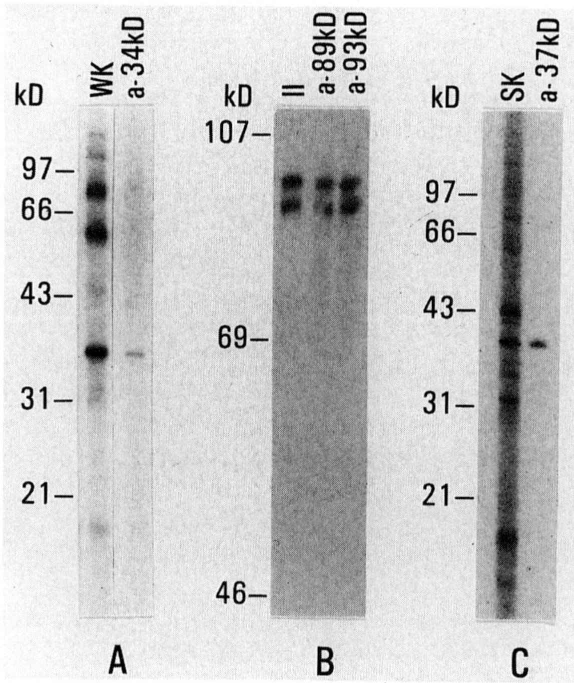

Fig. 2 Affinity-purified antibodies from specific bands on Western blots were used to show reactions. **A**: Whole serum W.K. demonstrated several bands against HEp-2 cell nuclear extract. Affinity-purified antibody from the 34 kDa band reacted only with this band in the whole nuclear extract. **B**: Lane I.I. shows reactivity of whole serum. Affinity-purified antibody from either the 89 kDa or 93 kDa band showed reactivity with both bands of this doublet, suggesting a shared epitope between the proteins. **C**: Serum S.K. also showed multiple reactivities but affinity-purified antibody from the 37 kDa band reacted only with this protein and no other antigens in the nuclear extract.

Table 3 Clinical data and antibody specificities in five cancer patients with antinucleolar antibodies

				Antibodies to cellular antigens Western blotting – M_r (kDa)	
Patient	*Sex*	*Age*	*Diagnosis*	*Identified*	*Unidentified*
W.K.	M	52	HCC	34 (fibrillarin)	56,80,99
I.I.	M	52	HCC	93/89 (NOR90)	
W.S.	M	45	HCC	37 (B23)	57
S.K.	M	70	Lung adenocarcinoma	37 (B23)	41
T.H.	F	65	Dysgerminoma	37 (B23)	

Currently, we are continuing studies to define the identity of other intracellular antigens which are targets of autoantibodies in HCC with the hypothesis that other activated intracellular particles might also be the target antigens. Defining the structure, and where possible the function, of such antigens might provide clues to intracellular proteins which are activated or enhanced in the process of malignant transformation. In this context, autoantibodies should be regarded as manifestations of an autoimmune reaction and as reporters of intracellular molecules involved in cellular activation.

Acknowledgements

This is publication No. 7617MEM of The Scripps Research Institute. Supported by NIH grants AR32063, CA56956 and AR41803.

References

1. Tan EM. Antinuclear antibodies: diagnostic markers for autoimmune diseases and probes for cell biology. Adv Immunol. 1989;44:93–151.
2. Tan EM. Autoantibodies in pathology and cell biology. Cell. 1991;67:841–2.
3. Kass S, Tyc K, Steitz JA, Sollner-Webb B. The U3 small nucleolar ribonucleoprotein functions in the first step of preribosomal RNA processing. Cell. 1990;60:897–908.
4. Chan EKL, Imai H, Hamel JC, Tan EM. Human autoantibody to RNA polymerase I transcription factor hUBF. Molecular identity of nucleolus organizer region autoantigen NOR-90 and ribosomal RNA transcription upstream binding factor. J Exp Med. 1991;174:1239–44.
5. Jantzen HM, Admon A, Bell SB, Tjian R. Nucleolar transcription factor hUBF contains a DNA-binding motif with homology to HMG proteins. Nature (Lond). 1990;344:830–4.
6. Ochs RL, Press RI. Centromere autoantigens are associated with the nucleolus. Exp Cell Res. 1992;20:339–50.
7. Prelich G, Stillman B. Coordinated leading and lagging strand synthesis during SV40 DNA replication *in vitro* requires PCNA. Cell. 1988;53:117–26.
8. Maniatis T, Reed R. The role of small nuclear ribonucleoprotein particles in pre-mRNA splicing. Nature (Lond). 1987;325:673–8.
9. Shero JH, Bordwell B, Rothfield NF, Earnshaw WC. Autoantibodies to topoisomerase I are found in sera from scleroderma patients. Science. 1986;231:737–40.
10. Reimer G, Rose KM, Scheer U, Tan EM. Autoantibody to RNA polymerase I in scleroderma sera. J Clin Invest. 1987;79:65–72.
11. Surh CD, Ahmed-Ansari A, Gershwin ME. Comparative epitope mapping of murine monoclonal and human autoantibodies to human PDH-E2, the major mitochondrial autoantigen of primary biliary cirrhosis. J Immunol. 1990;144:2647–52.
12. Huff JP, Roos G, Peebles CL, Houghten R, Sullivan KF, Tan EM. Insights into native epitopes of proliferating cell nuclear antigen using recombinant DNA protein products. J Exp Med. 1990;172:419–29.
13. Tan EM, Chan EKL, Sullivan KF, Rubin RL. Antinuclear antibodies (ANAs): Diagnostically specific immune markers and clues toward the understanding of systemic autoimmunity. Clin Immunol Immunopathol. 1988;47:121–41.
14. Popper H, Shafritz DA, Hoofnagle JH. Relation of the hepatitis B virus carrier state to hepatocellular carcinoma. Hepatology. 1987;7:764–72.
15. Imai H, Ochs RL, Kiyosawa K, Furuta S, Nakamura RM, Tan EM. Nucleolar antigens and autoantibodies in hepatocellular carcinoma and other malignancies. Am J Pathol. 1992;140:859–70.

19
Applications of molecular biology to the analysis of autoantigens

K. F. SULLIVAN

INTRODUCTION

Autoimmune diseases, both systemic and organ-specific, often present a humoral component in the form of circulating antibodies directed against normal self proteins[1]. In many instances these autoantibodies may be direct mediators of pathological processes, such as the anti-acetylcholine receptor antibodies of myasthenia gravis[2]. In other instances, however, the relationship of the B cell autoimmune response to the disease is unclear. What is clear in many systemic autoimmune diseases and autoimmune liver syndromes is that B cell responses can be very specific, focused on one or a few antigens. For diseases of unknown aetiology and pathological mechanism, characteristic autoantibody responses can be important diagnostic features and may represent the only feature of the disease amenable to focused experimental attack[3]. It has become possible, with advances in molecular cloning methodologies, to directly isolate cDNA clones that encode the autoantigens. This has moved our understanding of autoantibody responses from the phenomenological level to the molecular level, where it is possible to create reagents and experimental systems for dissection of the autoantibody response and analysis of the underlying biological systems targeted as autoantigens. Further, the ability to generate pure autoantigens using recombinant protein expression technology promises the development of serological diagnostic techniques that are based on defined molecular interactions. This chapter will examine the core technologies that have been used for molecular cloning and characterization of autoantigens, in theory and in practice, and some of the applications of recombinant proteins in autoimmune disease research.

Expression cloning was first applied to isolation of autoantigens in the laboratories of Keene[4] and Pederson[5] in 1985, who cloned human cDNAs encoding RNP antigens recognized by lupus sera. These original reports documented the utility of cloned autoantigens for diagnostic autoantibody determination, for molecular analysis of autoimmune epitopes and as tools for molecular characterization of autoimmune processes. These methods have been applied to the molecular analysis of numerous autoantigens in the ensuing years[6,7] and this volume contains current reports on many autoantigens of interest in hepatic disease.

METHODS

In order to isolate a recombinant DNA molecule representing a sequence of specific interest it is necessary to have a library of recombinant molecules to screen, and an assay system that allows one to detect a clone of interest. Prior to development of expression cloning methods, the only generally applicable way to screen libraries of recombinant DNA molecules was by hybridization with nucleic acid probes. This limited the range of sequences that could be cloned to those for which a probe could be physically isolated, such as naturally abundant mRNAs coding for histones[8] or cytoskeletal proteins[9], or mRNAs expressed as in specialized systems such as the globins in reticulocytes[10] and immunoglobulins in myelomas[11]. A second approach, independent of the ability to isolate a probe from a natural source, required at least partial knowledge of the amino acid sequence of a protein. The sequence of the DNA required to encode a peptide sequence can be calculated by 'back-translation' using the genetic code, and an oligonucleotide of this sequence can be chemically synthesized for use as a probe[12]. These approaches required considerable knowledge of the protein mRNA of interest, and thus limited molecular cloning to fairly well characterized proteins.

Expression cloning

The technique of expression cloning was perfected in the early 1980s with the introduction of the vector λgt11 by Young and Davis[13]. In expression cloning the transcription and translation apparatus of the host bacterial cell is used to synthesize proteins encoded by recombinant DNA segments. This allows for selection of clones on the basis of the properties of the encoded polypeptide rather than the nucleic acid sequence. The λgt11 vector combined the biological properties of two extensively studied systems, the *lac* operon and bacteriophage λ, to provide a general and experimentally straightfoward approach to the isolation of molecular clones based on assays for the encoded polypeptides (Fig. 1). The greatest utility of this system has been isolation of clones using antibodies, but more recently functional properties of the expressed polypeptide have been used to assay for specific recombinants, as in the isolation of specific DNA binding proteins, for example[14].

The principles of cloning with λgt11 are based on the biological properties of the vector components and are outlined in Fig. 1. Three important features provide for the synthesis and detection of polypeptides encoded by exogenous DNA: the regulated activity of the *E. coli lac* operon, the placement of the cloning site within the coding sequence of a bacterial gene, *lac*Z, and the lytic life cycle of phage λ. Regulation of recombinant protein expression by

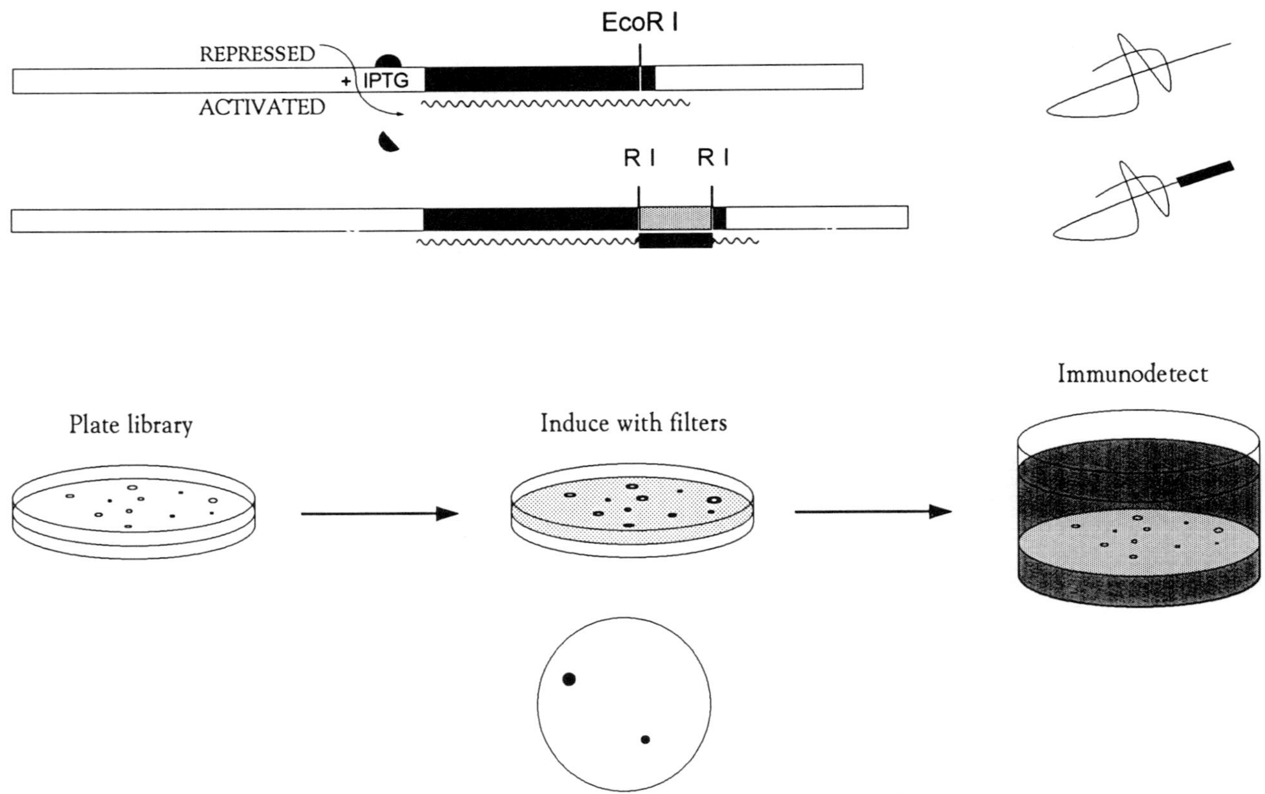

Fig. 1 Diagrammatic illustration of expression cloning with λgt11. The structure of the vector is shown at the top, showing the regulated *lac* operator, *lac*Z gene (black) and the Eco RI cloning site at the 3′ end of the *lac*Z gene. The wavy line beneath indicates mRNA transcribed in the presence of IPTG and the polypeptide is symbolized at the right. A recombinant molecule containing inserted DNA is shown below. The insert sequence is transcribed with the *lac*Z gene and, as indicated at the right, is translated as a fusion protein. At the foot, the screening process is illustrated. Phages are plated on a bacterial lawn and allowed to form. Nitrocellulose filters impregnated with a solution

the *lac* operator is essential for the construction and propagation of representative libraries. Certain eukaryotic proteins are toxic when expressed in bacteria. Using a constitutive expression system the sequences encoding these proteins cannot be isolated, since the bacteria expressing them are not viable. The *lac* operator regulates the expression of genes required for metabolism of lactose and represents one of the most thoroughly understood genetic regulatory systems[15]. λgt11 contains a segment of the *lac* operon, including the *lac* promoter and the *lacZ* gene, the structural gene encoding *E. coli* β-galactosidase. Transcription from the *lac* promoter is repressed by endogenous *lac* repressor under normal physiological conditions and can be specifically induced with a synthetic derivative of lactose, isopropyl-β-thiogalactopyranoside (IPTG). Induction results in the synthesis and translation of mRNA from the *lacZ* gene. The cloning site for foreign DNA is a unique Eco RI restriction endonuclease recognition site engineered into the *lacZ* gene so that recombinant peptides are fused to the coding region of the bacterial polypeptide. Recombinant sequences are thus expressed as fusion proteins containing 115 kDa of β-galactosidase linked at the N-terminus of the insert polypeptide. Expression of foreign genes as fusion proteins obviates the need to engineer protein translation initiation signals and stabilizes the foreign polypeptides within the *E. coli* cytoplasm. Thus, adaptation of the *lac* operon provides a means for regulated expression of even fragments of proteins encoded by cloned exogenous DNA sequences. Finally, the life cycle of phage λ results in lysis of the bacterial host to form a plaque on a bacterial lawn that contains the cytoplasmic contents of the host cells in addition to replicated bacteriophage. This delivers the expressed proteins in the medium in a form that allows sampling by adsorption onto nitrocellulose filters, which are then processed for immunodetection by standard techniques. λgt11 combines a well-characterized bacterial expression system with the advantages of lytic phage vector to provide a generally applicable approach to cloning genetic sequences on the basis of the properties of their encoded protein products.

Since the introduction of λgt11, a number of modified vectors have been introduced. One important modification has been the introduction of directional cloning methods[16]. In the original procedure, cDNA was cloned in a random orientation with respect to the *lacZ* gene because Eco RI restriction endonuclease recognition sites were added to both ends of the cDNA by ligation of synthetic linkers, synthetic oligonucleotide restriction recognition sequences. As a result, any given sequence could be inserted in any of six translational reading frames within the *lacZ* gene, three in the correct orientation 5′ to 3′ and three in the opposite orientation, so that only 1/6 cDNAs are capable of expressing the correct protein. With directional cloning the primer used to initiate cDNA synthesis, at the 3′ end of mRNA, contains a restriction endonuclease recognition site. After cDNA synthesis a second, different restriction site is added by linker ligation. When digested with both restriction enzymes the resulting cDNA possesses two different termini. The phage also possesses both restriction sites oriented so that the cDNA is inserted in the proper orientation within the *lacZ* gene. In the resulting libraries, 1/3 of cDNAs are theoretically capable of expressing protein.

Obtaining a cDNA library that is suitable for a given experimental purpose is an important consideration. It is crucial to choose a library prepared from a cell or tissue type known to express the protein of interest. Many autoantigens are expressed in a variety of cell types, so this is not a critical consideration. A large number of cDNA libraries, representing a variety of human tissue and cell types as well as other species, can be obtained commercially from companies such as Stratagene (La Jolla, CA) and Clontech (Palo Alto, CA). In addition, individual researchers will generally make libraries available to colleagues, referred to as the 'clone by phone' approach. The widespread commercialization of methodologies in kit format has rendered even complex experimental procedures that once required considerable expertise, such as mRNA isolation or cDNA synthesis, into simple and reproducible procedures. Thus, the major empirical methodological consideration in cDNA library construction is the selection of biological starting material.

Sera

Almost any well-characterized serum or immunoglobulin preparation can be used to screen a library, provided that certain constraints are met. The serum should be as specific for the antigen of interest as possible, to simplify identification of clones. The serum should not react with *E. coli* proteins, or should be preadsorbed with an *E. coli* lysate prior to use. Finally, it is nearly essential that the serum works in an immunoblot, with SDS-denatured antigen, to facilitate characterization of the cloned antigen. Since the screening process is fairly large scale, there must be sufficient serum available to provide 50–100 ml of working serum dilution for detection. This need not be a large amount if the serum is of sufficiently high titre; we have carried out cloning and characterization projects using serum samples as small as 400 μl.

Characterization of clones

Once a clone is isolated it must be critically characterized to verify its relationship with the autoantigen. An important methodological aspect of cDNA cloning, discussed above, is the random insertion of cDNA into the cloning site. Only a minor subset of sequences will be inserted in frame, capable of expression of bona-fide cDNA-encoded polypeptide sequences. A great deal of the library will express peptide sequences derived from nonsense reading frames. It is possible that random peptides may present crossreactive epitopes in the library that have no biological relevance. As a result it is particularly important to be able to characterize the identity of the cloned autoantigen using criteria other than crossreactivity with the original selecting serum. There are several approaches to this. If the antigen is a protein for which amino acid sequence data are known, it can be identified on the basis of sequence[17]. Another approach is to generate experimental antibodies using the recombinant fusion protein[18]. While it is possible that a random peptide sequence may crossreact with an antibody, it is exceedingly unlikely that two such random epitopes would be linked on a single polypeptide, so demonstrating that the cloned antigen and the cellular antigen share two or more primary structural epitopes is convincing demonstration of identity. Similarly, peptide mapping can be used to examine the relationship between expressed recombinant protein and the cellular antigen[19]. A supporting approach is to correlate reactivity of the cloned protein with a panel of sera, to determine whether it is specifically associated with a characteristic autoantibody[17,19–20].

Recombinant protein expression systems

A major application for cloned autoantigen sequences is to produce protein products for immunological, biochemical and molecular analysis. While protein expression technology is continually advancing, essentially two methods have been used for most experiments with expressed antigens. Expression *in vitro* is possible using vectors that contain bacteriophage promoters for efficient *in-vitro* transcription of synthetic mRNA[21]. *In-vitro* translation, generally in rabbit reticulocyte lysate[22], can be used to provide small amounts of radiolabelled proteins. Protein translated *in vitro* is sufficient for analysis by immunoprecipitation, peptide mapping and, in some instances, function. *In-vitro* expression also allows rapid and easy dissection of proteins by generation of nested C-terminal deletions[23]. *In-vitro* transcription requires linear DNA templates, which are prepared by restriction endonuclease digestion to form molecules with unique, defined termini. If a cDNA is linearized at a site within the coding region, the corresponding synthetic mRNA will be truncated and, upon translation, peptide synthesis will terminate at that point. Thus, a series of molecules with defined C-terminal ends can be prepared. This has been useful for mapping epitopes and functional regions of autoantigens (e.g. ref. 23). A methodological limitation of the *in-vitro* translation system is that the sequence must contain a proper ribosome initiation site for translation, and so it is technically much more difficult to perform the complementary experiment of N-terminal deletions. Nevertheless, it is possible to introduce these sequences easily by PCR[24] or *in-vitro* mutagenesis[25], allowing essentially any specific peptide fragment to be translated *in vitro*.

The second approach is *in-vivo* expression in an exogenous host, usually bacteria. This method has been the workhorse for molecular analysis of a great many proteins, the autoantigens included, and an array of systems has been developed with specialized properties to suit specific applications. A few of these are listed in Table 1. The methodological principles are essentially the same in each, e.g. the vectors contain a cloning site or sites within the coding region of a bacterial gene and expression of the hybrid gene is regulated experimentally using highly characterized gene regulatory systems of *E. coli*. The differences between systems that lead to suitability for different types of experiments are in the regulatory properties of the expression unit,

Table 1 Vector systems for protein expression in bacteria

Vector	*Fusion partner*	*Properties*	*Ref.*
pATH	*trp*E	First inducible vector system with multiple frame polylinker	27
pET	T7 gene 10	Highly regulated, highly inducible, ATG cloning site for non-fusion protein expression	28
pGEX	Glutathione-*S*-transferase	Fusion with GST for purification by glutathione affinity chromatography	29
pUC, pBluescript	*β*-Galactosidase	Widely available, inducible	13

the functionality of the fusion partner and the availability and distribution of cloning sites within the bacterial coding region. Expression of *β*-galactosidase fusion proteins is common because *λ*gt11 is a primary cloning vector, so the first recombinant polypeptide that becomes available during a cloning project is a > 115 kDa *β*-galactosidase fusion protein. In addition, many cloning vectors incorporate the *α*-peptide of *β*-galactosidase for use as an indicator in cloning experiments[26]. Thus, fusion proteins can be prepared in a number of common vectors that contain a small amount of amino terminal *β*-galactosidase sequence. Commercially available monoclonal antibodies are available that allow affinity purification or immunodetection of fusion proteins through the *β*-galactosidase fusion partner.

The pATH vector system[27] was the first widely used multi-frame vector system, incorporating the *trp* operator for regulation and the *trp*E gene as a fusion partner. Cloning for expression requires that the translational reading frame of the fusion partner and the fusion target be matched, otherwise expression would lead to production of a nonsense polypeptide. The multi-frame vector system incorporates multiple plasmids that have cloning sites offset from one another with respect to the translational reading frame of the fusion partner. The result is that specific restriction endonuclease sites are available in each of three possible translational phases, and so there is no barrier to expressing any sequence bounded by an available restriction site. This property has made pATH an ideal system for epitope mapping, discussed below, because essentially any element of a protein coding sequence can be expressed as a fusion with a uniform fusion partner.

The pET vector system[28] is optimized for high levels of expression coupled with very tight regulation, to allow even highly toxic proteins to be expressed in bacteria. It depends on elements of bacteriophage T7 which are optimized for high levels of protein synthesis during the short time of phage replication in *E. coli* cells. A phage-encoded RNA polymerase recognizes a phage-specific promoter sequence that regulates the genes of bacteriophage T7. The expression system combines these in the form of a complementary host and plasmid combination. Suitable hosts contain a copy of the T7 RNA polymerase gene integrated into the bacterial genome and under the genetic control of the *lac* promoter. Expression plasmids contain a copy of the structural gene, gene 10, that is transcribed by T7 RNA polymerase at very high rates to achieve high levels of mRNA in induced cells. T7 gene 10 contains a natural recognition site for the restriction endonuclease Nde1 which recognizes a sequence, CATATG, spanning the ATG codon for translation initiation. This allows foreign proteins to be expressed as non-fusion proteins, sharing only the universal initiator methionine residue with T7 gene 10, but utilizing the efficient upstream signals for ribosome binding. Thus, T7 gene 10 is a natural donor of transcription and translation signals, providing a free open reading frame optimized for translation initiation. Proteins can also be expressed as traditional fusions with the pET vector system. The system has been thoroughly developed to provide a variety of fusion partners of varying functionality, incorporating secretion signals, affinity tags and 'restriction' protease cleavage sites to allow separation of a eukaryotic peptide from its fusion partner after purification.

The second major aspect of the T7 system is an extensive set of biological reagents for maintaining low levels of endogenous expression. The host system has, as described above, an integrated copy of the T7 RNA polymerase gene that is regulated by the *lac* promoter. However, small amounts of expression, promoter leakage, occur in the absence of induction, allowing synthesis of a tiny amount of T7 RNA polymerase. RNA synthesis due to this leakage is suppressed by inclusion of natural inhibitors of T7 RNA polymerase function in the host or by use of a hybrid promoter that contains the *lac* repressor binding sequence coupled to the T7 promoter. This promoter is nearly leakproof, since the hybrid T7-*lac* promoter must be de-repressed in order to be transcribed. This extensive system of regulators allows the handling of proteins that are toxic to bacteria. Taken together, this system provides high levels of protein production through the use of phage gene expression mechanisms, allowing eukaryotic proteins to be expressed as up to 50% of total bacterial protein.

The purification of fusion proteins is often a limiting methodological step, and a great many experiments are performed using only crude bacterial lysates. While this is sufficient for many purposes, the availability of purified protein for biochemical analysis is always advantageous. To overcome the need for empirical determination of protein purification strategy for individual fusion proteins, the pGEX system was developed[29]. This vector utilizes the gene for Sj26, a 26 kDa glutathione *S*-transferase (GST; EC2.5.1.18) encoded by the parasitic helminth *Schistosoma japonicum*, as the fusion partner. Fusion proteins produced in this way are generally soluble and can be purified in a single step by affinity chromatography on immobilized glutathione. The vectors also contain recognition sites for highly specific proteases thrombin or factor Xa, allowing the expressed polypeptide to be removed from the GST fusion partner. The primary advantage of this system is the rapid and uniform purification strategy that can be applied to yield consistent preparations of a variety of expressed proteins.

Protein expression technology is one of the primary areas of development in molecular biotechnology and is continually being refined, adapted and extended for new applications or improvement of old ones. A major advance has been the development of the high-level insect cell expression system based on baculovirus as a cloning vector[30]. These advances will continue, refining our ability to manipulate eukaryotic proteins in exogenous biological environments. The basic principles and major approaches to important technological aspects of expression are, however, adequately represented by the cross-section of systems described above. The facility of recombinant protein expression has freed the investigator to focus on applications of the technology rather than implementation of the technology itself.

APPLICATIONS OF CLONED AUTOANTIGENS

Diagnostic antibody detection

For a number of systemic autoimmune diseases as well as hepatic diseases, the presence of characteristic autoantibodies in patient sera is a valuable diagnostic feature[1]. For example, autoantibodies to cytochrome P450 proteins are characteristic of idiopathic autoimmune hepatitis and also of acute, drug-induced hepatitis and their detection helps in distinguishing these syndromes from other non-viral inflammatory liver diseases[31]. Previously, identification of these autoantibodies has relied on immunofluorescence microscopy[32]. While this is the traditional assay method for many autoantibodies, the procedure is labour-intensive, requires interpretation by skilled personnel and, ultimately, provides a very low-resolution analysis of antibody specificity. The availability of recombinant fusion proteins provides a means for accurate, objective and methodologically simple determination of autoantibodies in patient sera. Thus Manns and coworkers[17] used immunoblot analysis with bacterially expressed fusion proteins to identify anti-LKM-1 autoantibodies in patient sera. This assay provided greater sensitivity than the immunofluorescence assay alone. Similarly, sera from patients with primary biliary cirrhosis react specifically with cloned mitochondrial antigens shown to be dihydrolipoamide acetyltransferases[20,33]. Use of recombinant peptides from two related antigens, the dihydrolipoamide acetyltransferases of pyruvate dehydrogenase and of branched-chain α-keto acid dehydrogenase, in an enzyme-linked immunoassay allowed detection of $> 95\%$ of patients with primary biliary cirrhosis with no false-positive results from among 124 control sera[34]. It is clear from these and other studies with autoantigens from a diverse group of autoimmune diseases that the use of expressed recombinant antigens has significant potential for development of simple, standardized, quantitative assays for detection of autoantibodies in patient sera[35].

Application of recombinant protein-based immunodiagnostic assays for autoantibodies has yet to be developed for routine clinical use. One of the barriers to commercialization of this technology is the rarity of autoimmune syndromes and the correspondingly small population of patients that require diagnosis at this level for any given disease. An approach that may overcome this limitation is to develop immunodiagnostic panels that contain reagents capable of detecting multiple antibodies. For example, a hepatic serodiagnostic panel could include viral antigens as well as specific autoantigens. Such a test would be informative for a number of different diseases, obviating the need to develop independent diagnostic systems for rare syndromes and distributing the cost of diagnosis across a larger patient population. Further, a multiparameter assay may prove useful for long-term correlative studies of immune system activity in hepatic disease.

Epitope mapping

Another major area of investigation that has been greatly stimulated by the availability of cloned autoantigens is analysis of the epitopes targeted by autoantibodies. This work is motivated by several objectives, both research-oriented and practically oriented. A significant unknown for most autoimmunity is the immunological stimulus that elicits autoimmune response. Are autoantibodies crossreactive antibodies elicited by pathogens, or are they primarily directed at the antigens themselves? Are there any distinguishing features of the types of structures targeted by autoantibodies? How are autoantibodies related to the disease process? A practical goal in identifying epitopes is to develop very sensitive and selective reagents for antibody detection. These experiments are facilitated by the relative ease with which molecular structures can be dissected and modified using molecular biological techniques. This has provided a fairly uniform methodology for structure–activity analysis of the interaction of antigen with antibody.

Three major methods provide a pathway for analysis of the structure of epitopes down to the level of individual amino acids. These are deletion-type experiments, in which defined segments of a protein are specifically expressed by methods discussed above; direct chemical peptide synthesis, which allows the production of peptides of defined sequence; and mutagenesis experiments, in which the role of individual amino acids can be tested by specific alteration. A review of results obtained by molecular autoepitope analysis is beyond the scope of this chapter, but it is of value to examine selected experiments to understand the logic of the experimental approach and some of the important findings that may be of general importance. In addition, other chapters in this volume detail recent results with specific autoantigens of interest for hepatic disease.

One of the hypotheses regarding the generation of autoantibodies is that the original autoimmune response is initiated by a foreign agent – a pathogen or foreign compound – and that the autoimmune reaction is a byproduct of 'molecular mimicry', a putative structural relationship between the eliciting agent and a normal cellular protein[36]. One way to evaluate the potential for molecular mimicry is to determine whether an autoepitope bears a primary structural relationship with any known pathogens. A major epitope of the LKM-1 autoantigen cytochrome P450 IID6 was mapped to a short linear peptide segment using a combination of bacterially expressed fusion proteins and synthetic peptides[37]. Within the epitope is a hexapeptide sequence identical to a segment of the IE175 protein of HSV-1 as well as elements with similarity to portions of the HCV polyprotein. Investigation of the significance of these findings is under way, and this could contribute to our understanding of the aetiology of idiopathic autoimmune hepatitis.

An important finding based on epitope analysis has been the clear demonstration that the cellular antigen is the immunogen in elicitation of autoantibodies in at least some systems. This conclusion is based on the demonstration of polyclonal autoimmune responses against centromere antigens[38] and lamin B[39]. Further, the fact that many autoimmune responses are directed at multiple components of supramolecular assemblies argues strongly that the immune system sees endogenous antigen[1]. Nevertheless, it is possible that antigen-specific antibodies represent a secondary immune response initiated by an original crossreactive antibody that, by formation of immune complex, targeted the fortuitous self-antigen for further immune attack (see N. R. Rose, this volume). Clearly, the use of cloned autoantigens will contribute to our further understanding of the genesis of autoantibodies.

The structures of the epitopes recognized by autoantibodies appear to be correlated with functionally important segments of autoantigens. Analysis of the epitopes recognized by the anti-mitochondrial acetyltransferases of primary biliary cirrhosis revealed that they correspond to relatively large segments ($\sim$75–100 residues) of the conserved lipoate binding domains of these proteins[40]. Functional analysis demonstrated that many human autoantisera inhibit the catalytic function of the acetyltransferases[41]. Similarly, autoantibodies against cytochrome P450 IID6 inhibit the function of the protein[42]. In both cases the relatively large peptide sequence required for optimal reactivity with antibodies suggests that some elements of structure are required beyond the primary sequence level. Analysis of epitopes recognized by autoantibodies against PCNA was carried out using three different types of reagents: a series of C-terminal deletion products prepared by *in-vitro* translation and assayed by immunoprecipitation; bacterial fusion proteins representing amino terminal deletions and internal segments of the polypeptide were analysed by western blotting; and a set of overlapping 15-mer peptides used in ELISA assays[23]. This work revealed that, unlike monoclonal antibodies to PCNA, the short linear peptide segments were unreactive with autoantibodies. Rather, a majority of sera were unreactive even in western blot, although all reacted with *in-vitro* translated protein by immunoprecipitation. The data are consistent with a single immunodominant region in the centre of the molecule that elicits primarily conformation-sensitive antibodies. Like the cytochrome P450 and mitochondrial acetyltransferase antibodies described above, autoantibodies to PCNA inhibit the function of the protein[43]. Thus it appears that autoantibodies are often directed against higher order – 2° and 3° – structural components of proteins, and that these often correspond to essential functional components of autoantigens.

One practical endpoint of these investigations is the development of reagents for autoantibody detection that will be useful in the clinical setting. By understanding the details of autoantibody reactivity it will be possible to develop optimized detection systems. A creative example of this strategy is the construction of a chimeric fusion protein that incorporates epitopes from two different mitochondrial acetyltransferases which, together, allow accurate determination of anti-mitochondrial antibodies in patients with primary biliary cirrhosis using an enzyme-linked immunoassay[44].

SUMMARY

Analysis of autoantigens has been a central element in the description and diagnosis of many human diseases and hepatic diseases in particular. The application of molecular biological methods and strategies has advanced the state of the art from morphological description of the structures containing autoantigens to molecular description of the genes that encode them. Identification of the molecules targeted in autoimmunity has been important for development of experimental approaches to analysing the autoimmune process and of reagents and assay systems that improve the ability to diagnose autoimmune disease. By understanding autoantigens at the molecular level it is hoped that clues will be found that provide aetiological links between autoimmune phenomenology and clinical pathology.

References

1. Tan EM. Antinuclear antibodies: diagnostic markers for autoimmune diseases and probes for cell biology. Adv Immunol. 1989;44:93–151.
2. Lindstrom J, Dau P. Biology of myasthenia gravis. Annu Rev Pharmacol Toxicol. 1980;20:337–62.
3. Tan EM, Chan EKL, Sullivan KF, Rubin R. Antinuclear antibodies (ANA); diagnostically specific immune markers and clues towards the understanding of systemic autoimmunity. Clin Immunol Immunopathol. 1988;47:121–30.
4. Chambers JC, Keene JD. Isolation and analysis of cDNA clones expressing human lupus La antigen. Proc Natl Acad Sci USA. 1985;82:2115–19.
5. Wieben ED, Rohleder AM, Nenninger JM, Pederson T. cDNA cloning of a human autoimmune nuclear ribonucleoprotein antigen. Proc Natl Acad Sci USA. 1985;82:7914–18.
6. Manns MP. Cytoplasmic autoantigens in autoimmune hepatitis: molecular analysis and clinical relevance. Semin Liver Dis. 1991;11:205–14.
7. Leung PS, Gershwin ME. The molecular structure of autoantigens. Curr Opin Immunol. 1989;2:567–75.
8. Kedes LH. Histone genes and histone messengers. Annu Rev Biochem. 1979;48:837–70.
9. Cleveland DW, Lopata MA, MacDonald RJ, Cowan NJ, Rutter WJ, Kirschner MW. Number and evolutionary conservation of α- and β-tubulin and β- and γ-actin genes using specific cloned cDNA probes. Cell. 1980;20:95–105.
10. Lawn RM, Fritsch EF, Parker RC, Blake G, Maniatis T. The isolation and characterization of a linked δ- and β-globulin gene from a cloned library of human DNA. Cell. 1978;15:1157–67.
11. Hozumi N, Tonegawa S. Evidence for somatic rearrangement of immunoglobulin genes coding for variable and constant regions. Proc Natl Acad Sci USA. 1976;73:3628–32.
12. Yang JH, Ye JH, Wallace DC. Computer selection of oligonucleotide probes from amino acid sequences for use in gene library screening. Nucl Acids Res. 1984;12:837–43.
13. Young RA, Davis RW. Efficient isolation of genes by using antibody probes. Proc Natl Acad Sci USA. 1983;80:1194–8.
14. Singh H, LeBowitz JH, Baldwin AS, Sharp PA. Molecular cloning of an enhancer binding protein: Isolation by screening of an expression library with a recognition site DNA. Cell. 1988;52:415–23.
15. Lewin B. Genes IV. Oxford: Oxford University Press; 1990.

16. Palazzolo MJ, Meyerowitz EM. A family of lambda phage cDNA cloning vectors, lambda SWAJ, allowing the amplification of RNA sequences. Gene. 1987;52:197–206.
17. Manns MP, Johnson EF, Griffin KJ, Tan EM, Sullivan KF. Major antigen of liver kidney microsomal autoantibodies in idiopathic autoimmune hepatitis is cytochrome P450dbl. J Clin Invest. 1989;83:1066–72.
18. Earnshaw WC, Sullivan KF, Machlin PS, Cooke CA, Kaiser DA, Pollard TD, Rothfield NF, Cleveland DW. Molecular cloning of cDNA for CENP-B, the major human centromere autoantigen. J Cell Biol. 1987;104:817–29.
19. Ben Chetrit E, Gandy BJ, Tan EM, Sullivan KF. Isolation and characterization of a cDNA clone encoding the 60-kD component of the human SS-A/Ro ribonucleoprotein autoantigen. J Clin Invest. 1989;83:1284–92.
20. Gershwin ME, Mackay IR, Sturgess A, Coppel RL. Identification and specificity of a cDNA encoding the 70 kd mitochondrial antigen recognized in primary biliary cirrhosis. J Immunol. 1987;138:3525–31.
21. Melton DA, Kreig PA, Rebagliati MR, Maniatis T, Zinn K, Green MR. Efficient *in vitro* synthesis of biologically active RNA and RNA hybridization probes from plasmids containing a bacteriophage SP6 promoter. Nucl Acids Res. 1984;12:7057–70.
22. Pelham HRB, Jackson RJ. An efficient mRNA-dependent translation system from reticulocyte lysates. Eur J Biochem. 1976;67:247–56.
23. Huff JP, Roos G, Peebles CL, Houghten R, Sullivan KF, Tan EM. Insights into native epitopes of Proliferating Cell Nuclear Antigen using recombinant DNA protein products. J Exp Med. 1990;172:419–29.
24. Innis MA, Gelfand DH, Sninsky JJ, White TJ (eds.) PCR protocols. San Diego: Academic Press; 1990.
25. McPherson MJ (ed). Directed mutagenesis. A practical approach. Oxford: IRL Press; 1991.
26. Messing J. New M13 vectors for cloning. Methods Enzymol. 1983;101:20–78.
27. Koerner TJ, Hill JE, Myers AM, Tzagoloff A. High-expression vectors with multiple cloning sites for construction of trpE fusion genes: pATH vectors. Methods Enzymol. 1991; 194:477–90.
28. Studier FW, Rosenberg AH, Dunn JJ, Dubendorf JW. Use of T7 RNA polymerase to direct expression of cloned genes. Methods Enzymol. 1990;185:60–89.
29. Smith DB, Johnson KS. Single-step purification of polypeptides expressed in *Escherichia coli* as fusions with glutathione *S*-transferase. Gene. 1988;67:31–40.
30. Summers MD, Smith GE. A manual of methods for baculovirus vectors and insect cell culture procedures. Texas Agricult Exp Sta Bull. 1987;1555.
31. Manns MP, Johnson EF. Identification of human cytochrome P450s as autoantigens. Methods Enzymol. 1991;206:210–20.
32. Rizzeto M, Swana G, Doniach D. Microsomal antibodies in active chronic hepatitis and other disorders. Clin Exp Immunol. 1973;15:331–44.
33. Surh CD, Danner DJ, Ahmed A, Coppel RL, Mackay IR, Dickson ER, Gershwin ME. Reactivity of primary biliary cirrhosis sera with a human fetal liver cDNA clone of branched-chain alpha-keto acid dehydrogenase dihydrolipoamide acyltransferase, the 52 kD mitochondrial autoantigen. Hepatology. 1989;9:63–8.
34. Van de Water J, Cooper A, Surh CD, Coppel R, Danner D, Ansari A, Dickson R, Gershwin ME. Detection of autoantibodies to recombinant mitochondrial proteins in patients with primary biliary cirrhosis. N Engl J Med. 1989;320:1377–80.
35. Williams DG. Recombinant autoantigens. Ann Rheum Dis. 1990;49:445–51.
36. Oldstone MBA. Molecular mimicry and autoimmune disease. Cell. 1987;50:819–20.
37. Manns MP, Griffin KJ, Sullivan KF, Johnson EF. LKM-1 autoantibodies recognize a short linear sequence in P450IID6, a cytochrome P-450 monooxygenase. J Clin Invest. 1991;88:1370–8.
38. Earnshaw WC, Machlin PS, Bordwell BJ, Rothfield NF, Cleveland DW. Analysis of the anticentromere autoantibodies using cloned autoantigen CENP-B. Proc Natl Acad Sci USA. 1987;84:979–83.
39. Chou CH, Reeves WH. Recognition of multiple epitopes in the coiled-coil domain of lamin B by human autoantibodies. Mol Immunol. 1992;29:1055–64.
40. Van der Water J, Gershwin ME, Leung P, Ansari A, Coppel RL. The autoepitope of the

74-kD mitochondrial autoantigen of primary biliary cirrhosis corresponds to the functional site of dihydrolipoamide acetyltransferase. J Exp Med. 1988;167:1791–9.
41. Van de Water J, Fregeau D, Davis P, Ansari A, Danner D, Leung P, Coppel R, Gershwin ME. Autoantibodies of primary biliary cirrhosis recognize dihydrolipoamide acetyltransferase and inhibit enzyme function. J Immunol. 1988;141:2321–4.
42. Manns M, Zanger U, Gerken G, Sullivan KF, Meyer zum Buschenfelde KH, Meyer UA, Eichelbaum M. Patients with type II autoimmune hepatitis express functionally intact cytochrome P-450 db1 that is inhibited by LKM-1 autoantibodies *in vitro* but not *in vivo*. Hepatology. 1990;12:127–32.
43. Tan C-K, Sullivan KF, Li X, Tan EM, Downey KM, So AS. Autoantibody to the proliferating cell nuclear antigen neutralizes the activity of the auxiliary protein of DNA polymerase delta. Nucl Acids Res. 1987;15:9299–309.
44. Leung PS, Iwayama T, Prindiville T, Chuang DT, Ansari AA, Wynn RM, Dickson R, Coppel R, Gershwin ME. Use of designer recombinant mitochondrial antigens in the diagnosis of primary biliary cirrhosis. Hepatology. 1992;15:367–72.

20
Immunological derangements in autoimmunity

N. R. ROSE

SELF VERSUS NON-SELF

The responsibility of distinguishing self from non-self resides in the populations of lymphocytes, the cells of the body that are specialized for antigen-specific recognition. Some of the mechanisms that have been suggested to explain the tolerance to self on the part of T cells and B cells are given in Table 1.

B-Cell tolerance

With respect to B-cell tolerance we still have very little information on deletional mechanisms. If clonal deletion of B cells takes place it can occur in the bone marrow during the genesis of B cells or in the periphery where predominantly mature B cells are found. Experimental evidence is based primarily on the findings of Nossal, who first described clonal abortion[1]. The encounter of an immature B cell with antigen of prescribed valency and concentration aborts the B cell and thereby prevents the development of an antigen-specific clone. The mechanism has been demonstrated both *in vitro* and *in vivo*. Whether fully matured B cells, as they are found in the peripheral circulation, can be aborted by this mechanism is still an open question.

An alternative mechanism for inducing tolerance at the B-cell level is clonal anergy[2]. Unlike abortion, anergy implies that antigen-specific B cells persist and can be stimulated to proliferate if a non-specific signal is delivered. Non-specific signals include the B-cell-stimulating cytokines. Recent experiments by Goodnow and his colleagues have taken advantage of transgenic mice to show that clonal anergy can be induced by surrogate self-antigens[3]. Anergized B cells can be found in both bone marrow and peripheral circulations.

Like anergy, receptor blockade implies that a B cell binds its respective antigen. Excessive quantities of antigen or their stereochemical arrangement

Table 1 Mechanisms of self tolerance

B-cell tolerance
Clonal deletion in bone marrow
Peripheral deletion
Anergy in bone marrow
Anergy in periphery
Receptor blockade
Suppression by:
T cells
idiotype/anti-idiotype network
Fc-mediated suppression
Absence of T-cell help
T-cell tolerance
Intrathymic negative deletion
Peripheral selection
Anergy
Non-specific immunosuppression:
TGF-β
T_H1 vs T_H2 balance
Specific immunosuppression:
idiotypic
anti-idiotypic

on a backbone or scaffolding prevent B-cell receptors from aggregating and thereby avoid the intracellular signals for antibody synthesis[4]. The classic demonstrations of immunological paralysis due to pneumococcus polysaccharides or soluble L-amino acid polypeptides may also be examples of receptor blockade[5,6].

Active suppression of antibody synthesis by T cells has been demonstrated in a variety of experimental protocols[7]. The subject of T-cell-mediated suppression, however, has remained controversial because of problems in isolating a phenotypically distinct population of T cells with suppressive properties. It seems likely that the same population of T cells can serve as inducers or inhibitors of antibody production depending upon the particular circumstance of their interaction with B cells.

Anti-idiotypic antibodies can also suppress or enhance antibody production depending upon as yet poorly defined conditions[8]. On the one hand, anti-idiotypes can abrogate production of antibodies, but under other conditions anti-idiotypes can serve as immunizing agents.

Antibody production is also regulated by feedback inhibition through the Fc portion of the immunoglobulin molecule[9]. The mechanism depends upon the production of antigen–antibody complexes and binding to the Fc γ-receptor on the B cell.

Even though any or all of the mechanisms described above are in place, B cells reactive with self-antigens are easily identified in peripheral circulation. Such B cells are the source of the low-affinity IgM autoantibodies to many self-antigens found naturally. In the absence of T-cell help the B cells fail to undergo somatic mutation to produce antibodies of higher affinities and fail to undergo class switch to IgG. The presence of these naturally occurring IgM antibodies, therefore, is generally not indicative of autoimmune disease.

T-Cell tolerance

In the case of T cells, clonal deletion in the thymus has been definitively demonstrated[10,11]. The clearest demonstrations have utilized histocompatibility antigens and superantigens, because they delete T cells in a sufficient proportion to be readily measurable. Whether self-antigens induce intrathymic negative selection probably depends upon their presence in the thymus medulla during T-cell generation and their presentation by thymic dendritic cells in conjunction with the appropriate class II major histocompatibility complex (MHC) product.

Some evidence for negative selection of T cells in the periphery has recently been presented; however, it is difficult to distinguish such selection from anergy in which T cells remain in a quiescent state[12]. It is now clear that T cells can be anergized, if they contact antigen 'presented' by fixed macrophages or by lipophilic membranes[13]. In most, but not all, instances the anergy can be overcome by addition of appropriate T-cell stimulating factors such as interleukin-2 (IL-2).

Non-antigen-specific suppression of T cells can readily be demonstrated both in the test tube and the living animal. Perhaps the most potent suppressive factor yet described is transforming growth factor beta (TGF-β)[14]. Its action, however, appears to depend upon the stage in T-cell cycling where it operates.

A great deal of attention has recently been paid to the concept of alternative subpopulations of CD4-helper T cells. T_H1 cells produce such proinflammatory cytokines as IL-2 and interferon-γ (IFN-γ) and mediate cell-mediated immune responses. T_H2 cells produce the B-cell-stimulating cytokines, IL-4, IL-5 and IL-6, and play an important role in antibody production and class switching. The balance of T_H1 and T_H1 subpopulations may itself be determined by the cytokine population present at induction. Therefore, cell-mediated immunity and humoral immunity can be viewed as alternative expressions of the immune response. In terms of many autoimmune disorders, the presence of cell-mediated immunity is often of greater pathological significance than is antibody-mediated immunity.

Finally, the question of antigen-specific immunosuppression arises in explaining T-cell tolerance. One proposal is the generation of a specialized population of regulatory T cells during induction of the immune response. These regulatory T cells may recognize the same or different epitopes on the immunogenic molecule, but their effect is to prevent the proliferation of other T cells directed to the same antigen[15]. Although there is indirect evidence that such populations of cells exist, a distinct population of suppressor T cells has not been cloned and therefore the issue remains in doubt.

Another possibility is that T cells can be induced to the antigen-specific receptor of other T cells representing an anti-idiotypic or anti-receptor immunity. Such a phenomenon is believed to be the basis of the 'vaccines' composed of inactivated T cells to self-antigens. Under experimental conditions such vaccines have been shown to prevent the development of particular autoimmune diseases[16].

In brief, many mechanisms have been proposed to explain the lack of reactivity to self-antigens on the part of B and T lymphocytes. It is, in fact, likely that more than one mechanism is involved in maintaining self-tolerance. Redundancy is a common feature of the immune response and it is not surprising that a property as important as self-tolerance depends upon a series of defensive mechanisms.

AUTOIMMUNITY VERSUS AUTOIMMUNE DISEASE

Despite the panoply of mechanisms described above, autoimmunity is a relatively common phenomenon. Natural autoantibodies to self-antigens are, as mentioned previously, a feature of all but the most severely immunologically crippled animals. Perhaps such naturally occurring autoantibodies serve a physiological function in eliminating effects or sequestered antigens. Natural autoantibodies may also be an early measure of defence against invading microorganisms. Such antibodies are mainly the product of B cells without the benefit of T-cell help.

Many self-reactive T cells are also found normally in healthy individuals. The relative ease with which autoimmunity to self-antigens such as thyroglobulin can be induced is evidence that such self-reactive T cells are available. They may, however, be of relatively low affinity and require the assistance of a potent adjuvant[17]. As an alternative they may require activation by a related crossreactive antigen.

Since both self-reactive B cells and T cells are often present, how can autoimmune disease, a pathogenetic autoimmune response, be defined? Some of the criteria that are useful for recognizing a human autoimmune disease are listed in Table 2.

Primary evidence of autoimmune disease – direct

The first step in establishing a disease as autoimmune in origin is to demonstrate the presence of a relevant immune response. In most cases an autoantibody to the target cell or organ, e.g. the red blood cell in haemolytic anaemia or the thyroid gland in chronic thyroiditis, can be demonstrated[18,19]. Sometimes autoantibodies are present but do not appear to have much relationship with the site of disease. Antibodies to smooth muscle are characteristic of chronic active hepatitis, whereas autoantibodies to mitochondria are often encountered in cases of primary biliary cirrhosis[20,21]. It may take special effort to establish the connection between the particular autoantibody and disease, as in the case of antibody to double-stranded DNA (ds-DNA) in systemic lupus erythematosus, where complexes of antibody and ds-DNA are occasionally found in the kidney[22].

In many autoimmune diseases, cell-mediated immunity is believed to be of greater importance than humoral antibody. In multiple sclerosis there is evidence of T-cell proliferation to myelin basic protein (MBP) in the absence of any demonstrable antibody[23]. It is still not known, however, if MBP is the ‘pathogenic’ antigen in multiple sclerosis.

Table 2 Criteria of autoimmune disease

Primary evidence
Direct
Immunological response to self
antibody-mediated
cell-mediated
Pathogenetic effector mechanism
destruction of target cell
binding to receptor
transfer of disease by antibody
Indirect
Reproduction of disease in experimental animal by immunization with analogous antigen
Genetically determined disease in experimental animal simulating human disease
Secondary evidence
Clinical
Association with other autoimmune diseases
MHC association
Female preponderance
Episodic course
Immunopathological
Depositis of immunoglobulin and complement
Infiltrates of activated T cells
Restricted TCR V-gene usage
Expression of MHC class II determinants

The demonstration of a relevant autoimmune response, humoral or cell-mediated, is only the first step in establishing the autoimmune aetiology of a human disease. The second, and equally critical, requirement is the demonstration of an effect of autoimmunity in the body. A suitable immune effector mechanism must be in place. In addition, the target antigen must be accessible.

Sometimes these requirements are easily met. In the haemolytic anemias, for example, antibodies to red cell surface antigens produce sequestration and destruction of the erythrocytes. A number of other diseases of the blood (including some of the leukopenias and thrombocytopenias as well as clotting defects) are mediated directly by antibodies. Several other diseases are also attributable to autoantibodies to receptors, including myasthenia gravis and Graves' disease[24,25]. In the former instance the antibody interferes with acetylcholine receptor function, whereas in the latter situation antibodies may actually stimulate the thyrotropin receptors.

When it comes to solid tissues it is more difficult to demonstrate that antibodies are responsible for disease. In some examples it is possible to transfer the essential lesions of the disease by injections of patient serum directly into the site of disease. Bullous skin disease, pemphigus vulgaris, can essentially be reproduced in experimental animals by such passive transfer of patient serum into animal skin[26]. In most other autoimmune diseases such autoantibody transfers have not been possible. Perhaps the antibody is unable to penetrate the tissue and reach the requisite antigen in sufficient quantity. Sometimes the absence of auxiliary factors, such as complement, prevents effective passive transfer.

Indirect evidence

Most observers feel that autoimmune diseases of solid tissue are produced by cytotoxic T cells rather than antibodies. T-cell transfer experiments from man to man or man to animal are not feasible, however, because the donor and recipient must be matched at the MHC.

In the absence of direct proof one must turn to indirect means. The most feasible approach to establish the autoimmune aetiology of a human disease is to reproduce the essential features of the disease in an experimental animal by immunization with the analogous antigen identified by the initial autoimmune response. The major autoantibody in human chronic thyroiditis, for example, is directed to thyroglobulin. The analogous antigen can be isolated from mice and shown to produce inflammatory lesions of the mouse thyroid that closely resemble the original human disease[27]. Although indirect, the reproduction in an experimental model is usually strong evidence for the autoimmune aetiology of the human disease.

An alternative approach is to identify a spontaneous disease of animals that resembles a human disease and then go through the steps necessary to demonstrate the autoimmune origin of the disease. An example of this approach is insulin-dependent diabetes, a human disease marked by the production of autoantibodies to islet cells[28]. The pathological effects of the disease are attributable to the loss of β cells, but the requisite antigen has not yet been identified. It is, however, possible to study the NOD mouse, which develops a disease closely similar to human diabetes. The insulitis and, to some extent, the hypoglycaemia characteristic of human diabetes mellitus can be transferred between mice by T cells, showing that the murine disease is autoimmune[29].

Secondary evidence

Many human diseases are commonly believed to be due to autoimmune responses, but direct or indirect proof is lacking. A number of clues, taken together, strengthen the inference that a human disease is of autoimmune origin. These clues are also included in Table 2. There is, for example, a genetic predisposition to the development of autoimmune diseases so that patients or members of their family will frequently show another autoimmune disease. Relatives of patients with chronic thyroiditis frequently develop atrophic gastritis, pernicious anaemia, Addison's disease of the adrenal, or insulin-dependent diabetes, all autoimmune diseases affecting endocrine organs.

The strongest genetic determinant of autoimmune diseases in the human are genes of the MHC (HLA complex), especially the class II (HLA-DR, -DQ, or -DP) gene segments. In most cases the relative risks associated with any HLA haplotype are rather modest although, as the fine structure of the genetic locus is more clearly defined, the associations become more immediate. Insulin-dependent diabetes in the human, for example, is now closely associated with particular nucleotide base sequences[30]. Our own studies have shown that within certain families it may be possible to predict the development of thyroid disease among brothers and sisters of parents with juvenile thyroiditis or Graves' disease, if they share both HLA haplotypes with the proband.

Most, but not all, autoimmune diseases are more common in females than males. In general, however, this biased ratio is seen only in diseases that start after puberty, and the ratio tends to return to 1:1 in older ages. Therefore, the difference between the sexes is probably due mainly to steroid hormones.

Clinically, most autoimmune diseases are episodic with periodic exacerbations and remissions. This course may reflect the homeostatic mechanisms of the immune system. From the clinical point of view, the most important criterion of an autoimmune disease is its response to immunosuppressive treatment. In fact, many clinicians consider any disease of unknown origin which responds to immunosuppression as autoimmune.

Autoimmune diseases have a number of immunopathological characteristics which provide important clues. For example, the deposition of immunoglobulin and complement in the respective organ indicates an immunological reaction. Even more persuasive are the occasions when antibody can be eluted from the respective target organ, e.g. the kidney in cases of glomerulonephritis, and transferred to a primate recipient where the essential features of the disease recur[31]. Such experiments have established the autoimmune basis of many types of glomerulonephritis.

The presence of a predominantly T-cell infiltrate in an organ is sometimes suggestive of an autoimmune response, but the appearance of activation markers on the T cell is even more persuasive. These markers include IL-2 receptor and MHC class II products.

Going one step further, some experimental evidence suggests that the T cells infiltrating an organ are clonally restricted. Therefore, the families of the V_α or V_β genes comprising the T-cell receptor are limited. The best example is the experimental disease, allergic encephalomyelitis, in the mouse and the rat, where the V_β gene segments of T cells directed to MBP are limited to one or two families[32]. Recent work suggests that the T cells in the cerebrospinal fluid of patients with multiple sclerosis may be similarly restricted[33].

Finally, a number of observers have reported that the organs involved in autoimmune responses aberrantly express class II MHC determinants[34]. Examples are seen in the islet cells of patients with insulin-dependent diabetes, and the thyroid epithelial cells of patients with chronic thyroiditis. This aberrant expression of class II MHC may be responsible for initiation of the disease process, although firm evidence to support this view is still lacking. In any case, the presence of these MHC class II markers can be taken as indirect support for the presence of a pathological autoimmune response.

CAUSE VERSUS EFFECT

Infection and autoimmunity

A major dilemma in the investigation of human disease is the distinction between autoimmunity as the cause of disease and harmless autoimmunity as a consequence. For example, a number of viral infections are associated with autoimmune responses, but there is little evidence that autoimmunity plays any pathological role. To establish that autoimmunity following virus infection is actually pathogenic requires the same stringent proof as any other human autoimmune disease. In our laboratory, for example, we have been studying the myocarditis produced by Coxsackievirus B3 in certain strains of mice[35,36]. Whereas this disease is generally limited and self-resolving, some strains develop a progressive form of myocarditis. We have been able to demonstrate that this progressive form of disease is reproduced by autoimmunization with cardiac myosin. Our current hypothesis is that the virus infection provides both release of the intracellular antigen and the necessary non-specific immunological signals to induce an autoimmune response. There are unfortunately very few other examples where it can actually be shown that a virus infection induces pathological autoimmunity.

Specific therapy

What is the importance of knowing whether a disease has an autoimmune aetiology? A first principle of medicine is to correctly assign a diagnosis, and from it infer a natural history or prognosis. It is, moreover, the aetiological diagnosis that leads to specific therapy. As the genetic basis of autoimmune diseases is progressively unravelled it will become more and more possible to identify individuals at increased risk of developing autoimmune disease. Early, effective treatment can then be instituted before irreversible tissue destruction occurs. Precise diagnosis also allows the performance of better epidemiological studies, so that environmental or infectious contributions to autoimmunity can be identified along with the genetic determinants.

The most important reason for establishing the autoimmune basis of a disease is the oncoming availability of specific therapies. They are based on the identification of the requisite antigen and, if possible, the actual peptide responsible for initiating the pathological autoimmune process. Under experimental conditions this information already allows the basic immunologist to prevent or even reverse an experimentally induced autoimmune disease, such as allergic encephalomyelitis[34]. Combining information about risk factors as obtained from genetic and epidemiological studies with data on the pathogenic peptides or their counterpart T-cell receptors holds great promise for antigen-specific therapy by clinical immunologists of the future.

Acknowledgements

The author's research was supported by NIH research grants DR-31632 and HL-33878.

References

1. Nossal GVJ. Autoimmunity and self-tolerance. In: Rose NR, Mackay IR, editors. The autoimmune diseases – II. San Diego: Academic Press; 1992;27–46.

2. Nossal GVJ, Pike BL. Clonal anergy: persistence in tolerant mice of antigen-binding B lymphocytes incapable of responding to antigen or mitogen. Proc Natl Acad Sci USA. 1980;77:1602–6.
3. Goodnow CC, Crosbie J, Adelstein S *et al.* Altered immunoglobulin in expression and functional silencing of self-reactive B lymphocytes in transgenic mice. Nature. 1988;334: 676–82.
4. Dintzis HM, Dintzis RZ. A molecular basis for immune regulation: the immunon hypothesis. In: Perelson AS, editor. Theoretical immunology. New York: Addison-Wesley; 1988: 83–103.
5. Felton LD. Significance of antigen in animal tissues. J Immunol. 1949;61:107–17.
6. Bonavida B, Mozes E, Shearer GM, Sela M. Immunological unresponsiveness induced in adult mice to synthetic polypeptides built on multichain polyproline and multichain polyalanine. Immunochemistry. 1974;11:347–53.
7. Gibson J, Basten A, Walker KZ, Loblay RH. A role for suppressor T cells in induction of self tolerance. Proc Natl Acad Sci USA. 1985;82:5150.
8. Pollok BA, Kearney JF, Stohrer RS. Selective alteration of humoral response to alpha-1-3 dextran and phosphorylcholine by early administration of monoclonal anti-idiotype. In: Kohler H, Urbain J, Cazenave P-A, editors. Idiotypy in biology and medicine. New York: Academic Press; 1984:187–202.
9. Sinclair NRStC, Panoskaltsis A. Immunoregulation by Fc signals. Immunol Today. 1987;8:76–9.
10. Kappler JW, Roehm N, Marrack P. T cell tolerance by clonal elimination in the thymus. Cell. 1987;49:273–80.
11. MacDonald HR, Schneider R, Lees RK *et al.* T-cell receptor V_β use predicts reactivity and tolerance to Mls^a-encoded antigens. Nature. 1988;332:40–5.
12. Gammon G, Dunn K, Shastri N *et al.* Neonatal T-cell tolerance to minimal immunogenic peptides is caused by clonal inactivation. Nature. 1986;319:413–15.
13. Quill H, Schwartz RH. Stimulation of normal inducer T cell clones with antigen presented by purified Ia molecules in planar lipid membranes: specific induction of a long lived state of proliferative nonresponsiveness. J Immunol. 1987;138:3704.
14. Kehrl J, Wakefield L, Roberts A *et al.* Production of TGFβ by human T lymphocytes and its potential role in the regulation of T cell growth. J Exp Med. 1986;163:1037.
15. Dohi I, Nisonoff A. Suppression of idiotype and generation of suppressor T cells with idiotype conjugated thymocytes. J Exp Med. 1979;150:909.
16. Cohen IR. Regulation of autoimmune disease: Physiological and therapeutic. Immunol Rev. 1986;94:5.
17. Ada GL, Rose NR. The initiation and early development of autoimmune diseases. Clin Immunol Immunopathol. 1988;41:3–9.
18. Pirofsky B. Autoimmune hemolytic anemia. In: Rose NR, Mackay IR, editors. The autoimmune diseases. Orlando: Academic Press; 1985;161–99.
19. Bigazzi PE, Rose NR. Autoimmune thyroid disease. In: Rose NR, Mackay IR, editors. The autoimmune diseases. Orlando: Academic Press; 1985:161–99.
20. Mackay IR. Autoimmune diseases of the liver: chronic active hepatitis and primary biliary cirrhosis. In: Rose NR, Mackay IR, editors. The autoimmune diseases. Orlando: Academic Press; 1985:291–337.
21. Gershwin ME, Manns MP, Mackay IR. Molecular analysis of cytoplasmic autoantigens in liver disease. In: Rose NR, Mackay IR, editors. The autoimmune diseases – II. San Diego: Academic Press; 1992:213–33.
22. Ferrell PB, Tan EM. Systemic lupus erythematosus. In: Rose NR, Mackay IR, editors. The autoimmune diseases. Orlando: Academic Press; 1985:29–57.
23. Hafler DA, Benjamin DS, Burks J *et al.* Myelin basic protein and proteolipid protein reactivity of brain and CSF-derived T cell clones in multiple sclerosis and post-infectious encephalomyelitis. J Immunol. 1987;139:68.
24. Lindstrom J. Immunobiology of myasthenia gravis, experimental autoimmune myasthenia gravis and Lambert–Eaton syndrome. Annu Rev Immunol. 1985;3:109.
25. Manley SW, Knight A, Adams DD. The thyrotrophin receptor. Springer Semin Immunopathol. 1982;5:413.
26. Anhalt GJ, Labib RS, Voorhees JJ *et al.* Induction of pemphigus in neonatal mice by

passive transfer of IgG from patients with the disease. N Engl J Med. 1982;306:1189.
27. Rose NR, Witebsky E. Studies on organ specificity. V. Changes in the thyroid glands of rabbits following acute immunization with rabbit thyroid extracts. J Immunol. 1956;76:417.
28. Prochazka M, Leiter EH, Serreze DV *et al.* Three recessive loci required for insulin dependent diabetes in non-obese diabetic mice. Science. 1987;237:286.
29. Bendelac A, Carnaud C, Boitard C *et al.* Syngeneic transfer of autoimmune diabetes from diabetic NOD mice to healthy neonates. Requirement for both L3T4 and Lyt-2^+ cells. J Exp Med. 1987;166:823.
30. Nepom GT, Concannon P. Molecular genetics of autoimmunity. In: Rose NR, Mackay IR, editors. The autoimmune diseases – II. San Diego: Academic Press; 1992:127–52.
31. Noble B, Brentjens JR, Andres GA. Autoimmune kidney diseases. In: Rose NR, Mackay IR, editors. The autoimmune diseases. Orlando: Academic Press; 1985:339–70.
32. Urban JL, Kumar V, Kono DH *et al.* Restricted use of T cell receptor V genes in murine autoimmune encephalomyelitis raises possibilities for antibody therapy. Cell. 1988;54:577.
33. Seboun E, Robinson MA, Doolittle TH *et al.* A susceptibility locus for multiple sclerosis is linked to the T cell receptor β chain complex. Cell. 1989;57:1095–100.
34. Gaur A, Wiers B, Liu A, Rothbard J, Fathman CG. Amelioration of autoimmune encephalomyelitis by myelin basic protein synthetic peptide-induced anergy. Science. 1992;258:1491–4.
35. Rose NR, Beisel KW, Herskowitz A *et al.* Cardiac myosin and autoimmune myocarditis. In: Evered D, Whelan J, editors. Autoimmunity and autoimmune disease. CIBA Foundation Symposium 129. Chichester: John Wiley & Sons; 1987;3–24.
36. Neu N, Rose NR, Beisel KW *et al.* Cardiac myosin induces myocarditis in genetically predisposed mice. J Immunol. 1987;139:3630–6.

Section VI
Autoimmune Chronic Active Hepatitis

21 Clinical spectrum and heterogeneity of autoimmune hepatitis: an overview

I. G. McFARLANE

INTRODUCTION

The earliest description of what later became known as autoimmune chronic active hepatitis (AI-CAH) is usually attributed to Waldenstrom in 1950[1], but there are at least two reports[2,3] suggesting that the disorder may have been recognized much earlier. Nevertheless, Waldenstrom is rightly credited with drawing attention to the marked female preponderance, young age of onset, fluctuating nature of the condition, hypergammaglobulinaemia (due mainly to elevated serum IgG concentrations), and associated features of arthralgia/myalgia, hepatosplenomegaly, amenorrhoea, and skin rashes (usually acne-form).

The 1950s were a period of intense research into what were becoming recognized as autoimmune conditions, such as rheumatoid arthritis and systemic lupus erythematosus (SLE), and Joske and King[4] noted the similarity with SLE with the finding that AI-CAH patients often had circulating LE cells. Indeed, this and other findings[5–10], including circulating antinuclear (ANA) and smooth muscle autoantibodies (SMA)[11–13], led to the adoption of the term 'lupoid hepatitis' – although it gradually became clear that the condition is distinct from SLE.

During the next two decades there were many significant developments. The discovery of the hepatitis A and B viruses and development of serological tests for infections due to these viruses made it possible to distinguish the condition from acute or chronic hepatitis A and B, and much progress was made in the histopathological classification of chronic hepatitis[14–20]. Nevertheless, there was a certain reluctance to formally recognize the disease in its own right and, for a long time, it was often included within various 'catch-all' categories such as HBsAg-negative or idiopathic or cryptogenic chronic active hepatitis, or non-A–non-B chronic active liver disease.

However, the finding that, in common with other autoimmune diseases, the condition is associated with inheritance of the HLA A1-B8-DR3 haplotype[21 23] and the controlled clinical trials of the early 1970s showing that it responds to immunosuppressive therapy[24–26], gradually reinforced the impression that this is an autoimmune liver disorder, and it became more commonly known as 'autoimmune chronic active hepatitis'. However, since the word 'autoimmune' already implies chronicity, and since the disease can become relatively inactive for long periods during treatment-induced or spontaneous remissions, the tendency now is to call it simply 'autoimmune hepatitis (AIH)'.

SPECTRUM OF FEATURES AT PRESENTATION

The following is an analysis of the features at presentation in 145 patients with AIH who have been regularly attending the Institute of Liver Studies at King's College Hospital, London, during the past 5 years.

Onset

The disease usually has an insidious onset, with most patients giving a history of various signs or symptoms fluctuating over a period of anything from a few months to more than 2 years. Indeed, many authorities used to require duration of symptoms of at least 3 months to establish chronicity. However, it is now well recognized that the disease can have an acute or subacute, occasionally fulminant, onset that can be very difficult to distinguish from acute viral hepatitis. Conversely, there is now ample evidence (see below) to indicate that the condition may be entirely asymptomatic for long periods before it reveals itself.

Age and gender

Although females still predominate (80% in our series), it is now known that the disease also affects males, and that it can present at any age. In our patients the age distribution at presentation is typical of that seen in any large series of caucasian AIH patients, showing a bimodal pattern (Fig. 1) with a peak around puberty and a second peak in the fourth and fifth decades (perimenopausally in women). The disease tends to be somewhat more severe in younger patients and more difficult to control with corticosteroids, whereas in older patients it tends to follow a rather milder course and is usually easier to control with immunosuppression.

As mentioned above, AIH is significantly associated with inheritance of the HLA A1-B8-DR3 haplotype, and particularly with the DR3 allotype. However, DR3 accounts for only about half of the patients, the disease in the remainder being associated with inheritance of DR4[27]. Comparison of the percentages of patients with DR3 or DR4 in each age group shows that, in the younger age groups, the patients are mainly DR3 while DR4 is much more strongly represented among the older age groups (Fig. 2). Since DR3

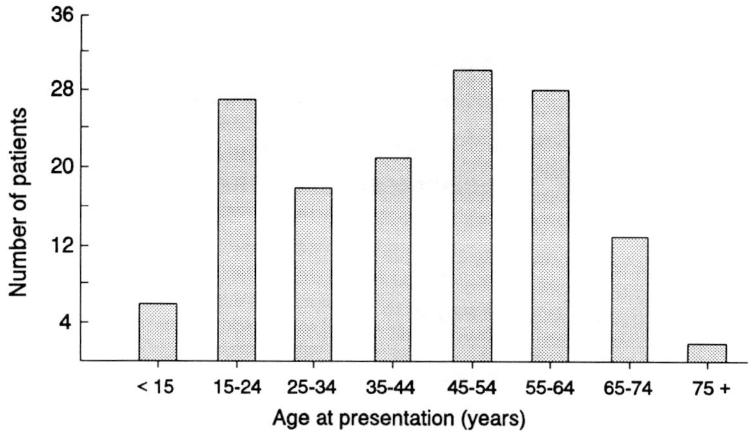

Fig. 1 Ages at presentation of the 145 patients with autoimmune hepatitis regularly attending the Institute of Liver Studies at King's College Hospital, London, during the past 5 years

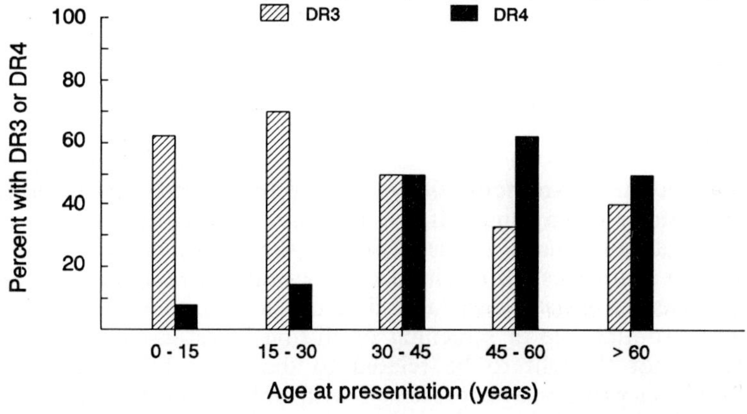

Fig. 2 Comparison of frequency of distribution of HLA DR3 and DR4 with age at presentation of the 145 patients with autoimmune hepatitis regularly attending the Institute of Liver Studies at King's College Hospital, London, during the past 5 years

and DR4 are only rarely inherited together as a haplotype, it is possible that these may be two genetically distinct groups. Interestingly, in Japan, where they see very few of the classical young female autoimmune hepatitis patients and most of their patients are older, there is no association with DR3 (which is very rare in the normal Japanese population) but a very strong association with DR4[28].

Symptoms

Lethargy, often extreme fatigue, was the most common complaint at presentation among our patients (Fig. 3), usually in combination with generalized malaise and/or nausea and loss of appetite, together with one or

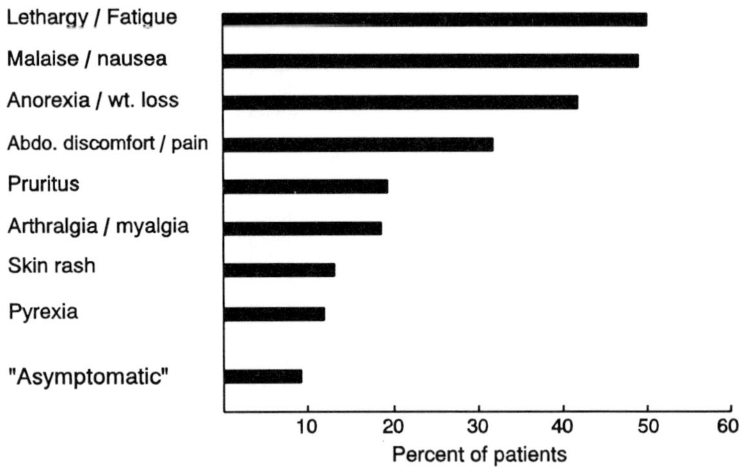

Fig. 3 Symptoms at presentation in the 145 patients with autoimmune hepatitis regularly attending the Institute of Liver Studies at King's College Hospital, London, during the past 5 years. 'Asymptomatic' patients were those who either had no symptoms at all or whose symptoms did not immediately suggest liver disease, and who were referred for investigation of the incidental finding of abnormal biochemical liver tests at routine health screening or during investigation of rheumatological or dermatological conditions

more of the other symptoms shown. This often preceded by several weeks the appearance of any signs. It is important to note, however, that about 10% were asymptomatic, in the sense that they either had no symptoms at all, or their symptoms did not immediately suggest liver disease. These were referred because of the incidental finding of abnormal biochemical liver tests either on routine health screening or during investigation of some other condition not thought to be related to the liver. The latter was most commonly in patients who presented with only a single symptom such as severe arthralgia, or skin lesions, and were referred by rheumatologists or dermatologists.

A further 10% of patients were referred because of the development of signs or symptoms or abnormal liver tests during management of some other condition. About half of these were being treated for autoimmune thyroid disease, and most of the remainder either had inflammatory bowel disease or presented following surgical procedures unrelated to the gastrointestinal tract. In all, therefore, some 20% either had no symptoms directly suggestive of liver disease or initially presented with other conditions.

Signs

Of the signs at presentation, again one sees a spectrum. The most common feature was jaundice (Fig. 4). This was often quite marked, as reflected in the high proportion with pale stools and/or dark urine, but it is worth noting that 25% were not clinically jaundiced. Most also had only one of these

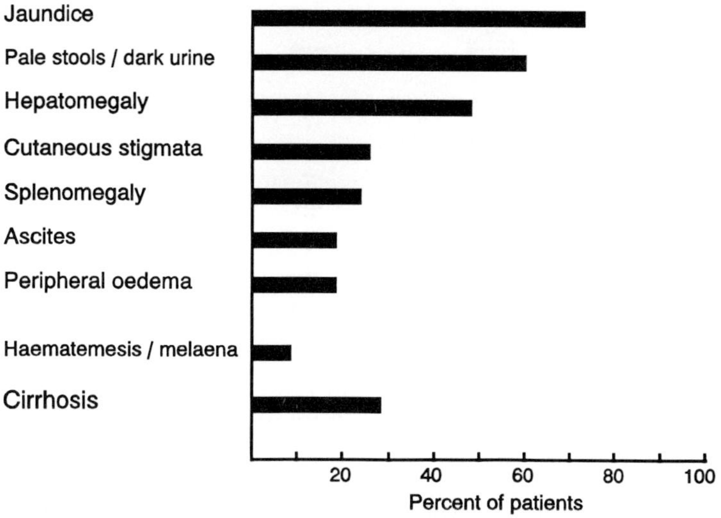

Fig. 4 Signs of liver disease at presentation in the 145 patients with autoimmune hepatitis regularly attending the Institute of Liver Studies at King's College Hospital, London, during the past 5 years. Note that 8% of patients presented with haematemeses and/or melaena as the first sign of their underlying liver disease and, including these, 29% had cirrhosis at presentation

signs. This includes the 8% who presented with haematemeses and/or melaena as the first evidence of their liver disease – without any other signs or symptoms.

It is significant that nearly 30% (including the 8% who presented with haematemeses or melaena) were found to have cirrhosis at presentation. This re-inforces the impression that a sizeable proportion of patients have the disease for some considerable time before they develop signs or symptoms.

Biochemical liver tests

The biochemical liver tests at presentation show a typically hepatitic picture but with a very wide variation – the aminotransferase and bilirubin levels ranging from just above normal to more than 50 times the upper normal limit (Fig. 5). Note that these are all patients with moderate or severe CAH on liver biopsy, and that these values therefore bear no direct relationship to histological severity. Occasionally, a slightly more cholestatic picture was seen, with a moderately raised alkaline phosphatase, high bilirubin and moderately elevated AST but, overall, the picture was still a hepatitic one.

Autoantibodies

As mentioned above, the first autoantibodies found in association with the disease were the ANA and SMA. In our series 77% had one or both of these antibodies at presentation.

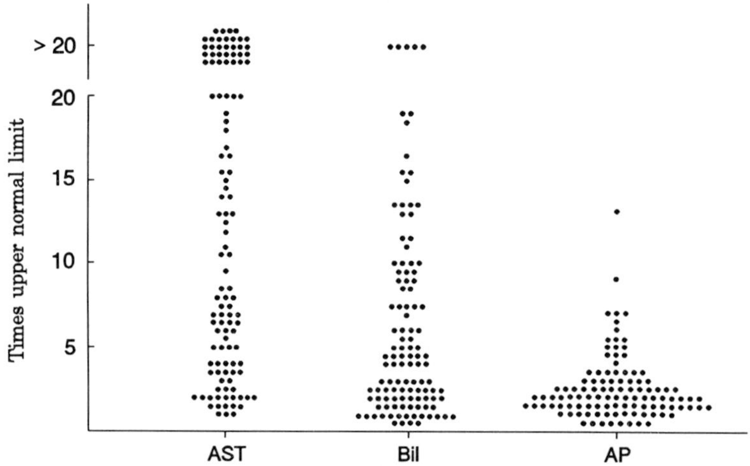

Fig. 5 Serum aspartate aminotransferase (AST), bilirubin (Bil) and alkaline phosphatase (AP) values at presentation in 145 patients with autoimmune hepatitis regularly attending the Institute of Liver Studies at King's College Hospital, London, during the past 5 years. Note the marked 'hepatitic' pattern of these abnormalities

In 1973 Rizetto described a new autoantibody, now known as LKM-1, reacting with an antigen in liver and kidney[29,30]. Patients with LKM-1 comprise only 3% of our cases, but it is difficult to say whether this is typical of the situation worldwide because there is wide geographic variation. LKM-1 was initially described as being associated with a severe form of the disease, particularly in young females, and this is still true in northern Europe[31], but in Mediterranean countries it is often seen in older subjects and in association with hepatitis C virus (HCV) infection[32].

It is important to note, also, that about 20% of patients have none of these antibodies at presentation. This is true also of our own series, although about half of our 'autoantibody-negative' patients subsequently developed ANA and/or SMA later in the course of their disease – with only 10% remaining persistently negative throughout.

SUBTYPES OF AIH

During the past 20 years many groups around the world have been searching for autoantibodies other than ANA, SMA or LKM that might be more specific to the liver and, particularly, to AIH. There is no shortage of candidates. Indeed, for those who are interested in humoral autoimmunity this is a disease *par excellence*. It seems that almost any autoantibody sought will be found in at least some of the patients. Those that have been more extensively studied are listed in Table 1 under the heading of 'liver' autoantibodies, since they are generally more specific to the liver and/or to liver disease and to distinguish them from the 'conventional' autoantibodies (ANA, SMA and LKM-1). Of these, anti-LSP and the liver membrane

Table 1 Some of the more extensively characterized 'liver' autoantibodies that have been described in association with autoimmune hepatitis

Antibody	*Target antigen*
Anti-LSP	'Liver-specific membrane lipoprotein' (LSP) preparation
Liver membrane antibody (LMA)	'26 kDa liver membrane antigen'
Anti-ASGP-R	Hepatic asialoglycoprotein receptor
Anti-SLA	'Soluble liver antigen' (cytokeratins 8 and 18)
Anti-LC1	'Liver cytosolic antigen 1'
Anti-LP	'Liver–pancreas antigen'
Anti-HHPM	60 kDa human hepatocyte plasma membrane antigen
Anti-sulphatide	Sulphated galactoceramide

Table 2 'Sub-types' of autoimmune hepatitis

Sub-type	*Characteristics*
1	Antinuclear (ANA) and/or smooth muscle (SMA) antibody positive
2	Liver–kidney microsomal (LKM-1) antibody positive 2a, Younger, anti-HCV negative 2b, Older, anti-HCV positive
3	'Autoantibody negative' (i.e. for ANA, SMA and LKM-1) Anti-SLA positive (see text)

antibody, LMA, are now largely of historic interest, although we still use anti-LSP routinely for monitoring patients on an empirical basis[33].

Eight years ago we found that the vast majority of these patients also have autoantibodies against the asialoglycoprotein receptor[34], and this was confirmed by Professor Meyer zum Buschenfelde's group a few years ago[35]. These anti-ASPG-R antibodies are particularly interesting because the asialoglycoprotein receptor seems to be an important target antigen in AIH – in that it is absolutely specific to hepatocytes, is preferentially expressed on the surfaces of periportal liver cells, and patients show both T and B cell responses to it[36,37].

Anti-SLA is an antibody against a soluble liver antigen which, although not liver-specific, is found at highest concentration in the liver and is now known to be cytokeratins 8 and 18[30]. Anti-LC are antibodies against another cytosolic liver antigen[30] and anti-LP react with an antigen present in liver and pancreas, the liver–pancreas antigen[30].

Antibodies against a 60 kDa human hepatocyte plasma membrane antigen have been described by an Australian group[38]. The precise nature of the antigen is not yet known, but it seems to be distinct from the above, while anti-sulphatide antibodies, being studied by a Japanese group, are directed at a glycosphingolipid in hepatocyte plasma membranes[39].

There has been a trend towards subdividing the disease according to the different autoantibody profiles: type 1 being the classical ANA and/or SMA positive group and type 2 defining those with LKM-1 antibodies (Table 2). With the recent finding that, in certain countries, many of these patients have evidence of chronic HCV infection[32], it has been suggested that this group should be further subdivided into type 2a, the younger patients without

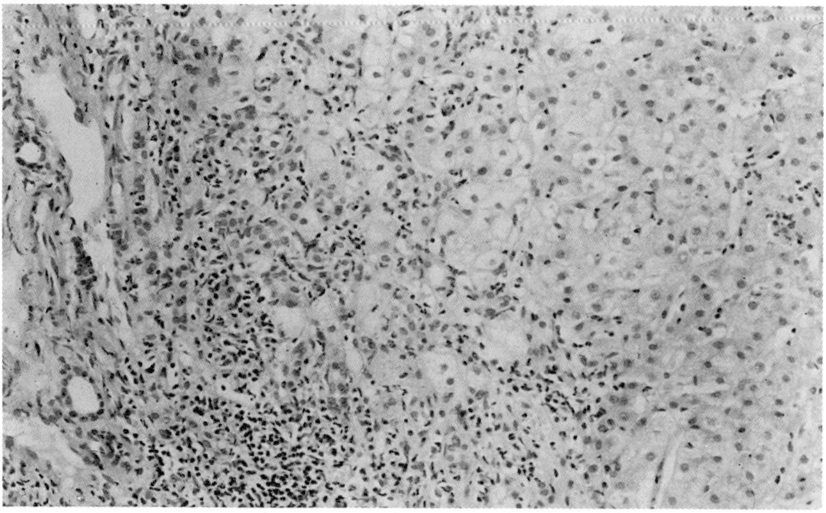

Fig. 6 Section of liver biopsy showing features of chronic active hepatitis (CAH) typical of that seen in autoimmune hepatitis, namely dense lymphoplasmacytic infiltrate of the portal tract spilling out into the periportal area with piecemeal necrosis and rosetting of hepatocytes. Note, however, that this biopsy was taken from a patient with CAH due to chronic hepatitis B virus infection, and is shown to illustrate the point that it can be very difficult with simple histology to distinguish between CAH of different aetiologies. Section stained with haematoxylin and eosin. Magnification × 260

HCV, and type 2b – the older patients with anti-HCV antibodies[40]. It has also been suggested that the so-called 'autoantibody negative' patients, many of whom are seropositive for anti-SLA, be defined as type 3[30]. It is worth noting, however, that anti-SLA is not exclusive to type 3 but is also found in types 1 and 2, and that the majority of patients in all three types have anti-ASGP-R autoantibodies[41].

HISTOLOGICAL FEATURES OF AIH

The histological features of AIH are those of chronic active hepatitis (CAH). Typically, as shown in Fig. 6, there is a dense lympho-plasmacytic infiltrate in the portal tract spilling out into the surrounding parenchyma, with disruption of the limiting plate and piecemeal necrosis and rosetting of periportal hepatocytes. However, the picture shown in Fig. 6 is actually of a section of a liver biopsy from a patient with chronic hepatitis B virus (HBV) infection – the point being that, with simple histology alone, it can be very difficult to distinguish between CAH of different aetiologies. In fact there are no particular morphological features unique to AIH.

OVERLAPPING CONDITIONS

In addition to HBV-CAH a very similar histological picture can be seen at various stages in a wide range of other chronic liver disorders (Table 3) as

Table 3 Some of the liver disorders that are often associated with histological features of chronic active hepatitis (CAH) and may have other features that overlap with autoimmune hepatitis

Chronic hepatitis B (HBV-CAH)
Primary biliary cirrhosis
Primary sclerosing cholangitis
Wilson's disease
Acute hepatitis A
α_1-Antitrypsin deficiency
Chronic non-A–non-B viral hepatitis (including hepatitis C)
Alcoholic liver disease

well as in acute hepatitis A[42]. Most of these conditions can now be fairly confidently diagnosed on the basis of other histological features together with serological and clinical findings, but within each disorder there is a small proportion of patients with clinical, biochemical and immunological features that overlap with those of autoimmune hepatitis.

Thus, whereas the vast majority of patients with primary biliary cirrhosis present with antimitochondrial autoantibodies, about 5% do not, and some of these will have ANA and/or SMA with elevated serum IgG levels. Conversely, a small proportion of AIH patients (2% in our series) have antimitochondrial antibodies.

In primary sclerosing cholangitis, between 10% and 80% of patients will have ANA, SMA or other autoantibodies and, at certain stages of the disease, it can be very difficult to distinguish it from AIH on histological criteria – particularly in children[43–45]. Cholangiography is essential for the diagnosis of these cases.

Patients with Wilson's disease may also have ANA and/or SMA and, conversely, occasionally AIH patients present with high serum copper and low caeruloplasmin concentrations reminiscent of Wilson's disease[46,47]. However, the two disorders can usually be distinguished by the fact that the AIH patients do not have ocular Kayser–Fleischer rings, and do not show a marked increase in urinary copper excretion following challenge with D-penicillamine.

Alcoholic liver disease can be a particularly difficult problem. This condition is associated with a wide range of cellular and humoral immunological abnormalities that in many respects resemble those seen in AIH and some patients respond to corticosteroid therapy[48–50]. Indeed, at the present time it is almost impossible to distinguish with any degree of confidence between alcoholic liver disease and autoimmune hepatitis in a patient who admits to moderate alcohol consumption and presents with antinuclear antibodies, an elevated serum IgG and a histological picture of chronic active hepatitis with some steatosis.

INTERNATIONAL AIH GROUP RECOMMENDATIONS

In view of the wide spectrum of features associated with the disease, this year a group of 27 investigators from 11 countries, who between them had expertise in the clinical management, histopathology, immunology and biochemistry of adult and paediatric AIH, got together to discuss criteria for diagnosis of the condition. During the period January to June 1992, members of this panel corresponded with each other about the various issues and a subcommittee of the pathologists on the panel met separately to consider the histological criteria. The panel then met in June in an open session attended by about 40 observers who contributed to the discussion, which then continued by correspondence during July and August, leading to a report of these discussions[51], of which the following is a brief summary.

The panel recommends that a diagnosis of AIH should be considered in any patient, particularly but not necessarily female, who presents with a hepatitic picture of liver test abnormalities together with hyperglobulinaemia (especially if this is due to a raised IgG), and who is seronegative for markers of active HAV and HBV infection, and for other common hepatotropic viruses such as CMV or EBV, but not necessarily excluding HCV.

If at all possible a liver biopsy should be obtained and this should show 'pure' chronic active hepatitis. This is defined as a dense portal and periportal lymphoplasmacytic infiltrate with periportal piecemeal necrosis, with or without features of lobular hepatitis and either portal–portal or central–portal bridging necrosis. Lobular involvement was previously thought to be more typical of viral hepatitis, but it is now recognized that this is often seen in patients with severe AIH.

It is strongly recommended that syndromes in which these features of CAH are seen, but in which there are also biliary changes, siderosis, copper deposits or any other changes suggestive of other aetiologies, should not be considered within the definition of AIH. This excludes most of the conditions that overlap with AIH, and which the panel feels should be considered as separate entities. A move in this direction has already been started by some groups of investigators, who have suggested the term 'autoimmune cholangitis' to describe one such overlapping condition associated with biliary lesions in patients who are seronegative for AMA but have circulating ANA[52]. These criteria will also exclude many patients with HCV infections, which are often associated with biliary and other changes in liver biopsies[53–55].

The panel felt that it could not recommend the current trend to subdivide the disease into the various subtypes according to autoantibody profiles, although these are clearly very interesting. With the possible exception of patients with HCV infections, it was felt that there is not yet sufficient evidence that these subtypes define different pathogenetic groups and, since the majority of patients of all subtypes seem to respond to corticosteroid therapy, they do not define different therapeutic subgroups. So, at the present time, they seem to have no practical clinical advantage. Instead, the panel proposes that patients with idiopathic CAH, as defined above, should be described as having 'definite' or 'probable' AIH according to the following criteria.

'Definite' AIH should be used to describe those patients who have circulating ANA, SMA or LKM-1 antibodies at titres of greater than 1:80, together with serum globulin or IgG concentrations greater than 1.5 times the upper normal limit. They should also be seronegative for anti-HCV antibodies and have no recent history of exposure to hepatotoxic drugs or of moderate to heavy alcohol intake.

'Probable' AIH could include patients with ANA, SMA or LKM-1 at lower titres, and serum globulin or IgG concentrations elevated to a lesser extent than for definite AIH. This category would also include the so-called 'autoantibody-negative' cases, provided that they fulfil all other criteria or are seropositive for one of the other defined 'liver' autoantibodies. By 'defined' is meant that there is published data on the methodology for detection of the antibody and its possible relevance to AIH. In addition, patients with a positive history of moderate alcohol consumption or recent hepatotoxic drug usage may be included, if there is clear evidence of continuing liver damage after cessation of drinking or of drug use. Patients with positive anti-HCV antibody tests who fulfil all of the other criteria may also be included until it is confirmed, preferably by demonstration of HCV-RNA in the serum by use of the polymerase chain reaction (PCR) method, that these reflect active HCV infection.

Liver histology is strongly recommended for all cases, but is considered mandatory for a diagnosis of 'definite' AIH. If it is impossible to perform a liver biopsy within a given time frame, a provisional diagnosis of 'probable' AIH may be made. For these and other difficult cases a scoring system has been devised as an adjunct to the descriptive criteria to aid in diagnosis. Corticosteroid responsiveness is considered to be an additional criterion which can be used to confirm the initial diagnosis and/or to upgrade a patient from 'probable' to 'definite'.

SUMMARY

In summary, autoimmune hepatitis (AIH) is a disease associated with hypergammaglobulinaemia that mainly affects females but also occurs in males and may present at any age.

In the majority of patients the onset is insidious with a range of signs and symptoms, some of which are fairly non-specific and may not immediately suggest liver disease. On the other hand, it can present acutely or, conversely, may be entirely asymptomatic.

Other than showing a hepatitic pattern, there are no biochemical features that are pathognomonic of the disease and, while the majority have ANA and/or SMA or LKM-1, about 20% may have none of these at presentation, and there is a wide range of other autoantibodies associated with the condition. Patients typically have the HLA DR3 or DR4 allotypes.

The histological features are those of chronic active hepatitis, which is also seen in a large number of other liver disorders, but, if the recommendations of the international panel are adopted, many of these so-called 'overlapping syndromes' and many cases of hepatitis C virus infections associated with autoantibodies will be excluded from the definition of autoimmune hepatitis on histological criteria.

References

1. Waldenstrom J. Leber, blutproteine und Nahrungsweiss. Deutsch Gesellschaft Z. Verdau Stoffwechselkr. 1950;15:113–19.
2. Amberg S. Hyperproteinaemia associated with severe liver damage. Proc Staff Meet Mayo Clin. 1942;17:360–2.
3. Cullinan ER. Idiopathic jaundice (often recurrent) associated with subacute necrosis of the liver. St Barthol Hosp Rep. 1936;69:55–142.
4. Joske RA, King WE. The 'L.E.-cell' phenomenon in active chronic viral hepatitis. Lancet. 1955;2:477–9.
5. Mackay IR, Taft LI, Cowling DC. Lupoid hepatitis. Lancet. 1956;2:1323–6.
6. Bartholomew LG, Hagedorn AB, Cain JC, Baggenstoss AH. Hepatitis and cirrhosis in women with positive clot tests for lupus erythematosus. N Engl J Med. 1958;259:947–56.
7. Aronson AR, Montgomery MM. Chronic liver disease with a 'lupus erythematosus-like syndrome'. Arch Intern Med. 1959;104:544–52.
8. Mackay IR, Taft LI, Cowling DC. Lupoid hepatitis and the hepatic lesions of systemic lupus erythematosus. Lancet. 1959;2:65–9.
9. Bartholomew LG, Cain JC, Baggenstoss AH, Hagedorn AB. Further observations on hepatitis in young women with positive clot tests for lupus erythematosus. Gastroenterology. 1960;39:730–6.
10. Mackay IR, Wood IJ. Lupoid hepatitis: a comparison of 22 cases with other types of liver disease. Q J Med. 1962;31:485–507.
11. Doniach D, Roitt IM, Walker JG, Sherlock S. Tissue antibodies in primary biliary cirrhosis, active chronic (lupoid) hepatitis, cryptogenic cirrhosis and other liver diseases and their clinical implications. Clin Exp Immunol. 1966;1:237–62.
12. Whittingham S, Mackay IR, Irwin J. Autoimmune hepatitis: immuno-fluorescence reactions with cytoplasm of smooth muscle and glomerular cells. Lancet. 1966;1:1333–5.
13. Whittingham S, Irwin J, Mackay IR, Smalley M. Smooth muscle autoantibody in 'autoimmune' hepatitis. Gastroenterology. 1966;51:499–505.
14. Geall MG, Schoenfield LJ, Summerskill WHJ. Classification and treatment of chronic active liver disease. Gastroenterology. 1968;55:724–9.
15. De Groote J, Desmet VJ, Gedigk P *et al.* A classification of chronic hepatitis. Lancet. 1968;1:626–8.
16. Bulkley BH, Heizer WD, Goldfinger SE, Isselbacher KJ. Distinctions in chronic active hepatitis based on circulating hepatitis associated antigen. Lancet. 1970;2:1323–6.
17. Dudley FJ, Scheuer PJ, Sherlock S. Natural history of hepatitis-associated antigen-positive chronic liver disease. Lancet. 1972;2:1388–93.
18. Baggenstoss AH, Soloway RD, Summerskill WHJ *et al.* Chronic active liver disease: the range of histologic lesions, their response to treatment and evolution. Human Pathol. 1972;3:183–98.
19. Sherlock S. Chronic hepatitis. Gut. 1974;15:581–97.
20. Bianchi L, de Groote J, Desmet VJ *et al.* Acute and chronic hepatitis revisited. Review by an international group. Lancet. 1977;2:914–19.
21. Galbraith RM, Eddleston ALWF, Smith MGM *et al.* Histocompatibility antigens in active chronic hepatitis and primary biliary cirrhosis. Br Med J. 1974;3:604–5.
22. Opelz G, Vogten AJ, Summerskill WH *et al.* HLA determinants in chronic active liver disease: possible relation of HLA-DW3 to prognosis. Tissue Antigens. 1977;9:36–40.
23. Mackay IR, Tait DB. HLA associations with autoimmune type chronic active hepatitis: identification of B8-DRw3 haplotype by family studies. Gastroenterology. 1980;79:95–9.
24. Cook GC, Mulligan R, Sherlock S. Controlled prospective trial of corticosteroid therapy in active chronic hepatitis. Q J Med. 1971;40:159–85.
25. Soloway RD, Summerskill WHJ, Baggenstoss A *et al.* Clinical, biochemical and histological remission in severe chronic active liver disease: a controlled study of treatments and early prognosis. Gastroenterology. 1972;63:820–33.
26. Murray-Lyon IM, Stern RB, Williams R. Controlled trial of prednisolone and azathioprine in active chronic hepatitis. Lancet. 1973;1:735–7.
27. Donaldson PT, Doherty DG, Hayllar KM *et al.* Susceptibility to autoimmune chronic active hepatitis: human leukocyte antigens DR4 and AI-B8-DR3 are independent risk

factors. Hepatology. 1991;13:701–6.

28. Seki T, Kiyosawa K, Inoko H, Ota M. Association of autoimmune hepatitis with HLA-Bw54 and DR4 in Japanese patients. Hepatology. 1990;12:1300–4.
29. Rizzetto M, Swana G, Doniach D. Microsomal antibodies in active chronic hepatitis and other disorders. Clin Exp Immunol. 1973;15:331–44.
30. Manns MP. Cytoplasmic autoantigens in autoimmune hepatitis: molecular analysis and clinical relevance. Semin Liver Dis. 1991;11:205–14.
31. Homberg J-C, Abauf N, Bernard O *et al.* Chronic active hepatitis associated with antiliver/kidney microsome antibody type 1: a second type of 'autoimmune' hepatitis. Hepatology. 1987;7:1333–9.
32. Lenzi M, Johnson PJ, McFarlane IG *et al.* Antibodies to hepatitis C virus in autoimmune liver disease: evidence for geographical heterogeneity. Lancet. 1991;338:277–80.
33. McFarlane IG, Hegarty JE, McSorley CT *et al.* Antibodies to liver specific protein predict outcome of treatment withdrawal in autoimmune chronic active hepatitis. Lancet. 1984;2:954–6.
34. McFarlane BM, McSorley CG, Vergani D *et al.* Serum autoantibodies reacting with the hepatic asialoglycoprotein receptor protein (hepatic lectin) in acute and chronic liver disorders. J Hepatol. 1986;3:196–205.
35. Treichel U, Poralla T, Hess G *et al.* Autoantiodies to human asialoglycoprotein receptor in autoimmune-type chronic hepatitis. Hepatology. 1990;11:606–12.
36. Poralla T, Treichel U, Lohr H, Fleischer B. The asialoglycoprotein receptor as target structure in autoimmune liver diseases. Semin Liver Dis. 1991;11:215–22.
37. McFarlane BM, Sipos J, Gove CD *et al.* Antibodies against the hepatic asialoglycoprotein receptor perfused in situ preferentially attach to periportal liver cells in the rat. Hepatology. 1990;11:408–15.
38. Swanson NR, Reed WD, Yarred LJ *et al.* Autoantibodies to isolated human hepatocyte plasma membranes in chronic active hepatitis. II. Specificity of antibodies. Hepatology. 1990;11:613–21.
39. Toda G, Ikeda Y, Kashiwagi M *et al.* Hepatocyte plasma membrane glycosphingolipid reactive with sera from patients with autoimmune chronic active hepatitis: its identification as sulfatide. Hepatology. 1990;12:664–70.
40. Lunel F, Abuaf N, Frangeul L *et al.* Liver/kidney microsome antibody Type 1 and hepatitis C virus infection. Hepatology. 1992;16:630–6.
41. Johnson PJ, McFarlane IG, McFarlane BM, Williams R. Autoimmune features in patients with idiopathic chronic active hepatitis who are seronegative for conventional autoantibodies. J Gastroenterol Hepatol. 1990;5:244–51.
42. Scheuer PJ. Viral hepatitis. In: MacSween RNM, Anthony PP, Scheuer PJ, editors. Pathology of the liver. Edinburgh: Churchill Livingstone; 1987:202–23.
43. Zauli D, Schrumpf E, Crespi C *et al.* An autoantibody profile in primary sclerosing cholangitis. J Hepatol. 1987;5:14–18.
44. Mieli-Vergani G, Lobo-Yeo A, McFarlane BM *et al.* Different immune mechanisms leading to autoimmunity in primary sclerosing cholangitis and autoimmune chronic active hepatitis of childhood. Hepatology. 1989;9:198–203.
45. Bedlow AJ, Donaldson PT, McFarlane BM *et al.* Autoreactivity to hepatocellular antigens in primary biliary cirrhosis and primary sclerosing cholangitis. J Clin Lab Immunol. 1989;30:103–9.
46. Hodges S, Lobo-Yeo A, Donaldson P *et al.* Autoimmune chronic active hepatitis in a family. Gut. 1991;32:299–302.
47. Ilan Y, Hillman M, Oren R *et al.* Undetectable caeruloplasmin values in a patient with autoimmune chronic active hepatitis. Gut. 1991;32:549–50.
48. Johnson RD, Williams R. State of the art: immune responses in alcoholic liver disease. Alcoholism Clin Exp Res. 1986;10:471–86.
49. Hofer T, McMahon L. Corticosteroids and alcoholic hepatitis. Hepatology. 1991;13: 199–201.
50. Ishak KG, Zimmerman HJ, Ray MB. Alcoholic liver disease: pathologic, pathogenetic and clinical aspects. Alcoholism Clin Exp. Res. 1991;15:45–66.
51. Johnson PJ, McFarlane IG. International Autoimmune Hepatitis Group Meeting Report. Autoimmune Hepatitis: Criteria for Diagnosis and Response to Therapy. Hepatology 1992:

submitted for publication.
52. Michieletti P, Bassendine MF, Heathcote EJ *et al.* Antimitochondrial antibody (AMA) negative primary biliary cirrhosis (PBC) or autoimmune cholangitis. Proceedings of the Biennial Scientific Meeting of the International Association for the Study of the Liver, Brighton, UK, 3–6 June 1992; Abstract No. 0-33.
53. Bach N, Thung SN, Schaffner F. The histological features of chronic hepatitis C and autoimmune chronic hepatitis: a comparative analysis. Hepatology. 1992;15:572–7.
54. Gerber MA. Chronic hepatitis C: The beginning of the end of a time-honoured nomenclature? Hepatology. 1992;15:733–4.
55. Scheuer PJ, Ashrafzadeh P, Sherlock S *et al.* The pathology of hepatitis C. Hepatology. 1992;15:567–71.

22 Nuclear antigens in autoimmune hepatitis

M. NISHIOKA

INTRODUCTION

Antibodies specific for nuclear macromolecules (ANA) are frequently observed in sera from patients with autoimmune hepatitis (AIH), as well as collagen diseases. Considerable information is now available as to the nuclear autoantigens seen in collagen diseases[1,2], but little is known about nuclear proteins reacting with sera from patients with liver diseases. In this chapter ANA profiles of AIH are presented on the basis of immunofluorescent studies and western blot analysis. In addition, some antibodies to recombinant nuclear proteins and to transfer (t) RNA in patients with chronic liver diseases are shown.

ANA APPEARANCE IN AUTOIMMUNE HEPATITIS

In recent years substrates being used in the indirect immunofluorescence (IF) method have changed, and HEp-2 cells are most frequently used. In this case the incidence of ANA is high and the fluorescent staining pattern of ANA can be analysed clearly. Figure 1 shows immunofluorescent patterns of ANA commonly present in sera from AIH patients. The fluorescent patterns of ANA are known to be divided into many patterns such as homogeneous, speckled, centromere, peripheral/rim, nuclear dots and others.

The diagnostic criteria for AIH in the present study are as follows: (a) persistent liver dysfunction, (b) hypergammaglobulinaemia more than 2.0 g/dl, (c) positive for ANA and anti-DNA antibody, (d) negative for HBs antigen, and (e) histologically proven CAH. AIH was divided into two groups based on presence or absence of HCV viraemia. HCV-RNA was detected by two-stage polymerase chain reaction with two pairs of primers deduced from the 5′-non-coding regions.

In our study of 34 Japanese patients with AIH, the most common pattern of ANA was homogeneous (56%). Table 1 presents incidence and

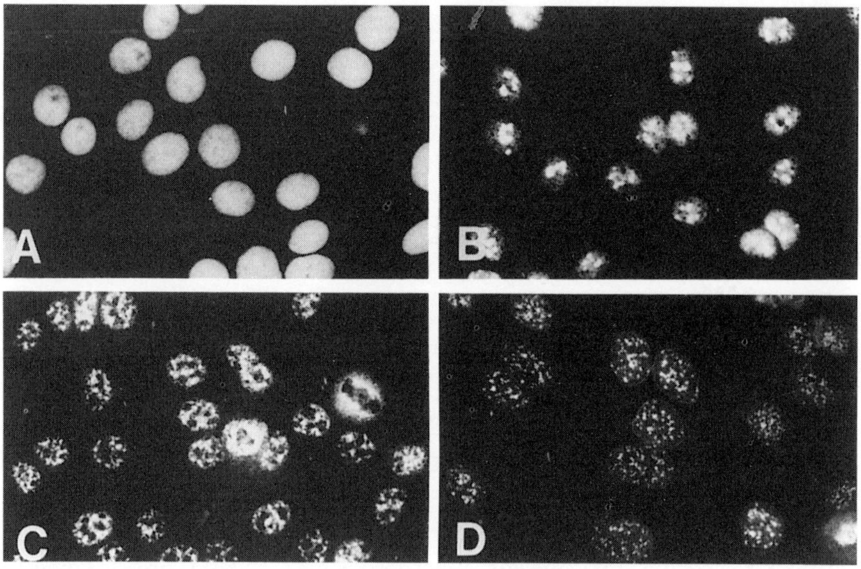

Fig. 1 Immunofluorescent patterns common in autoimmune hepatitis. **A**: Homogeneous pattern, **B**: nuclear dots pattern, **C**: speckled pattern, **D**: centromere pattern

immunofluorescent patterns of ANA in AIH comparing with those in collagen diseases. The speckled pattern was found in 18%, and centromere in 9%. The homogeneous pattern of ANA seems to be more common in AIH[3]. Bernstein *et al.*[4] also reported a high frequency of the homogeneous pattern in patients with HBs antigen-negative chronic active hepatitis. They did not mention the presence of centromere pattern of ANA in HBs-negative and positive chronic active hepatitis (CAH) patients. However, in our studies the centromere pattern of ANA was found in 23% of AIH patients positive for HCV. It is notable that the centromere pattern of ANA is sometimes present in sera of patients with AIH as well as progessive systemic (PSS) and primary biliary cirrhosis (PBC).

It is tempting to evaluate the clinical relevance of ANA patterns in AIH patients. Clinical characteristics of our patients with AIH have already been reported in relation to fluorescent patterns of ANA[3]. Patients with anti-centromere antibody had a mild course and a long duration of disease after the onset. They had a good prognosis because of the long duration of disease. Complication by other autoimmune diseases is known in patients with AIH. Golding *et al.* reported that as many as 63% of patients with AIH had diseases of various organs other than the liver[5]. In our study about half of the patients had complications with some other autoimmune diseases. Patients positive for homogeneous and speckled ANAs seem to have complications such as rheumatoid arthritis (RA), Sjögren's syndrome (SjS) and dermatitis.

A very rare case in our present study is a 41-year-old female patient with

Table 1 Incidence and immunofluorescent patterns of ANA in various diseases

		Immunofluorescent pattern						
	No. of cases	*Homogeneous*	*Perinuclear*	*Speckled*	*Centromere*	*Nucleolar*	*Homogeneous speckled*	*Homogeneous perinuclear*
AIH	34	19 (56)	0	6 (18)	3 (9)	0	3 (9)	2 (6)
HCV(−)[a]	19	11 (58)	0	4 (21)	0	0	2 (10)	1 (5)
HCV(+)	15	8 (53)	0	2 (13)	3 (23)	0	1 (7)	1 (7)
SLE	36	6 (16.6)	0 (0)	19 (52.7)	0 (0.0)	0 (0.0)	11 (30.5)	0 (0.0)
MCTD	14	0 (0.0)	0 (0)	14 (100)	0 (0.0)	0 (0.0)	0 (0.0)	0 (0.0)
PSS	16	0 (0.0)	0 (0)	4 (25)	3 (18.7)	1 (6.2)	8 (50.0)	0 (0.0)
SjS	11	0 (0.0)	0 (0)	6 (54.5)	0 (0.0)	0 (0.0)	4 (36.3)	1 (9.0)
RA	3	1 (33.3)	0 (0)	2 (66.6)	0 (0.0)	0 (0.0)	0 (0.0)	0 (0.0)

[a]HCV-RNA; figures in parentheses are percentages.

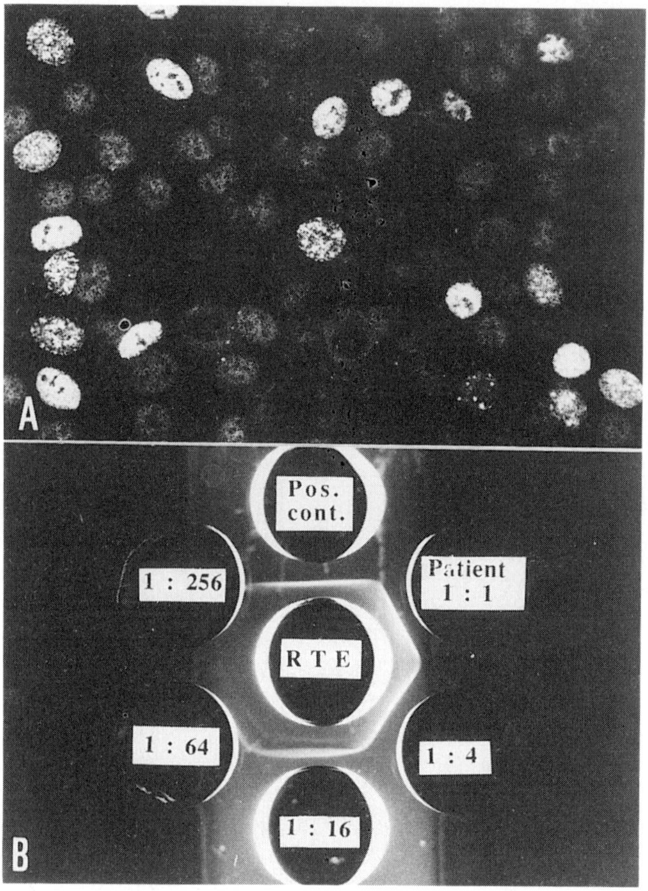

Fig. 2 Immunofluorescent pattern (**A**) and immunodiffusion tests (**B**) for anti-PCNA antibody

chronic persistent hepatitis, RA, and membranous nephropathy. Anti-PCNA (proliferating cell nuclear antigen) antibody was positive in her serum by immunofluorescent test (Fig. 2a). The presence of anti-PCNA was confirmed by the immunodiffusion method using soluble extracts of rabbit thymus (RTE) as target antigens (Fig. 2b). The incidence of anti-PCNA seems to be very low. Even in patients with SLE, anti-PCNA was found in only 3%[1].

Recent studies[6] showed that PCNA is the auxiliary protein of DNA polymerase δ. Interestingly,[7] anti-PCNA is inhibitory to oligonucleotide synthesis mediated by DNA polymerase δ. Although anti-PCNA has little clinical significance as a diagnostic marker, this might be a useful probe for the study of DNA replication as well as for understanding the mechanism of cell replication.

Table 2 Incidence of antinuclear antibodies in autoimmune diseases (percentages)

	AIH	*HCV(−)*	*HCV(+)*	*SLE*	*MCTD*	*PSS*	*SjS*	*RA*
ANA[a]	94	100	88	75	100	89	79	75
Anti-SS-A[b]	23	42	0	61	38	47	86	75
Anti-SS-B[b]	6	11	0	8	0	0	50	0
Anti-RNP[b]	6	12	0	33	100	21	14	21
Anti-ds-DNA[c]	19	21	18	38	36	90	50	75
Anti-ss-DNA[c]	97	100	94	94	94	32	7	75

[a]Immunofluorescent
[b]Ouchterlony
[c]ELISA (IgG)

ANTIBODIES TO NUCLEAR ANTIGENS

Recently, immunodiffusion and enzyme immunoassay techniques have been routinely carried out with partially purified nuclear antigens and are providing more reliable data on ANA subsets. Those antibodies are useful in differentiating autoimmune diseases[2] including autoimmune liver diseases (Table 2).

Antibodies to SS-A and SS-B

Antibodies designated SS-A (anti-SS-A) and SS-B (anti-SS-B) were first identified in patients with SjS and SLE[8,9], and have been shown to react with intracellular proteins which are involved in regulation of RNA polymerase III function[10].

Anti-SS-A was seen in 23% of AIH patients. Four of the patients, positive for anti-SS-A, had a complication of SjS. Interestingly, these antibodies were not found in AIH patients positive for HCV.

Anti-SS-B is known to be a specific diagnostic marker of SjS[1]. Anti-SS-B was very rare in AIH patients. One of the patients with anti-SS-B had been diagnosed for SjS for a long time before a diagnosis of AIH was made. In such a case a common pathogenic mechanism may be involved in both disorders. Histological analysis of the liver in this case revealed endoarteritis obliterans in medium-sized vessels, in addition to severe lymphoid infiltrations and severe piecemeal necrosis in the liver. A healing stage of vasculitis, presenting as endoarteritis obliterans, was often seen in skin and kidney from patients with SjS[11].

Antibodies to nuclear RNP

Antibodies to nuclear RNP (anti-RNP) were also found in patients with SLE[12] as well as antibodies to Sm. In patients with mixed connective tissue disease (MCTD), anti-RNP is commonly seen. Target antigens of anti-RNP are a species of small nuclear RNAs (U-RNAs) complexed with proteins. They are involved in the splicing of precursor messenger RNAs[1]. In the

Table 3 Molecular characterizations of recombinant antigens expressed in plasmids

Antinuclear antibodies	*Source*	*Amino acid no.*	*Expression plasmid*	*Fusion partner*	*Expression molecular weight (kDa)*
RNP-70	Human	1 ~ 437	pEX-2	cro-β-gal	158
RNP-A	Human	1 ~ 282	pEX-2	cro-β-gal	144
52K SS-A/Ro	Human	1 ~ 475	pGEX-2	GST	74
60K SS-A/Ro	Human	1 ~ 538	pUC-19	none	60
CENP-B	Human	528 ~ 599	pEX-2	cro-β-gal	123

Medical and biological laboratory, T. Hachiya

present study, anti-RNP was found in two out of 34 AIH patients. In one of the two patients, PSS was found.

In this context, it is noteworthy that autoantibodies such as anti-SS-A, anti-SS-B, and anti-RNP were more frequently seen in AIH patients negative for HCV. Anti-HCV is known to be found in 50% of AIH patients. A high incidence of anti-HCV has been reported in AIH type I[13] as well as AIH type II[14]. The present studies indicate that AIH patients negative for HCV may have the same immunological backgrounds as other autoimmune diseases such as SjS, SLE, and MCTD.

Antibodies to single- and double-stranded DNA

Antibodies reactive with single-stranded DNA (anti-ss-DNA) recognize polymers of purine and pyrimidine bases. Antibodies reactive with double-stranded DNA (anti-ds-DNA) recognize mainly the deoxyribose phosphate backbone[1]. These antibodies play an important role in the pathogenesis of SLE[15]. In general, detection of these antibodies is useful for the diagnosis of autoimmune diseases. Anti-ss-DNA was found in almost all AIH patients, but anti-ds-DNA was seen in only 19% of our patients. Wood *et al.*[16] reported that anti-ds-DNA is a non-specific manifestation of inflammatory activity.

ANTIBODIES TO RECOMBINANT PROTEINS IN AUTOIMMUNE LIVER DISEASES

Recent advances of recombinant DNA technology made it possible to synthesize recombinant proteins. Detection of ANA subtypes will be replaced by more reliable enzyme immunoassay using the recombinant proteins. In the present study, RNP-70 and RNP-A, which are autoantigens of anti-U1 snRNP[17,18], 52K and 60K SS-A/RO which are recognized by anti-SS-A.Ro[19–21], and cenp-B which is an 80 kDa centromere antigen[22] were synthesized. Table 3 presents molecular characterizations of recombinant antigens expressed in plasmids. Figures 3 and 4 show electrophoretic patterns of the recombinant antigens on sodium dodecylsulphate polyacrylamide gels (SDS-PAGE). The antigenicity of each peptide was evaluated using specific

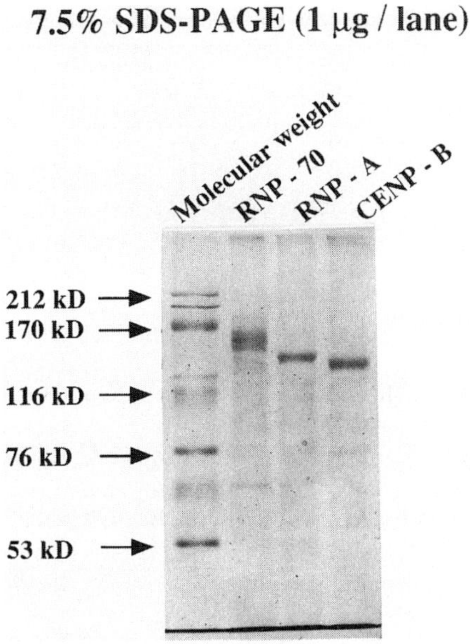

Fig. 3 Electrophoretic patterns of RNP-70, RNP-A and Cenp-B

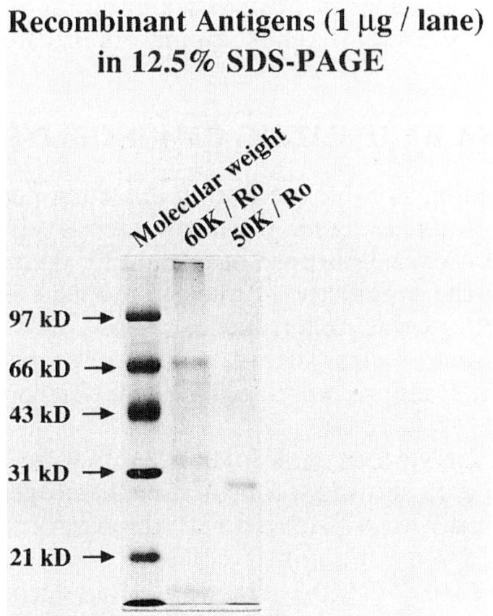

Fig. 4 Electrophoretic patterns of 52 K SS-A/Ro and 60 K SS-A/Ro

antibodies such as anti-SS-A, anti-U1-RNP and anti-centromere antibody as probes, and individual recombinant peptides were used as target antigens for ELISA.

The incidence of antibodies to recombinant proteins is shown in Table 4. The frequency of antibodies to U1-RNP-A and -70 in AIH patients became

Table 4 Incidence of antibodies to recombinant proteins in liver diseases

	No. of cases	*Antibodies to*				
		U1-RNP-A	*U1-RNP-70*	*SS-A-60*	*SS-A-52*	*Cenp-B*
AIH	35	5 (14)	6 (17)	4 (11)	7 (20)	5 (14)
HCV(−)	18	4 (22)	5 (28)	4 (22)	7 (39)	2 (11)
HCV(+)	17	1 (6)	1 (6)	0 (0)	0 (0)	3 (18)
PBC	10	0 (0)	1 (10)	2 (20)	7 (70)	4 (40)
Normal	20	0 (0)	0 (0)	0 (0)	0 (0)	0 (0)

Figures in parentheses are percentages

Table 5 Molecular weights (kDa) of target peptides of various types of ANA

Homogeneous	33, 36, 50, 55, 60, 62, 64, 80, 100
Speckled	12, 29, 33, 50, 60, 70, 80
Centromere	17, 25, 30, 80, 100, 120, 140
Peripheral	70, 90, 100

high, as compared with that of anti-RNP. In the cases of antibodies to SS-A-60 and -52, the incidence was almost similar to that of anti-SS-A, although there were some discrepancies in positivity among them. Anti-SS-A-52 and anti-cenp-B seem to be useful diagnostic markers in PBC patients.

ANALYSIS OF ANA BY UTILIZING IMMUNOBLOTTING

Western blot is the most suitable method in detecting peptides according to molecular size, but it still remains at the research level, particularly in the field of liver disease. For the purpose of estimating the molecular weight of peptides, as well as the specificity of nuclear antigens in liver disease, the western blotting method was undertaken.

Purified nuclear fractions from HeLa cells were prepared by the method of Penner[23]. Nuclear fractions were analysed by electrophoresis on 4–20% SDS-PAGE[3].

Nuclear proteins for various molecular weights were found in sera from AIH patients. These data showed a considerable heterogeneity of the nuclear antigens which reacted with ANA, even with the ANA that showed a similar fluorescent pattern. Similar findings have been reported in the sera from connective tissue diseases[24]. In the sera with a homogeneous ANA pattern, nine bands of nuclear proteins of 33–100 kDa were detected. There were 14 bands of 12–80 kDa in speckled pattern, seven bands of 17–140 kDa in centromere pattern, and three bands of 70–100 kDa in the peripheral pattern. A peptide of 17 kDa was found specifically in all the patients positive for anti-centromere antibody. Molecular weights observed by this western blot method in AIH patients are summarized in Table 5.

The characteristics of these proteins were analysed by immunoblotting patterns of reference ANA sera[25]. Penner *et al.*[26] have found antibodies to lamins A (70 kDa) and C (60 kDa) in patients with active classical AIH, but not in patients in remission. However, these anti-lamins antibodies have also been observed in other connective tissue disorders including acute or chronic hepatitis[27–29]. It was shown that 12 out of 51 patients (24%) were positive for anti-lamin antibodies[26]. In the present study, antibodies to 70 and 60 kDa polypeptides were seen in sera with peripheral, homogeneous and speckled ANA, but whether these polypeptides are identical to lamin A and C is unclear. The clinical significance of anti-lamin antibodies is not well established. It seems likely that this antibody is a marker of autoimmune disease associated with AIH and PBC. The clinical relevance of these antibodies, in particular with regard to therapy and prognosis, remains to be clarified by further studies.

In the present study, AIH sera also reacted with low molecular weight polypeptides such as 17, 25, 30, 33, 36 and 50 kDa. The speckled pattern of ANA is often seen in these cases. In western blot, nuclear antigens of 12, 29, 33, 50, 60, 70 and 80 kDa were seen. They may be target antigens of anti-U1-RNP. Anti-U1-RNP recognizes unique proteins of 33 and 22 kDa of the U1 small ribonucleoprotein. Anti-Sm antibodies are capable of recognizing the small nuclear ribonucleic acid U1-6 and two proteins of 25 and 13 kDa[30]. These antibodies are known to be involved in the splicing of precursor mRNA. On the other hand, antibodies to La antigen recognize a 48 kDa protein involved in the termination of RNA polymerase III transcription, and recently the La antigen has been identified as part of the nucleic acid-dependent ATPase/dATPase[31]. Antibody to La antigen was also present in 4% of AIH patients, but such antibody was absent in all PBC patients[32].

The present studies suggest that apparent target peptides of ANA common to AIH are the proteins of 25 (doublet), 33 (doublet), 55, 60, 80, 100 and 140 kDa. A peptide of 140 kDa has been thought to belong to the nuclear matrix. But, proteins of 25, 33, 80 and 100 kDa seem to be composed of unknown nuclear portions, whereas peptides of 60 and 70 kDa could be anti-lamin antibody. It is unclear how these antibodies relate to the pathogenesis, but those antibodies may serve as valuable probes for characterization of some nuclear antigens as well as diagnostic markers in AIH patients.

AUTOANTIBODIES SPECIFIC FOR TRANSFER RIBONUCLEIC ACID (tRNA) IN AIH PATIENTS

Autoantibodies which precipitate snRNP (ribonucleoprotein) are found to be induced in some autoimmune diseases. Anti-Sm antibodies are capable of recognizing snRNA such as U1-6. However, most of these epitopes are proteins complexed with RNA. In the process of determining whether the patients with autoimmune liver diseases elicit an antibody to RNA itself as well as RNP, these autoantibodies were identified by immunoprecipitation of HeLa cell extracts[33].

As shown in Fig. 5, sera from patients with AIH were found to contain antibody directed against gel-purified tRNA in HeLa cell extract immunoprecipitated by anti-tRNA sera. Antiserum was incubated with HeLa cell

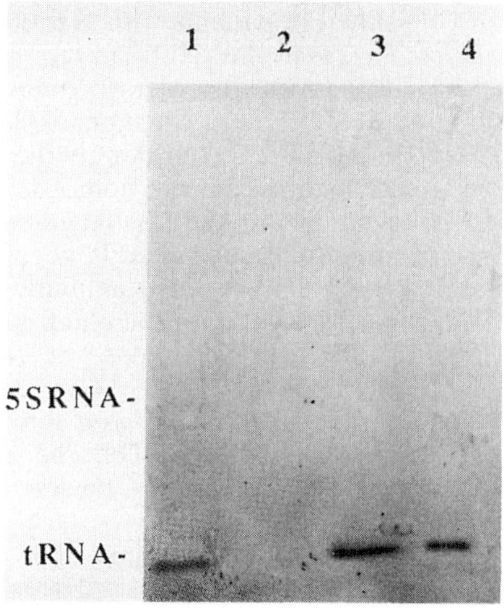

Fig. 5 Polyacrylamide gel elecrophoresis of tRNA immunoprecipitated by an anti-RNA serum. An antiserum was incubated with: HeLa cell extract (lane 1), HeLa cell extract digested by RNAase (lane 2), HeLa cell extract digested by DNAase (line 3), and HeLa cell extract digested by proteinase K (lane 4)

Table 6 Incidence of antibodies to sn-RNA in chronic hepatitis identified by immunoprecipitation

			Antibodies specific for									
			Small nuclear RNA						*Ribosomal RNA*			
Disease	*No.*	*tRNA*	*U1*	*U2*	*U3*	*U4*	*U5*	*U6*	*5s*	*5.8s*	*7s*	*> 7s*
Autoimmune CH	35	4 (3[a])	2	1	0	0	2	2	2	1	2	5
CH type B	10	0	0	0	0	0	0	0	0	0	0	0
NANB	10	0	0	0	0	0	0	0	0	0	0	0
Normal controls	10	0	0	0	0	0	0	0	0	0	0	0

[a]Antibodies, directed against purified tRNA
Shirai and Nishioka, *Hepatogastroenterology*. 1991;36:543

extracts, HeLa cell extract digested by RNAase, HeLa cell extract digested by DNAase, and HeLa cell extracts digested by proteinase K. Target antigens in sera from patients are sensitive to RNAase but not DNAase and proteinase. Four out of 35 sera from AIH showed the same reaction, but no sera obtained from CAH type B, CAH non-A–non-B or healthy volunteers reacted with HeLa cell RNA (Table 6).

A further study on these anti-tRNA sera disclosed, as shown in Fig. 6, that three of four sera that immunoprecipitated tRNA from HeLa cell extract, reacted with purified tRNA derived from calf liver, but reacted with neither 5 sRNA nor ribosomal RNA. After proteinase K and DNAase digestion of HeLa cell extract, the epitope for these three sera was conserved, and the antigen was sensitive to ribonuclease. It suggests that this epitope consists

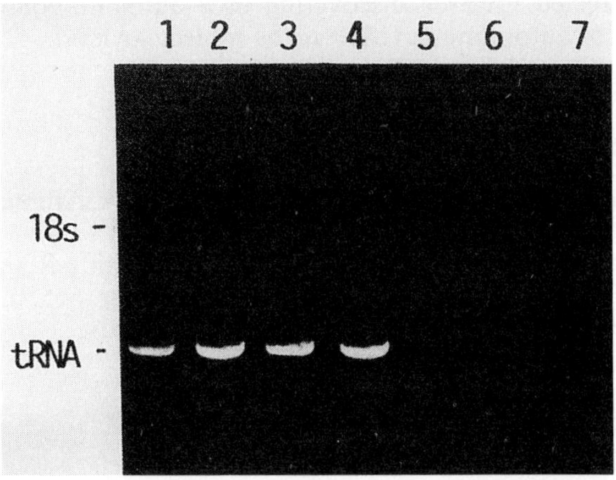

Fig. 6 tRNA immunoprecipitated by an anti-tRNA serum. An antiserum was incubated with: HeLa cell extract (lane 1), HeLa cell extract digested by proteinase K (lane 2), HeLa cell extract digested by DNAase (lane 3), purified calf liver tRNA (lane 4), HeLa cell extract digested by RNAase (lane 5), 5sRNA (E. coli) (lane 6), and rRNA (rabbit) (lane 7)

of tRNA. Antibodies to sn-RNA and ribosomal RNA were found in some sera from AIH patients.

Antibodies precipitating tRNA have been previously noted by immunoblotting in sera from patients with polymyositis[34] and SLE[35]. In the former report the antibody to Jo-1 antigen was found in 25% of polymyositis patients. The antigen was reported to be cytoplasmic histidyl-tRNA synthetase, resistant to digestion with RNAase. In the latter report, Hardin *et al.*[35] noted that patients with SLE had antibodies to two subsets of tRNA (anti-tRNA1, anti-tRNA2). These antibodies were thought to react with antigenic determinants that contain RNA only. We used deproteinized RNA as antigens and found that three sera from AIH were capable of precipitating RNA free from proteins. The antigens precipitated by these sera possibly contain tRNA only, or tRNA bound to other molecules rather than proteins. This antigen revealed a single sharp band, so it might be an unreported novel antigen which has a unique structure.

The patients exhibiting this antibody presented with severe hepatitis, but it was not clear how the antibody was related to the pathogenesis of this disease. Liver cell damage in autoimmune liver diseases is probably caused by cytotoxicity mediated by lymphocytes. It remains to be shown whether autoantibodies penetrate the cell membrane and exert a cytotoxic effect. However, some studies have suggested increased permeability of cell membranes to IgG-ANA in some patients[36] and IgG-ANA penetration of the membrane through the Fc receptor[37].

It is very important to investigate whether these antibody or antibody–RNA complexes play a role in cellular metabolisms such as RNA splicing or messenger RNA transcription. It is reasonable to expect that anti-tRNA antibodies participate in the synthesis of amino acids. Further research should be directed towards discovering how autoantibodies relate to the pathogenesis of autoimmune CAH at the molecular level.

Acknowledgements

This study was carried out in collaboration with Dr K. Arima, Dr M. Shirai, Dr S. A. Morshed, Dr H. S. Hong, Mrs S. Inoue and Mrs E. Ichikawa. The research was supported by a Grant in Aid for Scientific Research from the Ministry of Education, Science and Culture of Japan (61570345, 01570402) and from the Ministry of Health and Welfare of Japan.

References

1. Tan EM. Antinuclear antibodies. Diagnostic markers for autoimmune diseases and probes for cell biology. Adv Immunol. 1989;44:93–151.
2. Akizuki T. Collagen disease – laboratory tests and diagnosis. Tokyo: SRL; 1990.
3. Terada S, Hong HS *et al.* Analysis of antinuclear antibodies (ANA) in autoimmune hepatitis. In: Tsuchiya M, editor. Frontiers of mucosal immunology. Amsterdam: Elsevier; 1990: 39–42.
4. Bernstein RM, Neuberger JM *et al.* Diversity of autoantibodies in primary biliary cirrhosis and chronic active hepatitis. Clin Exp Immunol. 1984;55:553–60.
5. Golding PL, Smith M *et al.* Multisystemic involvement in chronic liver disease. Studies of the incidence and pathogenesis. Am J Med. 1973;55:772–82.
6. Bravo R, Rainer F, Blundell RA, Macdonald Bravo H. Cyclin/PCNA is the auxiliary protein of DNA polymerase delta. Nature. 1987;326:515–17.
7. Tan CK, Sullivan K, Li X *et al.* Autoantibody to the proliferating cell nuclear antigen neutralizes the activity of the auxiliary protein for DNA polymerase delta. Nucl Acids Res. 1987;15:9299–308.
8. Mattioli M, Reichlin M. Heterogeneity of RNA protein antigens reactive with sera of patients with systemic lupus erythematosus. Arthritis Rheum. 1974;17:421–9.
9. Alspaugh MA, Tan EM. Antibodies to cellular antigens in Sjögren's syndrome. J Clin Invest. 1975;55:1067–73.
10. Lerner MR, Boyle JA, Hardin JA, Steizz JA. Two novel classes of small ribonucleoproteins detected by antibodies associated with lupus erythematosus. Science. 1981;211:400–2.
11. Tsokos M, Lazarou AS, Haralampos M, Moutsopoulos M. Vasculitis in primary Sjogren's syndrome. Am J Clin Pathol. 1987;88:26–31.
12. Mattioli M, Reichlin M. Physical association of two nuclear antigens and mutual occurrence of their antibodies: the relationship of the Sm and RNA protein (Mo) systems in SLE sera. J Immunol. 1973;110:1318–24.
13. Esteban JI, Esteban R, Viladomiu L *et al.* Hepatitis C virus antibodies among risk groups in Spain. Lancet. 1989;2:294–7.
14. Lenzi M, Ballardini G, Fusconi M *et al.* Type 2 autoimmune hepatitis and hepatitis C virus infection. Lancet. 1990;1:258–9.
15. Swaak AJG, Aarden LA, van Epps LWS. Anti-ds DNA and complement profiles as prognostic guides in systemic lupus erythematosus. Arthritis Rheum. 1979;22:226–35.
16. Wood JR, Czaja AJ, Beaver SJ *et al.* Frequency and significance of antibody to double-stranded DNA in chronic active hepatitis. Hepatology. 1986;6:976–80.
17. Hinterberger M, Pettersson I, Steitz JA. Isolation of small nuclear ribonucleoprotein containing U1, U2, U4, U5 and U6 RNAs. J Biol Chem. 1983;258:2604–13.
18. Query CC, Bentley CR, Keene DJ. A common RNA recognition motif identified within a defined U1 RNA binding domain of the 70 K U1 snRNP protein. Cell. 1989;57:89–101.
19. Ben-Chetrit E, Chan EKL, Sullivan KF, Tan EM. A 52 kD protein is a novel component of the SS-A/Ro antigenic particle. J Exp Med. 1988;167:1560–71.

20. James AJ, Dickey DW, Fujisaku A *et al.* Antigenicity of a recombinant Ro (SS-A) fusion protein. Arthritis Rheum. 1990;33:102–6.
21. Deutscher LS, Harley BJ, Keene DJ. Molecular analysis of the 60-kDa human Ro ribonucleoprotein. Proc Natl Acad Sci USA. 1988;85:9479–83.
22. Earnshaw WC, Sullivan KF, Machlin PS *et al.* Molecular cloning of cDNA for CENP-B, the major human centromere autoantigen. J Cell Biol. 1987;104:817–29.
23. Penner E, Kindas-Mugge I *et al.* Nuclear antigens recognized by antibodies present in liver disease sera. Clin Exp Immunol. 1985;63:428–33.
24. Tan EM. Autoantibodies to nuclear antigen (ANA): their immunology and medicine. Adv Immunol. 1982;33:167–240.
25. Tan EM, Feltamp TEW *et al.* Reference agents for antinuclear antibodies. Arthritis Rheum. 1988;31:1331.
26. Wesierka-Gader J, Penner E *et al.* Antibodies to nuclear lamins in autoimmune liver disease. Clin Immunol Immunopathol. 1988;49:107–15.
27. Lassoued K, Guilly MN *et al.* Antinuclear antibodies specific for lamins. Characterization and clinical significance. Ann Intern Med. 1988;108:829–33.
28. Lozano F, Pares A *et al.* Autoantibodies against nuclear envelope-associated proteins in primary biliary cirrhosis. Hepatology. 1988;8:930–8.
29. McKeon FD, Tuffanelli DKL *et al.* Autoimmune response directed against conserved determinants of nuclear envelope proteins in a patient with linear scleroderma. Proc Natl Acad Sci USA. 1983;80:4374–8.
30. Lerner MR, Sleig JA. Antibodies to small nuclear RNAs complexed with proteins are produced by patients with systemic lupus erythematosus. Proc Natl Acad Sci USA. 1979;7:5495–9.
31. Bachmann M, Pfeifer K *et al.* Characterization of the antigen La as a nucleic acid-dependent ATPase/dATPase with melting properties. Cell. 1990;60:85–93.
32. Szostecki C, Krippner H *et al.* Autoimmune sera recognize a 100 KD nuclear protein antigen (sp-100). Clin Exp Immunol. 1987;68:108–16.
33. Shirai M, Watanabe S *et al.* Autoantibody specific for transfer ribonucleic acid in patients with autoimmune chronic active hepatitis and primary biliary cirrhosis. Hepatogastroenterology. 1991;3:543–6.
34. Mathews MB, Benestein RM. Myositis autoantibody inhibits histidyl-tRNA synthetase: a model for autoimmunity. Nature. 1983;304:177–9.
35. Hardin AJ, Rahn RD, Shen C *et al.* Antibodies from patients with connective tissue diseases bind specific subsets of cellular RNA–protein particles. J Clin Invest. 1982;70:141–7.
36. Izuno GT. Observations on the *in vitro* reaction of antinuclear antibodies with epidermal cells. Br J Dermatol. 1978;98:391–8.
37. Alarcon-Segovia D, Ruiz-Arguelles A, Fishbein E. Antibody to nuclear ribonucleoprotein penetrates live human mononuclear cells through Fc receptors. Nature. 1978;271:67–9.

23
Cytoskeleton antibodies in chronic active hepatitis

P. KURKI

INTRODUCTION

Autoantibodies to intracellular autoantigens are present in a wide variety of chronic inflammatory and 'autoimmune' diseases. Interestingly, antibodies in different diseases seem to be directed against different cellular compartments, such as the cell nucleus, cytosolic enzyme systems, endoplasmic reticulum, cytoskeleton, and cell membranes. The pathogenetic significance of these antibodies is usually not known. However, some autoantibodies serve as unique fingerprints of the underlying immunopathogenetic mechanisms. As such they are useful diagnostic markers for many diseases, including chronic active hepatitis (CAH). Johnson *et al.*[1] and Whittingham *et al.*[2] demonstrated high titres of antibodies to smooth muscle cells in sera from patients with 'lupoid' hepatitis. Subsequently, these antibodies were shown to be targeted against ubiquitous components of the cytoskeleton, notably the actomyosin system[3].

THE CYTOSKELETON

Extraction of the cells attached to a solid phase with detergent-containing buffers will remove most cellular constituents. The remaining structures are composed of adhesion sites, microfilaments attached to them, intermediate filaments surrounding the nuclear lamina, and in certain conditions also microtubules[4,5]. This structure is called the cytoskeleton – not only because of its resemblance to remnants of an unfortunate traveller in the desert but also because of the function in the normal cell[6]. The cytoskeleton of a muscle cell is very well developed owing to the contractile function. The main components of the microtubules and microfilaments are the same in all cells but intermediate filaments display more heterogeneity (Table 1). In cultured cells the microfilaments may occur in thick parallel bundles traversing the cytoplasm – the sheet filaments or 'stress fibres' (Fig. 1). Poisoning of the

Table 1 Cytoskeleton and cytoskeleton antibodies

Structure	*Main subunit protein(s)*	*Disease association of autoantibodies*
Microfilament	Actin	Liver diseases
Microtubule	Tubulin	Acute infections
Intermediate filaments in		
Mesenchymal cells	Vimentin	Acute and chronic inflammation
Muscle cells	Desmin	Myocarditis
Epithelial cells	Cytokeratins	Rheumatic diseases
Glial cells	GFA protein	Unknown
Neurones	Neurofilament protein triplet	Certain neurological disorders

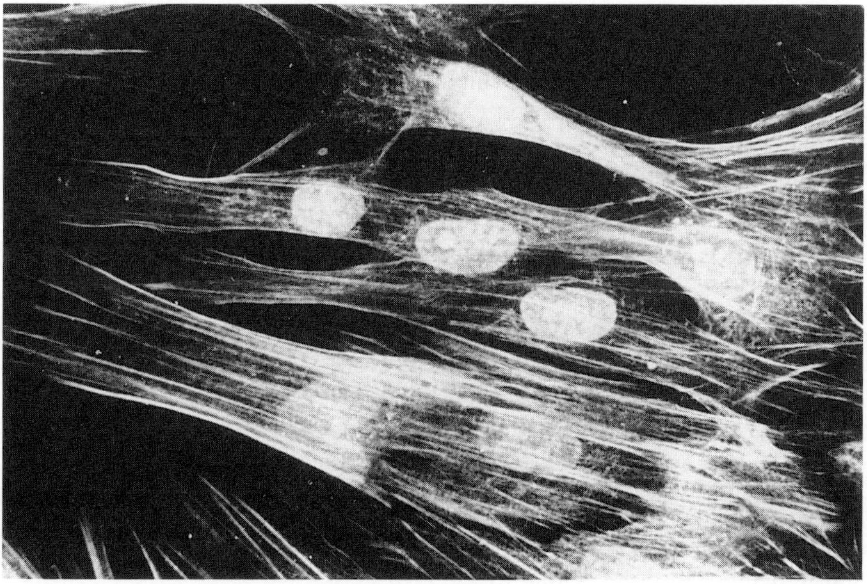

Fig. 1 Indirect immunofluorescence staining of human embryonic fibroblasts by serum from a patient with autoimmune chronic active hepatitis. The cells were grown on glass coverslips and fixed with acetone. Note the staining of actin-containing parallel sheet filaments and the homogeneous staining of the nuclei

cells with phalloidin leads to an irreversible polymerization of actin, the subunit protein of microfilaments[7]. There are several microfilament-associated 'contractile' proteins such as troponin, tropomyosin, and α-actinin. Vinca alkaloids, such as vinblastine, act by disrupting microtubules and inducing the formation of tubulin-containing paracrystals[8]. Intermediate filaments seem to regulate the spatial organization within the cell by providing the framework for various cellular structures[9]. Some but not all intermediate filaments can be collapsed into perinuclear filament bundles by the mitotic inhibitors[10]. The typical changes in the cytoskeletal organization induced by phalloidin and vinblastine help in the identification of the cytoskeleton structures labelled by human autoantibodies[11].

Table 2 Prevalence of SMA in liver disease (percentages)

CAH	
Idiopathic[2,12,42]	50–70
'Lupoid'[2]	80
Viral[15,42]	8–10
Drug[15]	34
PBC[12]	50
Alcoholic liver disease[43]	49

SMOOTH MUSCLE ANTIBODIES (SMA) IN CHRONIC ACTIVE HEPATITIS

The indirect immunofluorescence test for smooth muscle antibodies is still the standard cytoskeleton antibody test. This assay is difficult to standardize since it is based on subjective interpretation of the immunofluorescence staining pattern. Thus, there is a wide variation in reported prevalences among healthy individuals[12,13]. The lack of standardization makes it difficult to compare the prevalences of SMA in different CAH patient groups. Furthermore, it is probable that CAH patients in different parts of the world have a different prevalence of SMA due to the geographical differences in the proportion of various subtypes of CAH[14]. It is generally accepted that the highest prevalence of SMA, about 80%, can be found in the antinuclear antibody-positive, 'lupoid' type of CAH. Patients with drug-induced CAH may also have very high SMA titres[15]. Approximately 50–70% of patients with the cryptogenic CAH are SMA-positive. Some patients have high titres of SMA whereas in other diseases, such as virus-induced CAH, CAH associated with alcoholic liver injury, α-antitrypsin deficiency or Wilson's disease, as well as in primary biliary cirrhosis, the titres tend to be low (Table 2). Low-titre SMA are frequently seen in patients with acute and chronic infections, malignant diseases and rheumatic diseases[11]. SMA in CAH belong almost exclusively to the IgG class, whereas SMA in primary biliary cirrhosis and in acute infections belong to the IgM class[16–18].

CLASSIFICATION OF THE CYTOSKELETON ANTIBODIES IN CAH

Unfixed cryostat sections of rat, mouse and rabbit tissues are generally used as substrate in the assay for smooth muscle and other autoantibodies. Soon after the discovery of SMA it was observed that some sera reacted not only with smooth muscle but also with the glomerular mesangium, renal peritubular fibres and with bile canaliculi of rat and rabbit liver. These staining patterns were almost exclusively associated with sera from patients with CAH, whereas SMA from other patients reacted only with smooth muscle tissue. Absorption experiments revealed that the broad reacting (SMA-G and SMA-T) SMA and the bile canalicular antibodies were in fact actin antibodies[19,20].

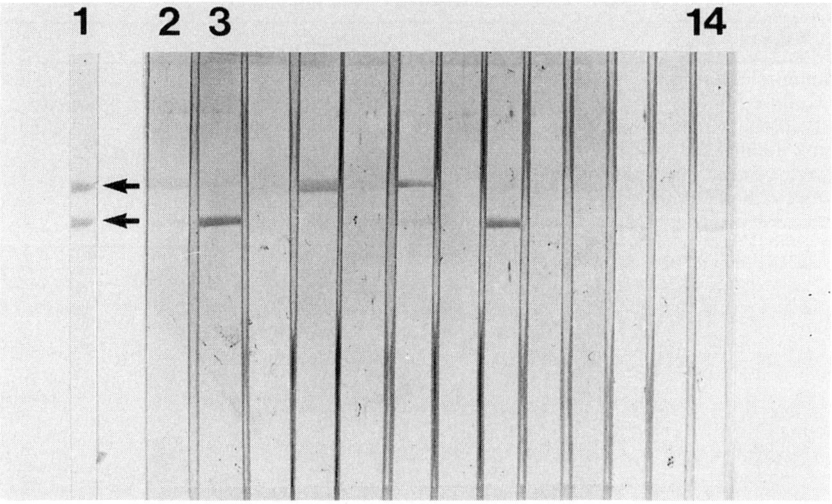

Fig. 2 Immunoblotting assay for human tropomyosin antibodies. Lane 1 shows the protein staining of tropomyosin preparation on a nitrocellulose strip. Lanes 2–14 show the immunoblotting with human sera. Lane 2 shows a normal human serum, and lanes 3–14 sera from patients with chronic hepatitis. Note the labelling of tropomyosin bands by sera on lanes 3, 5, 7 and 9

The use of tissue sections as substrate does not allow the identification of the subcellular target structures for SMA. This is achieved by using cultured cells such as embryonic fibroblasts as targets. The actin type SMA label the actin-containing microfilaments (Fig. 1) whereas the non-actin SMA bind to other fibrous and filamentous structures[21]. These structures were identified as intermediate filaments and microtubules[22,23]. Sera reacting with these structures often come from patients with viral infections including viral hepatitis[11].

DIFFERENT TYPES OF CYTOSKELETON ANTIBODIES IN CAH

Absorption experiments have shown that SMA in virtually all sera from CAH patients can be inhibited by purified actin[20,21,24,25]. The inhibition is usually defined by the lowering of the SMA titre by at least two steps. Thus, it is not excluded that the same sera may contain low titres of other SMA types; in fact, SMA-positive sera from patients with CAH may contain antibodies to other 'contractile' or microfilament-associated proteins, such as myosin, troponin, tropomyosin and α-actinin[26] (Kurki and Vuoristo, unpublished results; Fig. 2).

The cytoskeleton antibody assay with cultured fibroblasts as substrate has shown that patients with CAH may also have antibodies to vimentin intermediate filaments and microtubules[27]. The vimentin filament antibodies seem to be more prevalent in patients with virus-induced CAH as compared

Table 3 Alternative methods for the detection of actin antibodies[27,44–48]

Technique	*Comment*
Immunofluorescence	
Cultured cells	Insensitive; loss of diagnostic specificity
Phalloidin-treated liver tissue	Cumbersome in routine use
Immunodiffusion	False-positive reactions; insensitive
Enzyme-linked immunosorbent technique and radioimmunoassay	Loss of diagnostic specificity
Immunoblotting	Insensitive

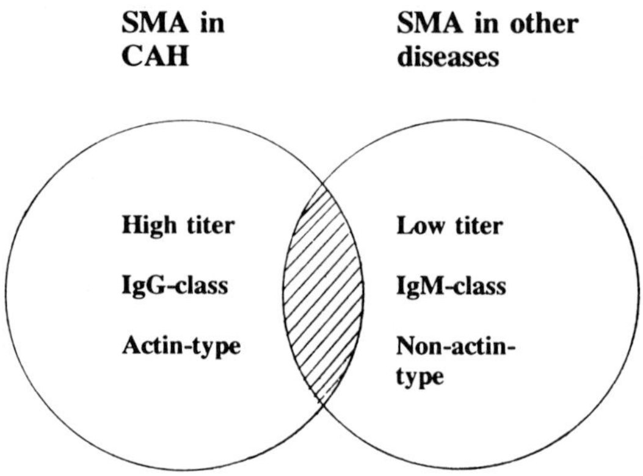

Fig. 3 Differences of the smooth muscle antibodies (SMA) in autoimmune chronic active hepatitis (CAH) and in other diseases

to the cryptogenic, autoimmune type I CAH that is associated with microfilament antibodies[14]. A fraction of autoimmune CAH patients have antibodies to a soluble antigen from the cytoplasm of the hepatocyte. These anti-SLA antibodies seem to react with cytokeratins[28]. The anti-SLA-positive patients may comprise a clinically distinct subgroup of the autimmune CAH[29].

THE ASSAY OF ACTIN ANTIBODIES

The routine indirect immunofluorescence assay for SMA offers a convenient and simple way of recognizing actin-type SMA[19,30]. There are several reports on alternative tests for actin antibodies. This is understandable because a specific and quantitative anti-actin assay could potentially be an important improvement in the screening and differential diagnostics as well as in the classification of CAH. Unfortunately, none of these assays has gained wide clinical acceptance (Table 3). It is obvious that the new assays may detect overlapping or entirely different antibody populations that may not have the same diagnostic specificity as the antibodies to 'native' actin detected by the immunofluorescence test.

THE NATURE OF THE HUMAN ACTIN ANTIBODIES

The human actin type SMA react with antigenic determinants that are well conserved in the evolution. It has been difficult to produce experimental antibodies to the same epitopes[30] (Fig. 3). The fact that in the tissues and in cultured cells human actin antibodies react with polymerized F-actin but not with unpolymerized G-actin is in contrast to the finding that the reaction can be inhibited by both F- and G-actin. This discrepancy can be explained by the high density of epitopes in F-actin. However, it is also possible that the antigenic sites are blocked by actin binding proteins that regulate actin polymerization, notably gelsolin and GC protein. It is of interest that gelsolin and actin are also present in the plasma[31].

THE ORIGIN OF ACTIN ANTIBODIES IN CAH

Attempts to produce actin antibodies in experimental animals have shown that the tolerance is very difficult to overcome. This tolerance is not due to the lack of B cells recognizing actin and other cytoskeleton antigens. B cells from healthy individuals can be triggered to produce cytoskeleton antibodies. Healthy individuals also have minute amounts of actin antibodies[32,33]. These antibodies are called ‘natural antibodies’ that are usually polyreactive and are coded for by germline genes[34].

The production of cytoskeleton antibodies, including actin antibodies, can be triggered by acute infections[11]. This may be explained by the fact that the viral antigens and the associated increase in cytokines will stimulate B lymphocytes with germline repertoire. The administration of interferon-α to patients with chronic hepatitis will induce the production of certain autoantibodies[35,36]. During the normal maturation of the immune response the autoreactivity is lost and antiviral activity becomes stronger[37].

The reason why IgG-class actin antibodies are produced in CAH in high titres cannot yet be explained. It can be suggested that the abnormal production of actin antibodies is due to a failure to redirect the initial immune response away from the self antigen actin. This situation can arise if actin is complexed with an agent, such as a viral component, that helps actin to bypass the T cell tolerance[38]. It should be noted that viruses may well be involved in the pathogenesis of the ‘idiopathic’ autoimmune type of CAH[39]. It is obvious that actin-containing structures themselves are contributing to the production of actin antibodies because the patients can simultaneously have antibodies of different antibody classes and also against different epitopes of actin molecule, as well as against antigens in the actin-associated proteins[26].

CONCLUSIONS

Cytoskeleton antibodies occur in a variety of inflammatory conditions. Cytoskeleton antibodies in the idiopathic autoimmune (type I) CAH are directed mainly against actin (Fig. 3). These actin antibodies react with antigenic determinants exposed in smooth muscle tissue. Antibodies to purified and partly denatured actin can be demonstrated in many chronic inflammatory conditions. The classification of CAH on the basis of autoantibody profiles, including actin antibodies, may become important in assessment of the prognosis and in the choice of the therapy for CAH[40,41]. The circulating anti-actin antibodies may derive from actin-specific lymphocytes with a germline repertoire. This anti-actin response may be triggered by exogenous antigens and 'mature' under the pressure of cytokines and self antigens. The mechanisms that lead to the strong anti-actin response in CAH are obviously closely related to the aetiology and pathogenesis of the disease.

References

1. Johnson GD, Holborow EJ, Glynn LE. Antibody to smooth muscle in patients with liver disease. Lancet. 1965;2:878–9.
2. Whittingham MB, Mackay IR, Irwin J. Autoimmune hepatitis. Immunofluorescence reactions with cytoplasm of smooth muscle and glomerular cells. Lancet. 1966;1:1333–5.
3. Farrow LJ, Holborow EJ, Brighton WD. Reaction of human smooth muscle antibody with liver cells. Nature New Biol. 1971;232:186–7.
4. Brown S, Levinson W, Spudich J. Cytoskeletal elements of chick embryo fibroblasts revealed by detergent extraction. J Supramol Structure. 1976;5:119–30.
5. McKeon FD, Kirschner MW, Caput D. Homologies in both primary and secondary structure between nuclear envelope and intermediate filament proteins. Nature. 1986;319:463–8.
6. Porter KR. The cytomatrix: a short history of its study. J Cell Biol. 1984;99:3–12.
7. Cooper JA. Effects of cytochalasin and phalloidin on actin. J Cell Biol. 1987;105:1473–8.
8. Bensch KG, Malawista S. Microtubule crystals: A new biophysical phenomenon induced by vinca alcaloids. Nature. 1968;218:1176–7.
9. Lazarides E. Intermediate filaments as mechanical integrators of cellular space. Nature. 1980;283:249–56.
10. Goldman RD, Knipe DM. Functions of cytoplasmic fibres. Cold Spring Harbor Symp Quant Biol. 1972;37:523–34.
11. Kurki P, Virtanen I. The detection of human antibodies against cytoskeletal components. J Immunol Meth. 1984;67:209–23.
12. Kurki P. Human smooth muscle antibodies. Thesis, Helsinki University; 1979.
13. Toh BH. Smooth muscle autoantibodies and autoantigens. Clin Exp Immunol. 1979;38: 621–8.
14. Pedersen JS, Toh BH, Mackay IR, Tait BD, Gust ID, Kastelan A, Hadzic N. Segregation of autoantibody to cytoskeletal filaments, actin and intermediate filaments with two types of chronic active hepatitis. Clin Exp Immunol. 1982;48:527–32.
15. Lindberg J, Lindholm A, Lundin P, Iwarson S. Trigger factors and HLA-A-antigens in chronic active hepatitis. Br Med J. 1975;4:77–79.
16. Kurki P, Miettinen A, Linder E, Pikkarainen P, Vuoristo M, Salaspuro M. Different types of smooth muscle antibodies in chronic active hepatitis and primary biliary cirrhosis: their diagnostic and prognostic significance. Gut. 1980;21:878–84.
17. Holborow EJ. Smooth-muscle autoantibodies, viral infections and malignant disease. Proc R Soc Med. 1972;65:481–4.
18. Mead GM, Cowin P, Whitehouse JMA. Antitubulin antibody in healthy adults and patients with infectious mononucleosis and its relationship to smooth muscle antibody (SMA). Clin Exp Immunol. 1980;32:328–36.
19. Bottazzo GF, Florin-Christensen A, Fairfax A, Swana G, Doniach D, Gröschel-Stewart U. Classification of smooth muscle autoantibodies detected by immunofluorescence. J Clin Pathol. 1976;29:403–10.
20. Kurki P, Linder E, Miettinen A, Alfthan O. Smooth muscle antibodies of actin and 'non-actin' specificity. Clin Immunol Immunopathol. 1978;9:443–53.

21. Gabbiani G, Ryan GB, Lamelin JP, Vassali P, Majno G, Bouvier CA, Cruchaud A, Lüscher EF. Human smooth muscle autoantibody. Its identification as antiactin antibody and a study of its binding to 'nonmuscular' cells. Am J Pathol. 1973;72:473–88.
22. Kurki P, Virtanen I, Stenman S, Linder E. Human smooth muscle antibodies reacting with intermediate (100Å) filaments. Nature. 1977;268:240–1.
23. Kurki P, Virtanen I, Stenman S, Linder E. Smooth muscle antibodies reacting with microtubular antigens. Protides Biol Fluids. 1979;26:629–32.
24. Lidman K, Biberfeld G, Fagraeus A, Norberg R, Thorstenson R, Utter G, Carlsson L, Luca, Lindberg U. Anti-actin specificity of human smooth muscle antibodies in chronic active hepatitis. Clin Exp Immunol. 1976;24:266–72.
25. Andersen P, Small JV, Sobieszek A. Studies on the specificity of smooth-muscle antibodies. Clin Exp Immunol. 1976;26:57–66.
26. Dighiero G, Lymberi P, Monot C, Abuaf N. Sera with high levels of anti-smooth muscle and anti-mitochondrial antibodies frequently bind to cytoskeleton proteins. Clin Exp Immunol. 1990;82:52–6.
27. Kurki P, Miettinen A, Salaspuro M, Virtanen I, Stenman S. Cytoskeleton antibodies in chronic active hepatitis, primary biliary cirrhosis and alcoholic liver disease. Hepatology. 1983;3:297–302.
28. Wachter B, Kyriatsoulis A, Lohse AW, Gerken G, Meyer zum Büschenfelde KH, Manns M. Characterization of liver cytokeratin as a major target antigen of anti-SLA antibodies. J Hepatol. 1990;11:232–9.
29. Manns M, Gerken G, Kyriatsoulis A, Staritz M, Meyer zum Büschenfelde KH. Characterization of a new subgroup of autoimmune chronic active hepatitis by antibodies against a soluble liver antigen. Lancet. 1987;1:292–4.
30. Kurki P. Determination of anti-actin antibodies by a solid phase immunoenzymatic assay and by indirect immunofluorescence technique. Clin Immunol Immunopathol. 1978;11: 328–38.
31. Lee WM, Galbraight RM. The extracellular actin-scavenger system and actin toxicity. N Engl J Med. 1992;326:1335–41.
32. Guilbert RD, Dighiero G, Avrameas S. Naturally occurring antibodies against nine common antigens in human sera. I. Detection, isolation and characterization. J Immunol. 1982;128:2779–87.
33. Bijlsma JWJ, Plater-Zyberk C, Mumford P, Maini RN. Lack of natural antibodies in rheumatic diseases. Rheumatol. Int. 1990;10:107–17.
34. Dighiero G, Hart S, Lim A, Borche L, Levy R, Miller RA. Autoantibody activity of immunoglobulins isolated from B-cell follicular lymphomas. Blood. 1991;3:581–5.
35. Fattovich G, Betterle C, Brollo L, Pedini B, Giustina G, Realdi G, Alberti A, Ruol A. Autoantibodies during α-interferon therapy for chronic hepatitis. Br J Med Virol. 1991;34:132–5.
36. Mayet WJ, Hess G, Gerken G, Felde KH. Treatment of chronic type B hepatitis with recombinant α-interferon induces autoantibodies not specific for autoimmune chronic hepatitis. Hepatology. 1989;1:24–8.
37. Avrameas S. Natural autoantibodies: from 'horror autotoxicus' to 'gnothi seauton'. Immunol Today. 1991;12:154–9.
38. Anomasiri WT, Tovell DR, Tyrrell DLJ. Paramyxovirus membrane protein enhances antibody production to new antigenic determinants in the actin molecule: a model for virus-induced autoimmunity. J Virol. 1990;64:3179–84.
39. Friedman LS, Patel KP, Munoz SJ. Hepatitis C virus and autoimmune chronic active hepatitis: closing the ring. Gastroenterology. 1992;102:1436–8.
40. Maddrey WC. Subdivisions of idiopathic autoimmune chronic active hepatitis. Hepatology. 1987;7:1372–5.
41. Manns M. Autoantibodies and antigens in liver diseases – updated. J Hepatol. 1989;9: 272–80.
42. Doniach D, Roitt IM, Walker JG, Sherlock S. Tissue antibodies in primary biliary cirrhosis and other liver diseases and their clinical implications. Clin Exp Immunol. 1966;1:237–62.
43. Gluud C, Tage-Jensen M, Bahnsen M, Dietrichson O, Svejgaard A. Autoantibodies, histocompatibility antigens and testosterone in males with alcoholic liver cirrhosis. Clin Exp Immunol. 1981;44:31–7.

44. Cassani F, Fusconi M, Bianchi FB, Selleri L, Baffoni L, Lenzi M, Pisi E. Precipitating antibodies to rabbit thymus extractable antigens in chronic liver disease: relationship with anti-actin antibodies. Clin Exp Immunol. 1987;68:588–95.
45. Fagraeus A, Norberg R, Biberfeld G. Anti-actin antibodies of human and rabbit origin. Ann Immunol. 1978;129C:245–54.
46. Fusconi M, Cassani F, Zauli D, Lenzi M, Ballardini G, Volta U, Bianchi FB. Anti-actin antibodies: a new test for an old problem. J Immunol Meth. 1990;130:1–8.
47. Louzir H, Ternynck T, Gorgi Y, Tahar S, Ayed K, Avrameas S. Autoantibodies and circulating immune complexes in sera from patients with hepatitis B virus-related chronic liver disease. Clin Immunol Immunopathol. 1992;62:160–7.
48. Mayet WJ, Press AG, Herrman E, Moll R, Manns M, Ewe K, Mayer zum Büschenfelde KH. Antibodies to cytoskeletal proteins in patients with Crohn's disease. Eur J Clin Invest. 1990;20:516–24.

24
Anti-liver cytosol antibodies in hepatology: autoimmune hepatitis, viral hepatitis C and graft-versus-host disease

N. ABUAF, C. JOHANET, E. SOULIE, J. LOEPER
and J.-C. HOMBERG

INTRODUCTION

During the 1980s it was our experience that 15% of sera yielding cytoplasmic immunofluorescence on the rat liver/kidney/stomach composite blocks used for autoantibody detection in liver disorders gave results that were difficult to interpret. These difficulties were partially resolved by the use of immunodiffusion and immunoabsorption, and were due to various causes:

1. new antibodies such as anti-liver-cytosol antibodies (anti-LC);
2. known autoantibodies giving atypical fluorescence, such as anti-liver/kidney microsome type 1 (anti-LKM1) which, contrary to initial reports[1,2], stains renal distal tubules in 10% of cases;
3. variations in the immunofluorescence pattern during the titration, suggesting an association of autoantibodies;
4. monoclonal immunoglobulins which stick to the cytoplasm of cells and mimic autoantibodies;
5. heteroantibodies against a rat or rodent antigen;
6. individual antibodies with special patterns, that are not present in other patients with the same disorder.

After the short paper limited to anti-LC1[3], we shall give here details of the different anti-rat liver cytosol antibodies. Immunodiffusion remains the reference method in our laboratory (because of the useful reaction of identity it allows) and will therefore be described first. As anti-LKM1 is frequently associated with anti-LC1, data on both autoantibodies will be given.

Table 1 Precipitating antibodies against the liver microsomal and cytosolic fractions in 2857 patients (Eric Martini, medical thesis, Paris, 1983)

	Microsomal fraction		*Cytosolic fraction*	
Positive sera	99		49	
Systems	Anti-LKM1	91	Anti-LC1	22
	Anti-ribosome	3	Anti-LC2	3
	Individual Ab	5	Anti-rat LKC	10
			Individual Ab	14

IMMUNODIFFUSION WITH RAT LIVER CYTOSOL

In 1982 Ouchterlony double-immunodiffusion with rat liver subcellular fractions was compared with immunofluorescence. Sera from 2857 patients were tested undiluted against the microsomal and cytosolic fractions containing 20 mg of protein/ml. The clinical diagnoses were as follows: primary biliary cirrhosis with anti-mitochondria type 2 (anti-M2) > 1/100 ($n = 100$), autoimmune hepatitis 1 with anti-actin antibody ($n = 100$), disorders with anti-LKM1 ($n = 65$), which can now be divided into 43 cases of autoimmune hepatitis 2 and 22 of viral hepatitis C after RIBA-2 testing for anti-HCV, drug-induced hepatitis ($n = 157$), chronic viral hepatitis B ($n = 100$), chronic viral hepatitis D with anti-LKM3 ($n = 4$), syphilitic hepatitis with anti-M1 ($n = 6$), and 925 miscellaneous liver disorders including non-A–non-B hepatitis, alcoholic hepatitis and malignant hepatic tumours, 1300 sera sent to our laboratory for autoantibody detection, and 100 samples from healthy blood donors. Since 1983 all sera staining the hepatocyte cytoplasm in the immunofluorescence test have been checked by means of immunodiffusion. More than 2000 sera from patients with liver diseases have been tested each year.

Liver subcellular fractions were prepared according to de Duve's method, as described by Martini *et al.*[3]. Good separation of the microsomal and cytosolic fractions requires a centrifuge speed of 105 000*g* for 90 min (not 60 min) and the top of the microsomal pellet must be washed with buffer. The latter fraction is dissolved in buffer by squashing it carefully against the container, without initially adding buffer. When the pellet becomes smoother, buffer is added drop by drop, each drop being mixed thoroughly with the pellet. The cytosolic fraction, initially diluted with 9 volumes of saccharose, is then concentrated by dialysis (PEG 20 000) overnight. All the steps are carried out at 4 °C. Finally the subcellular fractions are adjusted to a concentration of 20 mg protein/ml. The Ouchterlony double-immunodiffusion micromethod was carried out with 0.4% agarose in phosphate buffer, pH 7.4, without polyethyleneglycol. The reaction was read 24 and 48 h later. Positive reactions of identity were clearer the next day.

The immunodiffisuion method identified the three following precipitating anti-rat liver cytosol antibodies (Table 1):

1. Anti-LC1. This previously described antibody[3] reacted with rat liver but not with kidney, stomach, spleen and thymus cytosolic fractions in the

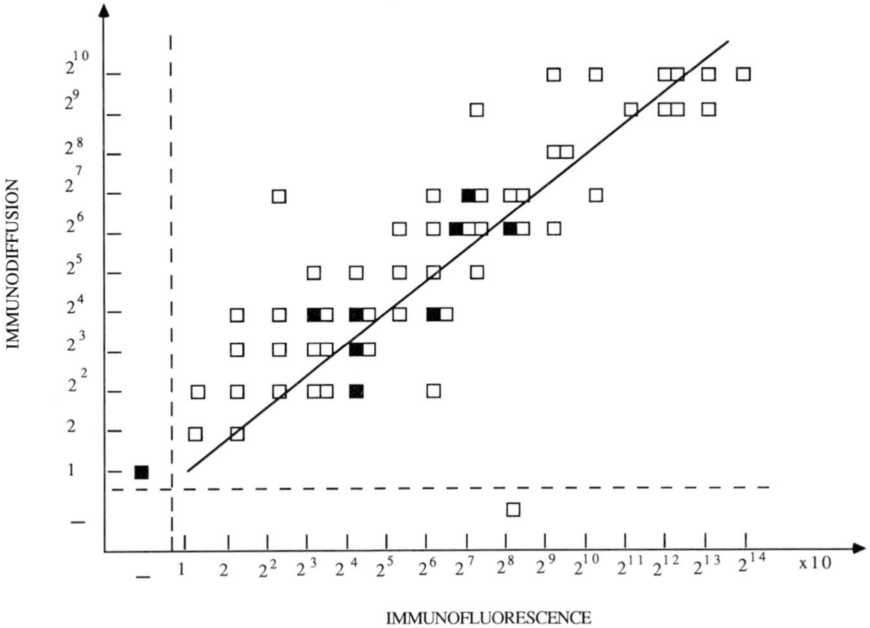

Fig. 1 Correlation between the titres of the antibodies detected by immunofluorescence and by immunodiffusion. Results are expressed as the reciprocal to the titres of anti-LC1 (■) and anti-LKM1 (□) found by immunofluorescence and immunodiffusion (correlation coefficient = 0.68). Eric Martini, medical thesis, Paris, 1983

immunodiffusion assay. A reaction of identity was obtained with liver from mouse, monkey and humans. The liver specificity was checked by means of immunofluorescence with a large number of rat organs.

2. Anti-LC2. This antibody was similar to anti-LC1 with regard to organ and species specificity but showed a reaction of non-identity with anti-LC1.
3. Anti-rat liver/kidney cytosol heteroantibody (anti-rat LKC). Contrary to the previous antibodies, anti-rat LKC precipitated with the cytosolic fractions of other rat organs (kidney, pancreas, spleen and thymus). In immunodiffusion and immunofluorescence tests, anti-rat LKC did not react with livers of other species and was considered a heteroantibody. Identification of this antibody avoids possible confusion with anti-LKM1.

The sensitivity of immunodiffusion for anti-LC1 and anti-LKM1 was 10–20 times lower than that of immunofluorescence (Fig. 1). Nevertheless, immunodiffusion involves undiluted sera, whereas immunofluorescence requires sera to be diluted 1/10. There was a good correlation between the two methods. Sometimes a serum was positive in only one method, e.g. the two cases indicated in Fig. 1. In a young girl with autoimmune hepatitis 2, all sera were negative by immunodiffusion during the course of the disease, in spite of a high titre by immunofluorescence at onset. In contrast, the

Table 2 Precipitating and non-precipitating autoantibodies in hepatology

Precipitating autoantibodies	*Non-precipitating autoantibodies*
Essential autoimmune disorders	Viral hepatitis
PBC anti-M2	Virus D anti-LKMδ
AH2 anti-LKM1	
anti-LC1	
Graft versus host disease	Drug-induced hepatitis
anti-M2	halothane anti-LKM1
anti-LKM1	tienilic acid anti-LKM2
anti-LC2	iproniazid anti-M6
Virus C hepatitis	
anti-LKM1	
anti-LC1	

serum of a 3-year-old girl was positive undiluted only by immunodiffusion at the onset of hepatitis. The great advantage of immunodiffusion over immunofluorescence is that immunodiffusion can be used to detect two associated autoantibodies: a mixture of microsomal and cytosolic fractions frequently gave two precipitating lines corresponding to anti-LKM1 and anti-LC1 in a given serum. With immunofluorescence, anti-LC1 was usually masked by anti-LKM1. In contrast, immunodiffusion detects only precipitating antibodies. Table 2 shows the disorders in which these latter antibodies are found. In essential autoimmune disorders most antibodies are detectable by immunodiffusion, and also in 60% of graft-versus-host disease (GVHD). Autoantibodies do not precipitate in viral and drug-induced hepatitis, with the exception of viral hepatitis C (anti-LKM1 and rare anti-LC1). A positive immunoprecipitation reaction requires the recognition of antigen by at least three distinct antigenic determinants. So precipitating autoantibodies argues for the self-antigen-driven hypothesis and is against crossreacting antibodies induced by foreign antigen.

IMMUNOFLUORESCENCE WITH IMMUNOABSORPTION

The classical indirect immunofluorescence method was used with rat liver/kidney/stomach composite tissue block cryostat sections from 2–3-month-old male rats (Wistar strain). As the third portion of proximal tubules (P3) was poorly reactive in the female rat, anti-LKM1 detection required kidney from a male rat[2]. At the first step rat organs are better than mouse organs because the different renal zones (outer cortex, inner cortex, outer medulla) could be clearly distinguished and gave better distinction between the different anti-LKMs. In addition, anti-M5 present in the anti-phospholipid syndrome was better distinguished from other anti-mitochondria antibodies such as anti-M1 and anti-M2. In a second step, mouse organs should be used to confirm anti-M5 (immunofluorescent change from proximal tubules (P1 and P2) in rat to distal tubules in mouse and anti-LKM2[4] (centrilobular fluorescence in only male mouse).

Anti-liver cytosol antibodies showed a uniformly homogeneous fluorescence pattern over the whole hepatocyte cytoplasm. Under a high-power

Table 3 Antibodies showing a rodent hepatocyte heterogeneity

		Centrilobular	
	Periportal hepatocytes	*Non-juxtavenous hepatocytes*	*Juxtavenous hepatocyes*
With zonal distribution			
Anti-juxtavenous hepatocytes	−	−	+
Anti-LC1	+	+	−
Anti-LM (cytochrome P450 IA2)	−	+	+
Anti-LKM2 (cytochrome P450 IIC)	−[a]	+	+
Anti-LC2	+	−	−
With non-zonal distribution			
Anti-proliferating cell nuclear antigen		< 1% hepatocytes	
Anti-M[b] with heterogeneity		60% hepatocytes	
Anti-C of few hepatocytes			
With panlobular distribution		5% hepatocytes	
With centrilobular distribution		5% hepatocytes	

[a]Anti-LKM2 gives a centrilobular pattern only on male mouse liver and a panlobular pattern on rat and human livers of both sexes and on female mouse liver[4]
[b]Anti-M = anti-mitochondria antibody

microscope the fluorescence could be distinguished from the granular pattern of anti-mitochondria antibodies, the perinuclear location of anti-ribosome antibodies, the localized staining of rare anti-Golgi apparatus and anti-lysosome antibodies. Five of the six homogeneous cytoplasmic fluorescence patterns suggestive of anti-LC were easily identified through rat hepatocyte heterogeneity as anti-rat juxtavenous hepatocytes, anti-LC1, anti-LC2, anti-few rat hepatocytes with a panlobular distribution and another with a centrilobular distribution (Table 3). In this way, anti-LC1, which spared the juxtavenous hepatocytes present only in rat and mouse livers, is easy to recognize when it is alone. When faced with an anti-LKM1 pattern, a weaker fluorescence of juxtavenous hepatocytes suggests a hidden anti-LC1. A periportal hepatocyte location in livers of different species (rat, mouse, monkey, humans) strongly indicates a rare antibody, the anti-LC2. Anti-rat LKC shows weak fluorescence which is stronger on proximal tubules (P1, P2, P3) than on hepatocytes which can appear negative. This antibody was confused with anti-LKM1 before the use of immunodiffusion (see fig. 5 of ref. 2).

The main advantage of indirect immunofluorescence remains the ability to detect simultaneously all the autoantibodies of interest in hepatology without the need for very expensive materials and reagents (except for the fluorescence microscope) and in a relatively short time. Precipitating and non-precipitating antibodies are similarly detected. The main weakness of this assay is the failure to identify autoantibodies in a mixture: only the autoantibody with the widest cellular distribution appears. As a result, anti-M2 masks anti-LKM and anti-LC, and anti-LKM masks anti-LC. For example, at the first examination, the association of anti-LKM1 and anti-LC1 in the sera of 32 patients was detected in only one case, in which the anti-LC1 titre was higher than the anti-LKM1 titre. A mixture of anti-

Table 4 Diagnosis of anti-liver cytosol antibodies and anti-LKM1

	Anti-LC1	*Anti-LC2*	*Anti-rat LKC*	*Anti-LKM1*
Autoimmune hepatitis 2	41			68
Idiopathic hepatitis		2		
Virus C hepatitis	2			53
Graft versus host disorder		3	1	8
Halothane hepatitis				4
Miscellaneous disorders			26	47

cytoplasmic autoantibodies was found in autoimmune hepatitis 2 (42%), hepatic GVHD (15%), and sometimes in viral hepatitis C and in primary biliary cirrhosis superinfected by viral hepatitis C associated with anti-LKM1 or anti-LC1.

Immunoabsorption with the different subcellular liver fractions is helpful to identify the different antibodies in a mixture. The serum is diluted 1:5 or more in phosphate buffer for immunofluorescence and added to an equal volume of mitochondrial, microsomal or cytosolic fractions (or buffer for control). After incubation for 48 h at 4 °C the tubes are centrifuged at a low speed (600*g* for 10 min) and dilutions of the supernatants are tested relative to the control. We tried to quantify this immunoabsorption by calculating 'the minimal amount of the corresponding subcellular fraction expressed in mg of protein/ml which completely absorbs the autoantibody with equal volumes of the serum and the subcellular fraction and with antibody diluted to the sixth dilution under the titer which gave final titer of 1/16 after adding the subcellular fraction'. According to this definition, anti-LC1 required a cytosolic fraction containing 40 mg of protein/ml, anti-LKM1 required a microsomal fraction with 2 mg, and anti-M2 a mitochondrial fraction with 5 mg. For some sera patients with GVHD, double-absorption with the mitochondrial and microsomal fractions was necessary to detect anti-LC. When the autoantibody titre is high in immunofluorescence, immunoabsorption became impossible at dilutions less than 1/10, and the hidden antibody could be missed at the chosen dilution.

DIAGNOSTIC VALUE OF ANTI-LC

In our laboratory, anti-LC have been detected over the past 12 years by means of immunofluorescence and immunodiffusion in a great number of patients with liver diseases (> 20 000 cases). Such antibodies were rare or very rare, but were found only in three circumstances, meaning they had great diagnostic value (Table 4).

1. Autoimmune hepatitis. The incidence of anti-LC1 detected by immunodiffusion in autoimmune hepatitis 2 was 52% (41/78), which is lower than anti-LKM1 with 87% (68/78). The detection of anti-LC1 alone increased the diagnostic yield for autoimmune hepatitis 2 to 13% (10/78). The value of anti-LC1 for follow-up, as well as the significance of the anti-LKM1/LC1 association, will be discussed in the next section. Anti-

Table 5 Autoantibodies in 100 syngeneic and allogeneic bone marrow grafts (Roumi, medical thesis, Paris, 1984)

	No. of cases	*ANF*[b]	*ASMA*[b]	*anti-M*[b]	*anti-LKM*[b]	*anti-LC*[b]
Syngeneic graft	17	0	1 (6%)	0	0	0
Allograft:						
GVHD = 0[a]	42	3 (7%)	6 (14%)	0	0	0
GVHD + (liver 0)[a]	17	11 (65%)	3 (18%)	0	2 (12%)	0
GVHD + (liver +)[a]	24	7 (29%)	7 (29%)	6 (25%)	5 (21%)	4 (17%)

[a]GVHD = graft versus host disease; 0 = absence, + = presence, liver 0 = without liver manifestation, liver + = with liver manifestation
[b]ANF = antinuclear factors ≥ 1/100; ASMA = anti-smooth muscle ≥ 1/100; anti-M = anti-mitochondria antibodies; anti-LKM = anti-liver/kidney microsome antibodies; anti-LC = anti-liver cytosol antibodies

LC2 was found in only two cases of idiopathic chronic hepatitis in young people, and was probably of the autoimmune type without other markers. Different heteroantibodies against rat liver, such as anti-rat LKC, anti-rat juxtavenous hepatocytes and the two anti-few rat hepatocytes had no diagnostic value at all.

2. Hepatic GVHD. Sera from about 200 patients with bone marrow or fetal hepatocyte allografts were tested in our laboratory before and after therapy. Table 5 shows the autoantibodies present in the first 100 cases after bone marrow grafting for aplastic anaemia or acute leukaemia. Various autoantibodies against mitochondria, microsomes and liver cytosol were found in 33% of patients with hepatic manifestations. Their titres were generally low (between 1/20 and 1/2000). Some sera contained three or four autoantibodies, which required double absorption by two liver cytoplasm subcellular fractions to characterize antibodies against the third. Three antibodies were confirmed as anti-LC2 by immunodiffusion. Anti-M2 similar to those found in primary biliary cirrhosis, and anti-LKM1 identical to those present in autoimmune hepatitis 2 were found together with unknown autoantibodies such as anti-mitochondria with hepatocyte heterogeneity among liver lobules. The small quantity of serum available to us limited this study.
3. Viral hepatitis C. Anti-LC1 seemed to be absent in viral hepatitis C[5], in contrast to anti-LKM1 that have been described by several authors[6–9]. In a prospective study of 374 sera from patients with viral hepatitis C, we found 16 anti-LKM1 by means of immunofluorescence and immunodiffusion (4%) and one anti-LC1 by immunodiffusion (0.2%). This last serum contained a strongly reactive anti-LKM1 immunofluorescence (titre: 1/1000). Another anti-LC1 was found in a blood donor with positive ELISA and RIBA test results for anti-HCV. Two other cases may be suspected but clinical or anti-HCV data were not available. Thus, anti-LC1 can be present in rare cases of viral hepatitis C. It is very strange that the two rare autoantibodies which characterize autoimmune hepatitis 2 can also be found in this viral disease, but this will be discussed in the last section.

Table 6 Comparison of the predicted frequency of the association of anti-LKM1 and anti-LC1 antibodies to observed cases (no. of positive cases = 78; anti-LKM1 = 68; anti-LC1 = 41)

	Anti-LKM1 + anti-LC1	*Anti-LKM1 alone*	*Anti-LC1 alone*	*No detectable antibodies*
Frequency[a]	$p\,q$	$p - p\,q$	$q - p\,q$	$1 - p - q + pq$
Calculated frequency[b]	0.35	0.41	0.11	0.13
Calculated cases[c]	31.4	36.7	9.8	11.5
Observed cases	31	37	10	?

[a] p is the frequency of anti-LKM1 in autoimmune hepatitis 2; q corresponds to anti-LC1
[b] The calculated frequencies p and q were calculated from the two equations: $p/p + q - pq = 68/78$ and $q/p + q - pq = 41/78$, which gave $p = 0.76$ and $q = 0.46$
[c] The calculated cases were found from the above values p and q and the equation: no. of positive and negative cases/$p + q - pq = 78$

SIGNIFICANCE OF THE ANTI-LKM1/ANTI-LC1 ASSOCIATION

Like most essential autoimmune disorders, autoimmune hepatitis 2 is associated with several autoantibodies. The prevalences of anti-LKM1 and anti-LC1 are indicated above. Other autoantibodies should also be considered, such as an antibody against a 64–66 kDa microsomal protein detected by immunoblotting[10,11] and an anti-gastric parietal cell antibody found in 30% of cases (unusual in young people). The proportion of patients with two antibodies can be compared with the expected occurrence corresponding to two independent phenomena in a closed system. A greater number of cases with two autoantibodies suggests a positive interference between the two autoimmunizations, e.g. a common antigenic determinant found in two autoantigens or the presence of the two antigens in the same complex structure. The absence of a statistical difference between the numbers of observed and expected cases with two antibodies suggests two independent autoimmunizations in one disorder. Finally, a lower than expected prevalence of patients with two autoantibodies suggests two frequently associated disorders with independent immunization. Using the data given above for the 78 cases of autoimmune hepatitis 2 with 68 anti-LKM1 and 41 anti-LC1, it is possible to calculate the expected number of cases with both anti-LKM1 and anti-LC1. The number of observed cases ($n = 31$) is not statistically different from the 35.7 expected cases (chi-square n.s.; $p > 5\%$). This calculation does not take into account possible cases of autoimmune hepatitis 2 with undetectable or undetected anti-LKM1 and anti-LC1. Table 6 gives a prevalence of 13% for such cases. In one patient, anti-LKM1 was detected only at the second relapse and, as indicated above, anti-LC1 was found only by immunodiffusion with undiluted serum at the beginning of the disease. In practice the two independent autoimmunizations against the LKM1 and LC1 antigens in autoimmune hepatitis 2 are confirmed during immunosuppressive treatment by the dissociation of the curves for anti-LKM1 and anti-LC1 (Fig. 2). Anti-LKM1 is a better immunological marker for the clinical course with improvements and relapses than is anti-LC1, which takes several further years to diminish.

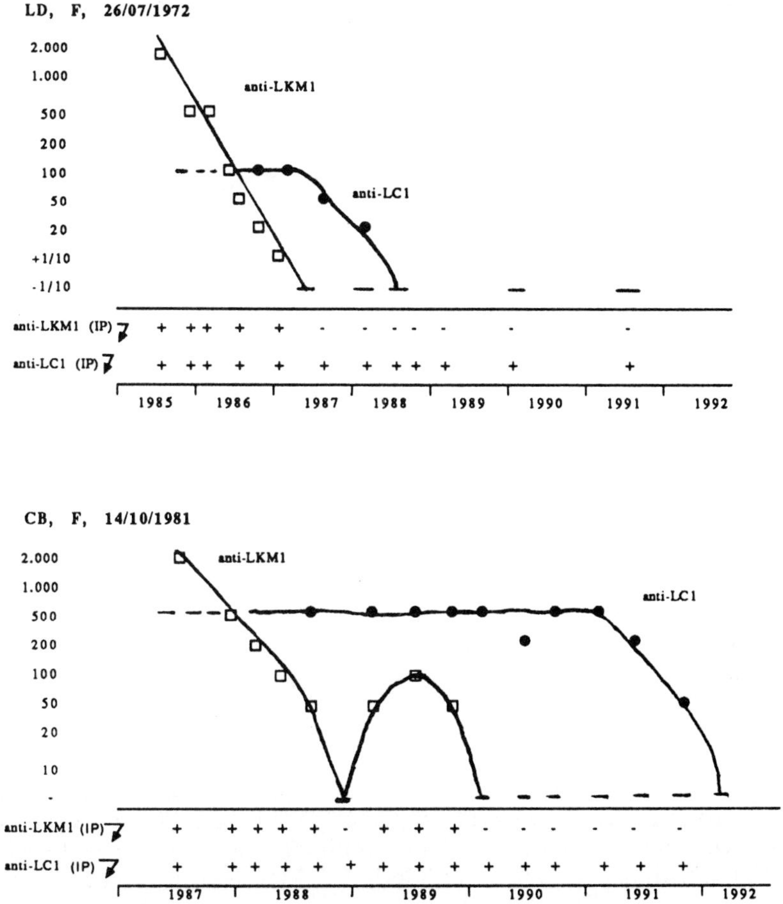

Fig. 2 Evolution of anti-LC1 (●), anti-LKM1 (□) and anti-gastric parietal cells (○) antibodies in four cases of autoimmune hepatitis 2 during immunosuppressive treatment

POSSIBLE RELATION BETWEEN AUTOIMMUNE HEPATITIS 2 AND VIRAL HEPATITIS C

The presence of autoantibodies such as anti-LKM1 has been reported in viral hepatitis C by many authors[6–9] and is astonishing. In our first description of 65 cases of autoimmune hepatitis 2[12], retrospective controls of anti-HCV by RIBA testing distinguished 43 autoimmune hepatitis 2 and 22 viral hepatitis C associated with anti-LKM1. This explains why we wrote: 'the results of treatment (immunosuppressors) tended to be good in young patients and doubtful in older patients. In adults, 12 cases were detected at the inactive cirrhotic stage when treatment was unnecessary: some patients spontaneously evolved towards clinical remission with complete disappearance of anti-LKM1 in five cases'[12]. As differences have been reported between

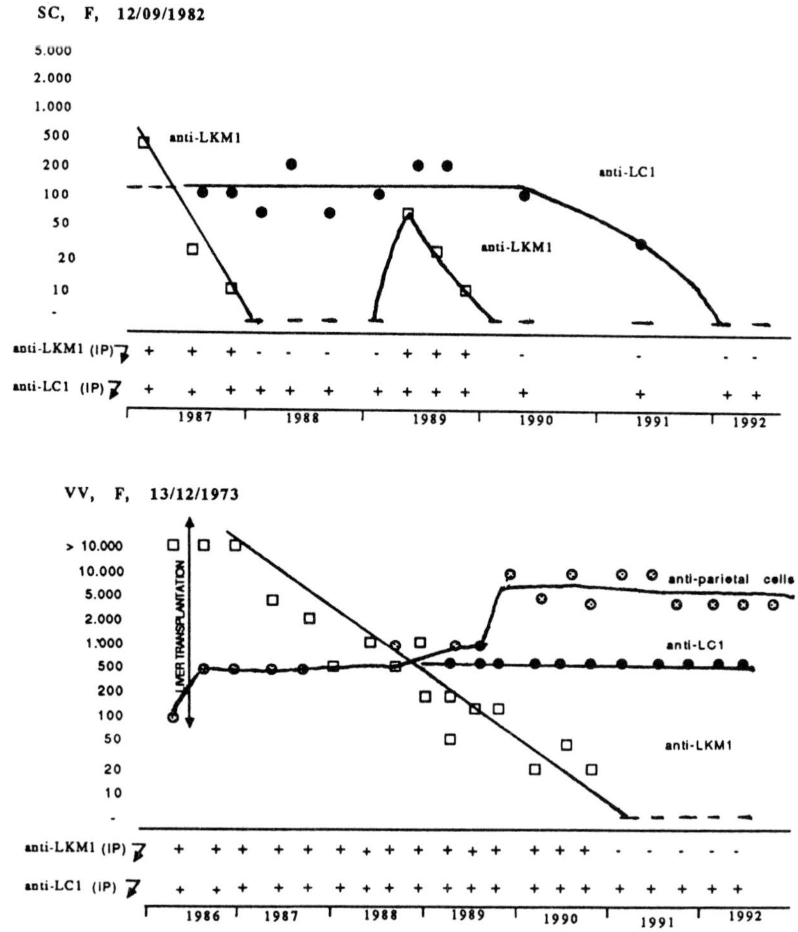

Fig. 2 *continued*

countries[8], it is important to consider epidemiological data with the relative prevalences of anti-LKM1 and anti-LC1 due to autoimmune hepatitis 2 and those corresponding to viral hepatitis C. The first disorder was considered as very rare, with 47 patients living in Ile de France (Paris and the five surrounding suburbs), that included 10 760 625 inhabitants[12]. Elsewhere, a prevalence of 0.85% among blood donors was found in the same region for viral hepatitis C, and pointed to 50 000 cases, taking into account the lower prevalence of infection in young people. With the frequencies given above for anti-LKM1 and anti-LC1 in the two disorders, we would expect to find 43 anti-LKM1 and 24 anti-LC1 corresponding to autoimmune hepatitis 2 and 1500 anti-LKM1 and 100 anti-LC1 due to viral hepatitis C. As viral hepatitis C is now screened for, our laboratory now found a ratio of 5 viral hepatitis C associated with these autoantibodies, for only one case of autoimmune hepatitis 2, which does not correspond with the previous

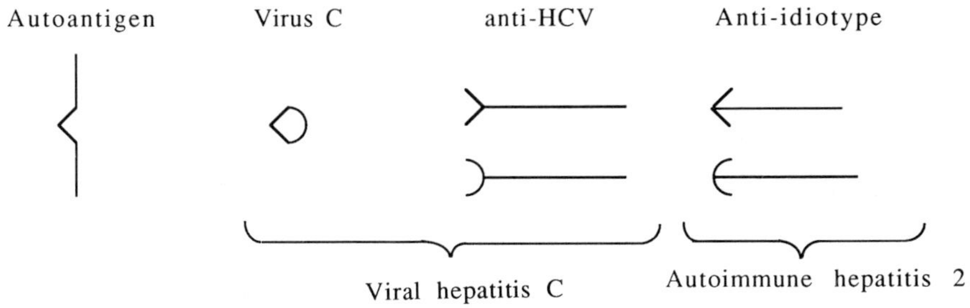

Fig. 3 An hypothesis: the autoimmune hepatitis 2 would be due to anti-idiotype antibodies against the anti-hepatitis C virus antibodies (anti-HCV)

study[12], where autoimmune hepatitis 2 was predominating. From a clinical point of view, autoimmune hepatitis 2 and viral hepatitis C associated with anti-LKM1 and anti-LC1 remain very different, and the latter condition does not differ from viral hepatitis C without autoantibodies. The most important epidemiological datum is the age difference. Autoimmune hepatitis 2 mainly occurs in 2–14-year-old patients; the oldest patient was 37 in our series and 38 in the literature[9]. Viral hepatitis C shows a maximum prevalence between 45 and 65 years, but some cases can occur in young people, most of whom have received donor blood.

The presence of the same two markers considered specific for autoimmune hepatitis 2 in some cases of viral hepatitis C is fascinating. We speculated how to link viral hepatitis C and autoimmune hepatitis 2. As shown in Fig. 3, autoimmune hepatitis 2 might be due to anti-idiotype antibodies against anti-HCV, and these antibodies could also thus recognize some complementary hepatocyte structures, e.g. the point at which HCV penetrates into these cells. We studied whether anti-HCV inhibited the reaction between anti-LKM1 or anti-LC1 with their corresponding autoantigens, but failed to confirm this hypothesis; further tests are now being undertaken. Several epidemiological and virological observations[5,9,13] argue against a connection between the two disorders. Today there is no explanation why the same two autoantibodies are present in autoimmune hepatitis 2 and viral hepatitis C.

Acknowledgements

We thank Thierry Ocwieja, Véronique Bon-Durand, Mariama Kantara, Boniface Absalon and Jacqueline Grégeois for their technical assistance, and Pascale Perrin for typing the manuscript.

References

1. Rizetto M, Swana G, Doniach D. Microsomal antibodies in active chronic hepatitis and other disorders. Clin Exp Immunol. 1973;15:331–44.

2. Homberg JC, Micouin C, Peltier A *et al.* Un nouvel anticorps non spécifique d'organe au cours d'hépatite chronique. Méd Chir Dig. 1974;3:82–5.
3. Martini E, Abuaf N, Cavalli F *et al.* Antibody to liver cytosol (anti-LC1) in patients with autoimmune chronic active hepatitis type 2. Hepatology. 1988;8:1662–6.
4. Homberg JC, Andre C, Abuaf N. A new anti-liver/kidney microsome antibody (anti-LKM2) in tienilic acid-induced hepatitis. Clin Exp Immunol. 1984;55:561–70.
5. Lunel F, Abuaf N, Frangueul L *et al.* Liver/kidney microsome antibody type 1 and hepatitis C virus infection. Hepatology. 1992;16:630–6.
6. Lunel F, Homberg JC, Valla D *et al.* Autoimmune liver disease and hepatitis C virus infection. Second international symposium on HCV, Los Angeles 1990;21:53 (Abstract).
7. Todros L, Touscoz G, D'Urso N *et al.* Hepatitis C virus-related chronic liver disease with autoantibodies to liver-kidney microsomes (LKM). Clinical characterization from idiopathic LKM-positive disorders. J Hepatol. 1991;13:128–31.
8. Lenzi M, Johnson PJ, McFarlane IG *et al.* Antibodies to hepatitis C virus in autoimmune liver disease: evidence for geographical heterogeneity. Lancet. 1991;338:277–80.
9. Michel G, Ritter A, Gerben G *et al.* Anti-GOR and hepatitis C virus in autoimmune liver diseases. Lancet. 1992;339:267–9.
10. Codoner-Franch P, Paradis K, Gueguen M *et al.* A new antigen recognized by anti-liver-kidney-microsome antibody (LKMA). Clin Exp Immunol. 1989;75:354–8.
11. Manns MP, Johnson EF, Griffin KJ *et al.* Major antigen of liver kidney microsomal autoantibodies in idiopathic autoimmune hepatitis is cytochrome P450db1. J Clin Invest. 1989;83:1066–72.
12. Homberg JC, Abuaf N, Bernard O *et al.* Chronic active hepatitis associated with anti-liver/kidney microsome antibody type 1: a second type of 'autoimmune' hepatitis. Hepatology. 1987;7:1333–9.
13. Magrin S, Craxi A, Fabiano C *et al.* Hepatitis C virus replication in 'autoimmune' chronic hepatitis. J Hepatol. 1991;13:364–7.

25 The asialoglycoprotein receptor (ASGPR) as hepatic autoantigen

U. TREICHEL and T. PORALLA

BACKGROUND

Autoimmune liver diseases are typically associated with circulating autoantibodies. The pathophysiological significance of target structures recognized by these antibodies, however, remains unclear so far. Efforts to define molecules which are abundantly expressed on the liver cell surface as candidates for organ-specific autoimmune attack were based on studies with the so-called liver-specific protein (LSP). This crude preparation was shown to exhibit relevant components for both disease induction[1] and clinical follow-up observation[2]. Further progress was achieved when the asialoglycoprotein receptor (ASGPR) was detected as a constituent of LSP[3].

The ASGPR is a major glycoprotein present on the hepatocellular surface[4]. Assembly of two ASGPR subunits (H1 and H2) on the liver cell membrane provides a high capacity system for hepatic endocytosis of D-galactosyl residues exposing glycoproteins[5]. Based on cDNA sequences ASGPR-H1 and -H2 proteins exhibit approximately 50% homology between the two subunits and nearly 80% homology between the same subunit of different species[6]. In adults the ASGPR is exclusively expressed on differentiated liver cells while cellular transformation causes at least different splicing of the encoding DNA sequence[7].

REGULATION OF THE ASGPR IN CHRONIC LIVER DISEASE AND INFLAMMATION

Morphological changes of ASGPR expression due to chronic liver disease were demonstrated recently[8]. In normal liver ASGPR protein is expressed on the sinusoidal and basolateral surface of hepatocytes. In contrast, the ASGPRs were shifted to the canalicular membrane in 67% of patients with liver cirrhosis due to different disorders. This might explain strikingly increased concentrations of circulating asialoglycoproteins which were observed in the blood of patients with cirrhosis[9].

Previously, reduced uptake of ASGPR ligands after experimental induction of acute-phase response was demonstrated[10] by both increased survival time in blood and suppressed binding to isolated plasma membranes. In more detail, cytokines as major mediators of acute and chronic liver inflammation were shown as potent inhibitors of ASGPR function and expression *in vitro*[11]. In HepG2 cells and isolated hepatocytes interferon-α (IFN-α) and interferon-γ, interleukin-2 and tumour necrosis factor completely suppress both binding and uptake activity by phosphorylation of the ASGPR. Furthermore, total ASGPR synthesis is reduced due to cytokine action which was shown on the protein and RNA level.

CLINICAL SIGNIFICANCE OF ANTI-ASGPR AUTOANTIBODIES

Radio- and enzyme immunoassays were established to analyse sera from patients suffering from various hepatic and non-hepatic inflammatory disorders for anti-ASGPR autoantibodies[12,13]. In essence a close linkage of anti-ASGPR antibodies to chronic liver diseases was observed (Table 1). Furthermore, if patients were suffering from autoimmune hepatitis with severe inflammatory activity nearly 90% were anti-ASGPR-positive. Interestingly, if human-derived ASGPR was used as substrate, sera from patients with viral hepatitis lacked anti-ASGPR reactivity while in autoimmune hepatitis binding activity was even more pronounced. These findings indicate a close link of anti-human ASGPR antibodies and autoimmune hepatitis. After initiation of immunosuppressive therapy patients with autoimmune hepatitis titres of anti-ASGPR decreased and, moreover, in approximately 50% anti-ASGPR antibodies were completely eliminated. Anti-ASGPR antibodies could also be detected in a few patients with chronic viral hepatitis after beginning treatment with IFN-α. In these cases, however, with one exception anti-ASGPR autoantibody occurred only transiently, and lacked any relationship to the course of the disease. It is noteworthy that two cases of liver failure during IFN-α therapy for non-A–non-B hepatitis were reported recently which exhibited anti-ASGPR reactivity[14]. Another report on autoimmune hepatitis and anti-ASGPR reactivity after hepatitis A virus infection supports both virus-induced autoimmunity in certain patients and a linkage to anti-ASGPR reactivity[15]. While subtypes of autoimmune hepatitis can be defined by its autoantibody profile anti-ASGPR antibodies are not restricted to the known marker autoantibodies[13].

CHARACTERIZATION OF ANTI-ASGPR AUTOANTIBODIES

Nearly 90% of patients with inflammatory active autoimmune hepatitis exhibit high-titred anti-ASGPR from IgG- and IgM-type (Table 1)[16]. Anti-ASGPR IgG may persist over years in nearly 40% of the patients. However, anti-ASGPR IgM are eliminated within a short time frame from the

Table 1 Anti-asialoglycoprotein receptor autoantibodies in liver diseases

	Prevalence (%)	*Immunoglobulin class*	*ASGPR fragment recognition*
Acute viral hepatitis	14	IgG, IgM	–
HbsAg+ chronic hepatitis, active	12	IgG, IgM, IgG_4	–
HbsAg+ chronic hepatitis, inactive	6	IgG, IgM	–
Anti HCV positive hepatitis, active	16	IgG, IgM, IgG_4	–
Anti HCV positive hepatitis, inactive	2	IgG, IgM	–
Autoimmune hepatitis, active	87	IgG, IgM, IgG_2	+
Autoimmune hepatitis, inactive	50	IgG	+
Primary biliary cirrhosis	13	IgG (IgM)	–(+)
Primary sclerosing cholangitis	0	–	n.d.
Alcoholic liver disease	8	IgG, IgM	n.d.
Liver cancer	10	IgG, IgM	n.d.

circulation. IgG subclass IgG_2 is the predominant isotype in autoimmune hepatitis, while IgG_4 is more restricted to viral hepatitis.

Peripheral blood lymphocytes exclusively from patients with autoimmune hepatitis, but not with viral hepatitis or from normal controls, showed spontaneous anti-ASGPR secretion after 7 days cell culture[17]. At least in part anti-ASGPR secretion is T-cell-dependent. This is shown by isolated T cells from sensitized patients which were capable of inducing specific autoantibody secretion by autologous B cells[18].

By using different derivatives of human ASGPR as target antigen anti-ASGPR autoantibodies were characterized as highly heterogeneous. A substantial number of anti-ASGPR-positive sera on animal substrate are low-titred or negative if human ASGPR was used as target antigen[13]. Furthermore, certain anti-ASGPR-positive sera only exhibited strong reactivity to the natural substrate purified by affinity chromatography. Once biochemically prepared peptide fragments were investigated, anti-ASGPR positive sera derived from patients with autoimmune hepatitis preserved avidity to the remaining ASGPR epitopes (Table 1)[19]. These sera reacted to virtually all components of ASGPR, as shown by immunoblotting of ASGPR fragments.

In-vivo binding of anti-ASGPR antibodies could be detected in isolated perfused livers[20]. *In vitro*, both anti-ASGPR-positive sera and IgG preparations showed inhibition of ligand binding and therefore uptake of asialoglycoproteins by the ASGPR[19].

THE ASGPR AS A TARGET FOR AUTOREACTIVE T-CELL RESPONSE

The ASGPR is a major target antigen for cellular autoimmune response. Lymphocyte migration inhibition (LIF) in the presence of ASGPR protein could be demonstrated mainly in peripheral blood lymphocytes from patients

Table 2 Cellular immune response against the asialoglycoprotein receptor

	Proliferative response		*Anti-ASGPR secretion*	
	Peripheral blood lymphocytes (%)	*Liver infiltrating lymphocytes*	*Spontaneous*	*Induced**
Viral hepatitis	5	–	–	–
Autoimmune hepatitis	40	+ HLA II restriction	+	+
Primary biliary cirrhosis	5	+ HLA II restriction	+	+

*By autologous, ASGPR-specific liver T-cell clones

with autoimmune liver diseases (Table 2)[21]. In addition some patients with viral hepatitis exhibited anti-ASGPR reactivity which, however, did not correlate to the presence of crossreactive anti-ASGPR autoantibodies. Furthermore, a so-called T-suppressor cell dysfunction was corrected by the addition of normal lymphocytes.

The proliferative response to purified ASGPR was investigated in both peripheral and liver infiltrating T lymphocytes[22]. Peripheral blood lymphocytes proliferated in the presence of ASGPR exclusively if they were prepared from patients with autoimmune chronic active hepatitis and from some patients with primary biliary cirrhosis. As mentioned above, anti-ASGPR reactive cultures of blood lymphocytes demonstrated anti-ASGPR autoantibody secretion into the culture medium[17]. In addition, a T-cell clone was established from peripheral blood capable of inducing anti-ASGPR autoantibody secretion *in vitro*[22].

T-cell clones responding to the ASGPR could also be isolated from liver specimens of patients with autoimmune liver diseases (Table 2)[23]. T-cell proliferation in the presence of ASGPR was thus shown to require antigen (ASGPR) presentation by autologous cells and, furthermore, was restricted to the human major histocompatibility complex class II. Phenotypic characterization revealed mainly T cells from the CD4-helper cell type. In parallel, addition of liver-infiltrating T-cell clones to autologous EBV-transformed B-cell lines was capable of inducing anti-ASGPR secretion *in vitro*[18].

CONCLUSION

The ASGPR was identified as a major target structure for immune response in humans. Its regulation under pathophysiological conditions such as inflammation or liver cirrhosis is an example for the specific pathobiology of the liver cell. Circulating autoantibodies directed against the ASGPR might implicate significance as both a disease-specific and an activity-related marker for autoimmune hepatitis. The recognition of the ASGPR by autoreactive T cells provides a useful tool for the study of the immunopathogenesis of autoimmune liver diseases.

References

1. Meyer zum Büschenfelde K-H, Hopf U. Studies on the pathogenesis of experimental chronic hepatitis in rabbits: induction of the disease and protective effect of allogenic liver specific protein. Br J Pathol. 1974;55:498–508.
2. McFarlane IG, Hegarty JE, McSorley CG, McFarlane BM, Williams R. Antibodies to liver-specific protein predict outcome of treatment withdrawal in autoimmune chronic active hepatitis. Lancet. 1984;2:954–6.
3. McFarlane IG, McFarlane BM, Major GN, Tolley P, Williams R. Identification of the hepatic asialoglycoprotein receptor (hepatic lectin) as a component of liver specific membrane lipoprotein (LSP). Clin Exp Immunol. 1985;55:347–54.
4. Harford J, Ashwell G. The hepatic receptor for asialoglycoproteins. In: Horowitz, M, ed. The glycoconjugates, vol. 4. New York: Academic Press; 1982;27–55.
5. Spiess M. The asialoglycoprotein receptor: a model for endocytotic transport receptors. Biochemistry. 1990;29:10009–18.
6. Spiess M, Lodish HF. Sequence of a second human asialoglycoprotein receptor: Conservation of two receptor genes during evolution. Proc Natl Acad Sci USA. 1985;82: 6465–9.
7. Paietta E, Stockert RJ, Racevskis J. Differences in the abundance of variably spliced receptor polypeptide, H2, in normal and transformed human liver. Hepatology. 1992;15:395–402.
8. Burgess JB, Baenziger JU, Brown WR. Abnormal surface distribution of the human asialoglycoprotein receptor in cirrhosis. Hepatology. 1992;15:702–6.
9. Sawamura T, Nakada H, Hazama H, Shiozaka Y, Sameshima Y, Tashiro Y. Hyperasialoglycoproteinemia in patients with liver diseases and/or liver cell carcinoma. Gastroenterology. 1984;87:2117–21.
10. Wong MWC, Jamieson JC. Evidence for reduced uptake of asialo-α1-acid glycoprotein during the acute phase response to inflammation. Life Sci. 1979;25:827–34.
11. Treichel U, Paietta E, Poralla T, Meyer zum Büschenfelde KH, Stockert RJ. Effects of cytokines on synthesis and function of the hepatic asialoglycoprotein receptor (ASGPR). J Clin Invest. 1992: submitted.
12. McFarlane BM, McSorley CG, Vergani D, McFarlane IG, Williams R. Serum autoantibodies reacting with the hepatic asialoglycoprotein receptor (hepatic lectin) in acute and chronic liver disorders. J Hepatol. 1986;3:1996–2005.
13. Treichel U, Poralla T, Hess G, Manns M, Meyer zum Büschenfelde K-H. Autoantibodies to human asialoglycoprotein receptor in autoimmune-type chronic active hepatitis. Hepatology. 1990;11,4:606–12.
14. Vento S, di Perri G, Garofano T, Cosco L, Concia E, Ferraro T, Basseti D. Hazards of interferon therapy for HBV-negative chronic active hepatitis. Lancet. 1989;2:926.
15. Vento S, Garofano T, Di Perri G, Dolci L, Concia E, Bassetti D. Identification of hepatitis A virus as a trigger for autoimmune chronic hepatitis type 1 in susceptible individuals. Lancet. 1991;1:1183–7.
16. Treichel U, Gerken G, Rossol S, Rotthauwe HW, Meyer zum Büschenfelde KH. Autoantibodies against the human asialoglycoprotein receptor: Effects of therapy in autoimmune and virus-induced chronic active hepatitis. J Hepatol. 1993; in press.
17. Treichel U, Löhr H, Poralla T, Manns M, Hess G, Fleischer B, Meyer zum Büschenfelde KH. The human asialoglycoprotein receptor. A specific target for autoimmune reactions in chronic liver diseases. J Hepatol. 1990;11:62 (abstract).
18. Löhr H, Treichel U, Poralla T, Manns M, Meyer zum Büschenfelde KH. Fleischer B liver-infiltrating T helper cells stimulate the production of autoantibodies against the human asialoglycoprotein receptor in autoimmune chronic active hepatitis *in vitro*. Clin Exp Immunol. 1992;88:45–9.
19. Treichel U, Poralla T, Meyer zum Büschenfelde KH, Stockert RJ. Significance of heterogeneous autoantibodies recognizing the asialoglycoprotein receptor. J Hepatol. 1992;16(1):59 (abstract).
20. McFarlane BM, Sipos J, Gove CD, McFarlane IG, Williams R. Antibodies against the hepatic asialoglycoprotein receptor perfused in situ preferentially attach to periportal liver cells in the rat. Hepatology. 1990;11:408–15.
21. Vento S, Hegarty JE, Bottazzo GF, Macchia W, Williams R, Eddleston ALWF. Antigen-

specific suppressor cell function in autoimmune chronic active hepatitis. Lancet. 1984;1: 1200 4.
22. Wen Li-Peakman M, Lobo-Yeo A, McFarlane BM, Mowat AP, Mieli-Vergani G, Vergani D. T-cell directed hepatocyte damage in autoimmune chronic active hepatitis. Lancet. 1990;336:1527–30.
23. Löhr H, Treichel U, Poralla T, Manns M, Meyer zum Büschenfelde KH, Fleischer B. The human hepatic asialoglycoprotein receptor is a target antigen for liver infiltrating T cells in autoimmune chronic active hepatitis and primary biliary cirrhosis. Hepatology. 1990;12:1314–20.

26 Autoimmune hepatitis: cellular immune reactions

D. VERGANI and G. MIELI-VERGANI

The concept that cellular immunity plays a role in the pathogenesis of autoimmune hepatitis (AH) was first suggested by the histological finding of a dense mononuclear cell infiltrate. This erodes the limiting plate and invades the parenchyma producing piecemeal necrosis and rosettes, lesions in which dying hepatocytes are surrounded by mononuclear cells[1,2]. The possible pathways that a cell-mediated immune attack can follow to inflict damage on the hepatocyte are summarized in Fig. 1. The first step is immune recognition[3,4]. For a hepatocyte to be recognized, an autoantigenic peptide must be presented within the groove of a human leucocyte antigen (HLA) class II molecule to a T helper cell. The cell presenting the peptide can be a professional antigen-presenting cell (APC) or the hepatocyte itself, if this has been induced to inappropriately express HLA class II molecules. When the autoantigenic peptide is presented in the correct form, the T helper cell will recognize it and become activated. This process of autoantigen recognition is, however, strictly controlled by regulatory mechanisms, here for convenience referred to as suppressor cells. If suppressor cells do not oppose, the T helper cell becomes activated and is in the position of masterminding the immune attack and recruiting effectors of damage. These include autoantibody-producing B lymphocytes, T cells specializing in the secretion of cytokines and T cytotoxic cells.

The evidence documenting involvement of the mechanisms described above, which has been accumulated over some 20 years, will be presented. The *afferent* and *efferent* components of the autoimmune response are summarized in Table 1. An impairment of immunomodulatory mechanisms, which would enable the autoimmune response to develop, has been described in several reports. Children and young adults with AH have low levels of T lymphocytes expressing the CD8 marker which is present on a population of T cells with a suppressor and cytotoxic function[5]. The hypothesis that these cells are suppressor is supported by the finding that suppressor cell function is also impaired in AH[5]. Nouri-Aria *et al.*[6,7] have shown: (1) that impairment of immunoregulation segregates with the possession of the HLA

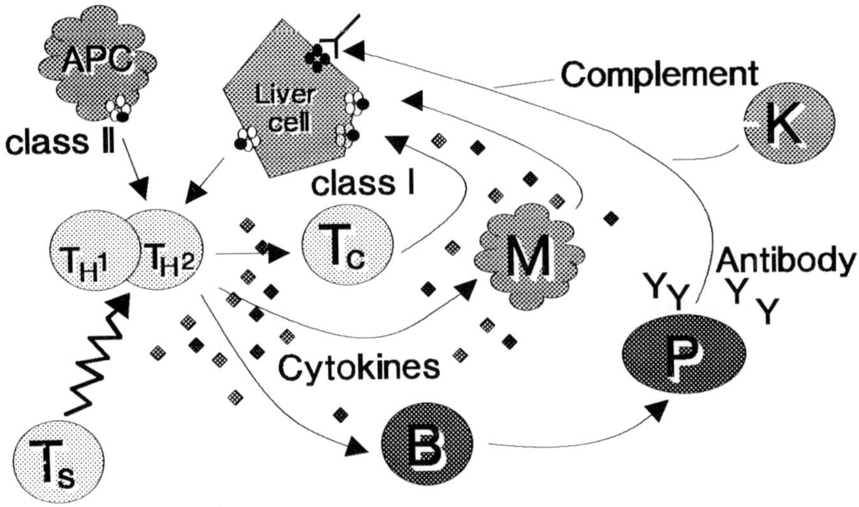

Fig. 1 Liver cell autoimmune attack. A normal component of the liver cell membrane is presented to helper (T_H1, T_H2) lymphocytes either directly on the hepatocyte or by an antigen-presenting cell (APC), in the context of class II HLA antigens. If there is no opposition from T suppressor (Ts) lymphocytes, then a variety of effector mechanisms are triggered. Liver cell destruction could derive from the action of: (a) T cytotoxic (Tc) lymphocytes which react with the self antigen(s) in the context of class I HLA antigens; (b) cytokines produced by T_H1 such as interferon-γ which recruits macrophages; or (c) autoantibody production by B lymphocytes with activation of complement and/or engagement of killer (K) lymphocytes, B lymphocyte (B); macrophage (M), plasma cell (P)

Table 1 Autoimmune hepatitis: pathogenic pathways

Afferent
Inappropriate HLA expression
Defective regulatory mechanisms
Activation of helper T lymphocytes
Efferent
Engagement of:
B-lymphocyte/autoantibody loop
Killer cells
Complement
Macrophage/cytokine loop
Cytotoxic T-lymphocyte loop

haplotype B8/DR3, the haplotype that predisposes to AH[6]; and (2) that this immunoregulatory defect is correctable by therapeutic doses of corticosteroids[7]. In addition, it has been shown that patients with AH also have a specific defect in a subpopulation of suppressor T cells controlling the immune response to liver-specific membrane antigens[8]. Impaired suppressor function appears to be liver antigen-specific, since patients with AH have been shown to have normal mechanisms regulating the antibody production against an exogenous antigen such as tetanus toxoid[9].

To summarize, there is persuasive evidence suggesting that mechanisms controlling the immune response to liver-specific antigens are defective in AH. Thus, there is a permissive environment for autoimmunity and autoimmune disease to occur. But do autoreactive T cells exploit this opportunity? Do they recognize a liver-specific autoantigenic peptide? If they recognize the peptide, do they do so when the peptide is presented by antigen-presenting cells or by hepatocytes? Hepatocytes do not normally express HLA class II antigens, and they would therefore be unable to act as antigen-presenting cells. Using anti-HLA class II monoclonal antibody in an immunoperoxidase technique, Lobo-Yeo *et al.*[10] have shown that hepatocytes from patients with AH do express HLA class II molecules.

Given the impaired regulatory function and the inappropriate expression of HLA class II antigens on hepatocytes, the question arises as to whether an autoantigenic peptide is presented to helper/inducer cells leading to their activation. Although we have no evidence, as yet, that an autoantigenic peptide is recognized, activation of helper cells has been documented in AH. Thus, patients with AH have a high level of activated T lymphocytes expressing interleukin-2 receptor (IL-2r) both in the circulation[11] and in the liver[12]. These activated cells possess the CD4 phenotype and their values are highest when the disease is most active.

Turning to the efferent loops of the autoimmune attack (Table 1), what is the evidence incriminating one or more of these pathways in generating liver injury in AH? The B lymphocyte/autoantibody loop will be analysed first. In the mid-1970s it was reported that antibodies to liver-specific lipoprotein (LSP) – a macromolecular complex present on the hepatocyte membrane and originally described by Meyer zum Büschenfelde and Miescher[13] – are not only present in AH but their titre correlates with the severity of the disease[14]. A similar relationship to disease severity has been observed for titres of an antibody to a well-characterized component of LSP, the asialoglycoprotein receptor (ASGPR)[15]. Immunofluorescence studies on monodispersed suspensions of liver cells obtained from patients with AH showed that these cells are coated with antibodies *in vivo*[16]. Do these antibodies recruit mediators of damage? Cytotoxicity assays showed that these antibody-coated hepatocytes are killed when incubated together with autologous[17] or allogeneic[16] lymphocytes. The cytotoxic effector cells were identified using purified populations of T and non-T lymphocytes and by blocking experiments[17]. It was found that non-T lymphocytes are responsible for the hepatocyte damage, and that the cytotoxic reaction is blocked by the addition of aggregated immunoglobulin, indicating that killer cells are involved through an antibody-dependent cell-mediated reaction in the destruction of the hepatocytes. An antibody-coated liver cell could also be killed through complement activation. When we investigated the complement profile in AH, however, we found no evidence of complement activation, but observed that these patients have genetically determined low levels of C4. We went on to demonstrate that this is due to the possession of a silent allele at the C4A locus (C4AQ0)[18]. Intriguingly, this allele is part of the 'autoimmune haplotype' A1,B8,DR3,C4AQ0, which confers susceptibility to AH.

What about the cytokine pathway? Study of cytokines in the circulation has given indication that the more active the disease, the more elevated are circulating levels of various cytokines including interleukin-1 (IL-1) and tumour necrosis factor (TNF)[19]. However, high levels of circulating cytokines could also be observed in liver diseases whose pathogenesis is unlikely to be immune, such as Wilson's disease or α_1-antitrypsin deficiency, possibly reflecting deficient hepatic catabolic function. The study of cytokine-containing cells in the liver tissue, on the other hand, shows that numerous cells of the portal tract infiltrate of patients with AH are positive for TNF-α and interferon-γ (IFN-γ), while this is not seen in the infiltrates of Wilson's disease and α_1-antitrypsin deficiency[20]. As mentioned earlier, microcytotoxicity assays suggest that cytotoxic T cells do not play a major role in causing hepatocellular damage in AH, at least when cells from the peripheral blood are investigated. To summarize the efferent pathways: B lymphocytes produce autoantibodies which engage killer cells but not complement; cytokines are likely to be involved in the pathogenic process, while early studies suggest that cytotoxic T lymphocytes are not.

For the fine characterization of the pathogenic pathways and mechanisms of liver damage it is necessary to have access to large numbers of cells. This can now be accomplished through cloning. Wen *et al.*[21,22] and Löhr *et al.*[23,24] exploiting the fact that the activated T cells from patients with AH express IL-2r, have stimulated their proliferation in the presence of IL-2. Once the cells are grown in number, they are seeded in limiting dilution in microculture plates to obtain clones. The majority of clones obtained from the peripheral blood of patients with AH by Wen *et al.*[21] were $CD4^+$ and used the conventional $\alpha\beta$ T cell receptor. Clones with similar characteristics were obtained from the liver of these patients both from Löhr *et al.*[23] and Wen *et al.*[22]. A proportion of these $CD4^+$ clones were found to react with partially purified antigens, such as crude preparations of liver cell membrane or LSP[21], and with purified ASGPR[21,24] or recombinant LKM-1[23]. Both groups showed that proliferation of these $CD4^+$ clones was antigen-specific and restricted by HLA class II molecules. Thus, these clones did not proliferate in the presence of antigenic preparations from other organs and reacted to liver-specific antigens, and only when these were presented by autologous antigen-presenting cells. The ability to block this latter reaction by addition of a monoclonal antibody directed against a monomorphic epitope of HLA DR indicated that the recognition was HLA class II restricted. Since CD4 is the phenotype of helper T cells, both Wen *et al.*[21] and Löhr *et al.*[24] investigated whether these clones were able to help autologous B lymphocytes in the production of immunoglobulin *in vitro*. B lymphocytes alone or in the presence of a liver membrane preparation produced negligible amounts of IgG. When a liver-specific $CD4^+$ clone was added to the B lymphocytes, IgG production increased dramatically (Fig. 2), demonstrating the clone's helper function. Investigation of the specificity of the antibody produced by the clone-stimulated B lymphocytes showed that a high proportion were liver-specific autoantibodies, some of which were specific for the ASGPR.

What should be done next? The process of immune recognition, the

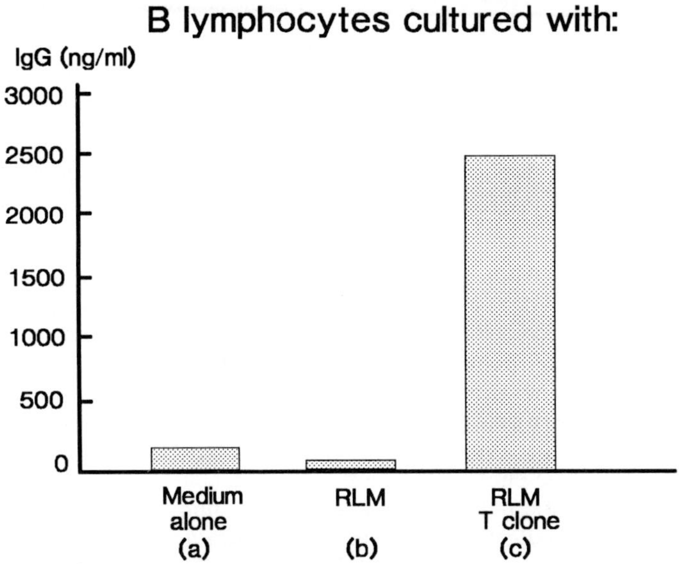

Fig. 2 B lymphocytes from patient L.B. cultured in (a) medium alone, (b) in the presence of a preparation of rabbit liver membrane (RLM) antigen and (c) in the presence of RLM plus a $CD4^+$ clone established from the peripheral blood of L.B. The addition of the helper clone promotes immunoglobulin production

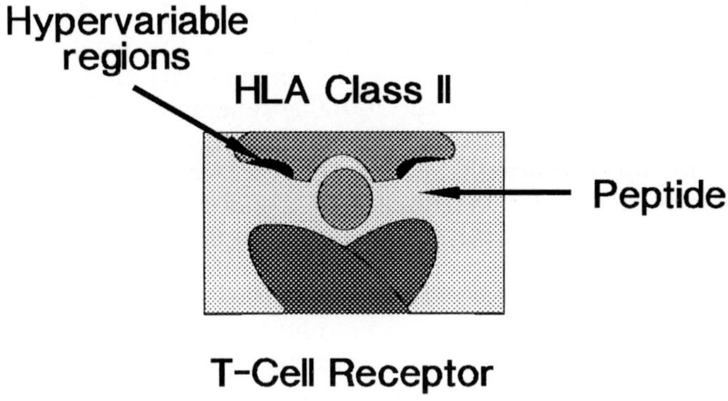

Fig. 3 A trimolecular complex composed of T-cell receptor (TCR), HLA molecule and autoantigenic peptide. Therapeutic approaches can be aimed at any of these three components

beginning of an immune attack, revolves around a trimolecular complex: the T cell receptor, the HLA molecule and the immunogenic peptide (Fig. 3). Future research should investigate the immunodominant epitopes, i.e. those sequences of 8–20 amino acids, recognized by autoreactive clones; characterize the fine composition of the HLA molecule that presents the autoantigenic peptide and the fine structure of the T cell receptor that reacts with the peptide/HLA complex. Once these structures are identified and demonstrated to be sufficiently disease-specific it will be possible to consider

Table 2 Immune intervention in autoimmune hepatitis

Anti-T cell receptor clonotype antibodies
Anti-HLA antibodies
Peptide immunotherapy
Anti-accessory molecule antibodies
Lymphocyte vaccination
Oral induction of tolerance

new modes of treatment of AH (Table 2), such as the manufacture and administration of: (1) antibodies directed against the T cell receptor, or the HLA molecule specifically involved in the autoimmune recognition; (2) competitive synthetic peptides very similar to the peptide that causes the disease but with higher affinity for the HLA molecule or the T cell receptor. Examples of the use of peptide therapy are already available. Specific peptides have been shown to abrogate autoimmune disease in animals, such as experimental allergic encephalomyelitis, a model of multiple sclerosis[25]. In the context of specific immune intervention the finding by Doherty *et al.*[26] appears to be particularly promising. The amino acid sequence Leu–Leu–Glu–Gln–Lys–Arg at position 67 to 72 on the DRβ polypeptide was found in 94% of patients with AH whether they were DR3- or DR4-positive, suggesting that this motif may be specific for AH and a possible target for immune manipulation.

In addition to investigation of patients with AH, useful insights into the pathogenetic mechanisms and possible treatments of the disease can be obtained with the use of suitable animal models. In this regard the murine model of AH established by Lohse *et al.*[27] mimics very closely the human condition. The administration of the 100 000*g* supernatant of syngeneic liver homogenate to C57BL/6 mice induces a cellular inflammatory liver infiltrate which lasts for up to 6 months. Importantly, splenocytes from an affected animal adoptively transfer the disease to a naive mouse. Such a model confirms the pivotal role of cellular immunity in the causation of AH, and will allow testing of the new immune therapeutic approaches described above.

References

1. De Groote J, Desmet VJ, Gedigk P *et al.* A classification of chronic hepatitis. Lancet. 1968;2:626–9.
2. Scheuer PJ. Chronic aggressive hepatitis. In: Liver biopsy interpretation, 2nd edn. London: Baillière Tindall; 1974:68.
3. Fremont DH, Matsumura M, Stura EA *et al.* Crystal structures of two viral peptides in complex with murine MHC class H-2K^b. Science. 1992;257:919–27.
4. Matsumura M, Fremont DH, Peterson PA, Wilson I. Emerging principles for the recognition of peptide antigens by MHC class I molecules. Science. 1992;257:927–34.
5. Nouri Aria K, Lobo-Yeo A, Vergani D *et al.* T suppressor cell function and number in children with liver disease. Clin Exp Immunol. 1985;61:283–9.
6. Nouri Aria KT, Donaldson PT, Hegarty JE *et al.* HLA A1-B8-DR3 and suppressor cell function in first degree relative of patients with autoimmune chronic active hepatitis. J Hepatol. 1985;1:235–41.

7. Nouri Aria KT, Hegarty JE, Alexander GJ *et al.* Effect of corticosteroids in suppressor cell activity in 'autoimmune' and viral chronic active hepatitis. N Engl J Med. 1982;307: 1301–4.
8. Vento S, Hegarty JE, Bottazzo G *et al.* Antigen specific suppressor cell function in autoimmune chronic active hepatitis. Lancet. 1984;1:1200–4.
9. Lobo-Yeo A, Mieli-Vergani G, Kenna G *et al.* Evidence of impaired antigen non-specific but normal antigen specific suppressor cell function in children with autoimmune chronic active hepatitis. Clin Exp Immunol. 1987;70:411–16.
10. Lobo-Yeo A, Senaldi G, Portmann B *et al.* Class I and class II major histocompatibility complex antigen expression on hepatocytes. A study in children with liver disease. Hepatology. 1990;12:224–32.
11. Lobo-Yeo A, Alviggi L, Mieli-Vergani G *et al.* Preferential activation of helper-inducer T lymphocytes in children with autoimmune chronic active hepatitis. Clin Exp Immunol. 1987;67:95–104.
12. Senaldi G, Portmann B, Mowat AP *et al.* Immunohistochemical features of the portal tract mononuclear cell infiltrate in chronic aggressive hepatitis of childhood. Arch Dis Child. 1992: in press.
13. Meyer zum Büschenfelde KH, Miescher PA. Liver specific antigens, purification and characterization. Clin Exp Immunol. 1972;10:89–102.
14. Jensen DM, McFarlane IG, Portmann B *et al.* Detection of antibodies directed against a liver-specific lipoprotein in patients with acute and chronic active hepatitis. N Engl J Med. 1978;299:1–7.
15. McFarlane BM, McSorley CG, Vergani D *et al.* Serum antibodies reacting with the hepatic asialoglycoprotein receptor (hepatic lectin) in acute and chronic liver disorders. J Hepatol. 1986;3:196–205.
16. Vergani D, Mieli-Vergani G, Mondelli M *et al.* Immunoglobulin on the surface of isolated hepatocytes is associated with antibody-dependent cell-mediated cytotoxicity and liver damage. Liver. 1987;7:307–15.
17. Mieli-Vergani G, Vergani D, Jenkins PJ *et al.* Lymphocyte cytotoxicity to autologous hepatocytes in HBsAg negative chronic active hepatitis. Clin Exp Immunol. 1979;38:16–21.
18. Vergani D, Wells L, Larcher VF *et al.* Genetically determined low C4: a predisposing factor to autoimmune chronic active hepatitis. Lancet. 1985;2:294–8.
19. Hussain MJ, Mowat AP, Mieli-Vergani G, Vergani D. Circulating levels of interleukin 1α, tumour necrosis factor, interferon γ and soluble interleukin-2 receptor are high in children with autoimmune chronic liver disease. Hepatology. 1990;12:937.
20. Hussain MJ, Mustafa A, Mowat AP *et al.* Immunohistochemical detection of TNF-α and IFN-γ in the liver of children with autoimmune chronic active hepatitis and primary cholangitis. J Hepatol. 1992;16:S59.
21. Wen L, Peakman M, Lobo-Yeo A *et al.* T-cell-directed hepatocyte damage in autoimmune chronic active hepatitis. Lancet. 1990;336:1527–30.
22. Wen L, Peakman M, Mieli-Vergani G, Vergani D. $\gamma\delta$ + ve T cell lines from liver biopsies of children with autoimmune chronic active hepatitis and primary sclerosing cholangitis are cytotoxic to human liver target cells. Hepatology. 1990;12:959.
23. Löhr H, Manns M, Kyriatsoulis A *et al.* Clonal analysis of liver-infiltrating T cells in patients with LKM-1 antibody-positive autoimmune chronic active hepatitis. Clin Exp Immunol. 1991;84:297–302.
24. Löhr H, Treichel U, Poralla T *et al.* Liver-infiltrating T helper cells in autoimmune chronic active hepatitis stimulate the production of autoantibodies against the human asialoglycoprotein receptor *in vitro*. Clin Exp Immunol. 1992;88:45–9.
25. Wraith DC, Smilek DE, Mitchell DJ *et al.* Antigen recognition in autoimmune encephalomyelitis and the potential for peptide-mediated immunotherapy. Cell. 1989;59:247–55.
26. Doherty DG, Donaldson PT, Underhill JA *et al.* Susceptibility to autoimmune hepatitis is associated with a specific amino acid substitution in the HLA-DR molecule. Hepatology. 1992;16:63A.
27. Loshe AW, Manns M, Dienes HP *et al.* Experimental autoimmune hepatitis: disease induction, time course and T-cell reactivity. Hepatology. 1990;11:24–30.

27
Immunogenetics of autoimmune chronic active hepatitis

E. L. KRAWITT and R. J. ALBERTINI

INTRODUCTION

Autoimmune chronic active hepatitis (ACAH) is included in a group of chronic necro-inflammatory disorders of unknown aetiology characterized by immunological and autoimmunological features, including the presence of circulating autoantibodies, without an antecedent viral infection[1]. The classification of these disorders has been based primarily on histopathological, clinical and immunological criteria, but overlaps occur which obscure classical boundaries and result in apparently contradictive morphological and serological findings. Moreover, the presence of autoantibodies in diseases of known aetiology, particularly chronic viral hepatitis, where histopathological features may mimic those in autoimmune liver disease, further blurs distinctions between disorders of known and unknown aetiologies.

Classical ACAH is a well-recognized disorder characterized by circulating antibodies to nuclei (ANA) and/or smooth muscle (ASMA) (the latter thought to be reflective of the more specific antibodies to actin [AAA]), a high serum globulin and a therapeutic response to glucocorticosteroid therapy. Classical ACAH is sometimes referred to as type 1 in recognition of other forms of ACAH that are characterized by antibodies to liver/kidney microsomes (ALKM) and/or soluble liver antigens.

For the most part, immunogenetic studies in ACAH have been performed in what has been presumed to be the classical form of disease. Genetic factors appear to play a major role in type 1 ACAH by predisposing to cirrhosis-producing immunopathogenic processes, although the interrelationships between genes and autoimmune processes remain largely undefined. Most genetic studies of this disease concern the HLA system. It has been postulated that the genes responsible for altered immune functions are either the HLA genes themselves, which constitute the major histocompatibility complex (MHC) in humans, or are other closely linked genes on chromosome 6. Many clinical studies have provided evidence for these hypotheses.

THE HLA SYSTEM

Before considering the many studies of HLA and type 1 ACAH, the HLA system itself, with some complexities that may be relevant to disease associations, will be briefly reviewed. It is useful to distinguish between the HLA genes and the proteins or antigens encoded by these genes. Furthermore, the normal functions of the HLA system are relevant in interpreting associations with autoimmune disease in that aberrations of these normal functions may mediate autoimmune processes.

Current understanding of the HLA system recognizes the fact that it is an extremely complex genetic region, consisting of a cluster of at least 35 genes (loci) on the short arm of chromosome 6[2]. There are, at present, 250 officially named alleles at these 35 loci, producing the most extensive polymorphism known for any human system[2]. The entire HLA region occupies more than 3.9 megabases of DNA and may be functionally divided into class I, class II and class III regions[3–5]. Class I and II genes encode molecules expressed as antigens on cell surfaces, i.e. the HLA antigens, while class III genes encode some of the complement factors.

The extreme polymorphism of HLA involves the class I A, B and C loci, and the class II D-region loci. There is less polymorphism for the class III loci. Fortunately, associations of autoimmune disease and HLA genes have been made for only a few of the 35 known loci. The loci that have been studied for disease associations are the A, B and C class I loci, the DR, DQ and DP class II or D-region loci, and a few of the class III or complement loci. However, the DR, DQ and DP loci themselves each include two or more loci, encoding for various α and β chains of the corresponding HLA antigens. The nomenclatures for these genes is therefore DRA, DRB1, DRB2, DRB3, etc. for DR; DQA1 DQB1, DQA2, etc. for DQ, etc.[6].

It is important to note that segregation of HLA genes is marked by the phenomenon of linkage disequilibrium, i.e. different alleles (different forms of the gene at a given locus) tend to be inherited together rather than randomly, as they would if segregation were totally independent. In fact, specific combinations of alleles tend to remain together in populations so that, if a particular allele at one locus is known for an individual, it is possible to predict alleles at other loci in linkage disequilibrium with the first. Specific combinations of HLA alleles at the different HLA loci (i.e. A, B and C class I loci, D-region loci, etc.) on chromosome 6 that are inherited together, except for infrequent recombinations, are termed haplotypes[7].

The HLA genes are related to other gene families that encode products that bind endogenous or exogenous peptides. These are the immunoglobulin genes on chromosomes 2, 14 and 22, and the T-cell receptor genes on chromosomes 7 and 14. The HLA, immunoglobulin and T-cell receptor genes, all important in immune processes, are believed to have evolved from a common genetic ancestor, and are referred to as a superfamily.

The molecules (antigens) encoded by the HLA genes are also termed class I (A, B and C), class II (DR, DQ and DP) or class III (complement factors), corresponding to their respective genes. The polymorphic portion of class I molecules is their α chain, which is a 45 kDa peptide. (The non-polymorphic

β chain of class I HLA antigens is β_2 microglobulin, which is encoded by a gene on chromosome 15.) Both the α (34 kDa heavy chains) and β (28 kDa light) chains of the class II molecules are polymorphic, except for the α chain of DR molecules, and all of these α and β chains are encoded by genes in the HLA D-region.

The structures formed by class I and II HLA molecules (antigens) on cell surfaces allow for antigen (polypeptide) binding and presentation. The tissue distribution of class I molecules includes all nucleated cells and platelets, whereas class II molecules are distributed more restrictively on B lymphocytes and macrophages/monocytes (antigen-presenting cells), and also on dendritic cells, activated T cells and perhaps melanoma and some epithelial cells.

Unlike class I and II HLA molecules, class III molecules are complement factors and are not cell bound. The complement components C2, C4 and factor B are encoded by class III HLA genes, with those for C2 and C4 being polymorphic.

It is now well recognized that most exogenous and endogenous protein antigens are presented to immunocompetent cells in the context of HLA. That is, foreign antigens are not recognized by themselves, but the immune system requires their presence with HLA antigens of the individual for a meaningful immune response to occur. Thus, one of the major functions of the HLA system is to 'process' and present antigens to the immune system. Protein antigens are presented as small peptides, which require cleavage within antigen-presenting cells (APCs), binding of the peptides to nascent HLA molecules, also produced in the APCs, and presentation on the cell surfaces. There is, in fact, a neat division of labour in that class I HLA molecules (antigens) present to $CD8^+$ T cells, i.e. to cytotoxic (and some suppressor) T cells, while class II HLA molecules present to $CD4^+$ helper (and some cytotoxic) T cells.

Understanding the HLA genetic region and its functions allows an informed speculation as to mechanisms by which HLA influences disease occurrences[5]. Results of clinical studies of HLA–disease associations may be interpreted in light of these possible mechanisms.

The first and perhaps most obvious potential mechanism by which HLA may influence disease susceptibility relates to its role in modulating specific immune responses. Disease susceptibility may be due to differential antigen processing by different HLA types, to some HLA antigens influencing T-cell repertoires during thymic selection more than others, or to some types of HLA antigens being expressed aberrantly on cells where others are not, thereby targeting an immune attack. In all instances the HLA genes are the disease genes. Another potential mechanism underlying HLA–disease associations is similarity between certain HLA antigens and those of one or another infectious agent. Therefore, individuals of this HLA type, by reacting aberrantly to antigens of the agent, develop an 'autoimmune disorder'. This possibility, called 'molecular mimicry', also incriminates the HLA genes as the disease genes. Finally, the association of an HLA type with a disease may be due not to the HLA genes themselves, but to other genes in the HLA region. (The 3.9 megabase long HLA region allows for the presence of many additional genes.) In this case the HLA genes merely serve as linkage markers, with the 'disease-susceptibility' and HLA genes being kept together by linkage disequilibrium. The disease-susceptibility genes may or may not be involved in immune processes. Any of these possibilities may underlie HLA–disease associations.

CLINICAL STUDIES OF HLA AND TYPE I ACAH

Clinical studies of HLA–disease associations usually involve comparison of HLA types between individuals with a given disease and normal controls (population studies), or an analysis of the co-segregation of HLA antigens and a disease within families. Both kinds of studies require that individuals be 'HLA typed', which in large part means serotyping. However, continuing improvements in antibody reagents have frequently revealed that what was thought to be a single HLA antigen is, in reality, two or more, encoded by two or more HLA alleles. These 'splits' lead to confusion in HLA disease studies because an inconsistent association with one HLA allele in an early study (erroneously determined) may lead to a more consistent association in a later study that uses a better-defined antibody reagent. Furthermore, some HLA alleles require T-cell responses or DNA-based methods for their definition. The former determines an individual's 'Dw' type, which cannot be assigned to any particular D-region allele but which may be shared by many; the latter clearly defines individual HLA alleles which may not differ serologically. The terminology for the HLA system is continually being revised to take account of this[2].

Serology appears to reflect the heterogeneity of class II alleles much more accurately than it does class I HLA alleles, although the DP class II alleles are not defined by serotyping but by cell typing and cloning[8,9]. Studies using DNA-based methods such as restriction fragment length polymorphisms (RFLPs) or sequencing should also further refine the associations between diseases and HLA genes. However, relevant to this review, Eckardt *et al.*[10] found no associations between type 1 ACAH and HLA type defined by RFLPs in 11 young women who were HLA type B8 DR3. The presence of undefined HLA alleles may greatly affect population-level studies of HLA–disease associations but the impact of family-based segregation analyses should be less.

POPULATION-LEVEL STUDIES

Type 1 ACAH is an example of an autoimmune disorder found in Caucasians in association with alleles identified by the class I HLA B8 antigen, one of the class II HLA DR3 antigens, and the lymphocyte-defined HLA Dw3 antigen(s)[11]. The relative risks for ACAH with B8, DR3 and Dw3 are of the order of 12. Preliminary data suggest that an association with HLA B8 and DR3 may also occur in Caucasians with type 2 (ALKM-1) ACAH[12]. In Japanese patients, population studies have given variable results, but associations between classical ACAH and alleles identified by HLA Bw54, and DR4, which occur in linkage disequilibrium, have been demonstrated[13,14]. Recent studies in Japanese subjects using DNA methods have confirmed the association with HLA DR4 found by serological typing[14,15]. In particular, there was an association with the DRB1*0405 allele, albeit, a weaker one than with the serologically determined DR4. Association with DQA1*0301 and DQB1*0404 was attributed to linkage disequilibrium of these alleles with those identified serologically as DR4[14].

It is quite possible that, in all of these studies, the class I allele associations with ACAH are secondary to the strong linkage disequilibrium that exists between class I alleles and the respective class II alleles, with the latter conferring the disease association. A study of United Kingdom Caucasian patients with classical ACAH who did not possess the HLA B8, DR3 haplotype has demonstrated a secondary association with HLA DR4[16]. In this group of patients onset of disease was later in life and appeared less likely to relapse and to be less severe than in young female HLA DR3 patients.

In an Australian study exploring possible associations of classical ACAH with extended haplotypes of HLA that include classes I, II, and III loci, and the glyoxalase locus (GLO1, GLO2 alleles) which maps 5–10 centimorgans centromeric to HLA, no greater associations were found for the extended haplotypes than for HLA B8 and DR3 alone[11]. Of 10 individuals who were HLA A1, B8 and DR3, seven were GLO1 and three were GLO2. Consistent with these results, Huot found that, of nine Caucasian ACAH patients who were HLA B8, four were GLO1, four were GLO2, and one was GLO1,2[17]. Thus, linked non-HLA loci between HLA and GLO probably do not play an important role in susceptibility to ACAH unless the 'susceptibility' alleles are quite common and not in strong linkage disequilibrium with HLA.

These studies of extended haplotypes must be examined in the light of Vergani's suggestion that the genetic predisposition for ACAH may also be associated with HLA class III complement alleles, in particular C2 and C4[18,19]. Because of the strong linkage disequilibrium between HLA B8 (class I) and the DR3 (class II) alleles, and the C4A (class II) null allele (no gene product detectable)[11,20], it is unlikely that the class III loci are independent disease-susceptibility loci. Nevertheless, it should be noted that in childhood-onset ACAH patients and their first-degree relatives, C4 phenotyping revealed a high incidence of C4 null phenotypes, as well as depressed serum C4 levels and function. To date, however, no family study characterizing the phenotypic expression and functional capacity of C4 has established a linkage relationship with childhood ACAH. A recent study of 24 Caucasian patients, however, using molecular techniques[20] in which a significantly higher percentage of ACAH patients had the C4A deletion compared to controls, also found the deletion in association with the HLA A1, B8, DR3 haplotypes and possibly with earlier onset and more severe disease.

In addition to studies of the MHC locus, population-level studies of genetic predisposition to autoimmune liver diseases have also sought association between disease and other 'immunoregulatory' genes. One of the studies seeking an association between ACAH and genes encoding for constant regions of the immunoglobulin heavy chains (chromosome 14) showed a weak association with the immunoglobulin allotype Gm (a,x)[21]. The effect of the immunoglobulin genes appeared to be interactive with the effect of the HLA genes in that this immunoglobulin allotype in the context of HLA B8 increased the relative risk of ACAH to greater than 39 over the population prevalence compared to a relative risk of ACAH of approximately 12 for individuals in whom HLA B8 and/or DR3 were present without immunoglobulin allotype Gm (a,x). We could not support these results, however, in family studies of classical ACAH patients[22].

FAMILY STUDIES

Family studies approach the question of genetic factors in ACAH in a different way. In such studies the intent is to define segregation of genes relevant to disease as they are distributed among family members. The analyses rely on Mendelian principles. A difficulty for a disease such as ACAH is that it is not known, *a priori*, if this disease in fact has a genetic basis but only infrequently affects multiple family members[23]. Although this is not surprising if the genetic trait is one that confers susceptibility rather than disease *per se* (i.e. a 10-fold increase in genetic susceptibility to a disease that is infrequent would only occasionally result in first-degree relatives being affected), it does make segregation analyses in families difficult. Attempts to circumvent this problem involve the use of 'surrogate phenotypes of disease'. These surrogate phenotypes are usually some identifiable trait that may be a marker for disease susceptibility. For autoimmune diseases these markers are usually immunological markers. The segregation analyses then relate the distribution of these markers among family members with the distribution of HLA alleles.

Family studies in classical ACAH using surrogate phenotypes for disease have been performed using antibodies to infectious agents and autoantibodies in disease-free first-degree relatives as the markers. Although the differential expression of antibodies implies some specificity, familial occurrences of antibody 'positivity' do not necessarily imply a genetic predisposition to antibody formations as presence of antibodies may reflect environmental factors.

An early study using the presence of circulating autoantibodies as surrogate phenotypes showed a significant increased prevalence of ANA in relatives of ACAH patients[24]. In another study[25] an increased prevalence of not only ANA, but also of anti-gastric parietal cell and anti-thyroglobulin antibodies was found in relatives of ACAH patients. Antibodies against infectious agents have also been studied in patients with ACAH. Although as a group, antibodies to rubeola and rubella in relatives of patients with autoimmune liver disease have not been found to differ from controls, clustering of antiviral titres has been observed in certain families in which the propositus had ACAH. In one family study evaluating levels of rubella antibodies in first-degree relatives of patients with ACAH, no associations with HLA class I antigens were found despite the association of elevated antibody titres in the index cases with HLA B8 and B12[26].

Using the strategy of assigning a surrogate phenotype, defined as the presence of ANA and/or ASMA in first-degree relatives, we searched for a postulated disease susceptibility gene in 10 families in which the index case had classical ACAH[22]. Patients and their first-degree relatives were genotyped for HLA A, B, and DR alleles and for immunoglobulin constant region allotypes G1m, G2m, G3m and A2m haplotypes. Segregation analysis did not support either single autosomal dominant or recessive inheritance for the antibody-positive phenotypes. Linkage between the postulated disease susceptibility locus and either HLA or immunoglobulin loci was excluded by several analyses and logistic regression indicated that neither immunogenetic marker was statistically associated with autoantibody positivity in these families. Therefore, despite the occurrence of autoantibody positivity in first-degree relatives of ACAH patients, there was no evidence that this trait has a simple genetic basis, or that it is an alternative manifestation of a postulated disease susceptibility gene conferring a predisposition to ACAH.

STUDIES OF IMMUNOREGULATORY DYSFUNCTION

Subsequent to Allison's hypothesis[27] that alterations of T-cell control play a role in the pathogenesis of autoimmune disorders, it was suggested[28] that suppressor cell dysfunction might be important in the pathogenesis of ACAH, and that the HLA B8 allele might serve as a genetic marker for such an immunoregulatory abnormality. Studies using an *in-vitro* assay of peripheral blood mononuclear cell suppression of T-cell proliferation in individuals provided no evidence that non-specific T-cell suppression differed in patients dependent on the presence or absence of HLA B8[29]. An investigation in nine families[30], ascertained by the presence of a single patient with classical ACAH, measured suppressor phenotypes by an *in-vitro* assay of peripheral blood mononuclear cell suppression of immunoglobulin secretion, and sought associations of this phenotype with inheritance of alleles at HLA and Gm loci. This study was designed to see if an abnormality of immune regulation represented a genetic phenotype, simply controlled by genes at putative disease susceptibility loci and if such loci were linked to either the HLA or the Gm loci. Although immunoregulatory dysfunction in ACAH was present as a familial abnormality, it occurred independent of circulating autoantibody allotypes. The clustering of decreased suppressor cell function seen in some families, reminiscent of clustering of antiviral antibodies noted above[26], indicated that it is possible that immunoregulatory dysfunction plays a role in the pathogenesis of ACAH in some families but not in others, supporting a concept of pathogenetic heterogeneity.

Similar studies have been undertaken in nine families with classical ACAH[31] investigating T-lymphocyte sensitization to the liver-specific asialoglycoprotein receptor (ASGPR), which has been implicated as a relevant antigen in ACAH, using an *in-vitro* indirect T-lymphocyte migration inhibitory factor assay. Although T cell sensitization to the crude fraction liver-derived lipoprotein complex (LSP) was observed in all ACAH index cases, and in 24% of first-degree relatives, it was also seen in 27% of tested spouses. Sensitization to the ASGPR was also present in the index cases, but in no first-degree relatives or spouses. In these families no linkage was demonstrated with T-cell sensitization to LSP nor to an antigen-specific T suppressor defect.

In summary, these studies in ACAH would indicate that abnormalities of specific and non-specific suppressor cell function do not serve as valid 'surrogate phenotypes for disease'. Environmental agents that are responsible for disease may also influence these immunological phenotypes, and immunological abnormalities may therefore be a response to the environment, and not primary to disease in affected individuals. For whatever reasons no family study today provides convincing evidence of linkage between HLA and a fundamental immunoregulatory defect that confers susceptibility to ACAH.

NATURAL HISTORY AND RESPONSE TO TREATMENT

Although a disease may be strongly associated with specific alleles of the MHC, implying genetic susceptibility, this does not necessarily imply any relationship to the natural history of disease or response to therapy. It is now 20 years since Mackay and Morris[32] first described the association between ACAH and HLA antigens which indicated the importance of the MHC locus in this disorder. A study in the mid-1970s[33] was the first to support an association between an HLA allele (identified by Dw3) and poor response to treatment for patients with ACAH and CAH patients with a hepatitis B surface antigen. Only half of the HLA Dw3 patients were HLA B8-positive, and two of the 17 had circulating hepatitis B surface antigen. From recent studies, however, it does appear that the presence of the HLA A1, B8, DR3 phenotype may mark a subgroup of classical ACAH which responds less well to treatment. The frequency of the HLA A1, B8, DR3 phenotype has been noted to be higher in patients referred for liver transplantation both in the United Kingdom[16] and in North America[34]. In a series from the Mayo Clinic, 70% of patients with ACAH who received liver transplants were HLA B8-positive. Similarly, of those patients who failed to respond to immunosuppressive therapy, 70% possessed the HLA B8 allele; only 46% of responders, however, were B8-positive[34]. It would appear, therefore, that these alleles may mark not only for predisposition to disease but also for more serious progression (i.e. those requiring transplantation) and lack of response to anti-inflammatory/immunosuppressive regimens. Because HLA A1, B8, DR3 ACAH patients are predominantly female and younger, however, factors of gender and age, as well as C4A gene deletion (see above), must also be considered.

Acknowledgement

The authors thank Karen Wright for preparation of the manuscript.

References

1. Krawitt EL, Wiesner RH, eds. Autoimmune liver diseases. New York: Raven Press; 1991.
2. Bodmer JG. Nomenclature 1991, Foreword. Hum Immunol. 1992;34:2–3.
3. Bell JI, Todd JA, McDevitt HO. The molecular basis of HLA–disease association. In: Harris H, Hirschhorn K, editors. Advances in human genetics. New York and London: Plenum Press, 1989;1:1–41.
4. Owen M. Major histocompatibility complex. In: Roitt IM, Brostoff J, Male DK, editors. Immunology. London: Gower; 1989:4.
5. Hansen JA, Nelson JL. Autoimmune diseases and HLA. Crit Rev Immunobiol. 1990;10:307–28.
6. Bodmer JG *et al.* Nomenclature for factors of the HLA system. Hum Immunol. 1991;34: 4–18.
7. Ceppellini R, Curtoni ES, Mattiuz PL *et al.* Genetics of leukocyte antigens: a family study of segregation and linkage. In: Curtoni ES, Mattiuz PL, Tosi RM, editors. Histocompatibility testing. Copenhagen: Munksgaard; 1967:149.
8. Shaw S, Kavathas P, Pollack MS *et al.* Family studies define a new histocompatibility locus, SB, between HLA-DR and GLO. Nature. 1981;293:745–7.
9. Kappes DJ, Arnot D, Okada K, Strominger JL. Structure and polymorphism of the HLA class II SB light chain genes. EMBRO J. 1984;3:2985–93.
10. Eckardt GS, O'Brien RM, Mackay IR *et al.* Lack of informative HLA restriction fragment length polymorphisms in autoimmune chronic active hepatitis. Tissue Antigens. 1989;34: 270–8.
11. Tait B, Mackay IR, Board P *et al.* HLA A1, B8, DR3 extended haplotypes in autoimmune chronic hepatitis. Gastroenterology. 1989;97:479–81.
12. Homberg J-C, Abuaf N, Bernard O *et al.* Chronic active hepatitis associated with antiliver/kidney microsome antibody type 1: a second type of 'autoimmune hepatitis'. Hepatology. 1987;7:1333–9.
13. Seki T, Kiyosawa K, Inoko H, Ota M. Association of autoimmune hepatitis with HLA-Bw54 and DR4 in Japanese patients. Hepatology. 1990;12:1300–4.
14. Seki T, Ota M, Furuta S *et al.* HLA Class II molecules and autoimmune hepatitis susceptibility in Japanese patients. Gastroenterology. 1992;103:1041–7.
15. Ota M, Seki T, Kiyosawa K *et al.* A possible association between basic amino acids of position 13 of DRB1 chains and autoimmune hepatitis. Immunogenetics. 1992;36:49–55.
16. Donaldson PT, Doherty DG, Hayllar KM *et al.* Susceptibility to autoimmune chronic active hepatitis: human leukocyte antigens DR4 and A1-B8-DR3 are independent risk factors. Hepatology. 1991;13:701–6.
17. Huot AE. The frequency of HLA and glyoxalase genes in patients with autoimmune chronic active hepatitis. Master of Science thesis. Burlington, VT: University of Vermont; 1987.
18. Vergani D, Larcher VF, Davies ET *et al.* Genetically determined low C4: a predisposing factor to autoimmune chronic active hepatitis. Lancet. 1985;2:294–8.
19. Senaldi G, Mieli-Vergani G, Mowat AO, Vergani D. C4 function in children with autoimmune chronic active hepatitis (Letter). Hepatology. 1989;9:345.
20. Goldstein R, Sengar DPS, Toze C, Scully LJ. C4A gene deletion and HLA associations in idiopathic autoimmune chronic active hepatitis. Hum Immunol. 1992;34:43 (Suppl 1) (abstract).
21. Whittingham S, Mathews JD, Schanfield MS *et al.* Interaction of HLA and Gm in autoimmune chronic active hepatitis. Clin Exp Immunol. 1981;43:80–6.
22. Krawitt EL, Kilby AE, Albertini RJ *et al.* Immunogenetic studies of autoimmune chronic active hepatitis: HLA, immunoglobulin allotypes and autoantibodies. Hepatology. 1987;7:1305–10.
23. Hodges S, Lobo-Yeo A, Donaldson P *et al.* Autoimmune chronic active hepatitis in a family. Gut. 1991;32:299–302.
24. Galbraith RM, Smith M, Mackenzie RM *et al.* High prevalence of seroimmunologic abnormalities in relatives of patients with active chronic hepatitis or primary biliary cirrhosis. N Engl J Med. 1974;290:63–9.
25. Salaspuro MP, Laitinen OI, Lehtola J *et al.* Immunological parameters, viral antibodies, and biochemical and histological findings in relatives of patients with chronic active hepatitis

and primary biliary cirrhosis. Scand J Gastroenterol. 1976;11:313–20.
26. Galbraith RM, Williams R, Pattison J *et al.* Enhanced antibody responses in active chronic hepatitis: relation to HLA-B8 and HLA-B12 and portosystemic shunting. Lancet. 1976;1:930–4.
27. Allison AC, Denman AM, Barnes RD. Cooperating and controlling functions of thymus-derived lymphocytes in relation to autoimmunity. Lancet. 1971;2:135–40.
28. Eddleston ALWF, Williams R. Inadequate antibody response to HBAg or suppressor cell defect in development of active chronic hepatitis. Lancet. 1974;1:1543–5.
29. Krawitt EL, Albertini RJ, Webb DD *et al.* Immune regulation and HLA types in chronic hepatitis. Hepatology. 1981;1:300–6.
30. Krawitt EL, Kilby AE, Albertini RJ *et al.* An immunogenetic study of suppressor cell activity in autoimmune chronic active hepatitis. Clin Immunol Immunopathol. 1988;46: 249–57.
31. O'Brien CJ, Donaldson PT, McFarlane IG *et al.* Cell-mediated immunity and suppressor-T-cell defects to liver-derived antigens in families of patients with autoimmune chronic active hepatitis. Lancet. 1986;350–3.
32. Mackay IR, Morris PJ. Association of autoimmune active chronic hepatitis with HL-A1,8. Lancet. 1972;793–5.
33. Opelz G, Vogten AJM, Summerskill WHJ *et al.* HLA determinants in chronic active liver disease: Possible relation of HLA-Dw3 to prognosis. Tissue Antigens. 1977;9:36–40.
34. Sanchez-Urdazpal L, Czaja AJ, van Hoek B *et al.* Prognostic features and role of liver transplantation in severe corticosteroid-treated autoimmune chronic active hepatitis. Hepatology. 1992;15:215–21.

28
Therapy of idiopathic autoimmune chronic active hepatitis

B. COMBES and W. C. MADDREY

Idiopathic autoimmune chronic active hepatitis (IACAH) is an inflammatory hepatocellular disease primarily affecting women and associated with abnormalities in immunoregulation[1,2]. It is usually present for 6 months or longer at the time of diagnosis, and is reflected in high values for serum transaminases. Histologically, the characteristic lesion is periportal and/or periseptal hepatitis (piecemeal necrosis)[3–5]. The spectrum of histological severity increases progressively with the presence of bridging necrosis, panlobular and multilobular necrosis, and active cirrhosis. All of the above precirrhotic lesions can progress to cirrhosis. A milder lesion without piecemeal necrosis, and referred to as persistent hepatitis, is relatively benign.

There appear to be several subgroups of patients with IACAH[6]. All are characterized by female predominance, the presence of polyclonal hypergammaglobulinaemia, and to varying degrees the coexistence of other autoimmune disorders. Differences exist in the type of autoantibodies present in serum. A classification based on serum antibodies is as follows: type I has a high incidence of ANA, and SMA (antiactin); type II is characterized by LKM_1 antibodies[7,8], and type III by anti-soluble liver antigen, SLA[9]. Serum antibodies to other liver components including the asialoglycoprotein receptor[10]; other liver membrane proteins and lipoproteins exist in varying degrees in some of the types outlined above, and in other patients with chronic hepatic disease of unknown aetiology[11]. The combination of the generic clinical features cited above, plus the presence of serum autoantibodies, leads us to call these disorders autoimmune. Response to corticosteroids supports the inference. There exist similar patients without identifiable autoantibodies who also respond to corticosteroids; we label their disorder cryptogenic. Until we discover the aetiology(ies) of these processes, we are restricted to clinical associations for these judgements, and recommendations for therapy are based on clinical trials in these disorders.

Before initiating treatment it is imperative that other chronic hepatic diseases that can present with similar symptoms, liver test abnormalities and histological appearance be recognized, since the approaches to their

Table 1 Causes of chronic hepatitis

Viral hepatitis B
Viral hepatitis C
Therapeutic drugs
Wilson's disease
Autoimmune chronic active hepatitis

Table 2 Disorders that may simulate chronic hepatitis

Primary biliary cirrhosis
Sclerosing cholangitis
Alcohol-induced liver disease
Non-alcoholic steatohepatitis
α_1-Antitrypsin deficiency
Iron storage disorders

therapy will differ considerably from those used in the management of autoimmune hepatitis. These disorders are listed in Table 1 as causes of chronic hepatitis, and in Table 2 as conditions that may simulate chronic hepatitis.

Controlled therapeutic trials in autoimmune chronic hepatitis have largely been confined to the most prevalent subgroup which is characterized by the presence of antinuclear and antismooth muscle (anti-actin) antibodies; so-called type I IACAH. These trials have demonstrated that corticosteroids with and without concomitant use of azathioprine are effective forms of therapy[12–15]. Much has been learned about the use of these compounds and their impact on the disease process. Although similar therapy is also used in other forms of IACAH, the relative rarity of these other subgroups and the lack of controlled trials in their management make drawing of inferences about their treatment both difficult and probably premature. Discussion of treatment in this presentation will be limited to type I IACAH.

The bases for therapy of IACAH include the observations that: (1) mortality is high in untreated disease; (2) there is a low incidence of spontaneous remission; and (3) corticosteroid-containing regimens improve survival and the incidence of remission.

Mortality data obtained for control patients in three prospective, randomized therapeutic trials suggest that close to 50% of patients will die in approximately 5 years. By contrast, patients receiving prednisolone or prednisone with or without azathioprine fared much better, with significant decreases in mortality[12–14,16].

Currently used corticosteroid regimens include: (1) prednisone or prednisolone alone, in which a high oral dose (30–60 mg/day originally) is lowered to a maintenance dose (7.5–20 mg/day) by predetermined schedule (Mayo) or in response to laboratory tests, aiming for the lowest daily dose that yields normal or near-normal values for serum transaminases; and (2) azathioprine plus prednisone or prednisolone (combined). Two types of regimen are used. In one, azathioprine and corticosteroid are started together and adjusted in a predetermined schedule, leading to a daily maintenance dose of 50 mg azathioprine and 10 mg prednisone (Mayo). In the other regimen(s), patients are usually started on corticosteroid alone. The dose is lowered as activity of the disease decreases. Azathioprine is introduced in doses of 75–150 mg/day at varying times along the way to improvement. In successfully treated patients, daily maintenance doses of 7.5–12.5 mg of corticosteroid and 75–150 mg of azathioprine are utilized.

Goals of such therapy include: (1) improvement in symptoms; (2) improvement in biochemical abnormalities; (3) improvement in histology with an additional aim of preventing cirrhosis; (4) prevention of complications of liver disease including ascites, encephalopathy and variceal bleeding; and (5) decrease in mortality.

It is important that one have some insight into what to expect in favourable responses to treatment. The prolonged experience which has undergone the most extensive analyses is the Mayo Clinic Experience. Because of different treatment regimens, exclusions of some patients who were subsequently found to be HBsAg-positive, incorrect initial diagnoses, changes in criteria for the histological diagnosis of cirrhosis, and increasing length of follow-up, it has been difficult at times to follow patients from one publication to another. This has now been made much easier by the publication in 1986 of a monograph of the Mayo Clinic Experience[17].

In patients treated with daily prednisone alone or prednisone plus azathioprine, symptoms improve first (87% by 6 months), followed by biochemical resolution (68% by 6 months), while histological resolution lags considerably (8% at 6 months, only 29% at 12 months)[18]. Complete remission requires attaining: (1) absence of symptoms; *and* (2) an AST less than twice the upper limit of normal, *and* a normal serum bilirubin and γ-globulin; *and* (3) absent or minimal piecemeal necrosis (with or without cirrhosis) on liver biopsy.

Utilizing these criteria for remission, of 111 patients treated with either of the two corticosteroid regimens, 82 (74%) remitted, 16 (14%) were treatment failures, and 13 (12%) had neither remitted nor failed therapy[19]. Achieving remission takes time. This was accomplished by 2 years in 61 (74%), by 3 years in 73 (89%) and 4 years in 78 (95%)[19]. Thus, it is important to be patient; complete remission may take several years of continuous treatment.

One aim of therapy is to arrest the disease, i.e. reach remission, and then stop treatment. Unfortunately, relapses occur commonly once treatment is halted[20–22]. They occur in up to 87% of patients within 1 year; the majority occur within 3 months. They cannot be predicted from pretreatment data. They are more likely to occur in non-cirrhotics when histology shows residual piecemeal necrosis, even when liver tests are completely normal. Some feel that relapses will occur almost invariably in cirrhotics even with little evidence of residual piecemeal necrosis.

Fortunately, most patients who relapse will respond to reinitiation of therapy. However, the likelihood of further relapse after subsequent remission appears to increase progressively with each subsequent relapse such that the likelihood of sustaining remissions off therapy after two or more relapses becomes relatively low[22]. Of the 82 Mayo patients who remitted, sustained remission was achieved in only 27[19]. Finally, patients who relapse more than

Table 3 Development of cirrhosis (all patients received prednisone)

	Morphology of initial liver biopsy			
	CAH	*SHB*	*SHMN*	*Total*
Cirrhosis	8	13	12	33
No cirrhosis	17	21	12	50
Total	25	34	24	83
Percentage developing cirrhosis	32	38	50	40

Adapted from ref. 23

once, and who require additional periods of higher dose corticosteroids to become recaptured, exhibit an increased incidence of corticosteroid-induced complications[22].

In precirrhotic patients treated with corticosteroids, cirrhosis continues to develop in a moderate number[18]. There is considerable interest in the potential for histological lesions of varying severity to progress to cirrhosis. Now that long-term follow-up is available, it seems clear that the pretreatment lesion of piecemeal necrosis alone (CAH), as well as this lesion complicated by bridging necrosis (SHB), panlobular or multilobular necrosis (SHMN) can all progress to cirrhosis[23] (Table 3).

A body of observations suggest that development of cirrhosis is related to both the duration and severity of the inflammatory activity in the liver. These observations include the following: (1) cirrhosis usually develops during the initial 2 years of treatment; (2) longer periods of treatment are required to suppress inflammation in patients who develop cirrhosis; (3) the risk of developing cirrhosis once remission is achieved is low (12% in 5 years) – such patients had commonly relapsed off therapy and before progressing to cirrhosis; and (4) treatment failures have an increased likelihood of developing cirrhosis[18] (Fig. 1).

Although it is clear, then, that cirrhosis develops on therapy, it is not clear whether treatment lowers the incidence or rate of development of cirrhosis that would develop in the absence of treatment.

The probability of survival in corticosteroid-treated patients who already had cirrhosis at initiation of therapy was 80% at 5 years and 65% after 10 years[18]. By contrast, those who developed cirrhosis while on treatment had a much better prognosis; it was as good as in those who did not develop cirrhosis[18]. This combination of findings has supported the notion that the severity of the inflammation accompanying cirrhosis is more important than cirrhosis *per se* in determining outcome of the disease. Thus, rapid suppression of inflammation would appear to be one of the most important goals of therapy (Fig. 2).

Serious complications may accompany the use of corticosteroids; to occur, they usually require that more than 10 mg of corticosteroid be administered per day and for more than 18 months. The incidence of complications appears to be more common in patients who relapse more than once and in those who are postmenopausal[22,24]. Complications are more common on maintenance prednisone of 20 mg/day than on half the dose when combined with azathioprine 50 mg/day. Since outcome is comparable with steroid alone

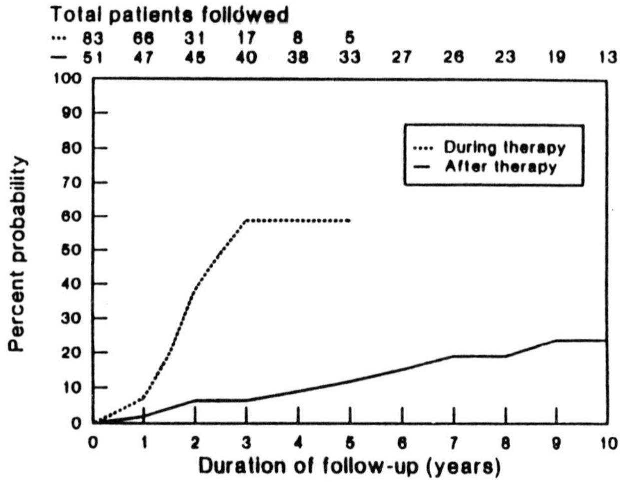

Fig. 1 Probability of developing cirrhosis during initial corticosteroid therapy and after remission and cessation of initial treatment (from ref. 3)

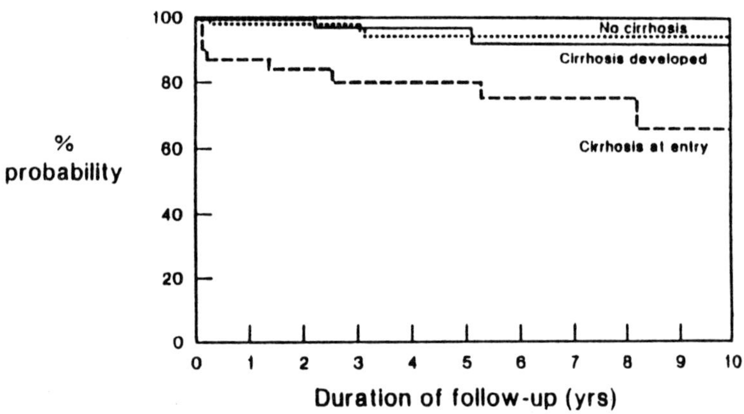

Fig. 2 Probability of survival in corticosteroid-treated chronic active hepatitis with and without cirrhosis (from p. 280 of ref. 18)

and steroid plus azathioprine, the reduced incidence of complications attributed to the steroid-sparing effect of azathioprine has led to the recommendation of combined therapy as the optimal one[15].

Indeed, this has now been carried even further. Low-dose corticosteroid alone may not maintain remission when azathioprine is removed from a combined regimen[25]. By contrast, when corticosteroids were removed from patients in remission, and azathioprine was instituted at a dose of 2 mg/kg per day, remission was maintained in the ensuing year[26]. Thus, even though azathioprine alone may not be effective in inducing remission, it may exert an important effect in maintaining remission. The incidence of complications of azathioprine has fortunately been low thus far in patients maintained on single therapy.

There is little available information on the value of other forms of therapy for management of IACAH. For the patient who fails medical therapy, liver transplantation offers a viable alternative. Recurrence of disease has not been a major problem in the relatively small number of cases transplanted to date[19].

References

1. Maddrey WC. Chronic hepatitis: In: Zakim D and Boyer TD, editors. Hepatology: a textbook of liver disease, 2nd edn. Philadelphia: WB Saunders; 1990:1025–62.
2. Czaja AJ. Natural history, clinical features, and treatment of autoimmune hepatitis. Semin Liver Dis. 1984;4:1–12.
3. DeGroote J, Desmet VJ, Gedigk P *et al.* A classification of chronic hepatitis. Lancet. 1968;2:626–8.
4. Baggenstoss AH, Soloway RD, Summerskill WHJ *et al.* Chronic active liver disease. The range of histologic lesions, their response to treatment, and evaluation. Hum Pathol. 1972;3:183–98.
5. Bianchi L and an International Group. Acute and chronic hepatitis revisited. Lancet. 1977;2:914–19.
6. Maddrey WC. Subdivisions of idiopathic autoimmune chronic active hepatitis. Hepatology. 1987;7:1372–5.
7. Homberg JC, Abuaf N, Bernard O *et al.* Chronic active hepatitis associated with anti-liver/kidney microsome antibody type 1: a second type of 'autoimmune' hepatitis. Hepatology. 1987;7:1333–9.
8. Manns M, Johnson E, Griffin K *et al.* Major antigen of liver kidney microsomal autoantibodies in idiopathic autoimmune hepatitis is cytochrome P450dbl. J Clin Invest. 1989;3:1066–72.
9. Manns M, Gerken G, Kyriatsoulis A *et al.* Characterization of a new subgroup of autoimmune chronic active hepatitis by autoantibodies against a soluble liver antigen. Lancet. 1987;1:292–4.
10. Poralla T, Treichel V, Löhr H, Fleischer B. The asialoglycoprotein receptor as target structure in autoimmune liver disease. Semin Liver Dis. 1991;11:215–22.
11. Manns MP. Cytoplasmic autoantigens in autoimmune hepatitis: molecular analysis and clinical relevance. Semin Liver Dis. 1991;11:205–14.
12. Cook GC, Mulligan R, Sherlock S. Controlled prospective trial of corticosteroid therapy in active chronic hepatitis. Q J Med. 1971;40:159–85.
13. Soloway RD, Summerskill WHJ, Baggenstoss AH *et al.* Clinical, biochemical and histologic remission of severe chronic active liver disease: A controlled study of treatments and early prognosis. Gastroenterology. 1972;63:820–33.
14. Murray-Lyon IM, Stern RB, Williams R. Controlled trial of prednisone and azathioprine in active chronic hepatitis. Lancet. 1973;1:735–7.
15. Summerskill WHJ, Korman MG, Ammon HV *et al.* Prednisone for chronic active liver disease: dose titration, standard dose and combination with azathioprine compound. Gut. 1975;16:876–83.
16. Kirk AP, Jain S, Pocock S *et al.* Late results of the Royal Free Hospital prospective controlled trial of prenisolone therapy in hepatitis B surface antigen negative chronic active hepatitis. Gut. 1980;21:78–83.
17. Czaja AJ, Dickson ER (eds). Chronic active hepatitis. The Mayo Clinic Experience. New York and Basel: Marcel Dekker; 1986.
18. Davis GL, Czaja AJ. Immediate and long term results of corticosteroid therapy for severe idiopathic chronic active hepatitis. In: Czaja AJ, Dickson ER, editors. Chronic active hepatitis. The Mayo Clinic Experience. New York and Basel: Marcel Dekker; 1986: 269–83.

19. Sanchez-Urdazpal L, Czaja AJ, Van Holk B *et al.* Prognostic features and role of liver transplantation in severe corticosteroid-treated autoimmune chronic active hepatitis. Hepatology. 1991;15:215–21.
20. Czaja AJ, Ammon HV, Summerskill WHJ. Clinical features and prognosis of severe chronic active liver disease (CALD) after corticosteroid-induced remission. Gastroenterology. 1980;78:518–23.
21. Hegarty JE, Nouri-Aria KT, Portmann B *et al.* Relapse following treatment withdrawal in patients with autoimmune chronic active hepatitis. Hepatology. 1983;3:685–9.
22. Czaja AJ, Beaver SJ, Shiels MT. Sustained remission after corticosteroid therapy of severe hepatitis B surface antigen-negative chronic active hepatitis. Gastroenterology. 1987;92: 215–19.
23. Davis GL, Czaja AJ, Ludwig J. Development and prognosis of histologic cirrhosis in corticosteroid-treated hepatitis B surface antigen-negative chronic active hepatitis. Gastroenterology. 1984;87:1222–7.
24. Wang KK, Czaja AJ. Prognosis of corticosteroid-treated hepatitis B surface antigen-negative chronic active hepatitis in postmenopausal women: a retrospective analysis. Gastroenterology. 1989;97:1288–93.
25. Stellon AJ, Hegarty JE, Portmann B *et al.* Randomized controlled trial of azathioprine withdrawal in autoimmune chronic active hepatitis. Lancet. 1985;1:668–70.
26. Stellon AJ, Keating JJ, Johnson PJ *et al.* Maintenance of remission in autoimmune chronic active hepatitis with azathioprine after corticosteroid withdrawal. Hepatology. 1988;8: 781–4.

Section VII
Autoimmunity against Cytochrome P450 Enzymes

29
The cytochrome P450 supergene family: a class of autoantigens

E. F. JOHNSON

INTRODUCTION

It is now recognized that at least five human cytochrome P450s are recognized by autoantibodies that are associated with autoimmune diseases. In this short review, general features of the P450 enzymes will be outlined. In addition, specific attributes of these proteins that may play a role in their occurrence as autoantigens will be discussed. These include the capacity of P450s to activate substrates to products that can bind covalently to cellular macromolecules. This may in turn elicit an immune reaction to the modified protein. In severe cases, the generation of reactive intermediates can lead to tissue necrosis. In addition, some P450s are induced by environmental chemicals. In some cases, prolonged exposure to inducing chemicals can lead to highly elevated expression of P450s as well as other proteins, and to a proliferation of endoplasmic reticulum. It is possible that changes that occur in protein processing during this process, or following the cessation of the insult, contribute in some way to the development of autoantibodies to these proteins.

SHARED PROPERTIES OF P450 ENZYMES

P450s are haem proteins. When the ferrous (reduced) enzyme binds to carbon monoxide it exhibits a distinctive chromophore that absorbs visible light maximally at around 450 nm leading to the designation P450 (pigment 450 nm)[1]. This distinctive spectrum reflects the ligation of the haem to a cysteinyl residue at the axial ligation site opposite from where carbon monoxide binds. This cysteine and adjacent residues form a distinctive amino acid sequence motif that is characteristic of P450s[2]. During catalysis the enzyme binds oxygen at the open coordination site and reductively cleaves dioxygen to form a molecule of water and an oxygen species that remains bound at the active site[3]. This is a powerful oxidant, and the different P450s have evolved to control the reactivity of this oxidant with a wide range of chemical substances. For the mammalian, microsomal P450s, the reduction of the enzyme to permit oxygen binding and the second reduction of the enzyme substrate complex to complete the reductive cleavage of oxygen is performed by a flavoprotein reductase that is also present in the endoplasmic reticulum[3]. The flavoprotein is reduced in turn by NADPH. There are also mitochondrial forms of P450s in mammals that utilize different protein partners to provide reducing equivalents. However, the P450s that are known to be recognized by autoantibodies are all microsomal enzymes.

CATALYTIC DIVERSITY

The cytochrome P450 enzymes are a diverse family of enzymes that are thought to have evolved from a common ancestral gene, and this relationship forms the basis for a widely used nomenclature based on sequence relatedness[4]. Although the relatedness of these enzymes is apparent when their amino acid sequences are compared, they can exhibit very low ($< 20\%$) amino acid sequence identity. This sequence diversity underlies a rich catalytic diversity that has evolved to serve many functions. In mammals, P450 enzymes are involved in many biosynthetic reactions that include the synthesis of androgens, steroid hormones, and the hormonal forms of vitamin D3. The P450 enzymes that have evolved to fill specific niches, like most enzymes, are distinguished by their specific catalysis of a single reaction. Autoantibodies to the adrenal steroid 21-hydroxylase (CYP21) have been found in patients with Addison's disease[5], and autoantibodies to the steroid 17α-hydroxylase/lyase have been detected in Addison's patients with autoimmune polyglandular disorder[6]. The 17α-hydroxylase (CYP17) is expressed in tissues such as testes and ovaries where it catalyses a specific step in the synthesis of androgens and oestrogens.

On the other hand, P450s play an important role in a variety of catabolic pathways for steroids and fatty acids as well as a wide range of foreign compounds. These catabolic enzymes are found at many sites where environmental chemicals might gain access to the body, and many are found at relatively high concentrations in the liver, which plays a central role in the detoxication of foreign compounds. The P450s that are recognized by autoantibodies associated with autoimmune hepatitis are members of this latter group of enzymes.

In general, the P450s that metabolize foreign compounds catalyse the formation of more polar compounds from generally hydrophobic substrates[7]. These products are often more readily excreted. The introduction of hydroxyl groups into the substrate or the unmasking of other functional groups by oxidation can lead to further metabolism by enzymes which can conjugate the product of the P450 catalysed reaction with glutathione, glucuronic acid, and other molecules which render the product more water-soluble and readily excreted.

The P450 enzymes that have evolved to function in the detoxication of foreign compounds and catabolism of endogenous fatty acids and sterols are

Table 1 Catalytic activities of P450 2C5 and functional overlap with other P450s

Substrate	*Also catalysed by*	*Reference*
Progesterone (21-OH)	CYP21	65
Pregnenolone (21-OH)		66
Benzo(*a*)pyrene	CYP1A1, CYP3A	67
2-Acetylaminofluorene (7-OH)	CYP1A1, CYP2C3	25

Table 2 Number of characterized P450s in the indicated subfamilies and species

	1A	*2A*	*2B*	*2C*	*2D*	*2E*	*3A*	*4A*	*4B*	*Total*
Rat	2	3	5	8	5	1	5	4	1	> 34
Rabbit	2	2	3	8	2	2	1	4	1	> 25
Human	2	2	1	4	1	1	3	1	1	> 16

not only numerous but, in contrast to the biosynthetic enzymes, they also readily metabolize numerous structurally dissimilar substrates. Moreover, there is often an overlap among different enzymes in the metabolism of a particular substrate. Thus, P450 enzymes are difficult to identify by the specific reactions that they catalyse. For example, P450 2C5 or CYP2C5 catalyses several activities that are also catalysed by other enzymes, which are listed in Table 1. For this reason a widely used nomenclature based on sequence relatedness and on likely evolutionary relationships is used to identify P450s by a number, letter, number combination.

Three simple rules guide the naming of a P450[4]. The first number, which was originally a Roman numeral but is now more widely denoted by an Arabic numeral, designates a family of P450s that share 40% or greater amino acid sequence identity. The following letter designates subfamilies within each family that generally exhibit greater than 65–75% amino acid sequence identity. Subfamilies may be simple or complex. As shown in Table 2, the number of members in each subfamily can vary between species. Moreover, many of these enzymes appear to reflect gene duplication and divergence that has occurred since the radiation of mammals. For example, the human P450 2C enzymes will exhibit roughly 75% amino acid sequence identity with any rabbit P450 2C protein, whereas the sequence identity among rabbit 2C enzymes ranges from 68% to > 95%. The third number in the designation is used to identify specific P450s. In subfamilies where there are multiple members for different species the numbers are generally unique for each enzyme in each species.

Interestingly, P450s with highly similar amino acid sequences can often exhibit pronounced differences in substrate specificity and catalytic properties. For instance, genetic polymorphisms affecting 2C5 and 2C3 greatly affect the capacity of rabbit liver microsomes to catalyse the 21-hydroxylation[8] and 6β-hydroxylation[9] of progesterone respectively, suggesting that other class 2C enzymes do not participate significantly in these reactions. On the other hand, P450s with very different sequences can catalyse the same reaction, as is indicated in Table 1.

Table 3 P450s recognized by autoantibodies associated with autoimmune hepatitis

P450s	*Aetiology*	*Reference*
CYP2C?	Tienilic acid-induced	17
CYP1A2	Idiopathic	68
	Dihydralazine-induced	18
CYP2D6	Idiopathic	14–16

The multiplicity of P450s is likely to reflect a process of gene duplication and divergence that generally expands the catalytic capacity of the P450 system to metabolize a wide range of structurally distinct substrates[10]. These include chemicals that may have been created by humans in recent time. The divergence of duplicated genes can also lead to the production of pseudo-genes. This has occurred for the CYP2D locus in humans. Most individuals contain a single functional CYP2D gene locus, 2D6, and two tandemly arranged pseudo-genes, 2D7P and 2D8P[11]. In addition, defective alleles of 2D6 occur with a high frequency leading to roughly 10% of Caucasians being deficient in this enzyme. This results in an impaired clearance of a wide variety of drugs including antihypertensives such as debrisoquine, β-blockers such as propranolol, and tricyclic antidepressants such as nortrip-tyline, among others[12]. In some cases this can lead to unexpected toxic side-effects. CYP2D6 also catalyses the conversion of codeine to morphine which is impaired in deficient individuals[13]. CYP2D6 is one of the P450 enzymes that is recognized by autoantibodies associated with autoimmune chronic active hepatitis[14–16].

GENERATION OF REACTIVE PRODUCTS

Of the three hepatic P450s that are recognized by autoantibodies associated with autoimmune chronic active hepatitis (Table 3), two are associated with exposure to specific drugs, tienillic acid[17] and dihydrazaline[18] respectively, that are substrates for the enzymes recognized by the autoantibodies. This suggests that a mechanistic relationship might exist between the autoimmune hepatitis, the drug and its metabolism by the P450. P450s have the capacity to generate electrophilic products that can covalently modify cellular macromolecules. This process underlies the carcinogenicity of many chemicals which are otherwise rather inert[19,20]. These reactive metabolites can also modify proteins, as described in other contributions to this volume, and their production can lead to cytotoxicity[21].

The cytochrome P450 monooxygenases can catalyse both the initial steps in either carcinogen activation or detoxification[22–24]. For instance, 2-acetylaminofluorene is metabolized by a number of rabbit P450s to ring-hydroxylated products[25]. These products are readily excreted and are not thought to be carcinogenic. On the other hand, CYP1A2 catalyses the *N*-hydroxylation of 2-acetylaminofluorene[25] which can be subsequently sulphated. Alternatively, the *N*-acetyl group may migrate to form the *N*-acetoxy compound. The hydroxyl, sulphate and acetoxy moieties are good

Table 4 Mechanisms of P450 induction

Gene	*Inducer*	*Mechanism*
CYP1A	TCDD, PAH	Gene transcription
CYP2B	Phenobarbital	Gene transcription
CYP3A	Rifampicin, dexamethasone	Gene transcription
CYP4A	Clofibrate, peroxisome proliferators	Gene transcription
CYP2E	Drug-induced diabetes	mRNA stabilization
CYP3A	Erythromycin and TAO	Protein stabilization
CYP2E	EtOH	Protein stabilization

leaving groups which are subject to nucleophilic displacement by cellular nucleophiles. This can include nucleic acids, and the resulting modification of cellular DNA is thought to lead to mutations that in turn lead to neoplastic growth.

The relative balance between the detoxication pathways catalysed by some P450s versus the activation pathway catalysed by other P450 enzymes is likely to contribute to the relative risk of carcinogenesis. Gillette[26] has provided a mathematical model for carcinogen metabolism, indicating that for the period of time following the complete metabolism/elimination of the carcinogen, the concentration of the covalent adduct is dependent on the initial concentration of the carcinogen, the rate of turnover of the adduct, and a set of multiplicative factors relating the formation of the adduct to the fractional conversion of the carcinogen and intermediates from their precursors at each step of the pathway leading to adduct formation. This model may approximate conditions *in vivo* because tissue concentrations resulting from environmental exposure to chemical carcinogens are likely to be low, and enzymatic metabolism of these compounds may therefore proceed in a first-order manner. The implication of this model is that, under appropriate conditions, the effect of altering reaction pathways available to the carcinogen and intermediates can be modulated independently at each step of the activation pathway. This balance often differs between cell types, tissues and with age and diet, due to the highly differentiated expression of various members comprising the P450 system. Moreover, this balance can be altered through the induction of specific P450s as a result of exposure to drugs and environmental chemicals.

INDUCTION OF P450s BY ENVIRONMENTAL CHEMICALS

A variety of foreign chemicals can selectively increase the abundance of specific P450s. As indicated in Table 3, the principal mechanism of induction appears to occur by increasing gene transcription. This has been shown experimentally by nuclear run-on assays for the induction of P450 2B enzymes by phenobarbital[27,28], of P450 1A enzymes by 2,3,7,8-tetrachlorodibenzo-*p*-dioxin (TCDD or dioxin)[29,30], of P450 3A enzymes by dexamethasone[31,32] and rifampicin[32] as well as of P450 4A enzymes by clofibrate[33]. In contrast, the induction of P450 2E enzymes by ethanol or heterocyclic compounds such as pyrazole or imidazole appears to reflect a stabilization of the enzyme to turnover because the accumulation of protein is not preceded by an elevation of mRNA concentration[34,35]. P450 2E is also elevated in diabetic states, and in this case the abundance of mRNA is increased but there is no evidence for an increase in transcription[36]. The induction of P450 3A enzymes by the antibiotics erythromycin and troleandromycin also reflects a contribution from protein stabilization as the half-life of P450 3A is increased by these drugs[37]. It is important to note that the spectrum of inducing agents may differ between species. For instance, rifampicin is an antibiotic that induces P450 3A enzymes in humans[38,39] and in rabbits[40], but it does not induce P450 3A in rats[41].

The mechanisms by which the transcription of P450 genes is selectively activated by foreign chemicals remains a fundamental question. However, recent work has substantially increased our understanding of these mechanisms. The transcriptional activation of CYP1A enzymes by aromatic hydrocarbons and TCDD reflects the actions of a cytosolic receptor, the dioxin or aryl hydrocarbon (Ah) receptor[42] that was first detected as a high-affinity, low-capacity binding protein in mouse cytosol[43]. The binding affinity of this cytosolic protein was shown to be lower in 'non-responsive' strains of mice[43] which differed from 'responsive' strains in that the cytochrome P450 IA1 gene was not induced by polynuclear aromatic hydrocarbons (PAH)[44]. In responsive strains of mice, PAH compete with dioxin for binding to the receptor, but their affinity for the receptor for PAH prevents its activation. The affinity toward dioxin remains sufficiently high, however, for dioxin to induce P450 IA1 in the 'non-responsive' strains[45].

The induction of IA1 gene transcription by dioxin is mediated by multiple copies of an upstream regulatory element[46–48] that binds the ligand–dioxin receptor complex[49–51]. This mechanism of action is similar to that of the glucocorticoid receptor and other membranes of the steroid hormone receptor family of ligand-activated transcription factors[52,53]. However, the dioxin-receptor is a distinct protein oligomer composed of two non-identical subunits that bear a basic helix–loop–helix motif[54–57].

Until recently there has been little direct evidence to indicate that receptors for foreign chemicals mediate the induction of other P450s. We have shown, however, that a member of the steroid hormone receptor family, the peroxisome proliferator activated receptor (PPAR)[58] mediates the induction of the CYP4A6 by peroxisome proliferators[59]. CYP4A6 is induced by the peroxisome proliferator, clofibric acid, in rabbit liver and kidney[60]. Gene transfer experiments were employed as a means of evaluating the role of PPAR in the regulation of the CYP4A6 gene[59]. The induction of luciferase expression driven by the promoter and 5′ flanking sequences of the rabbit cytochrome CYP4A6 gene by clofibric acid is dependent on co-transfection with expression plasmid for the PPAR. Deletion analysis was used to localize a responsive element to a 34 bp segment located 677 bp upstream of the transcription start site.

Peroxisome proliferators, such as clofibric acid, cause the numbers of liver peroxisomes to increase in some species such as rats and mice, where they are also carcinogenic but do not appear to be genotoxic[61]. Peroxisome proliferators have also been shown to be promoters of carcinogenesis[62].

These effects may be mediated by the PPAR[63]. Moreover, many of the toxic effects of dioxin are thought to be mediated by the dioxin receptor[64]. These events can include long-term changes in protein expression in hepatocytes. Following the cessation of this insult, the liver must remodel these changes as it returns to normal. It is possible that these changes alter the normal proteolytic processing of P450s and potentially lead to the presentation of new peptide fragments to the immune system that could contribute to the initiation of autoimmune hepatitis.

Acknowledgements

The author wishes to acknowledge the support of NIH grants GM31001 and HD04445, and Keith Griffin, Mei-Hui Hsu, Toby Richards, and Colin Palmer for helpful suggestions during the preparation of this manuscript.

References

1. Omura T, Sato R. The carbon monoxide-binding pigment of liver microsomes. I. Evidence for its hemoprotein nature. J Biol Chem. 1964;239:2370–8.
2. Kalb VF, Loper JC. Proteins from eight eukaryotic cytochrome P-450 families share a segmented region of sequence similarity. Proc Natl Acad Sci USA. 1988;85:7221–5.
3. White RE, Coon MJ. Oxygen activation by cytochrome P-450. Annu Rev Biochem. 1980;49:315–56.
4. Nebert DW, Nelson DR, Coon MJ, Estabrook RW, Feyereisen R, Fujii-Kuriyama Y, Gonzalez FJ, Guengerich FP, Gunsalus IC, Johnson EF, Loper JC, Sato R, Waterman MR, Waxman DJ. The P450 superfamily: update on new sequences, gene mapping, and recommended nomenclature. NDA Cell Biol. 1991;10:1–14.
5. Winqvist O, Karlsson FA, Kämpe O. 21-Hydroxylase, a major autoantigen in idiopathic Addison's disease. Lancet. 1992;339:1559–62.
6. Krohn K, Uibo R, Aavik E, Peterson P, Savilahti K. Identification by molecular cloning of an autoantigen associated with Addison's disease as steroid 17α-hydroxylase. Lancet. 1992;339:770–3.
7. Alvares AP, Pratt WB. Pathways of drug metabolism. In: Pratt WB, Taylor P, editors. Principles of drug action: the basis of pharmacology. New York: Churchill Livingstone; 1990:365–422.
8. Johnson EF, Finlayson M, Hujsak CM, Pendurthi UR, Tukey RH. Genetic contributions to the variation among rabbits of liver microsomal deoxycorticosterone synthesis. Arch Biochem Biophys. 1989;273:273–80.
9. Dieter HH, Johnson EF. Functional and structural polymorphism of rabbit microsomal cytochrome P-450 form 3b. J Biol Chem. 1982;257:9315–23.
10. Nebert DW, Gonzalez FJ. P450 genes: structure, evolution, and regulation. Annu Rev Biochem. 1987;56:945–93.
11. Heim MH, Meyer UA. Evolution of a highly polymorphic human cytochrome P450 gene cluster. *CYP2D6*. Genomics. 1992;14:49–58.
12. Caporaso NE, Shaw GL. Clinical implications of the competitive inhibition of the debrisoquin-metabolizing isozyme by quinidine. Arch Intern Med. 1991;151:1985–92.
13. Dayer P, Desmeules J, Leemann T, Striberni R. Bioactivation of the narcotic drug codeine in human liver is mediated by the polymorphic monooxygenase catalyzing debrisoquine 4-hydroxylation. Biochem Biophys Res Commun. 1988;152:411–16.
14. Zanger UM, Hauri H-P, Loeper J, Homberg J-C, Meyer UA. Antibodies against human cytochrome P-450db1 in autoimmune hepatitis type II. Proc Natl Acad Sci USA. 1988;85:8256–60.

15. Manns MP, Johnson EF, Griffin KJ, Tan EM, Sullivan KF. Major antigen of liver kidney microsomal autoantibodies in idiopathic autoimmune hepatitis is cytochrome P450db1. J Clin Invest. 1989;83:1066–72.
16. Gueguen M, Yamamoto AM, Bernard O, Alvarez F. Anti-liver kidney microsome antibody type 1 recognizes human cytochrome P450 db1. Biochem Biophys Res Commun. 1989;159:542–7.
17. Beaune P, Dansette PM, Mansuy D, Kiffel L, Finck M, Amar C, Leroux JP, Homberg JC. Human anti-endoplasmic reticulum autoantibodies appearing in a drug-induced hepatitis are directed against a human liver cytochrome P-450 that hydroxylates the drug. Proc Natl Acad Sci USA. 1987;84:551–5.
18. Bourdi M, Gautier J-C, Mircheva J, Larrey D, Guillouzo A, Andre C, Belloc C, Beaune PH. Anti-liver microsomes autoantibodies and dihydralazine-induced hepatitis: Specificity of autoantibodies and inductive capacity of the drug. Mol Pharmacol. 1992;42:280–5.
19. Miller EC. Some current perspectives on chemical carcinogenesis in humans and experimental animals: presidential address. Cancer Rs. 1978;38:1479–96.
20. Heidelberger C. Chemical carcinogenesis. Annu Rev Biochem. 1975;44:79–121.
21. Boobis AR, Fawthrop DJ, Davies DS. Mechanisms of cell death. TIPS. 1989;10:275–280.
22. Wattenberg LW. Inhibitors of chemical carcinogenesis. Adv Cancer Res. 1978;26:197–226.
23. Conney AH. Induction of microsomal enzymes by foreign chemicals and carcinogenesis by polycyclic aromatic hydrocarbons: G.H.A. Clowes Memorial Lecture. Cancer Res. 1982;42:4875–917.
24. Guengerich FP. Metabolic activation of carcinogens. Pharmacol Ther. 1992;54:17–61.
25. McManus ME, Minchin RF, Sanderson N, Schwartz D, Johnson EF, Thorgeirsson SS. Metabolic processing of 2-acetylaminofluorene by microsomes and six highly purified cytochrome P-450 forms from rabbit liver. Carcinogenesis. 1984;5:1717–23.
26. Gillette JR. Activation systems – characteristics and drawbacks – comparisons of different organs, tissues, problems with toxication-detoxication balance in various tissues, extrapolation from *in vitro* to *in vivo*. Pharmacokinetics, absorption, distribution, excretion, metabolism. In: deSerres FJ, Fouts JR, Bend JR, Philphot RM, editors. In vitro metabolic activation in mutagenesis testing. Amsterdam: Elsevier/North-Holland; 1976:13–54.
27. Hardwick JP, Gonzalez FJ, Kasper CB. Transcriptional regulation of rat liver epoxide hydratase, NADPH-cytochrome P-450 oxidoreductase, and cytochrome P-450b genes by phenobarbital. J Biol Chem. 1983;258:8081–5.
28. Pike SF, Shephard EA, Rabin BR, Phillips IR. Induction of cytochrome P-450 by phenobarbital is mediated at the level of transcription. Biochem Pharmacol. 1985;34: 2489–94.
29. Israel DI, Whitlock Jr. JP. Regulation cytochrome P1-450 gene transcription by 2,3,7,8-tetrachlorodibenzo-*p*-dioxin in wild type and variant mouse hepatoma cells. J Biol Chem. 1984;259:5400–2.
30. Gonzalez FJ, Tukey RH, Nebert DW. Structural gene products of the Ah locus. Transcriptional regulation of cytochrome P1-450 and P3-450 mRNA levels by 3-methylcholanthrene. Mol Pharmacol. 1984;26:117–21.
31. Simmons DL, McQuiddy P, Kasper CB. Induction of the hepatic mixed-function oxidase system by synthetic glucocorticoids. J Biol Chem. 1987;262:326–32.
32. Potenza CL, Pendurthi UR, Strom DK, Tukey RH, Griffin KJ, Schwab GE, Johnson EF. Regulation of the rabbit cytochrome P-450 3c gene: age dependent expression and transcriptional activation by rifampicin. J Biol Chem. 1989;264:16222–8.
33. Hardwick JP, Song B-J, Huberman E, Gonzalez FJ. Isolation, complementary DNA sequence, and regulation of rat hepatic lauric acid ω-hydroxylase (cytochrome P-450LAω). J Biol Chem. 1987;262:801–10.
34. Song B-J, Gelboin HV, Park S-S, Yang CS, Gonzalez FJ. Complementary DNA and protein sequences of ethanol-inducible rat and human cytochrome P-450s. J Biol Chem. 1986;261:16689–97.
35. Porter TD, Khani SC, Coon MJ. Induction and tissue-specific expression of rabbit cytochrome P450IIE1 and IIE2 genes. Mol Pharmacol. 1989;36:61–5.
36. Song BJ, Matsunaga T, Hardwick JP, Park SS, Veech RL, Yang CS, Gelboin HV, Gonzalez FJ. Stabilization of cytochrome P450j messenger ribonucleic acid in the diabetic rat. Mol Endocrinol. 1987;1:542–7.

37. Watkins PB, Wrighton SA, Schuetz EG, Maurel P, Guzelian PS. Macrolide antibiotics inhibit the degradation of the glucocorticoid-responsive cytochrome P-450p in rat hepatocytes in vivo and in primary monolayer culture. J Biol Chem. 1986;261:6264–71.
38. Combalbert J, Fabre I, Fabre G, Dalet I, Derancourt J, Cano JP, Maurel P. Metabolism of cyclosporin A. IV. Purification and identification of the rifampicin-inducible human liver cytochrome P-450 (cyclosporin A oxidase) as a product of P450IIIA gene subfamily. Drug Metab Dispos. 1989;17:197–207.
39. Ged C, Rouillon JM, Pichard L, Combalbert J, Bressot N, Bories P, Michel H, Beaune P, Maurel P. The increase in urinary excretion of 6β-hydroxycortisol as a marker of human hepatic cytochrome P450IIIA induction. Br J Clin Pharmacol. 1989;28:373–87.
40. Lange R, Larroque C, Balny C, Maurel P. Isolation and partial characterization of a rifampicin induced rabbit liver microsomal cytochrome P-450. Biochem Biophys Res Commun. 1985;126:833–9.
41. Wrighton SA, Schuetz EG, Watkins PB, Maurel P, Barwick J, Bailey BS, Hartle HT, Young B, Guzelian P. Demonstration in multiple species of inducible hepatic cytochromes P-450 and their mRNAs related to the glucocorticoid-inducible cytochrome P-450 of the rat. Mol Pharmacol. 1985;28:312–21.
42. Whitlock JP, Jr. Genetic and molecular aspects of 2,3,7,8-tetrachlorodibenzo-p-dioxin action. Annu Rev Pharmacol Toxicol. 1990;30:251–77.
43. Poland A, Glover E, Kende AS. Stereospecific, high affinity binding of 2,3,7,8-tetrachlorodibenzo-p-dioxin by hepatic cytosol. Evidence that the binding species is a receptor for induction of aryl hydrocarbon hydroxylase. J Biol Chem. 1976;251:4936–46.
44. Thomas PE, Kouri RE, Hutton JJ. The genetics of aryl hydrocarbon hydroxylase induction in mice: a single gene difference between C57BL/6J and DBA/2J. Biochem Genet. 1972;6: 157–68.
45. Poland AP, Glover E, Robinson JR, Nebert DW. Genetic expression of aryl hydrocarbon hydroxylase activity. Induction of monooxygenase activities and cytochrome P_1-450 formation by 2,3,7,8-tetrachlorodibenzo-p-dioxin in mice genetically ‘nonresponsive’ to other aromatic hydrocarbons. J Biol Chem. 1974;249:5599–606.
46. Fujisawa-Sehara A, Sogawa K, Yamane M, Fujii-Kuriyama Y. Characterization of xenobiotic responsive elements upstream from the drug-metabolizing cytochrome P-450c gene: a similarity to glucocorticoid regulatory elements. Nucl Acids Res. 1987;15:4179–91.
47. Jones PBC, Durrin LK, Fisher JM, Whitlock Jr. JP. Control of gene expression by 2,3,7,8-tetrachlorodibenzo-p-dioxin: Multiple dioxin-responsive domains 5′-ward of the cytochrome P_1-450 gene. J Biol Chem. 1986;261:6647–50.
48. Denison MS, Fisher JM, Whitlock JP. Inducible, receptor-dependent protein-DNA interactions at a dioxin-responsive transcriptional enhancer. Proc Natl Acad Sci USA. 1988;85:2528–32.
49. Fujisawa-Sehara A, Yamane M, Fujii-Kuriyama Y. A DNA-binding factor specific for xenobiotic responsive elements of P-450c gene exists as a cryptic form in cytoplasm: Its possible translocation to nucleus. Proc Natl Acad Sci. USA. 1988;85:5859–63.
50. Denison MS, Fisher JM, Whitlock JP Jr. Protein-DNA interactions at recognition sites for the dioxin-Ah receptor complex. J Biol Chem. 1989;264:16478–82.
51. Hapgood J, Cuthill S, Denis M, Poellinger L, Gustafsson J-Å. Specific protein-DNA interactions at a xenobiotic-responsive element: copurification of dioxin receptor and DNA-binding activity. Proc Natl Acad Sci USA. 1989;86:60–4.
52. O'Malley B. The steroid receptor superfamily: more excitement predicted for the future. Mol Endocrinol. 1990;4:363–9.
53. Evans RM. The steroid and thyroid hormone receptor superfamily. Science. 1988;240: 889–95.
54. Hoffman EC, Reyes H, Chu F-F, Sander F, Conley LH, Brooks BA, Hankinson O. Cloning of a factor required for activity of the Ah (dioxin) receptor. Science. 1991;252:954–8.
55. Reyes H, Reisz-Porszasz S, Hankinson O. Identification of the Ah receptor nuclear translocator protein (Arnt) as a component of the DNA binding form of the Ah receptor. Science. 1992;256:1193–5.
56. Ema M, Sogawa K, Watanabe N, Chujoh Y, Matsushita N, Gotoh O, Funae Y, Fujii-Kuriyama Y. cDNA cloning and structure of mouse putative Ah receptor. Biochem Biophys Res Commun. 1992;184:246–53.

57. Burbach KM, Poland A, Bradfield CA. Cloning of the Ah-receptor cDNA reveals a distinctive ligand-activated transcription factor. Proc Natl Acad Sci USA. 1992;89:8185–9.
58. Issemann I, Green S. Activation of a member of the steroid hormone receptor superfamily by peroxisome proliferators. Nature. 1990;347:645–50.
59. Muerhoff AS, Griffin KJ, Johnson EF. The peroxisome proliferator activated receptor mediates the induction of CYP4A6, a cytochrome P450 fatty acid omega-hydroxylase, by clofibric acid. J Biol Chem. 1992;267:19051–3.
60. Yokotani N, Bernhardt R, Sogawa K, Kusunose E, Gotoh O, Kusunose M, Fujii-Kuriyama Y. Two forms of ω-hydroxylase toward prostaglandin A and laurate. J Biol Chem. 1989;264:21665–9.
61. Rao MS, Reddy JK. Peroxisome proliferation and hepatocarcinogenesis. Carcinogenesis. 1987;8:631–6.
62. Kraupp-Grasl B, Huber W, Putz B, Gerbracht U, Schulte-Hermann R. Tumor promotion by the peroxisome proliferator nafenopin involving a specific subtype of altered foci in rat liver. Cancer Res. 1990;50:3701–8.
63. Green S. Peroxisome proliferators: a model for receptor mediated carcinogenesis. Cancer Surv. 1992;14:221–32.
64. Poland A, Knutson JC. 2,3,7,8-Tetrachlorodibenzo-*p*-dioxin and related halogenated aromatic hydrocarbons: examination of the mechanism of toxicity. Annu Rev Pharmacol Toxicol. 1982;22:517–54.
65. Dieter HH, Muller-Eberhard U, Johnson EF. Identification of rabbit microsomal cytochrome P-450 isozyme, form 1, as a hepatic progesterone 21-hydroxylase. Biochem Biophys Res Commun. 1982;105:515–20.
66. Trant JM, Lorence MC, Johnson EF, Shackleton CHL, Mason JI, Estabrook RW. Characterization of the steroid-metabolizing capacity of the hepatic cytochrome P450IIC5 expressed in COS-1 cells: 3β-Hydroxysteroid dehydrogenase/$\Delta^{5\to4}$ isomerase type activity. Proc Natl Acad Sci USA. 1990;87:9756–60.
67. Raucy JL, Johnson EF. Variations among untreated rabbits in benzo(a)pyrene metabolism and its modulation by 7,8-benzoflavone. Mol Pharmacol. 1985;27:296–301.
68. Manns MP, Griffin KJ, Quattrochi LC, Sacher M, Thaler H, Tukey RH, Johnson EF. Identification of cytochrome P450IA2 as a human autoantigen. Arch Biochem Biophys. 1990;280:229–32.

30 Cytochrome P450 IID6 in autoimmune hepatitis

M. P. MANNS

INTRODUCTION

Cytochrome P450 IID6 was the second cytochrome P450 isozyme that became identified as a hepatocellular autoantigen. It is highly polymorphic. A genetic polymorphism is responsible for the fact that 5–10% of Caucasians are poor metabolizers due to mutant genes[1]. Cytochrome P450 IID6 protein is not expressed in the livers of these individuals. This chapter gives an overview on the present knowledge of cytochrome P450 IID6 as human autoantigen. A historical retrospective describes the development of the molecular identification of cytochrome P450 IID6 as autoantigen. The effect of autoantibodies on cytochrome P450 IID6 function *in vitro* and on enzyme function *in vivo* will be elaborated. Furthermore it will be discussed whether sufficient evidence has been published concerning the membrane expression of this antigen on normal human hepatocytes. The question arises whether T lymphocytes infiltrating the liver specifically react with cytochrome P450 IID6 or parts of it. Furthermore data have been published that show the regulation of P450 IID6 gene expression by cytokines. Several of them are secreted locally. Autoimmune hepatitis associated with autoimmunity to cytochrome P450 IID6 is a rare disease[2]. A specific genetic background seems to be a prerequisite for the manifestation of this disease[3,4]; therefore the evaluation of the genetic background at the MHC locus and at the autoantigen locus itself is quite important. The aetiology of autoimmune hepatitis is unknown. However, viruses are always discussed as triggers of autoimmune diseases. In this context recent data are of particular interest that demonstrate a molecular mimicry between a herpes simplex virus protein and cytochrome P450 IID6. In addition markers of hepatitis C virus (HCV) infection are observed in a proportion of these patients. Therefore autoimmune hepatitis associated with autoimmunity to cytochrome P450 IID6 may become a model to study virus-induced autoimmunity in humans.

IDENTIFICATION OF CYTOCHROME P450 IID6 AS TARGET ANTIGEN OF LKM-1 AUTOANTIBODIES

LKM-1 autoantibodies were described first[5,6] due to their immunofluorescence pattern on rodent liver and kidney sections. The characteristic feature was the exclusive staining of the P3 portion of the proximal renal tubuli. In contrast mitochondrial antibodies in primary biliary cirrhosis react on kidney tissue with proximal, and even stronger with distal renal tubuli. Western blot experiments demonstrated the reaction of LKM-1 autoantibodies with a 50 kDa microsomal protein[7,8]. Some sera recognize antigens at 55 and 64 kDa[9,10]. Two independent approaches led to the identification of cytochrome P450 IID6 as the major antigen of LKM-1 autoantibodies. The laboratory of Urs Meyer has shown that LKM-1 autoantibodies specifically inhibit the function of cytochrome P450 IID6 in isolated human liver cytochromes *in vitro*[11]. Furthermore they showed that LKM-1 antibody-positive serum, as evidenced by immunofluorescence, immunoprecipitates cytochrome P450 IID6[11]. On the other hand, screening of human liver cDNA libraries with human serum containing LKM-1 autoantibodies revealed that the major antigen at 50 kDa is human cytochrome P450 IID6[9,12], which is immunologically distinct from the other 55 and 64 kDa microsomal autoantigens[9].

EFFECT OF LKM-1 AUTOANTIBODIES ON CYTOCHROME P450 IID6 FUNCTION *IN VITRO* AND *IN VIVO*

Zanger *et al.*[11] have shown that sera from patients with LKM-1 autoantibodies inhibit the hydroxylation of bufuralol in isolated human liver microsomes. Later this has also been shown for sparteine metabolism[13]. The capacity of cytochrome P450 IID6-mediated drug metabolism in isolated microsomes correlated with the amount of P450 IID6 protein in these microsomes as evidenced by Western blot analysis[11]. While bufuralol is an experimental β-blocker the antiarrhythmic drug sparteine can be used to measure the patient's phenotype for cytochrome P450 IID6-mediated drug metabolism. This means that for the first time the function of an autoantigen could be tested *in vivo*[13]. In this primary study the *in vivo* phenotype was evaluated in patients who had undergone a liver biopsy at the same time. The P450 IID6 content was measured semi-quantitatively by Western blotting. All patients in this first series were extensive metabolizers for drug metabolism mediated by P450 IID6. In the meantime this was confirmed by a larger series of more than 50 patients (own unpublished data). It can be concluded from these experiments that LKM-1 autoantibodies react with the active site of this P450 protein, and that the poor metabolizer phenotype does not select for the manifestation of autoimmune hepatitis type 2[14]. The poor metabolizer phenotype has a prevalence of 5–10% for Caucasians. These individuals carry two defective alleles which are responsible for a lack of P450 IID6 protein expression in their livers[1]. Finally it can be concluded that LKM-1 autoantibodies, despite their reaction with the active site of this enzyme, do not penetrate the intact liver cell membrane sufficiently to inhibit enzyme function *in vivo*.

MEMBRANE EXPRESSION OF CYTOCHROME P450 IID6

For many years the membrane expression of an autoantigen was postulated as a prerequisite for antigens of pathogenetic relevance. For a long time this was thought to be relevant for antigens as targets for humoral and cellular immune reactions. Loeper and co-workers[15,16] have presented data supporting a membrane expression of all three P450 enzymes that have been so far identified as autoantigens: P450 IIC9, P450 IID6 and P450 IA2. These authors used isolated rat and human hepatocytes as well as isolated plasma membrane fractions. Indirect immunofluorescence, Western blotting and immunoelectron microscopy with either patient serum or murine monoclonal antibodies were used as method. Several years ago Lenzi and co-workers[17] demonstrated a surface staining of isolated rabbit hepatocytes by LKM-1 antibody-positive serum. Others, including ourselves[18,19] had problems showing the expression of P450 IID6 epitopes on the surface of isolated hepatocytes using either fluorescence-activated cell sorting (FACS) analysis or indirect immunofluorescence on isolated rodent hepatocytes. It certainly needs to be evaluated whether and how these P450 enzymes are expressed on the hepatocyte surface during autoimmune liver disease. Possibly certain cytokines synthesized *in situ* may up-regulate the cellular and possible membrane expression of P450 IID6 protein, or parts of it. However, these key questions are difficult to approach experimentally.

CELLULAR IMMUNE RESPONSE TO CYTOCHROME P450 IID6

Since LKM-1 autoantibodies do not sufficiently penetrate through the intact liver cell membrane and inhibit enzyme function *in vivo*, and since the histological hallmark of this autoimmune liver disease is tissue-infiltrating T lymphocytes, it was logical to search for the antigen specificity of these liver-infiltrating T cells. Löhr and co-workers[20] have prepared 189 T lymphocyte clones from four different patients suffering from autoimmune hepatitis type 2 associated with LKM-1 antibodies. These T cell clones were isolated by limiting dilution and stimulated with recombinant IL-2 *in vitro*. Four of these 189 liver-derived T cell clones were shown to proliferate specifically in the presence of human recombinant cytochrome P450 IID6. These T lymphocytes expressed the CD4 helper cell phenotype and the stimulation was inhibited by addition of anti-MHC class II monoclonal antibodies. In order to really evaluate the significance of cellular immune reactions against P450 IID6 it will be necessary to develop an autologous cytotoxicity system possibly expressing the P450 IID6 gene in cultured autologous cells such as fibroblasts.

CYTOCHROME P450 IID6 GENE REGULATION

Little is known regarding how hepatocellular autoantigen gene expression is regulated. Cytochrome P450 enzymes are markers of highly differentiated cells. Therefore it is understandable that P450 expression is frequently absent in liver-derived tumour cells and in cultured hepatocytes. Special matrices may help to maintain the expression of P450 proteins in isolated cultured hepatocytes (Trautwein *et al.*, unpublished).

Furthermore it seems necessary to analyse whether cytokines synthesized systemically or locally up- or down-regulate P450 gene expression. We have chosen the acute-phase mediators IL-1, IL-6 and TNF-α[21]. We have found that the application of these recombinant cytokines in mice led to the suppression of P450 IID6 expression up to 75% after 6 h at the RNA level. Very recently this has been confirmed by a different approach[22]. These recombinant proteins were administered *in vivo* to mice and all three acute-phase mediators diminished the metabolic ratio, i.e. the mouse liver capacity of P450 IID6-dependent drug metabolism *in vivo*. In the meantime several members of the cytochrome P450 supergene family were shown to respond as negative acute-phase reactants[23]. Until now no cytokine has been identified that up-regulates the expression of cytochrome P450 proteins or any other autoantigen.

GENETICS IN AUTOIMMUNE HEPATITIS TYPE 2 ASSOCIATED WITH LKM-1 AUTOANTIBODIES

Limited data are available until now that give insight into the immunogenetic background of autoimmune liver disease associated with autoimmunity to P450 proteins. These studies are hampered by the rarity of these autoimmune liver diseases. The prevalence of LKM-1 autoantibody-associated autoimmune hepatitis type 2 is estimated to be around 20–30 per million population. Furthermore all HLA data available so far were obtained by serotyping. Homberg *et al.*[2] first presented some information. They reported an increased frequency of HLA DR3 in patients with autoimmune hepatitis type 2[2]; 75% of his patients were children. We also found an increased frequency of HLA DR3 alleles[3]. This finding, however, only became statistically significant for the hepatitis C virus (HCV)-negative population (see below). In contrast C4A-QO alleles are significantly increased in the whole group of patients with autoimmune hepatitis type 2 independent of HCV status[3]. Genes for complement factors C4, C2, and factor B (Bf) are localized on the short arm of chromosome 6 between HLA class I and class II genes. They are therefore called HLA class III molecules. An increased frequency of C4A-QO alleles has been reported in a number of different diseases believed to have an autoimmune background, or are regarded as a virus-induced immune-mediated disease. Among these diseases are systemic lupus erythematosus, rheumatoid arthritis, primary biliary cirrhosis and measle virus-induced subacute sclerosing panencephalitis (SSPE)[23]. Since C4 is involved in immune complex clearance and virus elimination this phenomenon may contribute to tissue destruction. The association of autoimmune hepatitis type 1 with complement factor C4 deficiency has been known for some time[24,25]. This C4 deficiency was recently identified to be due to a C4 gene deletion that is in linkage disequilibrium with the HLA haplotype A1-B8-DR3[26].

In Italy, where HCV prevalence is high, patients with LKM-1 antibody-positive autoimmune hepatitis type 2 show evidence of replicating HCV infection in up to 90%. In these Italian patients an increased incidence of HLA DR3 was also described[4]. However, the number of patients in all these series is low due to the limited number of patients in each centre. Immunogenetics in this autoimmune liver disease, and its relation to hepatotropic viral infection, will be clarified only if many patients from different parts of the world are analysed in a multicentre trial. In such a study MHC data should be obtained by DNA genotyping and the data should be analysed in relation to markers of infection with HCV or other viral infection (see below), age, disease activity and treatment response.

In this context we had the luck to analyse a family with identical twins at the age of 13[27]. Only one twin suffered from autoimmune hepatitis type 2, and in addition from ulcerative colitis. The other family members were healthy. Both children carried the autoimmune HLA haplotype: A1-B8-DR3-C4A-QO.

One further attractive approach is to study the genetic background at the autoantigen locus itself. We could take advantage of a PCR technology that can simply identify at the DNA level more than 80% of the defective alleles. More than 30 patients have been tested so far. Every patient carries at least one wild-type allele. Apart from two individuals all other patients carry, in addition, one defective allele. Thus the only allele that is associated with the disease seems to be the wild-type allele. These studies also extend our previous observation that poor metabolizers with no P450 protein expression in their livers do not develop this autoimmune liver disease[14]. No data are so far available on the genetics of the T cell receptor.

HEPATOTROPIC VIRUSES AND CYTOCHROME P450 IID6

Depending on the geographical origin of patients a different proportion of patients with autoimmune hepatitis type 2, i.e. patients with autoimmune liver disease and autoantibodies to cytochrome P450 IID6, have signs of HCV infection. More than 90% of the patients in Japan[28] and Italy[28], about 50% in France[29] and Germany[30] and less than 10% in England[28] are hepatitis C antibody (anti-HCV)-positive and the majority is also HCV RNA-positive. The involvement of HCV in immunopathogenesis is also supported by the observation that anti-GOR, an antibody to an HCV-associated nuclear antigen, is found only in autoimmune hepatitis type 2b, i.e. patients with HCV markers. Interestingly the two patient populations differ clinically[28,29].

The HCV-negative population of patients is young, female predominance is striking, inflammatory activity is high and response to immunosuppression is good. In contrast the HCV-positive patients rather resemble those with chronic hepatitis C. Age at onset is above 40 years, inflammatory activity is low, response to corticosteroids is not convincing and a majority of these patients does not require treatment since the disease is less severe.

Recently there has been a debate whether anti-LKM-1 antibodies in HCV-positive autoimmune hepatitis type 2 recognize the 50 kDa cytochrome P450 IID6 antigen[32]. An English group of investigators reported that the antigen is different from the 50 kDa antigen[31]. We reported that, apart from the 50 kDa P450 IID6 antigen, other proteins at 59 and 70 kDa are recognized in Western blot. They still need to be identified at their molecular level[33]. It seems that patients who react with the 50 and 70 kDa antigen have the best response to IFN-α treatment, if treated[33]. At present we evaluate whether specific HCV variants are associated with autoimmunity to microsomal proteins.

It is still unknown what triggers autoimmune hepatitis type 2a, i.e. the HCV-negative young females with high disease activity and good response to immunosuppression. One approach is to search for sequence homologies between cytochrome P450 IID6 and hepatotropic viruses. Therefore we identified the major B cell epitope on cytochrome P450 IID6[34]. This eight amino acid peptide has a high sequence homology with the immediate early protein of the herpes simplex virus type I. LKM-1 antibodies affinity-purified from a synthetic peptide with the sequence of this epitope react with the cellular cytochrome P450 and the viral protein. Indirect clinical evidence supports this hypothesis: we observed a family with identical female twins, 13 years old[27]. Only the child suffering from autoimmune hepatitis type 2, and in addition from ulcerative colitis, had signs of herpes simplex type I (HSV-1) infection. No other family member, including the healthy twin sister, had serological evidence of HSV or HCV infection. However, the twins both carried the autoimmune haplotype A1-B8-DR3-C4A-QO. Furthermore we observed a child with fulminant hepatic failure and LKM antibodies who was high titre positive for IgM herpes simplex virus antibodies[35]. Therefore herpes simplex virus could be a candidate to trigger this autoimmune liver disease.

References

1. Gonzales FJ, Skoda RC, Kimura S *et al.* Characterization of the common genetic defect in humans deficient in debrisoquine metabolism. Nature. 1988;331:442–6.
2. Homberg JC, Abuaf N, Bernard O *et al.* Chronic active hepatitis associated with anti-liver/kidney microsome antibody type I: a second type of 'autoimmune hepatitis'. Hepatology. 1987;7:1333–9.
3. Manns M, Jentzsch M, Mergener K *et al.* HLA class I–III in autoimmune hepatitis type 2 and its association with hepatitis C virus infection. J Hepatol. 1992;16(Suppl. 1):4.
4. Lenzi M, Mantovani W, Cataleta M *et al.* HLA typing in autoimmune hepatitis (AI-CAH) type 2. J Hepatol. 1992;15(Suppl 1):59 (abstract).
5. Rizzetto M, Swana D, Donaich D. Microsomal antibodies in active chronic hepatitis and other disorders. Clin Exp Immunol. 1973;15:331.
6. Storch W. Diagnostische Bedeutung von Antikörpern gegen Zellorganellen (Mitochondrien endoplasmatisches Retikulum und Ribosomen). Schweiz Med Wochenschr. 1983;113: 47–59.

7. Alvarez F, Bernard O, Homberg JC, Kreibich G. Anti-liver kidney microsome antibody recognizes a 550,000 molecular weight protein of the endoplasmatic reticulum. J Exp Med. 1985;161:1231–6.
8. Kyroatsoulis A, Manns M, Gerken G *et al.* Distinction between natural and pathological autoantibodies by immunoblotting and densitometric subtraction: liver–kidney–microsomal antibody (LKM) positive sera identify multiple antigens in human liver tissue. Clin Exp Immunol. 1987;70:53–60.
9. Manns M, Johnson EF, Griffin KJ *et al.* The major target antigen of liver and kidney microsomal autoantibodies in idiopathic autoimmune hepatitis in cytochrome P450 db1. J Clin Invest. 1989;83:1066–72.
10. Codonor-Franch P, Paradis K, Guegan M *et al.* A new antigen recognized by anti-liver–kidney–microsome antibody (LKMA). Clin Exp Immunol. 1989;75:354–8.
11. Zanger UM, Hauri HP, Loeper J *et al.* Antibodies against human cytochrome P450 db 1 in autoimmune hepatitis type III. Proc Natl Acad Sci USA. 1988;27:8256–60.
12. Guegen M, Meunioer-Rotival M, Bernard O, Alvarez F. Anti-liver kidney microsome antibody recognizes a cytochrome P450 from the second subfamily. J Exp Med. 1988;168:801–6.
13. Manns M, Zanger U, Gerken G *et al.* Patients with type II autoimmune hepatitis express functional intact cytochrome P450 db 1 that is inhibited by LKM-1 autoantibodies *in vitro* but not *in vivo*. Hepatology. 1990;12:127–32.
14. Manns M, Scheucher S, Jentzsch M *et al.* Genetics in autoimmune hepatitis type 2. Hepatology. 1991;14:60A.
15. Loeper J, Descatoire V, Maurice M *et al.* Presence of functional cytochrome P-450 on isolated rat hepatocyte plasma membrane. Hepatology. 1990;15:850–8.
16. Loeper J, Descatoire V, Maurice M *et al.* Cytochrome P450 in human hepatocyte plasma membrane: recognition by several autoantibodies. Gastroenterology. 1993;104:203–16.
17. Lenzi M, Bianchi FB, Cassani F, Pisi E. Liver cell surface expression of the antigen reacting with liver–kidney microsomal antibody (LKM). Clin Exp Immunol. 1984;55:36–40.
18. Trautwein C, Gerken G, Löhr H *et al.* Lack of surface expression for the B-cell autoepitope of cytochrome P450 IID6 evidenced by flow cytometry. Z Gastroenterol. 1993;31:in press.
19. Peakman M, Lobo Yeo A, Vergani G *et al.* Characterization of anti-liver–kidney microsomal antibody in childhood autoimmune chronic active hepatitis: evidence of IgG1 subclass restriction, polyclonality, and nonreactivity with hepatocyte surface antigen. Clin Exp Immunol. 1987;69:543–9.
20. Löhr H, Treichel U, Poralla T *et al.* The human hepatic asialoglycoprotein receptor is a target antigen for liver infiltrating T cells in autoimmune chronic active hepatitis and primary biliary cirrhosis. Hepatology. 1990;12:1314–20.
21. Trautwein C, Ramadori G, Gerken G *et al.* Regulation of cytochrome P450 IID6 by acute phase mediators in C3H/HeJ mice. Biochem Biophys Res Commun. 1992;182:617–23.
22. Orishiki M, Nishioka M, Tsuneoka Y *et al.* Human CYP2D6 gene in chronic liver disease. Falk Symposium no. 70, Immunologie und Leber, Basel, 18–20 October 1992; abstract no. 12.
23. Waterman MR, Johnson EF (editors) Methods in enzymology, 206: cytochrome P450. San Diego: Academic Press; 1991.
24. Manns MP, Bremm A, Schneider PM *et al.* HLA DRw8 and complement C4 deficiency as risk factors in primary biliary cirrhosis. Gastroenterology. 1991;101:1367–73.
25. Vergani D, Wells L, Larcher VF *et al.* Genetically determined low C4: a predisposing factor to autoimmune chronic active hepatitis. Lancet. 1985;2:294–8.
26. Toze C, Scilly LJ, Goldstein R. C4R gene deletion is associated with early onset autoimmune chronic active hepatitis. Hepatology. 1990;12:907 (abstract).
27. Manns M, Koletzko S, Löhr H *et al.* Discordant manifestation of LKM-1 antibody positive autoimmune hepatitis in identical twins: *in vivo* inhibition of the target antigen cytochrome P450 db1 and *in vivo* phenotype. In press.
28. Lenzi M, Johnson PJ, McFarlane IG *et al.* Antibodies to hepatitis C virus in autoimmune liver disease: evidence for geographical heterogeneity. Lancet. 1991;338:277–80.
29. Lunel F, Abuaf N, Franguel L *et al.* Liver/kidney microsome antibody type 1 and hepatitis C virus infection. Hepatology. 1992;16:630–6.
30. Michel G, Ritter A, Gerken G *et al.* Anti-GOR and hepatitis C virus in autoimmune liver disease. Lancet. 1992;339:267–9.

31. Lenzi M, Ballardini G, Fusconi M *et al.* Type 2 autoimmune hepatitis and hepatitis C virus infection. Lancet. 1990;1:258–9.
32. Ma Y, Lenzi M, Gäken J *et al.* The target antigen of liver kidney microsomal antibody is different in type II autoimmune chronic active hepatitis and chronic hepatitis C virus infection. J Hepatol. 1992;16(Suppl 1):S4 (abstract).
33. Durazzo M, Philipp Th, Lüttig B *et al.* Heterogeneity of microsomal autoantibodies (LKM) in chronic hepatitis V virus (HCV) infection. Falk Symposium no. 70, Immunologie und Leber, Basel, 18–20 October 1992; abstract no. 12.
34. Manns MP, Griffin KJ, Sullivan KF *et al.* LKM-1 autoantibodies recognize a short linear sequence in P450 IID6. J Clin Invest. 1991;88:1370–8.
35. Tillmann H, Michitaka K, Rodeck B *et al.* Fulminant hepatic failure in autoimmune hepatitis type 2 with markers of acute herpes simplex virus infection. Falk Symposium no. 70, Immunologie und Leber, Basel, 18–20 October 1992; abstract no. 175.

31
Mechanisms of adverse drug reactions directed against cytochromes P450

P. BEAUNE, M. BOURDI, S. LECOEUR, P. LOPEZ-GARCIA, P. DANSETTE, D. MANSUY, C. BELLOC, J.-C. GAUTIER, D. LARREY, D. PESSAYRE, R. CATINOT and F. BALLET

Because of its central role in xenobiotic metabolism, the liver is an important target for adverse drug reactions. Two main mechanisms of hepatotoxicity have been described; they are described in Fig. 1.

The drug or a reactive metabolite can either be detoxicated and excreted or lead to adverse cellular effects. In the latter case the toxicity may be

1. Direct: the drug or reactive metabolite interacts directly with cellular vital targets and triggers cell death or modifications leading to cancer, for instance.
2. Indirect: the reactive metabolite (or drug) binds to cellular protein(s) leading to a neonantigen which triggers an immune response.

These different pathways are controlled and variable. Depending upon the

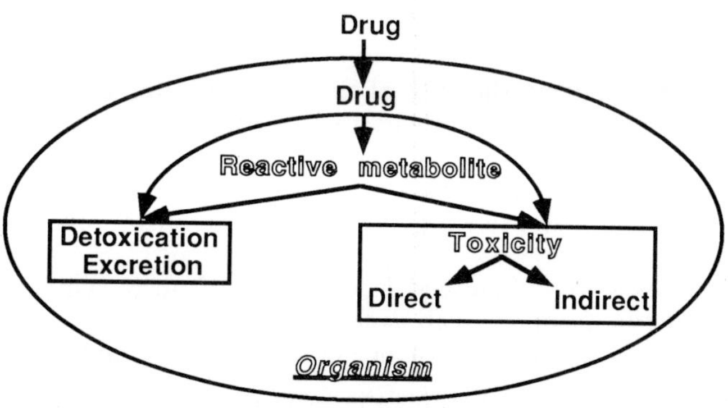

Fig. 1 Pathways of drug-induced diseases

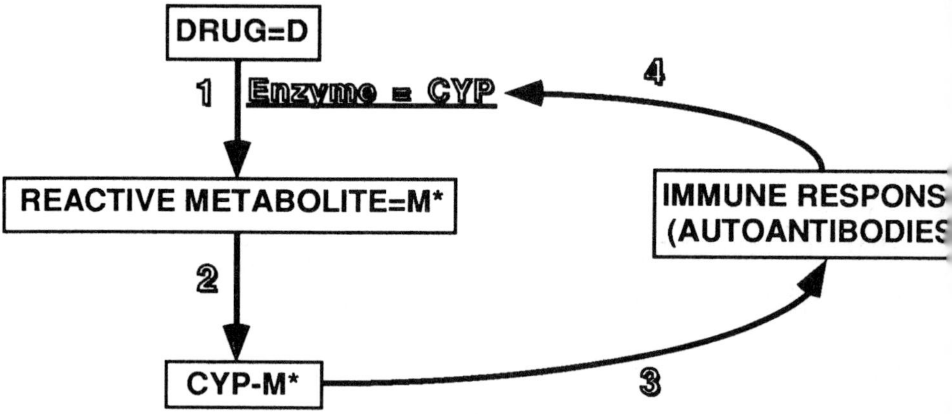

Fig. 2 Hypothetical steps leading to immunoallergic drug-induced diseases

nature and the activity of these pathways a drug can be either detoxicated or lead to an adverse effect.

In this chapter we will concentrate on the indirect type of toxicity, essentially immunoallergy. This kind of toxicity is also very dependent on genetic factors, and varies among individuals. It is therefore very difficult to predict. A better knowledge of the mechanisms underlying these kinds of adverse reactions should help in their prediction and early detection.

Drug-induced immunoallergic hepatitis has been reported. Halothane, tienilic acid, dihydralazine or iproniazide are examples of such diseases[1–6]. Their main characteristics were as follows:

1. Among all treated persons only a very small number developed the disease.
2. The disease appeared several days, weeks, or even months after the beginning of treatment.
3. In the case of rechallenge, the disease was generally more severe and appeared immediately.
4. These adverse drug reactions were apparently not dose-dependent.
5. Autoantibodies were found in the serum of the patients. These antibodies are the hallmark of the disease. Anti-LKM2 (liver kidney microsomes type 2) were found in the case of tienilic acid-induced hepatitis[5], anti-LM in dihydralazine-induced hepatitis[6,7], anti-M6 in iproniazide-induced hepatitis[3,4]. In the case of halothane anti-microsomes autoantibodies were also detected. Autoantibodies (anti-LKM1) were also found in chronic active hepatitis in which no drug or toxic effect could be identified as triggering cause[8].
6. These diseases are often accompanied by clinical symptoms of an immunoallergic response such as fever or eosinophilia.
7. Corticotherapy was generally efficient against the symptoms.

The hypotheses that have been initially proposed to explain the triggering of these diseases are presented in Fig. 2.

Step 1: the drug is metabolized into a reactive metabolite by an enzyme, here cytochrome P450 (CYP).

Step 2: the reactive metabolite then binds to proteins, and particularly to CYP which generated it, to form a neoantigen.

Step 3: the neoantigen triggers an immune response, including the production of autoantibodies.

Step 4: the immune response leads to liver inflammation and necrosis. It has been shown that the autoantibodies were directed against the neoantigen but also against the native protein. However, it must be emphasized that the physiopathological role of autoantibodies in the development of the immune response, as well as in liver injury, is still unknown.

In this chapter we will briefly summarize the data supporting these different steps, taking as examples two drugs inducing such immunoallergic hepatitis: tienilic acid and dihydralazine.

MATERIALS AND METHODS

Patient sera

Sera containing anti-LM (dihydralazine) or anti-LKM2 came from Hôpital Beaujon, or were the generous gift of Dr J.-C. Homberg and Dr C. André. Control sera were from patients taking the drug without any sign of disease, or from patients suffering from other hepatic diseases such as viral hepatitis B or C.

Human liver

This came from donors for kidney transplantation. Livers were removed shortly after circulatory arrest in compliance with French regulations. They were stored at $-80°C$. Microsomes were prepared as previously described[9].

Covalent binding

This was performed as previously described on fibreglass filters[10]. The specificity of the covalent binding was assessed as follows: after incubation with NADPH and radiolabelled substrates ([^{14}C]tienilic acid or dihydralazine), microsomes were submitted to SDS-PAGE and then electrotransferred to nitrocellulose (NC). The NC was then cut into small stripes perpendicular to the direction of migration, then each stripe was counted in a scintillation counter. This method allows identification of the protein(s) on which the reactive metabolite(s) was bound.

Heterologous expression

Human cytochromes P450 were expressed either in yeast or in bacteria[11–13].

Immunoblots

Immunoblots were performed as previously described. Human sera or rabbit antisera were used as probe[13,14] at 1/100 to 1/500.

RESULTS AND DISCUSSION

Steps 1 and 2

These two steps have to be studied together since the reactive metabolite was usually detected through its capacity to covalently bind to microsomal proteins. Both tienilic acid and dihydralazine were able to covalently bind on rat and human liver microsomes[10] (Bourdi *et al.*, manuscript in preparation). The covalent binding was much higher with tienilic acid than with dihydralazine (40–50 and 5–10 pmol min^{-1} $nmol^{-1}$ P450 respectively at 10 μmol/l substrate concentration). This indicates that both compounds might be activated to reactive metabolites by liver microsomes. The covalent binding of tienilic acid was inhibited by anti-LKM2 and anti-P450 2C[14], indicating that the formation of the reactive metabolite was dependent on P450 2C. This result was confirmed by the use of recombinant yeasts. Indeed, upon incubations of tienilic acid with NADPH and microsomes from yeast expressing pure cloned P450 2C9 and 2C10, covalent binding was observed, while very low covalent binding was detected with yeast expressing P450 3A4, 1A1 or 1A2 (Lopez-Garcia *et al.*, manuscript in preparation). Covalent binding with dihydralazine was increased by using liver microsomes from β-naphthoflavone-treated rats, and inhibited by antibodies directed against rat and human liver P450 1A (Bourdi *et al.*, manuscript in preparation). This result showed that P450 1A were responsible for the production of the dihydralazine-derived reactive metabolite. It was not possible to confirm this result with recombinant yeasts because of a very high background. The reactive metabolite of the tienilic acid isomer was identified as the sulphoxide on the thiophene ring[15]. It was not yet possible to identify the reactive metabolite of dihydralazine because this product is quite unstable under aerobic conditions.

Finally, by immunoblots, it was shown that the covalent binding was very specific for both products. Tienilic acid was bound on a protein comigrating with P450 2C and dihydralazine with P450 1A (Bourdi *et al.* and Lecoeur *et al.*, manuscripts in preparation).

In summary, for these steps tienilic acid and dihydralazine are metabolized to reactive metabolites by P450 2C and 1A, respectively. These reactive metabolites were specifically bound to the proteins which generated them, P450 2C and 1A, respectively.

Step 3

Very little is known on this step. It involves the presentation of the neoantigen to the immune cells. For halothane it has been shown that the neoantigen (protein-reactive metabolite, trifluoroacetic acid) was processed in Kupffer cells[16]. Moreover, when a liver biopsy is performed, liver inflammation and T lymphocyte infiltration is a common finding. Knowledge of this step, as well as step 4, could be greatly enhanced by the development of an animal model. However, the development of an animal model of drug-induced autoimmune hepatitis has not been reported so far.

Step 4

Autoantibodies have been found in the sera of all patients with tienilic acid- or dihydralazine-induced hepatitis. Their specificity was tested in both cases. Anti-LKM2 were directed specifically against P450 2C[14,17]. This was shown by immunoblots: anti-LKM2 recognized human liver microsomes as single band which comigrated with pure P450 2C; moreover they recognized pure P450 2C, either purified from human liver or expressed in yeast (Challine *et al.*, unpublished data). None of the other P450s tested were recognized. These autoantibodies were also able to inhibit P450 2C-dependent monooxygenase activities and tienilic acid metabolism[14]. These autoantibodies were also very specific since they were present only in patients and in none of the controls[14]. Anti-LM were directed specifically against P450 1A2[13]. In immunoblots they recognized human liver microsomes as a single band, comigrating with P450 1A; anti-LM recognized purified and yeast expressed human P450 1A2. It was also interesting to observe that these anti-LM were very specific for P450 1A2 since they did not recognize human P450 1A1, more than 80% similar to human P450 1A2 expressed in yeast and bacteria[13]. These autoantibodies were also specific for the disease since they were found in all tested patients and in none of the controls[7].

Finally it is interesting to observe that these autoantibodies recognized the native protein which did not need to be modified by the hapten to be recognized by the autoantibodies. Indeed the microsomes used in the above-described experiments came from patients who did not take dihydralazine or tienilic acid[7,14]. In the case of halothane-induced hepatitis the autoantibodies recognized only the microsomes from halothane-treated animals[2].

In summary, the autoantibodies found in these two diseases recognized very specifically one P450, probably the one responsible for the generation of the reactive metabolite. We have no indication that these antibodies play any role in the disease; they are present in all patients, but not in controls. The evolution of the titre is parallel to the disease: antibodies disappear after recovery. However, they could be only a marker of the disease without any physiopathological role.

CONCLUSION

Steps 1, 2, 4 of the simple initial scheme shown in Fig. 2 were clearly demonstrated for the two diseases taken as examples. In both cases a cytochrome P450 was able to generate a reactive metabolite which was then able to bind on this P450, producing a neoantigen. This neoantigen could trigger an immune response by an unknown mechanism. Finally, the response of the immune system was established through the presence of autoantibodies. Although the exact contribution of these autoantibodies in the immune response itself, or to the liver injury, is not clear, their presence can be considered as a hallmark of the disease.

Many questions remain unanswered, for instance:

1. Why do so few people develop the disease?
2. How is the neoantigen presented to the immune system?
3. Is there any P450 expressed at the membrane? Loeper *et al.* have shown that both rat and human hepatocyte membranes contain active P450[18] (Loeper *et al.*, manuscript accepted for publication).
4. Is the mechanism identical between the hepatitis induced by halothane on one hand and dihydralazine or tienilic acid on the other hand?
5. What is the mechanism of the disease, since we have no proof of the role of the autoantibodies in the triggering of the disease?

Many investigations are still necessary in order to address these questions, and among them we have undertaken the epitope mapping of anti-LKM2 and anti-LM (as described by Manns *et al.* for anti-LKM1[19]) and are attempting to develop an animal model with dihydralazine.

References

1. Homberg JC, Abuaf N, Helmy-Khalil S, Biour M, Poupon R, Islam S, Darnis F, Levy VG, Opolon P, Beaugrand M, Toulet J, Danan G, Benhamou JP. Drug induced hepatitis associated with anticytoplasmic organelle autoantibodies. Hepatology. 1985;5:722–7.
2. Kenna JR. The molecular basis of halothane-induced hepatitis. Autoimmunity. 1991;19: 191–5.
3. Danan G, Homber JC, Bernuau J, Roche-Sicot J, Pessayre D. Hépatite à l'iproniazide. Intérêt diagnostique d'un nouvel anticorps antimitochondrial l'anti-M6. Gastroentérol Clin Biol. 1983;7:529–32.
4. Homberg JC, Stelly M, Andreis I, Abuaf N, Saadoun F, André C. A new antimitochondrial antibody (anti-M6) in iproniazid-induced hepatitis. Clin Exp Immunol. 1982;47:93–103.
5. Homberg JC, André C, Abuaf N. A new anti-liver kidney microsome antibody (anti-LKM2) in tienilic acid induced hepatitis. Clin Exp Immunol. 1984;55:561–70.
6. Pariente EA, Pessayre D, Bernuau J, Degott C, Benhamou JP. Dihydralazine hepatitis: report of a case and review of the literature. Digestion. 1983;27:47–52.
7. Bourdi M, Larrey D, Nataf J, Bernuau J, Pessayre D, Iwasaki M, Guengerich FP, Beaune P. Anti-liver endoplasmic reticulum autoantibodies are directed against human cytochrome P-450 IA2. A specific marker of dihydralazine-induced hepatitis. J Clin Invest. 1990;85: 1967–73.
8. Manns MP, Meyer KH zum Büschenfelde. Nature of autoantigens and autoantibodies in autoimmune hepatitis, Springer Semin Immunopathol. 1990;12:57–65.
9. Kremers P, Beaune P, Cresteil T, De Graeve J, Columelli S, Leroux JP, Gielen JE. Cytochrome P450 monooxygenase activities in human and rat liver microsomes. Eur J Biochem. 1981;118:599–606.
10. Dansette P, Amar C, Valadon P, Pons C, Beaune P, Mansuy D. Hydroxylation and formation of electrophilic metabolites of tienilic acid and its isomer by human liver microsomes: catalysis by a cytochrome P-450 IIC different from that responsible for mephenytoin hydroxylation. Biochem Pharmacol. 1991;41:553–60.
11. Renaud JP, Cullin C, Pompon D, Beaune P, Mansuy D. Expression of human liver

cytochrome P450 NF in yeast: a functional model for the in vivo hepatic enzyme. Eur J Biochem. 1990;194:889–96.

12. Srivastava PK, Yun C, Beaune P, Ged C, Guengerich F. Separation of human liver microsomal tolbutamide hydroxylase and (S)mephenytoin 4′hydroxylase cytochrome P450 enzymes. Mol Pharmacol. 1991;40:69–79.
13. Bourdi M, Gautier JC, Mircheva J, Larrey D, Guillouzo A, André C, Belloc C, Beaune P. Anti-liver microsomes autoantibodies and dihydralazine induced hepatitis: specificity of autoantibodies and inductive capacity of the drug. Mol Pharmacol. 1992;42:280–5.
14. Beaune P, Dansette P, Mansuy D, Kiffel L, Finck M, Amar C, Leroux JP, Homberg JC. Human antimicrosome antibodies appearing in a drug induced hepatitis are directed against a cytochrome P-450 hydroxylating the drug. Proc Natl Acad Sci USA. 1987;84:551–5.
15. Mansuy D, Valadon P, Erdelmeier I, Lopez-Garcia P, Amar C, Girault JP, Dansette P. Thiophene S-oxides as new reactive metabolites: formation by cytochrome P450 dependent oxidation and reaction with nuclephiles. J Am Chem Soc. 1991;113:7825–6.
16. Christen U, Bürgin M, Gut J. Halothane metabolism: Kupffer cells carry and partially process trifluoroacetylated protein adducts. Biochem Biophys Res Commun. 1991;175: 256–62.
17. Beaune P, Dansette P, Mansuy D, Kiffel L, Amar C, Leroux JP, Homberg JC. Autoantibodies to anticytochrome P450 during autoimmune hepatitis. In: Guillozo A, editor. Liver cells and drugs. 1988;164:175–80.
18. Loeper J, Descatoire V, Maurice M, Beaune P, Feldmann G, Larrey D, Pessayre D. Presence of functional cytochrome P450 on isolated hepatocyte plasma membrane. Hepatology (Baltimore). 1990;11:145–53.
19. Manns MP, Griffin KJ, Sullivan KF, Johnson EF. LKM1 autoantibodies recognize a short linear sequence in P-450IID6, a cytochrome P-450 monooxygenase. J Clin Invest. 1991;88:1370–8.

32
Identification and characterization of protein adducts of reactive metabolites by the use of specific antibodies

L. R. POHL

INTRODUCTION

Drugs that cause hepatotoxicity have been classified into two categories: those that are intrinsic hepatotoxins and those that are idiosyncratic hepatotoxins[1]. The hepatotoxicity caused by intrinsic hepatotoxins, such as chloroform and acetaminophen, is generally characterized as being host-independent, dose-dependent, and reproducible in animals. The majority of drugs that cause hepatotoxicity, however, appear to be idiosyncratic hepatotoxins. Their reactions are host-dependent, often apparently dose-independent, and difficult to reproduce in animals. They are also hard to predict, and usually are not recognized as a potential medical problem until the drug has been in general use for some time.

Drug-induced hepatotoxicities, whether intrinsic or idiosyncratic, are believed to be caused in many cases by reactive metabolites[2,3]. In the case of intrinsically hepatotoxic agents, reactive metabolites are thought to cause cellular damage by covalently altering cellular macromolecules either directly, or possibly through the intermediacy of reactive endogenous oxygen species such as hydrogen peroxide, hydroxyl radical, or lipid peroxides that are formed from the reactions of reactive metabolites of drugs[2–4]. This may lead to the inactivation of enzymes, to the disruption of intracellular calcium homeostasis, or to a general loss of cellular membrane integrity by lipid peroxidation[2–6]. Idiosyncratic drug-induced hepatic damage might also be attributed to similar processes. If this were the case, then there would have to be some reason why the toxicities are host-dependent. It could be due to the presence of abnormally high levels of enzymes that activate the drug into a reactive metabolite or a mutant form of the enzyme that is catalytically more active than the normal enzyme. Alternatively, an individual may have an abnormally low level or activity of enzymes that detoxify reactive metabolites such as glutathione transferases, glutathione peroxidase, catalase, or superoxide dismutase. An alternative mechanism for idiosyncratic drug-induced hepatotoxicity is an allergic or hypersensitivity reaction against covalently altered tissue macromolecules[1].

One reason why very little progress has been made in the understanding of how drugs produce intrinsic or idiosyncratic hepatitis, or even other types of toxicity, is that little is known of the identity of the protein adducts associated with many of these diseases. In the past the major way in which macromolecular targets of reactive metabolites were detected was by the use of radiolabelled parent compounds. This approach, however, is frequently insensitive and involves the hazards of working with radioactive materials. However, because of our present knowledge of the structure and chemistry of reactive metabolites of many compounds it is now possible to prepare antibodies that will recognize these metabolites when they are covalently bound to tissue macromolecules. These reagents can be used as sensitive probes for detecting the target macromolecules of reactive metabolites in tissues and cells, and for purifying them. In this chapter I will discuss how antibodies directed against covalently bound reactive metabolites have been used to characterize the protein adducts associated with halothane ($CF_3CHClBr$) hepatitis and the protein adducts associated with the toxicities produced by other drugs and environmental chemicals.

PROTEIN ADDUCTS ASSOCIATED WITH HALOTHANE HEPATITIS

Several studies have suggested that the idiosyncratic hepatitis caused by the inhalation of anaesthetic halothane may be due to immune reactions against liver proteins that had been altered by halothane (for reviews see refs 7–10). The most informative findings that have led to this conclusion have come from immunoblotting studies. In these investigations, serum antibodies from halothane hepatitis patients were found to recognize polypeptide fractions of 100, 76, 59, 57, and 54 kDa in liver microsomes of humans[11] and animals[12–14] that had been treated with halothane. Patients' sera differed markedly in patterns of polypeptide recognition, with the 100 and 76 kDa antigens being recognized most commonly. Subcellular fraction studies revealed that the antigens recognized by the patients' sera were concentrated in the microsomal fraction of the liver[12]. The reactions with these protein fractions were not seen when the sera of control patients or patients suffering from other forms of hepatitis were used in place of the halothane hepatitis patients' sera. Moreover, very little, if any, reaction occurred when the liver microsomes used for the immunoblotting studies were from sources other than halothane-treated humans or animals. These findings indicated that halothane treatment had somehow altered the liver microsomal proteins to produce neoantigens that were recognized by the patients' serum antibodies.

Since halothane is not chemically reactive under physiological conditions, it appeared that a reactive metabolite of halothane was most likely responsible for the recognition of the liver microsomal proteins by the halothane patients' serum antibodies. In this regard, studies indicated that this metabolite was a trifluoroacetyl halide (CF_3COX, where X = Cl or Br), formed from the oxidative metabolism of halothane by cytochromes P450[15]. For example, it was found, with the use of an enzyme-linked immunosorbent assay (ELISA), that two of six patients diagnosed as having halothane-associated massive liver cell necrosis contained serum antibodies that reacted with trifluoroacetylated (TFA)-rabbit serum albumin[16]. This finding was consistent with the idea that the hapten–carrier conjugates recognized by the halothane–hepatitis serum antibodies might be formed by the reaction of endoplasmic microsomal proteins with CF_3COX. In order to test this idea an antibody was raised against the TFA hapten by immunizing rabbits with TFA-rabbit serum albumin[17]. Immunoblotting studies with microsomes from rats[13] and humans[9] that had been treated with halothane revealed that the protein fractions recognized by the patients' serum antibodies contained the TFA hapten. When the TFA hapten was removed from the liver microsomes by treatment with 1 mol/l piperidine, the patients' antibody recognition of the microsomal proteins was abolished[13]. This showed that the TFA moiety was required for antibody recognition by the patients' serum antibodies. The patients' antibodies, however, did not appear to be directed solely against the TFA hapten, but instead against epitopes that consisted of the TFA hapten and undefined specific structural features of the individual carrier proteins. This conclusion was based upon the finding that the patients' sera often differed in their patterns of protein recognition, and by the discovery that the reaction of the patients' antibodies with the TFA-microsomal proteins was only partially inhibited by the hapten derivative ε-*N*-TFA-L-lysine, whereas it nearly abolished the binding of the anti-TFA antibodies to the TFA-liver microsomal proteins[13,18]. These results also indicated that the TFA hapten was preferentially bound to lysine residues of microsomal proteins, a finding that was recently confirmed by ^{19}F nuclear magnetic resonance studies[19].

Purification and characterization of several of the TFA proteins from rat liver microsomes has been accomplished with the use of the anti-TFA antibodies. The 59 kDa target protein was purified by affinity chromatography on an anti-TFA column, and has been identified as a carboxylesterase[18]. The anti-TFA antibodies were used to monitor the purification of several other TFA proteins by traditional chromatographic procedures. The 100 kDa protein was identified as ERp99, which is identical to a 94 kDa glucose-regulated protein (GRP94), and endoplasmin[20]; the 76 kDa protein fraction was resolved into two protein targets of CF_3COX, an 80 kDa protein, which is identical to ERp72[21], and an 82 kDa protein, which corresponds to GRP78, also known as BiP[22]; the 57 kDa target protein is identical to protein disulphide isomerase[23]; and the 54 kDa protein target appears to correspond to an unidentified form of cytochromes P450[24]. Two additional protein targets of CF_3COX were discovered during the purification of the TFA proteins: a 63 kDa protein target, which corresponds to calreticulin[25], and a 58 kDa protein[26], which may be a member of the PDI family[27] or possibly a cellular protease[28].

The purified rat liver TFA proteins appear to correspond, at least in part, to the TFA-carrier proteins detected by the serum antibodies of the halothane hepatitis patients on immunoblots of liver microsomes from halothane-treated animals and humans. For example, it was found in an ELISA study that the sera of 10 halothane hepatitis patients reacted with several of the purified rat TFA proteins: TFA-100 kDa (9 of 10), TFA-80 kDa (5 of 10), TFA-63 kDa (1 of 10), TFA-59 kDa (2 of 10), TFA-58 kDa (5 of 10) and TFA-57 kDa (2 of 10)[24]. Recently, the ELISA study was repeated with sera from 40 halothane hepatitis patients. In this case the test antigens used for the assay were the purified TFA-80 kDa protein or the purified unlabelled native 80 kDa protein. It was found that the halothane hepatitis patients' serum antibodies reacted with both the TFA-80 kDa protein (12 of 40) and the native 80 kDa protein (10 of 40)[21]. These findings were in contrast to the results of the immunoblotting studies with liver microsomes, which showed very little, if any, reaction of halothane patients' serum antibodies with native proteins[11–13]. The reason for this discrepancy is not known at this time. It might be due to the patients' sera containing antibodies that reacted with conformational epitopes[29] of the native unmodified 80 kDa protein, which were destroyed by the denaturing conditions of immunoblotting, but were not altered appreciably by the relatively mild conditions of the ELISA[30–32]. In contrast, antibodies to the TFA-induced epitopes present only on the TFA-80 kDa protein might have recognized sequential epitopes that were not as susceptible to denaturation, and so were detectable by immunoblotting. Although these possibilities cannot be proven until epitope mapping of both the TFA-80 kDa and native 80 kDa proteins has been done, our findings are consistent with immunofluorescence studies, which have shown that 19 of 76 (25%)[33] and 2 of 6 (33%)[34] of halothane hepatitis patients had serum antibodies that reacted with native unmodified proteins present in frozen liver sections.

Since the carrier proteins of the TFA hapten appear to be highly conserved proteins, it is quite possible that they correspond to the immunogens that elicited the patients' immune responses. If this were the case it remains to be determined how these proteins, which all appear to be concentrated in the lumen of the endoplasmic reticulum[35], led to the patients' immune reactions and possibly hepatotoxicity. Several possibilities, however, have been discussed in detail elsewhere[36].

OTHER USES OF THE ANTI-TFA ANTIBODIES

The anti-TFA antibodies have been used to solve several additional problems. In immunohistochemistry studies the antibodies were employed to show that the perivenous region of the liver lobule was the major site of trifluoroacetylation of liver proteins and that surface macromolecules were also labelled by the trifluoroacetyl halide metabolite of halothane[17]. Western blotting and immunohistochemical studies have revealed that small levels of TFA proteins are formed in extrahepatic tissues including the testes[15], kidney[37], heart[38], and lung (unpublished results). Moreover, in the liver, low levels have been discovered in Kupffer cells, which may have a role in the development of the immune responses ot the halothane hepatitis patients against the TFA proteins[39].

The anti-TFA antibodies have been used to detect target proteins of reactive metabolites of other halogenated hydrocarbons that form TFA adducts or adducts that are structurally similar to the TFA group. For example, HCFC-123 (CF_3CHCl_2), which has been developed as a replacement for ozone depleting chlorofluorocarbons (CFCs), produced nearly identical patterns and levels of TFA-liver proteins as that of halothane[19]. Much lower levels of hepatic TFA proteins were found after rats were exposed to HCFC-124 (CF_3CHFCl) or HCFC-125 (CF_3CHF_2) treatments[40]. These results indicated that because HCFC-124 and HCFC-125 produced lower TFA-protein concentrations, they may be safer CFC alternatives than HCFC-123. Similarly, the protein targets of the reactive acyl halide metabolite (CHF_2OCF_2COX, where X = F or Cl) of the inhalation anaesthetic enflurane (CHF_2OCF_2CHFCl) have been found to be similar to those of halothane[41,42]. In this case the anti-TFA antibodies and serum antibodies of the halothane hepatitis patients crossreacted with CHF_2OCF_2CO adducts. Recently, the anti-TFA antibodies have been shown to crossreact with CHF_2CS adducts formed from the reaction of tissue proteins with the difluorothionoacetylating metabolite (CHF_2CSF) of the nephrotoxic agent S-(1,1,2,2-tetrafluoroethyl)-L-cysteine (TFEC). When rats were treated with TFEC, immunohistochemical analysis revealed that CHF_2CS adducts in the kidney were localized to the damaged areas of proximal tubules[43]. Immunoblotting of subcellular fractions showed that major targets of CHF_2CSF were mitochondrial proteins of apparent monomeric masses of 87, 79, 61, and 40 kDa[43,44].

OTHER EXAMPLES WHERE ANTIBODIES DIRECTED AGAINST COVALENTLY BOUND DRUG METABOLITES HAVE BEEN USED TO IDENTIFY CELLULAR PROTEIN TARGETS OF REACTIVE METABOLITES

The reactive metabolite that causes the hepatotoxicity produced by an overdose of acetaminophen (*N*-acetyl-*p*-aminophenol) is *N*-acetyl-*p*-benzoquinone imine (NAPQI)[45]. Antibodies have been raised to detect this reactive metabolite when it is bound to tissue proteins. The adducts have been studied by the use of several immunochemical techniques including immunohistochemistry[46,47], ELISA[48], and immunoblotting[47,49,50]. The immunoblotting studies have revealed that several proteins are targets of NAPQI. In mouse liver, major targets are a microsomal protein of 44 kDa and a cytosolic protein of 55–58 kDa[47,49,50]. Recently the 55–58 kDa protein target has been purified and identified as a selenium binding protein[51,52].

Acetaldehyde, a reactive metabolite of ethanol, has been implicated in alcoholic liver disease[36]. In order to develop antibodies that could detect acetaldehyde–protein adducts in liver, animals were immunized with products from the reaction of acetaldehyde with one of several different carrier proteins. Immunoblotting studies with the use of these antibodies have led to the detection of a 52 kDa adduct and a 37 kDa adduct in microsomal and cytosolic fractions of rat liver, respectively[36]. The 52 kDa protein target has been identified as cytochrome P450 2E1, while the identity of the 37 kDa target protein is not known. Although it is not clear what role these adducts have in alcoholic liver disease, they or others appeared to have induced immune responses in 38–74% of alcoholic patients[36].

Diclofenac (2-[(2,6-dichlorophenyl)amino]benzeneacetic acid) is a widely used non-steroidal anti-inflammatory drug (NSAID). Reports have indicated that it produces a mild hepatotoxicity in 15% of patients and, in rare instances, fulminant hepatic necrosis[53]. In order to investigate the possibility that diclofenac–protein conjugates might be involved in the severe form of hepatotoxicity, it was necessary to develop a method for detecting adducts of diclofenac in liver tissue. In order to do this the assumption was made that the covalent binding would be due, at least in part, to the acyl glucuronide metabolite of diclofenac, or possibly an acyl-CoA metabolite. In both cases this meant that the covalently bound product would be an acyl derivative of diclofenac. Therefore, diclofenac was coupled to carrier proteins through its carboxyl group and anti-hapten antibodies were raised against this product. With the use of these antibodies, several protein adducts were detected in immunoblots of liver homogenates of mice treated with diclofenac. A major adduct had an apparent monomeric mass of approximately 110 kDa[54] and was found to be concentrated in the plasma membrane fraction of liver cells[55]. This finding was corroborated by the immunohistochemical evidence of diclofenac adduct accumulation in canalicular plasma membranes in the perivenous region of the liver lobule[55]. The role that this adduct may have in the hepatotoxicity produced by diclofenac is currently being studied.

Acknowledgement

I thank Dr James R. Gillette for valuable suggestions in editing the manuscript.

References

1. Zimmerman HJ. Classification of hepatotoxins and mechanisms of toxicity. In: Hepatotoxicity: the adverse effecs of drugs and other chemicals on the liver. New York: Appleton-Century-Crofts; 1978;91–121.
2. Nelson SD, Pearson PG. Covalent and noncovalent interactions in acute lethal cell injury caused by chemicals. Annu Rev Pharmacol Toxicol. 1990;30:169–95.
3. Hinson JA, Roberts DW. Role of covalent and noncovalent interactions in cell toxicity: effects on proteins. Annu Rev Pharmacol Toxicol. 1992;32:471–510.
4. Reed DJ. Glutathione: toxicological implications. Annu Rev Pharmacol Toxicol. 1990;30:603–31.
5. Tirmenstein MA, Nelson SD. Acetaminophen-induced oxidation of protein thiols. Contribution of impaired thiol-metabolizing enzymes and the breakdown of adenine nucleotides. J Biol Chem. 1990;265:3059–65.
6. Nicotera P, Bellomo G, Orrenius S. The role of Ca^{2+} in cell killing. Chem Res Toxicol. 1990;3:484–94.
7. Satoh H, Davies HW, Takemura T, Gillette JR, Maeda K, Pohl LR. An immunochemical

approach to investigating the mechanism of halothane-induced hepatotoxicity. In: Bridges JW, Chasseaud LF, Gibson GG, editors. Progress in drug metabolism. Philadelphia: Taylor & Francis, 1987:187–206.
8. Neuberger J, Kenna JG. Halothane hepatitis: a model of immune mediated drug hepatotoxicity. Clin Sci. 1987;72:263–70.
9. Pohl LR, Kenna JG, Satoh H, Christ DD, Martin JL. Neoantigens associated with halothane hepatitis. Drug Metab Rev. 1989;20:203–17.
10. Kenna JG. The molecular basis of halothane-induced hepatitis. Biochem Soc Trans. 1991;19:191–5.
11. Kenna JG, Neuberger JM, Williams R. Evidence for expression in human liver of halothane induced neoantigens recognized by antibodies in sera from patients with halothane hepatitis. Hepatology. 1988;8:1635–41.
12. Kenna JG, Neuberger J, Williams R. Identification by immunoblotting of three halothane-induced liver microsomal polypeptide antigens recognized by antibodies in sera from patients with halothane-associated hepatitis. J Pharmacol Exp Ther. 1987;242:733–40.
13. Kenna JG, Satoh H, Christ DD, Pohl LR. Metabolic basis for a drug hypersensitivity: antibodies in sera from patients with halothane hepatitis recognize liver neoantigens that contain the trifluoroacetyl group derived from halothane. J Pharmacol Exp Ther. 1988;245:1103–9.
14. Pohl LR, Satoh H, Christ DD, Kenna JG. The immunologic and metabolic basis of drug hypersensitivities. Annu Rev Pharmacol Toxicol. 1988;28:367–87.
15. Kenna JG, Martin JL, Satoh H, Pohl LR. Factors affecting the expression of trifluoroacetylated liver microsomal protein neoantigens in rats treated with halothane. Drug Metab Dispos. 1990;18:788–93.
16. Satoh H, Gillette JR, Takemura T, Ferrans VJ, Jelenich SE, Kenna JG, Neuberger J, Pohl LR. Investigation of the immunological basis of halothane-induced hepatotoxicity. Adv Exp Biol Med. 1986;197:657–73.
17. Satoh H, Fukuda Y, Anderson DK, Ferrans VJ, Gillette JR, Pohl LR. Immunological studies on the mechanism of halothane-induced hepatotoxicity: immunohistochemical evidence of trifluoroacetylated hepatocytes. J Pharmacol Exp Ther. 1985;233:857–62.
18. Satoh H, Martin BM, Schulick AH, Christ DD, Kenna JG, Pohl LR. Human anti-endoplasmic reticulum antibodies in sera of halothane hepatitis patients are directed against a trifluoroacetylated carboxylesterase. Proc Natl Acad Sci USA. 1989;86:322–6.
19. Harris JW, Pohl LR, Martin JL, Anders MW. Tissue acylation by the chlorofluorocarbon substitute 2,2-dichloro-1,1,1-trifluoroethane. Proc Natl Acad Sci USA. 1991;88:1407–10.
20. Thomassen D, Martin BM, Martin JL, Pumford NR, Pohl LR. The role of a stress protein in the development of a drug-induced allergic response. Eur J Pharmacol. 1990;183: 1138–9.
21. Pumford NR, Martin BM, Thomassen D, Burris JA, Kenna JG, Martin JL, Pohl LR. Serum antibodies from halothane hepatitis patients react with the endoplasmic reticulum protein ERp72. Chem Res Toxicol. 1992: in press.
22. Davila JC, Martin BM, Pohl LR. Patients with halothane hepatitis have serum antibodies directed against glucose-regulated stress protein GRP78/BiP. Toxicologist. 1992;12:255.
23. Martin JL, Kenna JG, Martin BM, Thomassen D, Reed GF, Pohl LR. Halothane hepatitis patients have serum antibodies that react with protein disulfide isomerase. Hepatology. (in press).
24. Pohl LR, Thomassen D, Pumford NR, Butler LE, Satoh H, Ferrans VJ, Perrone A, Martin BM, Martin JL. Hapten carrier conjugates associated with halothane hepatitis. Adv Exp Biol Med. 1991;283:111–20.
25. Butler LE, Thomassen D, Martin JL, Martin BM, Kenna JG, Pohl LR. The calcium-binding protein calreticulin is covalently modified in rat liver by a reactive metabolite of the inhalation anesthetic halothane. Chem Res Toxicol. 1992;5:406–10.
26. Martin JL, Pumford NR, LaRosa AC, Martin BM, Gonzaga HM, Beaven MA, Pohl LR. A metabolite of halothane covalently binds to an endoplasmic reticulum protein that is highly homologous to phosphatidylinositol-specific phospholipase C-alpha but has no activity. Biochem Biophys Res Commun. 1991;178:679–85.
27. Srivastava SP, Chen NQ, Liu YX, Holtzman JL. Purification and characterization of a new isozyme of thiol: protein-disulfide oxidoreductase from rat hepatic microsomes. Relationship

of this isozyme to cytosolic phosphatidylinositol-specific phospholipase C form 1A. J Biol Chem. 1991;266:20337–44.

28. Urade R, Nasu M, Moriyama T, Wada K, Kito M. Protein degradation by the phosphoinositide-specific phospholipase C-alpha family from rat liver endoplasmic reticulum. J Biol Chem. 1992;267:15152–9.
29. Laver WG, Air GM Webster RG, Smith-Gill SJ. Epitopes on protein antigens: misconceptions and realities. Cell. 1990;61:553–6.
30. Waxman DJ, Lapenson DP, Krishnan M, Bernard O, Kreibich G, Alvarez F. Antibodies to Liver/Kidney Microsome in chronic active hepatitis recognize cytochrome P-450. Gastroenterology. 1988;95:1326–31.
31. Finke R, Seto P, Rapoport B. Evidence for the highly conformational nature of the epitope(s) on human thyroid peroxidase that are recognized by sera from patients with Hashimoto's thyroiditis. J Clin Endocrinol Metab. 1990;71:53–9.
32. Leedman PJ, Harrison PJ, Harrison LC. Immunoblotting for the detection of TSH receptor autoantibodies. J Autoimmun. 1991;4:529–42.
33. Walton B, Simpson BR, Strunin L, Doniach D, Perrin J, Appleyard AJ. Unexplained hepatitis following halothane. Br Med J. 1976;1:1171–6.
34. Homberg JC, Abuaf N, Helmy-Khalil S, Biour M, Poupon R, Islam S, Darnis F, Levy, VG, Opolon P, Beaugrand M *et al.* Drug-induced hepatitis associated with anticytoplasmic organelle autoantibodies. Hepatology. 1985;5:722–7.
35. Kenna JG, Martin JL, Pohl LR. The topography of trifluoroacetylated protein antigens in liver microsomal fractions from halothane treated rats. Biochem Pharmacol. 1992;44: 621–9.
36. Pohl LR. Drug-induced allergic hepatitis. Semin Liver Dis. 1990;10:305–15.
37. Huwyler J, Aeschlimann D, Christen U, Gut J. The kidney as a novel target tissue for protein adduct formation associated with metabolism of halothane and the candidate chlorofluorocarbon replacement 2,2-dichloro-1,1,1-trifluoroethane. Eur J Biochem. 1992;207:229–38.
38. Huwyler J, Gut J. Exposure to the chlorofluorocarbon substitute 2,2-dichloro-1,1,1-trifluoroethane and the anesthetic agent halothane is associated with transient protein adduct formation in the heart. Biochem Biophys Res Commun. 1992;184:1344–9.
39. Christen U, Burgin M, Gut J. Halothane metabolism: Kupffer cells carry and partially process trifluoroacetylated protein adducts. Biochem Biophys Res Commun. 1991;175: 256–62.
40. Harris JW, Jones JP, Martin JL, LaRosa AC, Olson MJ, Pohl LR, Anders MW. Pentahaloethane-based chlorofluorocarbon substitutes and halothane: correlation of *in vivo* hepatic protein trifluoroacetylation and urinary trifluoroacetic acid secretion with calculated enthalpies of activation. Chem Res Toxicol. 1992;5:720–5.
41. Christ DD, Satoh H, Kenna JG, Pohl LR. Potential metabolic basis for enflurane hepatitis and the apparent cross-sensitization between enflurane and halothane. Drug Metab Dis. 1988;16:135–40.
42. Christ DD, kenna JG, Kammerer W, Satoh H, Pohl LR. Enflurane metabolism produces covalently-bound liver adducts recognized by antibodies from patients with halothane hepatitis. Anesthesiology. 1988;69:833–8.
43. Hayden PJ, Ichimura T, McCann DJ, Pohl LR, Stevens JL. Detection of cysteine conjugate metabolite adduct formation with specific mitochondrial proteins using antibodies raised against halothane metabolite adducts. J Biol Chem. 1991;266:18415–18.
44. Hargus SJ, Anders MW. Immunochemical detection of covalently modified kidney proteins in *S*-(1,1,2,2-tetrafluoroethyl)-L-cysteine-treated rats. Biochem Pharmacol. 1991;42:R17–20.
45. Nelson SD. Molecular mechanisms of the hepatotoxicity caused by acetaminophen. Semin Liver Dis. 1990;10:267–78.
46. Roberts DW, Bucci TJ, Benson RW, Warbritton AR, McRae TA, Pumford NR, Hinson JA. Immunohistochemical localization and quantification of the 3-(cystein-*S*-yl)-acetaminophen protein adduct in acetaminophen hepatotoxicity. Am J Pathol. 1991;138:359–71.
47. Birge RB, Bartolone JB, Hart SG, Nishanian EV, Tyson CA, Khairallah EA, Cohen SD. Acetaminophen hepatotoxicity: correspondence of selective protein arylation in human and mouse liver *in vitro*, in culture, and *in vivo*. Toxicol Appl Pharmacol. 1990;105:472–82.
48. Pumford NR, Roberts DW, Benson RW, Hinson JA. Immunochemical quantitation of 3-

(cystein-*S*-yl)acetaminophen protein adducts in subcellular liver fractions following a hepatotoxic dose of acetaminophen. Biochem Pharmacol. 1990;40:573–9.
49. Pumford NR, Hinson JA, Benson RW, Roberts DW. Immunoblot analysis of protein containing 3-(cystein-S-yl)acetaminophen adducts in serum and subcellular liver fractions from acetaminophen-treated mice. Toxicol Appl Pharmacol. 1990;104:521–32.
50. Birge RB, Bulera SJ, Bartolone JB, Ginsberg GL, Cohen SD, Khairallah EA. The arylation of microsomal membrane proteins by acetaminophen is associated with the release of a 44 kDa acetaminophen-binding mouse liver protein complex into the cytosol. Toxicol Appl Pharmacol. 1991;109:443–54.
51. Pumford NR, Martin BM, Hinson JA. A metabolite of acetaminophen covalently binds to the 56 kDa selenium binding protein. Biochem Biophys Res Commun. 1992;182:1348–55.
52. Bartolone JB, Birge RB, Bulera SJ, Bruno MK, Nishanian EV, Cohen SD, Khairallah EA. Purification, antibody production, and partial amino acid sequence of the 58-kDa acetaminophen-binding liver proteins. Toxicol Appl Pharmacol. 1992;113:19–29.
53. Zimmerman HJ. Update of hepatotoxicity due to classes of drugs in common clinical use: non-steroidal drugs, anti-inflammatory drugs, antibiotics, antihypertensives, and cardiac and psychotropic agents. Semin Liver Dis. 1990;10:322–38.
54. Pumford NR, Myers TG, Davila JC, Highest RJ, Pohl LR. Immunochemical detection of liver protein adducts of the nonsteroidal anti-inflammatory drug diclofenac. Biochem Biophys Res Commun. 1992:in press.
55. Myers TG, Pumford NR, Davila JC, Pohl LR. Covalent binding of diclofenac to plasma membrane proteins of the bile canaliculi in the mouse. Toxicologist. 1992;12:253.

Section VIII
Primary Sclerosing Cholangitis

33
Advances in primary sclerosing cholangitis

R. H. WIESNER

INTRODUCTION

Primary sclerosing cholangitis (PSC) is a chronic, cholestatic syndrome of unknown aetiology which is characterized by diffuse inflammation and fibrosis of the entire biliary tree. The syndrome is most commonly progressive but at an unpredictable and variable rate. The syndrome usually advances to biliary cirrhosis, portal hypertension, and premature death from liver failure unless intervention with liver transplantation occurs[1–3]. In general, a diagnosis of PSC is based collectively on a combination of clinical, radiological, and biochemical abnormalities[4,5]. The term 'primary' indicates that this type of sclerosing cholangitis is idiopathic, and distinguishes this entity from secondary sclerosing cholangitis, a syndrome with similar clinical, radiological, and histological findings but with identifiable causes. Secondary sclerosing cholangitis can occur as a result of a number of associated conditions: choledocholithiasis, congenital abnormalities of the biliary tree, cholangiopathy associated with acquired immune deficiency syndrome, bacterial cholangitis, biliary infection with organisms such as *Cryptococcus*, *Cryptosporidium*, and *Cytomegalovirus*, toxicity related to intra-arterial infusion of floxuridine, toxicity related to caustic therapy for hydatid disease and, finally, cholangiocarcinoma which can occur independently or in association with primary sclerosing cholangitis.

DIAGNOSIS AND CLINICAL FEATURES

In the past, PSC was diagnosed most often in advanced histological stages when the patient was extremely ill and markedly jaundiced. More recently, non-surgical diagnostic tests, such as transhepatic cholangiography and endoscopic retrograde cholangiography, coupled with the increased awareness of PSC and its association with chronic ulcerative colitis, have led to

Table 1 Disease associated with primary sclerosing cholangitis

Inflammatory bowel disease	Chronic pancreatitis
Coeliac disease	Rheumatoid arthritis
Retroperitoneal fibrosis	Peyronie's disease
Thyroiditis	Bronchiectasis
Sjögren's syndrome	Systemic sclerosis
Autoimmune chronic active hepatitis	Membranous nephropathy
Lupus erythematosus	Pseudotumour of orbit
Vasculitis	Autoimmune haemolytic anemia
Immune thrombocytopenic purpura	Angioblastic lymphadenopathy
Histiocytosis X	Cystic fibrosis
Gallbladder disease	Eosinophilia
Intra-abdominal adenopathy	

an earlier diagnosis. Indeed, PSC is a cholangiographic diagnosis provided that other causes of secondary sclerosing cholangitis are excluded (see above).

The onset of PSC is most often insidious and usually occurs in middle-aged males[1,2]. The mean age at the time of diagnosis of PSC is 40 years, and two-thirds of patients are male. Most patients have had symptoms for 1 or 2 years before the diagnosis of PSC is made. The gradual onset of progressive fatigue and pruritus, followed by jaundice, is the most frequent symptom complex leading to the diagnosis. Clinical cholangitis marked by recurrent fever, right upper quadrant pain, and jaundice is uncommon except in patients who have had previous reconstructive biliary surgery, or in those patients who develop a dominant stricture of the extrahepatic bile duct. PSC may occur alone; however, 70% of cases are associated with inflammatory bowel disease, most commonly chronic ulcerative colitis (CUC) and rarely Crohn's disease[7]. CUC usually precedes the onset of PSC but can be diagnosed simultaneously and can occur after the diagnosis of PSC. Indeed, a number of patients have developed PSC 10 years or more following proctocolectomy for CUC. In general, CUC associated with PSC is quiescent; indeed, 80% are either asymptomatic or mildly symptomatic from CUC at the time PSC is diagnosed.

PSC is further associated with a number of other autoimmune disorders, including thyroiditis, arthritis, coeliac sprue, chronic pancreatitis, retroperitoneal fibrosis, and intra-abdominal lymphadenopathy[6]. A number of other associations have been made; however, whether these represent incidental associations or true associations remains undefined (Table 1).

BIOCHEMICAL ABNORMALITIES

PSC is usually manifested by the presence of a cholestatic biochemical profile. However, we and others have documented normal levels of serum alkaline phosphatase activity in PSC patients, even in the presence of advanced histological findings on liver biopsy[8]. The vast majority of PSC patients have a modest increase in serum levels of aminotransferases (five times normal) and about half of PSC patients have a modest increase in total serum bilirubin levels at the time the diagnosis of PSC is made[6]. As in other cholestatic liver diseases, hepatic copper and urine copper levels increase as PSC progresses, approaching levels seen in primary biliary cirrhosis, Wilson's disease, and Indian childhood cirrhosis[9].

In contrast to primary biliary cirrhosis, a cholestatic liver disease of middle-aged women, characterized by the destruction of only interlobular and septal bile ducts and the presence of serum antimitochondrial and other autoantibodies, the presence of traditional autoantibodies is infrequent in PSC. Testing for antimitochondrial antibodies is almost always negative, or they are found in low titres, and other antibodies such as antinuclear (6–34%) and antismooth muscle antibodies (11%) are found infrequently[10,11]. On the contrary, the presence of anticolon antibodies, antineutrophil nuclear antibodies, and neutrophil cytoplasmic antibodies is documented in the majority of patients with PSC[11]. However, these antibodies also occur in a high percentage of patients with ulcerative colitis without evidence of PSC, and thus appear to be non-specific findings.

RADIOLOGICAL AND HISTOLOGICAL FINDINGS

Biliary visualization by endoscopic or transhepatic cholangiography classically exhibits diffuse stricturing and beading of the intrahepatic and extrahepatic bile ducts[4]. Most commonly, strictures are short and annular with intermediate segments of slightly dilated bile ducts. Morphologically, we have shown that this beading represents cholangiectasis[12].

Hepatic histological abnormalities are found on liver biopsy in virtually all patients with PSC[13,14]. Early histological changes include enlargement of portal tracts characterized by oedema, increased connective tissue, and proliferation of interlobular bile ducts. Other changes include periductal inflammation and fibrosis, ductal obliteration, and loss of interlobular bile ducts. Although hepatic histological findings are rarely specific, the presence of the obliterative interlobular bile duct lesion appears to be most specific for PSC[15]. The end stages of PSC are marked by histological findings which include the loss of interlobular and septal bile ducts and biliary cirrhosis with or without the presence of cholestasis.

PATHOGENIC FACTORS

The aetiology of PSC remains unknown at this time. However, a number of clinical findings have shed some light on the potential aetiology of this syndrome. We have shown that there is an increased incidence of both PSC and CUC in families of patients who have PSC[16]. In addition, the frequency of human leukocyte antigen, HLA B8, DR2, DR3, and DRw52a, appears to be higher in patients with PSC than in controls, suggesting a hereditary nature of this syndrome[17]. It is now well known that the HLA B8 and DR3 loci appear to be associated with other autoimmune diseases and may potentially be associated with immune abnormalities which may predispose to the development of PSC[19]. Thus, currently, it is felt the pathogenesis of PSC is linked most closely to alterations in the immune system. In support of this view, we and others have found that PSC patients have increased serum levels of immunoglobulin M, the presence and a decreased hepatic clearance of circulating immune complexes, increased complement activation, and abnormalities in lymphocyte subsets in the peripheral blood[10,11]. Other studies have revealed aberrant expression of HLA class II antigen on bile duct epithelial cells in PSC[20]. However, all of these findings appear to be non-specific for PSC and, in particular, the expression of HLA class II antigen on bile duct epithelial cells is also seen in patients with hepatic allograft rejection, primary biliary cirrhosis and bacterial cholangitis.

Some have suggested that T lymphocytes may be involved in the destruction of bile ducts in PSC. Furthermore, we have found circulating autoreactive T lymphocytes to HLA class II antigens are increased in patients with PSC when compared to controls[21,22]. Thus these studies, in part, support the idea that immune alterations are potentially important in the pathogenesis of PSC in genetically predisposed individuals; indeed, it appears that PSC may be an autoimmune disease.

It is tempting to postulate that a viral infection involving the biliary tree might trigger immunological bile duct destruction. However, a search for such viruses, including the Rheo type III, cytomegalovirus, and other viruses, has so far been unsuccessfully linked to PSC. Finally, it appears that increases in hepatic copper levels merely result from prolonged cholestasis but do not play a major role in the overall pathogenesis or progression of PSC.

COMPLICATIONS

The management of PSC complications can be divided into (1) complications related to chronic liver disease and liver failure in general; and (2) complications relatively specific for PSC. In general, one may use conventional approaches to manage such problems as pruritus, ascites, and oesophageal variceal bleeding. Since PSC patients are susceptible to fat-soluble vitamin deficiencies in the advanced stages of the disease, night blindness related to vitamin A deficiency can occur, as can coagulopathy related to vitamin K deficiency and bone disease related to either osteoporosis or, rarely, to vitamin D deficiency in patients having marked steatorrhoea[23,24]. In such patients with steatorrhoea the aetiology is most often related to a decrease in the concentration of bile acids in the duodenum, but infrequently steatorrhoea can be associated with chronic pancreatitis, coeliac sprue, or to the administration of medications such as cholestyramine[25,26].

Complications specific for PSC include recurrent bacterial cholangitis, bacteraemia, dominant stricturing of the extrahepatic bile ducts, and cholangiocarcinoma. Although recurrent episodes of bacterial cholangitis are unusual initial symptoms in PSC, they are frequent in PSC patients who have undergone previous biliary surgery, or in those who have dominant stricture formation of the extrahepatic bile duct. Clinicians often treat these individuals with broad-spectrum antibiotics. Many clinicians favour monthly prophylactic antibiotics, but the effectiveness of prophylactic therapy is not yet clearly established. At the Mayo Clinic, Ciprofloxacin is used because of its high biliary concentrations and broad Gram-negative and broad Gram-positive bacterial coverage. The ability of Ciprofloxacin to reduce the frequency of bacterial cholangitis in PSC in patients who have a history of recurrent bacterial cholangitis seems impressive; however, controlled data remain unavailable.

Approximately 15–20% of PSC patients develop dominant strictures of the biliary tree during the course of their disease. These occur most often at the hilus, but they can also infrequently involve the common bile duct as well as the right and left hepatic ducts. Dominant strictures are frequently associated with the acute onset of jaundice, pruritus, and often bacterial cholangitis with fever and chills. In our opinion, balloon dilatation of dominant strictures by either a transhepatic or endoscopic retrograde approach, depending on the location, appears to be a reasonable approach to the problem. Our recent data suggest a long-term benefit using percutaneous balloon dilatation of dominant bile duct strictures in patients with PSC who presented with new onset of dominant stricture, jaundice, or bacterial cholangitis[27]. In 33 PSC patients, 18 presented with recurrent cholangitis and 15 had a recent onset of jaundice. In the 18 PSC patients presenting with cholangitis, 14 patients had symptomatic relief following percutaneous balloon dilatation of the biliary tree with stenting, but four patients experienced recurrent cholangitis. Of the 15 patients for whom balloon dilatation was carried out for jaundice, improvement (defined as a $> 50\%$ decline in total serum bilirubin level) occurred in 11 patients (73%). Overall, 25/33 (76%) patients had improvement in symptoms and/or liver function. The mean follow-up was 38.4 months (range 2–107 months). Stricture recurrence requiring repeat percutaneous balloon dilatation occurred in 10/33 (30%) patients, and in five patients, restricturing occurred a second time. Time to stricture recurrence was a mean 360 days from initial balloon dilatation. In summary, dominant strictures developing in patients with PSC can frequently be successfully treated with percutaneous balloon dilatation and long-term stenting. Thus, biliary surgical intervention can generally be avoided in this group of PSC patients. Balloon dilatation seems to be most effective in patients who had a recent increase in serum bilirubin levels or a recent onset of bacterial cholangitis, and appears less effective in patients with long-standing jaundice or with long-standing history of recurrent bouts of bacterial cholangitis.

CHOLANGIOCARCINOMA

In patients with PSC, 10–15% appear to develop cholangiocarcinoma during the course of their disease[28]. The highest incidence appears to occur in those patients with long-standing CUC and cirrhotic-stage PSC. Indeed, we consider PSC to be a premalignant condition of the biliary tree just as CUC is considered a premalignant condition of the colon. Because PSC patients often have long-standing, relatively quiescent colitis, they are at risk for developing both cholangiocarcinoma and colon cancer. Unfortunately, it has been difficult to diagnose bile duct cancer early in PSC patients, since fine-needle aspiration, brush cytology, and exfoliative cytology have been rather insensitive in detecting cholangiocarcinoma in the presence of PSC. The difficulty in making the diagnosis of cholangiocarcinoma in PSC is supported by the recent report from the University of Pittsburgh in which 10.6% of patients with PSC undergoing liver transplantation were found to have an unsuspected cholangiocarcinoma at the time of operation[29]. These findings attest to the difficulty of diagnosing this condition in PSC. However, a recent report has suggested that the measurement of serum concentrations of the glycoprotein CA-19-9 may be promising for the detection of cholangiocarcinoma complicating PSC. Indeed, eight of nine patients (89%) with PSC and cholangiocarcinoma had a significant elevation in CA-19-9 levels compared to a group of PSC patients without known cholangiocarcinoma[30]. Further prospective study to evaluate the usefulness of CA-19-9 as a screening test for PSC with early and potentially curable cholangiocarcinoma is presently under way.

NATURAL HISTORY

Information regarding the natural history of PSC continues to evolve. However, given our lack of knowledge of the pathogenesis of PSC, the unavailability of serological markers for diagnosis, and the unpredictable nature of the syndrome, defining the natural history and prognosis of PSC has been difficult. Nevertheless, on the basis of a number of prospective studies, there is growing evidence that PSC frequently is a progressive disease[23]. The largest of these studies, from the Mayo Clinic, reported on 174 patients with documented PSC who had a mean follow-up of 6.0 years[2]. The median survival from the time of diagnosis of PSC was 11.9 years, and both symptomatic and asymptomatic patients had a shorter survival as compared to a US population matched for age, sex, and race. In this study we found 31% of patients died as a result of underlying liver disease or the development of cholangiocarcinoma; an additional 10% were referred for liver transplantation. These findings have been confirmed by a number of other centres which have reported median survival from the time of diagnosis of PSC to be between 9 and 11 years.

A subgroup of patients with PSC without symptoms at the time of diagnosis has also been evaluated[31]. At the Mayo Clinic, 45 patients with PSC without symptoms had a mean follow-up of 6.25 years. During this follow-up period, 76% had evidence of progression of disease on the basis of clinical and pathological findings, and 31% developed liver failure resulting in death or the need for liver transplantation. However, other institutions have found PSC to be a more benign disease. Helzberg *et al.*, at Yale, reported a 75% 9-year survival, and studies from Norway estimated the mean survival of patients with PSC to be 17 years from the time of diagnosis[32,33]. Reasons for these differences have recently been put into perspective[34]. First, PSC progresses silently for a number of years and can be detected only by prospective follow-up of liver function tests and hepatic histology; observations which were not performed in a number of these studies. Second, early detection of the disease would be associated with prolonged survival, which seems to be the case in the Norwegian studies, in which patients with inflammatory bowel disease who had minimal abnormalities in liver function tests were aggressively evaluated with cholangiography. Third, the starting point for survival analysis is important in determining overall survival time. Comparing one group of patients in whom follow-up began at the time of cholangiographic diagnosis of PSC with a second group of patients in whom a diagnosis of PSC was backdated to the time of first onset of symptoms or biochemical abnormalities would obviously lead to differences in overall survival time. Therefore, if these differences in study design are taken into account, we believe the weight of evidence indicates that PSC is indeed a progressive disease, and that therapeutic intervention should be evaluated in the early as well as in the later stages of this syndrome.

PSC PROGNOSTIC SURVIVAL MODELS

One of the main purposes of analysing the natural history of PSC is to more accurately determine its rate of progression, and to be able to estimate survival for the individual patient at any particular point in the course of his/her disease. Predicting survival based on clinical, biochemical, and histological features of PSC is also very important for the timing of liver transplantation and for monitoring therapeutic intervention. The use of sophisticated statistical approaches, most notably the Cox multivariate regression analysis, has enabled us to develop a prognostic model based on five independent variables in which a risk score can be calculated and translated into a survival function to estimate survival for the individual patient with PSC[2]. In the Mayo PSC model the important clinical variables identified are age, serum bilirubin, haemoglobin, hepatic histological stage, and the presence or absence of inflammatory bowel disease. More recently, by combining data from a number of other clinical centres interested in PSC, a more refined model has been established in which age, bilirubin, presence or absence of splenomegaly, and histological stage represent the key diagnostic clinical variables[35].

A second PSC model was recently developed by the King's College group. Multivariate analysis revealed hepatomegaly, splenomegaly, serum alkaline phosphatase level, histological stage, and age to be independent predictors of prognosis[3]. While these and other models provide some objective evidence with regard to disease progression and estimation of survival in the individual PSC patient, additional studies are already under way to cross-validate these models, and to assess the application to the timing of liver transplantation and in monitoring the effect of experimental therapy on disease progression.

Table 2 Therapy for primary sclerosing cholangitis

Biochemical			
Cupruritic	*Immunosuppressive*	*Antifibrinogenic*	*Choleretic*
D-Penicillamine*	Corticosteroids	Colchicine	Ursodeoxycholic acid*
	Cyclosporin A*		
	FK506		
	Methotrexate*		
	Azathioprine		
Radiological			
Balloon dilatation with stenting			
Biliary lavage with steroids			
Surgical			
Biliary reconstructive surgery			
Proctocolectomy			
Liver transplantation			

*Controlled trial performed

MEDICAL THERAPY

Medical therapy to halt the progression of PSC has centred on the use of cupruretic, antifibrinogenic, immunosuppressive, and anticholestatic agents[36]. To date, four agents have been evaluated in controlled clinical trials, which include D-penicillamine, cyclosporin A, methotrexate, and ursodeoxycholic acid. In addition, uncontrolled studies have evaluated corticosteroids, azathioprine, biliary lavage with steroids, FK506, cholestyramine, and antibiotic therapy. While two of these therapies, namely ursodeoxycholic acid and methotrexate therapy, have been reported to be associated with temporary improvement in biochemical liver tests, and some have been associated with improvement in symptoms of fatigue and pruritus, none has had a major impact on histological progression of disease or on time to the development of complications related to portal hypertension. Furthermore, it appears that none of these agents has had a major impact on improving survival. Presently, drugs such as ursodeoxycholic acid and methotrexate have generated considerable enthusiasm.

With regard to ursodeoxycholic acid therapy there are a number of uncontrolled reports suggesting improvement in biochemical parameters of liver function, as well as improvement in symptoms. However, none of these therapies has had a major impact on halting histological progression or time to the progression of complications of portal hypertension. The most recent report from Oxford indicates, in fact, that ursodeoxycholic acid therapy had little or no effect on decreasing histological progression[37].

Other investigators have used low-dose methotrexate, 15 mg/week, and have claimed associated improvement in biochemical liver tests and stabilization of bile duct scarring and hepatic histological progression[38]. However, in carefully analysing these data it appears that methotrexate therapy may be effective only in the earlier stages of disease, and may have little or no effect on those patients who have cirrhotic stage disease. Clearly, other than showing improvement in biochemical liver studies, methotrexate has not been shown conclusively to decrease histological progression or to prevent complications of portal hypertension. Furthermore, the hepatotoxic potential and the demonstrated lung toxicity associated with methotrexate therapy mandates the use of this agent only in controlled trials, with careful follow-up until effectiveness and safety have been fully confirmed.

In summary, we continue to look for medical therapies which will conclusively improve symptoms related to PSC, improve biochemical liver function tests, halt histological progression of the disease, reverse biliary stricturing, prolong time to complications of portal hypertension, and prolong survival. While no single agent appears to have had a major impact on this disease, it is attractive to consider evaluating combinations of drugs, such as ursodeoxycholic acid and methotrexate, two drugs which independently have shown promising results.

RECONSTRUCTIVE BILIARY TRACT SURGERY

We consider choledochoduodenostomy or choledochojejunostomy for PSC in the same light as radiological balloon dilatation of dominant strictures: specifically, as palliative therapy to alleviate symptoms. Unfortunately, no good published data exist presenting confident evaluation of surgical procedures for the treatment of PSC. Our data suggest that surgery has no beneficial effect on the natural history of PSC, particularly if performed in patients with cirrhotic stage disease. In addition, bouts of bacterial cholangitis have developed postoperatively in more than 60% of patients undergoing such surgical procedures in some series. However, data from an uncontrolled trial suggest that patients with severe hilar or extrahepatic biliary stricturing and persistent jaundice or cholangitis, but without cirrhosis, may benefit from biliary reconstruction and long-term transhepatic stenting[39]. A second report describes PSC treated by creating a choledochojejunostomy or hepaticojejunostomy and a choledochojejunocutaneous fistula created for repeated postoperative balloon dilatation[40]. It is thought that this approach avoids the necessity of long-term transhepatic stenting. Of 16 patients treated with this procedure, 14 survived the operation, and there were two late deaths. However, cholangitis continued to be a major problem in the survivors, and at this time this procedure cannot be recommended without further evaluation.

PROCTOCOLECTOMY

The question of whether proctocolectomy in PSC patients with CUC may favourably affect hepatobiliary disease is important, because there is no beneficial therapy for PSC at this time. However, it is known that such surgery may be associated with considerable morbidity from the development of peristomal varices after ileostomy[41].

This question was recently addressed by a prospective follow-up of 45 PSC patients who had CUC, of whom 20 had undergone proctocolectomy[42]. In this study proctocolectomy had no apparent effect on clinical, biochemical, hepatic histological or radiological features of PSC. Additionally, proctocolectomy had no effect on overall survival. From this study we concluded that proctocolectomy of PSC is not beneficial for patients who had PSC. However, since most of our patients had advanced histological stage (stage 4 – cirrhotic stage disease) on liver biopsy, we cannot exclude the possibility that proctocolectomy performed earlier in the course of the disease might be beneficial.

At present we believe proctocolectomy should not be performed simply to remove the colon in a patient with PSC in anticipation of having a beneficial effect on liver disease. Obviously, if carcinoma or precancerous lesions develop in the colon, a proctocolectomy is indicated. We further believe that patients who require a proctocolectomy and are potential liver transplant candidates should undergo an ileal–anal anastomosis to avoid the potential formation of peristomal varices, and to eliminate the constant threat of bacterial contamination from the ileostomy at the time of liver transplantation. In our series of 40 patients with PSC who had an ileal–rectal pull-through procedure, with a mean follow-up of 45 months, none of the patients developed perianal bleeding or bleeding related to portal hypertension. In comparison, in a group of 32 patients having a Brooke ileostomy, 26% developed bleeding from peristomal varices. Thus, it appears that performing an ileal–anal pull-through procedure has major advantages over the traditional Brooke ileostomy in patients undergoing proctocolectomy who have PSC[29,43,44].

LIVER TRANSPLANTATION

The treatment of choice for patients with endstage PSC is liver transplantation. Recent results show that patients with PSC undergoing liver transplantation have an 85% 1-year survival and a 75% 3-year survival[29,44,45]. However, in our experience we have found that patients with primary sclerosing cholangitis have what appear to be an increased incidence of chronic ductopenic rejection and graft loss from rejection, and an increased incidence of biliary stricturing. We have found evidence of recurrence of PSC in five of 32 patients who have undergone liver transplantation at our institution[46]. However, it remains difficult to conclusively attribute the biliary stricturing to recurrent PSC since the bile duct strictures may be attributable to low-grade bacterial cholangitis, which could be related to the Roux-en-Y biliary anastomosis that is routinely performed in PSC patients as compared to a choledochocholedochostomy biliary anastomosis that is performed in other liver transplant patients. In addition, rejection, ischaemia, ABO mismatch, and possibly cytomegalovirus or other viral infections are known to be able to contribute to biliary stricturing after liver transplantation.

Therefore, the waters are muddy with regard to the question of whether PSC recurs following liver transplantation, and more long-term follow-up data will be needed.

References

1. Wiesner RH, LaRusso NF. Clinicopathic features of the syndrome of primary sclerosing cholangitis. Gastroenterology. 1980;79:200–6.
2. Wiesner RH, Grambsch PM, Dickson ER *et al.* Primary sclerosing cholangitis: natural history, prognostic factors, and survival analysis. Hepatology. 1989;10(4):430–7.
3. Farrant JM, Hayllar KM, Wilkinson ML *et al.* The natural history and prognostic variables in primary sclerosing cholangitis. Gastroenterology. 1991;100:1710–17.
4. MacCarty RL, LaRusso NF, Wiesner RH, Ludwig J. Primary sclerosing cholangitis: findings on cholangiography and pancreatography. Radiology. 1983;149:39–44.
5. Elias E, Summerfield JA, Dick R, Sherlock S. Endoscopic retrograde cholangiopancreatograph in the diagnosis of jaundice with ulcerative colitis. Gastroenterology. 1974;67: 907–11.
6. LaRusso NF, Wiesner RH, Ludwig J, MacCarty RL. Primary sclerosing cholangitis. N Engl J Med. 1984;310:899–903.
7. Fausa O, Schrumpf E, Elgjo K. Relationship of inflammatory bowel disease and primary sclerosing cholangitis. Semin Liv Dis. 1991;11:31–9.
8. Balasubramaniam K, Wiesner RH, LaRusso NF. Primary sclerosing cholangitis with normal serum levels of alkaline phosphatase. Gastroenterology. 1988;95:1395–8.
9. Gross JB, Ludwig J, Wiesner RH *et al.* Abnormalities in tests of copper metabolism in primary sclerosing cholangitis. Gastroenterology. 1985;8:272–8.
10. Wiesner RH, LaRusso NF, Ludwig J, Dickson ER. Comparison of clinicopathologic features of primary sclerosing cholangitis and primary biliary cirrhosis. Gastroenterology. 1985;88:108–14.
11. Crippin JS, Lindor KD. Primary sclerosing cholangitis: etiology and immunology. Eur J Gastroenterol Hepatol. 1992;4:261–5.
12. Ludwig J, MacCarty RL, LaRusso NF *et al.* Intrahepatic cholangiectases and large-duct obliteration in primary sclerosing cholangitis. Hepatology. 1986;6:560–8.
13. Ludwig J, LaRusso NF, Wiesner RH. The syndrome of primary sclerosing cholangitis. Prog Liv Dis. 1990;9:555–66.
14. Fleming KA. The hepatobiliary pathology of primary sclerosing cholangitis. Eur J Gastroenterol Hepatol. 1992;4:266–71.
15. Ludwig J. Small-duct primary sclerosing cholangitis. Semin Liver Dis. 1991;11:11–17.
16. Quigley EM, LaRusso NF, Ludwig J *et al.* Familial occurrence of primary sclerosing cholangitis and ulcerative colitis. Gastroenterology. 1983;85:1160–5.
17. Chapman RW, Varghese Z, Gaul R *et al.* Association of primary sclerosing cholangitis with HLA-B8. Gut. 1983;24:38–41.
18. Prochazka EJ, Terasaki PI, Park MS *et al.* Association of primary sclerosing cholangitis with HLA-DRW52a. N Engl J Med. 1990;32:1842–4.
19. Magrin S, Nouri-Aria KT, Donaldson PT *et al.* The relationship between HLA-DR3 and T-cell regulation of immunoglobulin production in primary sclerosing cholangitis. Clin Immunol Immunopathol. 1989;50:205–12.
20. Chapman RW, Kelly PM, Heryet A *et al.* Expression of HLA-DR antigens on bile duct epithelium in primary sclerosing cholangitis. Gut. 1988;29:422–7.
21. Lindor KD, Wiesner RH, LaRusso NF, Homburger HA. Enhanced autoreactivity of T-lymphocytes in primary sclerosing cholangitis. Hepatology. 1987;7:884–8.
22. Whiteside TL, Lasky S, Si L, Van Thiel DH. Immunologic analysis of mononuclear cells in liver tissues and blood of patients with primary sclerosing cholangitis. Hepatology. 1985;5:468–74.
23. Sartin JS, Wiesner RH, LaRusso NF. Fat-soluble vitamin deficiencies in primary sclerosing cholangitis. Gastroenterology. 1987;92:1615 (abstract).
24. Hay JE, Lindor KD, Wiesner RH *et al.* The metabolic bone disease of primary sclerosing cholangitis. Hepatology. 1991;14:257–61.

25. Hay JE, Wiesner RH, Shore RG *et al.* Primary sclerosing cholangitis and celiac disease. A novel association. Ann Intern Med. 1988;109:713–17.
26. Borkje B, Vetvik K, Odegaard S *et al.* Chronic pancreatitis in patients with sclerosing cholangitis and ulcerative colitis. Scand J Gastroenterol. 1985;20:539–42.
27. Bender CE, Wiesner RH, LeRoy AJ. Clinical improvements following percutaneous balloon dilatation of dominant bile duct strictures in primary sclerosing cholangitis. Gastroenterology. 1992;102:780 (abstract).
28. Rosen CB, Nagorney DM, Wiesner RH *et al.* Cholangiocarcinoma complicating primary sclerosing cholangitis. Ann Surg. 1991;213(1):21–5.
29. Marsh JW Jr, Iwatsuji S, Makowka L *et al.* Orthotopic liver transplantation for primary sclerosing cholangitis. Ann Surg. 1988;207:21–5.
30. Nichols JC, Gores GJ, LaRusso NF *et al.* Diagnostic role of CA 19-9 for cholangiocarcinoma in primary sclerosing cholangitis. Hepatology. 1992;16:62A (abstract).
31. Porayko MK, Wiesner RH, LaRusso NF *et al.* Patients with asymptomatic primary sclerosing cholangitis frequently have a progressive disease. Gastroenterology. 1990;98: 1594–602.
32. Helzberg JH, Petersen JM, Boyer JL. Improved survival with primary sclerosing cholangitis. A review of clinicopathologic features and comparison of symptomatic and asymptomatic patients. Gastroenterology. 1987;92:1869–75.
33. Aadland E, Schrumpf E, Fausa O *et al.* Primary sclerosing cholangitis: a long-term follow-up study. Scand J Gastroenterol. 1987;22:655–64.
34. Porayko MK, LaRusso NF, Wiesner RH. Primary sclerosing cholangitis: a progressive disease? Semin Liver Dis. 1991;11(1):18–25.
35. Dickson ER, Murtaugh P, Grambsch PM *et al.* Primary sclerosing cholangitis: refinement and validation of survival models. Gastroenterology. 1992; 103:1893–901.
36. Wiesner RH. Advances in therapy for primary sclerosing cholangitis. Eur J Gastroenterol Hepatol. 1992;4:276–83.
37. Chapman RW. Primary sclerosing cholangitis. J Hepatol. 1985;1:179–86.
38. Knox TA, Kaplan MM. Treatment of primary sclerosing cholangitis with oral methotrexate. Am J Gastroenterol. 1991;86:546–52.
39. Cameron JL, Pitt HA, Zinner MJ *et al.* Resection of hepatic duct bifurcation and transhepatic stenting for sclerosing cholangitis. Ann Surg. 1988;207:614–22.
40. Hutson DG, Russell E, Schiff E *et al.* Balloon dilatation of biliary strictures through a choledochojejuno-cutaneous fistula. Ann Surg. 1984;199:637–47.
41. Wiesner RH, LaRusso NF, Dozois RR, Beaver SJ. Peristomal varices after proctocolectomy in patients with primary sclerosing cholangitis. Gastroenterology. 1986;90:316–22.
42. Cangemi JR, Wiesner RH, Beaver SJ *et al.* Effect of proctocolectomy for chronic ulcerative colitis on the natural history of primary sclerosing cholangitis. Gastroenterology. 1989;96:790–4.
43. Kartheuser AH, Dozois RR, LaRusso NF *et al.* Peristomal variceal bleeding after proctocolectomy for ulcerative colitis in patients with primary sclerosing cholangitis can be avoided by ileal pouch-anal anastomosis. Gastroenterology. 1991;100:220 (abstract).
44. Langnas AN, Grazi GL, Stratta RJ *et al.* Primary sclerosing cholangitis: the emerging role of liver transplantion. Am J Gastroenterol. 1990;85:1136–41.
45. McEntee G, Wiesner RH, Rosen C *et al.* A comparative study of patients undergoing liver transplantation for primary sclerosing cholangitis and primary biliary cirrhosis. Transplant Proc. 1991;23:1563–4.
46. Hunter EB, Wiesner RH, MacCarty JL *et al.* Does primary sclerosing cholangitis recur after liver transplantation? Gastroenterology. 1989;96(5):A610.

34
Immunohistology of primary sclerosing cholangitis

P. VAN EYKEN and V. J. DESMET

INTRODUCTION

Primary sclerosing cholangitis (PSC) is a syndrome of unknown aetiology characterized by chronic inflammation and fibrosis of the biliary tree. Routine histological examination of liver biopsies is essential in the diagnosis and treatment of this disorder. The use of immunohistochemical techniques may help in diagnosing PSC. Moreover, they have provided more insight into the pathological mechanisms operative in this chronic cholestatic disease. This chapter is based upon data from the literature, supplemented by observations made by the authors on a small series (five cases) of liver biopsies of patients suffering from PSC. The biopsies were studied on paraffin as well as on cryostat sections using a broad panel of monoclonal and polyclonal antibodies directed against cytokeratins, lymphocyte surface antigens, extracellular matrix components and adhesion molecules.

HISTOPATHOLOGY AND STAGING OF PSC

PSC can be classified as 'large duct' or 'small duct' PSC[1]. In the former, large cholangiographically identifiable bile ducts are involved showing a typical 'beaded' appearance. The latter (formerly termed 'pericholangitis'[2,3]) is characterized by involvement of interlobular and septal bile ducts. Large duct PSC may be accompanied by small duct PSC and vice-versa[1]. Ducts of the calibre affected by large duct PSC are not comprised in liver biopsies. The diagnosis is based primarily on cholangiography (usually endoscopic retrograde cholangiopancreatography)[1]. Conversely, since interlobular and septal bile ducts cannot be evaluated on cholangiography, liver biopsy is needed to establish a diagnosis of small duct PSC[1].

The most suggestive histopathological lesion of PSC is a concentric periductal fibrosis that may lead to strangulation, progressive atrophy and eventual disappearance of the duct[4,5] (Fig. 1). This lesion corresponds to the

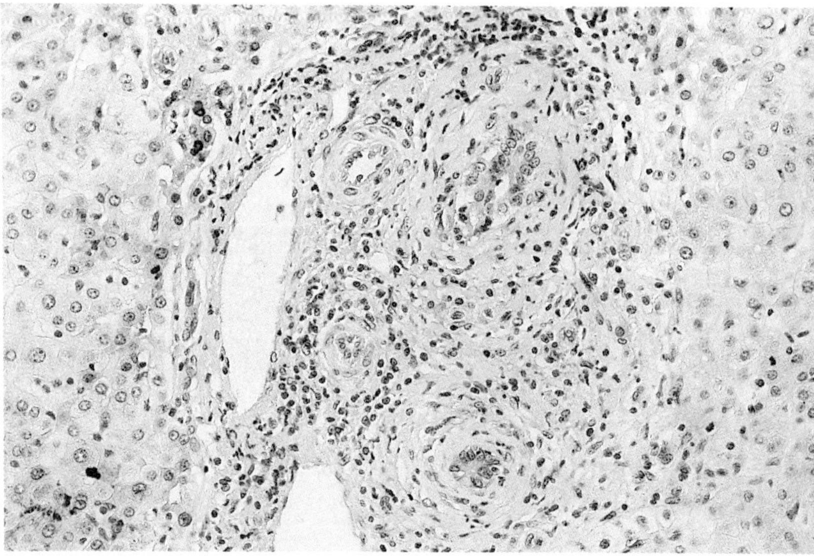

Fig. 1 PSC. A portal tract contains a predominantly mononuclear inflammatory cell infiltrate. Interlobular bile ducts are surrounded by concentric layers of connective tissue. Biliary epithelial cell damage is evidenced by vacuolation of the cytoplasm of some cells and the presence of a few pycnotic nuclei. (H&E, × 260)

'fibro-obliterating cholangitis'[6]. PSC thus leads to progressive disappearance of intrahepatic bile duct radicles and as such belongs to the group of 'vanishing bile duct diseases'[4,7,8]. It has to be emphasized that the above-described histological lesions are present in only 40–60% of cases and are non-specific. Indeed, concentric periductal fibrosis may also be seen in the later stages of primary biliary cirrhosis[9].

PSC is a progressive disease, even in asymptomatic patients[10]. Prognosis is determined primarily by the parenchymal changes seen in biopsy specimens; therefore staging is based on biopsy features[1]. The first stage (portal stage) is characterized by portal inflammation with some oedema and fibrosis and proliferation of ductules. Some ducts may show degenerative changes. Periportal hepatocytes rarely contain a few granules of copper or copper binding protein. In stage 2 (periportal stage), portal tracts become enlarged. There is ductular proliferation and focal ductopenia may already be noted. Stage 3 (septal stage) is characterized by portal-to-portal bridging by fibrous septa and corresponds to biliary fibrosis. Further disease progression leads to biliary cirrhosis with formation of regenerative nodules (stage 4, cirrhotic stage). In stage 4, ductopenia may be very pronounced. In stages 3 and 4, PSC and primary biliary cirrhosis often cannot be distinguished by histology alone[1,5]. The rationale for staging is based on the observation that clinical course and outcome are not determined by the bile duct changes *per se*. Especially in large duct PSC, severe cholangiographic abnormalities may coexist with only mild parenchymal abnormalities and clinical wellness. The course of PSC is indeed determined by the progression from a portal stage to a final cirrhotic stage, as described above. It should be mentioned that a recent study indicates that cholangiographic findings may also be of value in determining prognosis[11].

IMMUNOHISTOLOGY OF PSC

Identification of bile ducts in tissue sections

As discussed above, ductopenia is an important histological feature of PSC (and the other 'vanishing bile duct diseases'). When examining a liver biopsy one should keep in mind that normal portal tracts contain an interlobular bile duct, the diameter of which roughly corresponds to that of the adjacent branch of the artery[12]. However, it is often difficult to ascertain whether a bile duct is present or not in inflamed portal tracts.

Immunohistochemical staining techniques may be used to visualize to a better extent bile ducts in tissue sections. A widely used and reliable technique uses antibodies directed against cytokeratins (CK)[13,14]. The latter are the intermediate filament type characteristic of epithelial cells[15–17]. Using two-dimensional gel electrophoresis, Moll *et al.*[16,18] have identified and catalogued 20 different CK polypeptides which are expressed in different combinations by human epithelia. Human liver parenchymal cells contain only CK8 and 18, whereas biliary epithelial cells express in addition CK7 and 19. The latter two polypeptides can therefore be considered markers of the biliary cell lineage in the liver[19–21]. Monoclonal and polyclonal antibodies directed against single or several CKs are commercially available and can be used on cryostat and/or paraffin sections[13]. Since bile duct cells possess several phenotypic characteristics that distinguish them from hepatocytes (for review see refs 22 and 23), antibodies reactive with such proteins (e.g. tissue polypeptide antigen TPA, epithelial membrane antigen EMA[22,24]) or surface markers[19] can theoretically be used to stain bile ducts in histological sections.

Ductular proliferation and the concept of ductular metaplasia of hepatocytes

Various liver diseases, including PSC, are characterized by an increased number of ductular structures[25,26]. The origin of this ductular 'proliferation' has been, and continues to be, subject to debate (for review see refs 20, 21 and 27). Some authors claim that the ductules are derived from pre-existent ducts, whereas others claim that they are derived from hepatocytes through a process of 'transdifferentiation'. The latter concept is also referred to as 'ductular metaplasia of hepatocytes' (for review see refs 21 and 27). The two mechanisms are by no means mutually exclusive. The available evidence indicates that in acute bile duct obstruction (e.g. bile duct ligation in the rat) the increased number of ductules is indeed the result of actual cell proliferation[20,28]. In long-standing cholestatic conditions such as PSC and

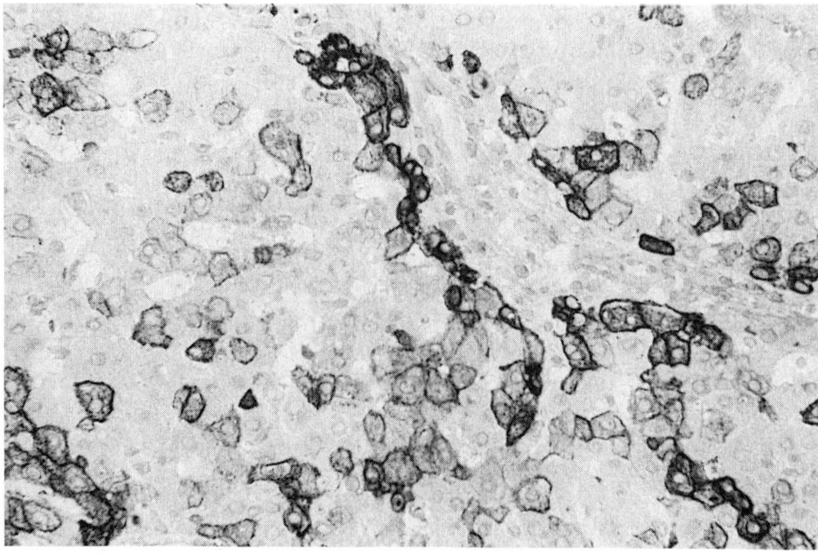

Fig. 2 PSC. Numerous liver parenchymal cells in acinar zone 1 are immunoreactive for CK7. Note the apparent continuity between some CK7-positive hepatocytes and ductular structures at the portal tract–parenchymal interface (cryostat section, indirect immunoperoxidase, counterstained with Mayer's haemalum, × 260)

primary biliary cirrhosis there is a large amount of evidence indicating that liver parenchymal cells can change their phenotype and can acquire phenotypic characteristics of bile duct cells[20,21,27]. We have previously shown that in chronic cholestasis, including PSC, hepatocytes of acinar zone 1 (periportal zone) can become immunoreactive for CK 7[29]. CK7-positive liver parenchymal cells were often in apparent continuity with ductules at the portal tract–parenchymal interface (Fig. 2). The number of hepatocytes showing a positive staining for CK7 also increased with the stage of the disease[29]. In advanced PSC and primary biliary cirrhosis, a few hepatocytes expressed in addition CK 19[29]. These observations provide strong arguments in favour of the gradual transformation of hepatocytes into bile duct cells. It should be emphasized that these changes are not unique to PSC, but occur in long-standing cholestasis regardless of aetiology. The factors inducing the gradual phenotypic transformation of hepatocytes into bile duct-type cells are unknown at present, but it is likely that the extracellular matrix plays an important – albeit not the only – role[20,30].

The role of immune mechanisms in PSC

Immunhistochemistry has been used to study the distribution of B and T lymphocytes and the expression of MHC molecules on bile ducts in PSC. Most of the mononuclear cells infiltrating the portal tracts in PSC livers belong to the T-cell lineage[31–34]. In a study on end-stage (cirrhotic) PSC livers, $CD8^+$ T cells (suppressor/cytotoxic subset) tended to localize in areas of bile duct proliferation and infiltrated the ductal epithelium[33]. $CD4^+$ T cells (helper/inducer subset) were generally found on the parenchymal side of fibrosed tissue[33]. Snook *et al.*[34] however, who studied pre-cirrhotic PSC patients, failed to find this differential distribution of both T-cell subsets. In a small series of PSC livers (five specimens) the vast majority of T cells were immunoreactive with the monoclonal antibody UCHL1 (CD45RO), indicating that they correspond to memory T cells (personal observation). 2H4 (CD45RA) positive 'naive' T cells were virtually absent (Fig. 3). Volpes *et al.*[35] have previously shown that, in chronic hepatitis, memory T cells represent the predominant subset.

In PSC the intrahepatic bile ducts show an enhanced expression of HLA class I antigen and a *de-novo* expression of HLA-DR[36,37]. The latter occurs from relatively early stages of histological damage on[36]. Using a monoclonal antibody directed to the α-chains of HLA-DR antigens on fixed, paraffin-embedded liver specimens, Nakanuma and Kono[38] found positive staining of interlobular bile ducts in PSC in only two out of five cases. Using cryostat sections, Broomé *et al.*[39] found immunoreactivity of the biliary epithelium for HLA-DR and HLA-DP in all cases studied. HLA-DQ was expressed less frequently and less intensely (only 3/8 cases positive). The aberrant expression of HLA-DR antigens on the biliary epithelial cells may enable the cell to present foreign or autoantigens to T lymphocytes[31,32,37]. The possibility remains that the expression of HLA-DR is only a secondary phenomenon, since it occurs in cholestatic liver disease of various aetiologies[31,32,38]. Interestingly, *de-novo* expression of class II molecules was also observed in an experimental model of sclerosing cholangitis involving the injection of formalin into the common bile duct of rats[40]. Treatment with ursodeoxycholic acid does not affect the expression of HLA class I or II molecules on biliary epithelial cells, but reduces HLA class I expression on hepatocytes[41].

Ballardini *et al.*[42] reported the presence of Langerhans cells around and among class II positive bile duct cells in PSC. Demetris *et al.*[43] found occasional intra-epithelial S-100 positive dendritic cells, but fewer in number and less prevalent than in primary biliary cirrhosis. This would indicate the presence of 'professional' antigen-presenting cells in PSC livers. However, only a small number of cases have been studied. Recently, attention has begun to focus on the expression of various adhesion molecules in liver diseases, including PSC. Adams *et al.*[44] found a strong expression of the intercellular adhesion molecule 1 (ICAM-1, which is the ligand for the leucocyte adhesion receptor lymphocyte function associated antigen 1 or LFA-1) on interlobular bile ducts and proliferating bile ductules in PSC. Surprisingly, another group of investigators reported a lack of expression of ICAM-1 on bile duct epithelial cells in PSC[45]. The reasons for this discrepancy are not clear.

The data discussed above are usually interpreted as indicative of the role of immune factors in the pathogenesis of PSC. However, various non-immune factors may also play a role (for review see ref. 46).

A

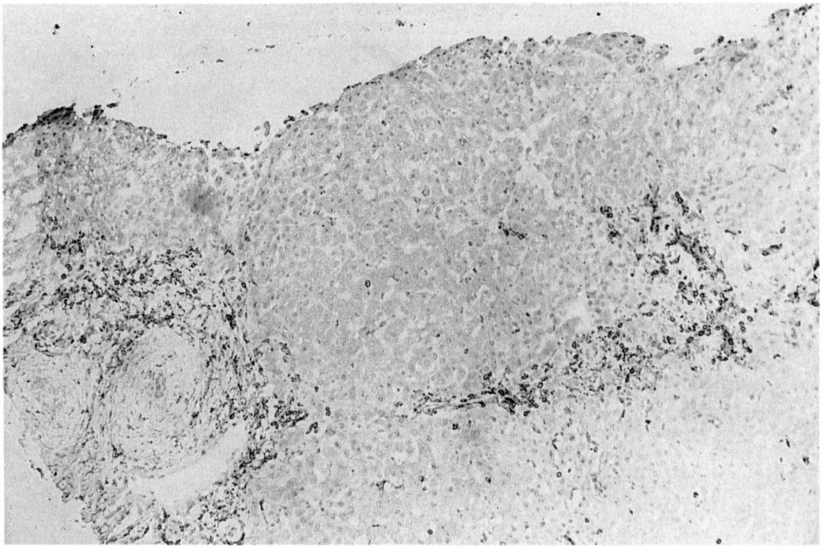

B

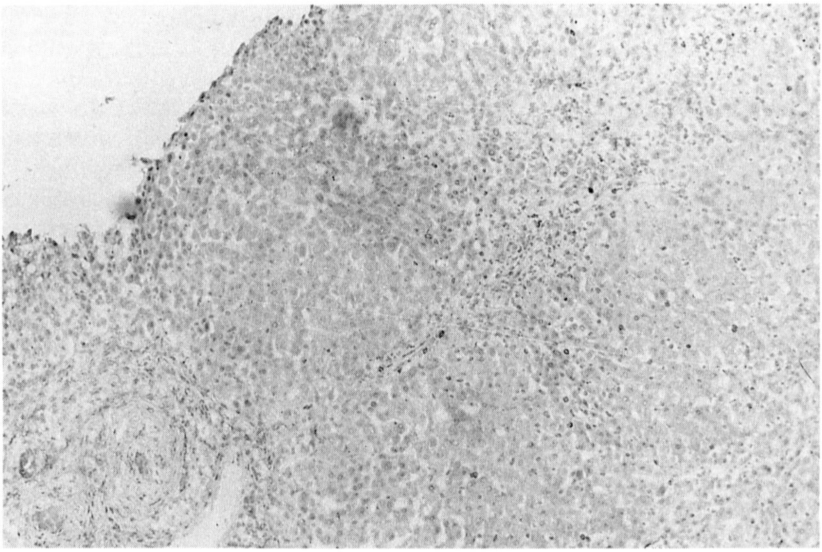

Fig. 3 Distribution of 'naive' and 'memory' T cells in PSC. Most mononuclear cells infiltrating the portal tracts are UCHL1-positive 'memory' T cells (**A**). A serially cut section reveals that 2H4 'naive' T cells are almost lacking (**B**) (cryostat sections, indirect immunoperoxidase, counterstained with Mayer's haemalum, × 260)

The extracellular matrix

Disease progression in PSC is accompanied by an increase in connective tissue components ('fibrogenesis') leading to liver fibrosis and culminating in cirrhosis. A large amount of information has accumulated on the biochemistry and *in-situ* distribution of the various constituents of the extracellular matrix (collagens, proteoglycans and non-collagenous glycoproteins) of both the normal and fibrotic liver[47–49]. We have recently reported that the extracellular matrix glycoprotein tenascin accumulates between the ductules at the portal tract–parenchymal interface in various diseases including PSC[50]. Interestingly, this protein is normally absent from portal tracts and is also absent from 'mature' fibrous septa. Therefore, tenascin might play a role in early matrix organization[50]. Tenascin also accumulates around interlobular bile ducts in PSC (personal observation, Fig. 4). In rat liver, fat-storing cells produce and secrete tenascin[51,52]. In PSC we have observed α-smooth muscle actin positive cells (probably corresponding to activated fat-storing cells and active portal fibroblasts[53]) between cells of the proliferating ductules as well as in concentric layers around interlobular bile ducts (Fig. 4). It is thus likely that, also in human liver, activated fat-storing cells and activated portal fibroblasts are the cellular source of tenascin. In rat liver, following bile duct ligation, tenascin rapidly appears around interlobular bile ducts and subsequently between ductular structures at the portal tract–parenchymal interface[54,55]. α-Smooth muscle actin positive cells are found in the areas where immunoreactive tenascin is demonstrable[54,55]. The observations made in PSC livers thus closely parallel the findings in rat liver.

PSC and cholangiocarcinoma

Patients with PSC are at an increased risk for developing cholangiocarcinoma (for review see refs 56–58). Cholangiocarcinoma arises in 5–10% of patients with pre-existing PSC and (less frequently) can also present in a synchronous fashion with PSC[56]. Tumours are often multifocal[57]. Areas of carcinoma *in situ* were found in seven out of eight cases by Wee *et al.*[57], and in 100% of cases by Miros *et al.*[58]. Dysplastic biliary epithelium showed both cytoplasmic and luminal staining for carcinoembryonic antigen CEA, whereas normal bile duct cells only display apical positivity[58]. Immunohistochemical staining may thus be of value in identifying dysplastic foci[58].

Acknowledgements

The secretarial assistance of Marjan Veulemans-Weckx, and the photographic assistance of Michel Rooseleers, are gratefully acknowledged. Thanks are due to Paula Aertsen and Suzanne Taelemans for performing the immunohistochemical stainings. The authors are indebted to Jos Mebis for help in editing the references.

A
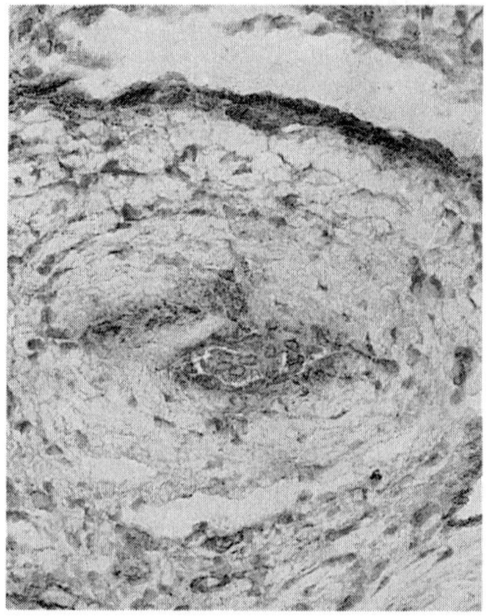

B
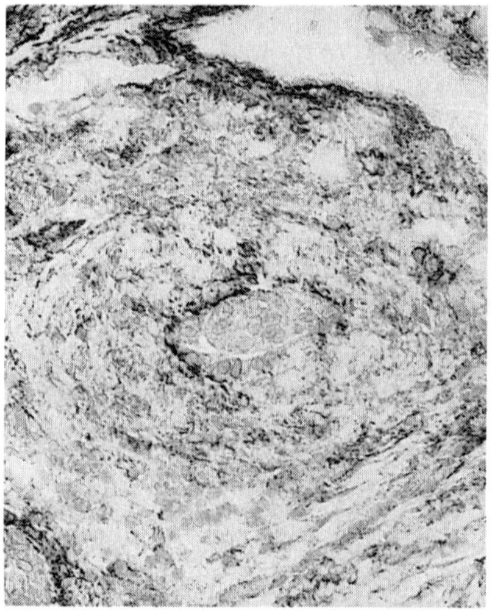

Fig. 4 PSC. Immunoreactivity for tenascin is found beneath the damaged epithelium of a bile duct showing concentric periduct fibrosis (**A**). A serially cut section shows layers of α-smooth muscle actin-positive cells surrounding the biliary epithelium (**B**) (cryostat sections, indirect immunoperoxidase, counterstained with Mayer's haemalum, × 300)

References

1. Ludwig J. Small-duct primary sclerosing cholangitis. Semin Liver Dis. 1991;11:11–17.
2. Mistilis SP. Pericholangitis and ulcerative colitis. I. Pathology, etiology and pathogenesis. Ann Intern Med. 1965;63:1–16.
3. Wee A, Ludwig J. Pericholangitis in chronic ulcerative colitis: primary sclerosing cholangitis of the small bile ducts? Ann Intern Med. 1985;102:581–7.

4. Desmet VJ. Cholangiopathies: past, present and future. Semin Liver Dis. 1987;7:67–76.
5. Desmet VJ. Vanishing bile duct disorders. Prog Liver Dis. 1992;10:89–121
6. Ludwig J, Czaja AJ, Dickson R, Larusso NF, Wiesner RH. Manifestations of nonsuppurative cholangitis in chronic hepatobiliary diseases: morphologic spectrum, clinical correlations and terminology. Liver. 1984;4:105–16.
7. Sherlock S. The syndrome of disappearing intrahepatic bile ducts. Lancet. 1987;2:493–5.
8. Desmet VJ. Pathologie der intrahepatischen Gallengänge. Z Gastroenterol. 1989;27: 638–48.
9. Nakanuma Y, Ohta G. Histometric and serial section observations of the intrahepatic bile ducts in primary biliary cirrhosis. Gastroenterology. 1979;76:1326–32.
10. Porayko MK, LaRusso NF, Wiesner RH. Primary sclerosing cholangitis: a progressive disease? Semin Liver Dis. 1991;11:18–25.
11. Craig DA, MacCarty RL, Wiesner RH, Grambsch PM, LaRusso NF. Primary sclerosing cholangitis: value of cholangiography in determining the prognosis. Am J Radiol. 1991;157:959–64.
12. International Group. Histopathology of the intrahepatic biliary tree. Liver. 1983;3:161–75.
13. Van Eyken P, Sciot R, Van Damme B, De Wolf-Peeters C, Desmet VJ. Keratin-immunohistochemistry in normal human liver. Cytokeratin pattern of hepatocytes, bile ducts and acinar gradient. Virchows Arch [A]. 1987;412:63–72.
14. De Lellis RA, Bhan I, Mueller J, Kwan P, Cho S, Hull D, Reinhold R, Fawaz K, Kaplan M. The use of keratin antibodies in the assessment of rejection in orthotopic liver transplants. Hepatology. 1986;6:1194.
15. Alberts B, Bray D, Lewis J, Raff M, Roberts K, Watson JD. The cytoskeleton. In: Alberts B, Bray D, Lewis J, Raff M, Roberts K, Watson JD, editors. Molecular biology of the cell. New York, London: Garland Publishing; 1989:613–80.
16. Moll R, Franke WW, Schiller DA, Geiger B, Krepler R. The catalog of human cytokeratins: patterns of expression in normal epithelia, tumors and cultured cells. Cell. 1982;31:11–24.
17. Steinert PM, Roop DR. Molecular and cellular biology of intermediate filaments. Ann Rev Biochem. 1988;57:523–5.
18. Moll R, Schiller DL, Franke WW. Identification of protein IT of the intestinal cytoskeleton as a novel type I cytokeratin with unusual properties and expression patterns. J Cell Biol. 1990;11:567–80.
19. Marceau N. Cell lineages and differentiation programs in epidermal, urothelial and hepatic tissues and their neoplasms. Lab Invest. 1990;63:4–20.
20. Van Eyken P, Desmet VJ. Development of intrahepatic bile ducts, ductular metaplasia of hepatocytes and cytokeratin patterns. In: Sirica AE, editor. The role of cell types in hepatocarcinogenesis. Ann Arbor: CRC Press; 1992:227–63.
21. Van Eyken P. Phenotypic modulation of hepatocytes: a cytokeratin-immunohistochemical study. Leuven: Acco, Ph.D. thesis, 1990.
22. Van Eyken P, Desmet VJ. Bile duct cells. In: Lebouton AV, editor. Molecular and cell biology of the liver. Ann Arbor: CRC Press; 1993:in press.
23. Sirica AE, Mathis GA, Sano N, Elmore LW. Isolation, culture, and transplantation of intrahepatic biliary epithelial cells and oval cells. Pathobiology. 1990;58:44–64.
24. Burt AD, Stewart JA, Aitchison M, MacSween RNM. Expression of tissue polypeptide antigen (TPA) in fetal and adult liver: changes in liver disease. J Clin Pathol. 1987;40: 719–24.
25. Desmet VJ. Cholestasis: extrahepatic obstruction and secondary biliary cirrhosis. In: MacSween RNM, Anthony PP, Scheuer PJ, editors. Pathology of the liver, 2nd edn. Edinburgh: Churchill Livingstone; 1987:364–423.
26. Desmet VJ. Intrahepatic bile ducts under the lens. J Hepatol. 1985;1:545–59.
27. Desmet VJ. Modulation of biliary epithelium. In: Bianchi L, Reutter W, editors. Modulation of liver cell expression. Lancaster: MTP Press; 1986;195–214.
28. Slott PA, Liu MH, Tavoloni N. Origin, pattern and mechanism of bile duct proliferation following biliary obstruction in the rat. Gastroenterology. 1990;99:466–77.
29. Van Eyken P, Sciot R, Desmet VJ. A cytokeratin immunohistochemical study of cholestatic liver disease: evidence that hepatocytes can express 'bile duct-type' cytokeratins. Histopathology. 1989;15:125–35.
30. Schulz R, Schuppan D, Hahn EG. Connective tissue and ductular metaplasia of hepatocytes.

In: Wolff JR, Sievers J, Berry M, editors. Mesenchymal–epithelial interactions in neural development. Berlin, Heidelberg: Springer Verlag; 1987:119–25.
31. Chapman RW. The immunology of primary sclerosing cholangitis. Springer Semin Immunopathol. 1990;12:121–8.
32. Chapman RW. Role of immune factors in the pathogenesis of primary sclerosing cholangitis. Semin Liver Dis. 1991;11:1–4.
33. Whiteside TL, Lasky S, Si L, Van Thiel DH. Immunologic analysis of mononuclear cells in liver tissues and blood of patients with primary sclerosing cholangitis. Hepatology. 1985;5:468–74.
34. Snook JA, Chapman RW, Sachdev GK, Heryet A, Kelly PM, Fleming KA, Jewell DP. Peripheral blood and portal tract lymphocyte populations in primary sclerosing cholangitis. J Hepatol. 1989;9:36–41.
35. Volpes R, Van den Oord JJ, Desmet VJ. Memory T-cells represent the predominant lymphocyte subset in acute and chronic liver inflammation. Hepatology. 1991;13:826–9.
36. Chapman RW, Kelly P, Heryet A, Jewell DP, Fleming KA. Expression of HLA-DR antigens on bile duct epithelium in primary sclerosing cholangitis. Gut. 1988;29:422–7.
37. Van den Oord JJ, Sciot R, Desmet VJ. Expression of MHC products by normal and abnormal bile duct epithelium. J Hepatol. 1986;3:310–17.
38. Nakanuma Y, Kono N. Expression of HLA-DR antigens on interlobular bile ducts in primary biliary cirrhosis and other hepatobiliary diseases. An immunohistochemical study. Hum Pathol. 1991;22:431–6.
39. Broomé U, Glaumann H, Hultcrantz R, Forsum U. Distribution of HLA-DR, HLA-DP, HLA-DQ antigens in liver tissue from patients with primary sclerosing cholangitis. Scand J Gastroenterol. 1990;25:54–8.
40. Bedossa P, Houry S, Bacci J, Martin E, Lemaigre G, Huguier MA. A longitudinal study of histologic and immunohistologic changes in an experimental model of sclerosing cholangitis. Virchows Arch [A]. 1989;414:165–71.
41. Beuers U, Spengler U, Kruis W, Aydemir U, Wiebecke B, Sauerbruch T, Paumgartner G. Ursodeoxycholic acid for treatment of primary sclerosing cholangitis: a placebo-controlled trial. Hepatology. 1992;16:707–14.
42. Ballardini G, Fallani M, Bianchi FB, Pisi E. Antigen presenting cells in liver biopsies from patients with primary biliary cirrhosis. Autoimmunity. 1989;3:135–44.
43. Demetris AJ, Sever C, Kakizoe S, Oguma S, Starzl TE, Jaffe R. S100 protein positive dendritic cells in primary biliary cirrhosis and other chronic inflammatory liver diseases. Relevance to pathogenesis? Am J Pathol. 1989;134:741–7.
44. Adams DH, Hubscher SG, Shaw J, Johnson GD, Babbs C, Rothlein R, Neuberger JM. Increased expression of intercellular adhesion molecule 1 on bile ducts in primary biliary cirrhosis and primary sclerosing cholangitis. Hepatology. 1991;14:426–31.
45. Hultcrantz B, Broomé U, Scheynius A. Lack of ICAM-1 expression on bile ducts from patients with primary biliary cirrhosis (PBC) and primary sclerosing cholangitis (PSC). Hepatology. 1991;14:63A.
46. Sherlock S. Pathogenesis of sclerosing cholangitis: the role of nonimmune factors. Semin Liver Dis. 1991;11:5–10.
47. Bissel DM, Choun MO. The role of extracellular matrix in normal liver. Scand J Gastroenterol [Suppl]. 1988;151:1–7.
48. Schuppan D. Structure of the extracellular matrix in normal and fibrotic liver: collagens and glycoproteins. Semin Liver Dis. 1990;10:1–10.
49. Gressner AM, Bachem MG. Cellular sources of noncollagenous matrix proteins: role of fat-storing cells in fibrogenesis. Semin Liver Dis. 1990;10:30–46.
50. Van Eyken P, Sciot R, Desmet VJ. Expression of the novel extracellular matrix component tenascin in normal and diseased human liver. An immunohistochemical study. J Hepatol. 1990;11:43–52.
51. Van Eyken P, Geerts A, De Bleser P, Lazou J-M, Vrijsen R, Sciot R, Wisse E, Desmet VJ. Localization and cellular source of the extracellular matrix protein tenascin in normal and fibrotic rat liver. Hepatology. 1992;15:909–16.
52. Ramadori G, Schwögler S, Veit T, Rieder H, Chiquet-Ehrismann R, Mackie EJ, Meyer zum Buschenfelde KH. Tenascin gene expression in rat liver and in rat liver cells; *in vivo* and *in vitro* studies. Virchows Arch [B]. 1991;60:145–53.

53. Schmitt-Gräff A, Krüger S, Bochard F, Gabiani G, Denk H. Modulation of alpha smooth muscle actin and desmin expression in perisinusoidal cells of normal and diseased human livers. Am J Pathol. 1991;138:1233–42.
54. Miyazaki H, Van Eyken P, Roskams T, De Vos R, Desmet VJ. Transient expression of tenascin in experimentally induced cholestatic fibrosis in rat liver: an immunohistochemical study. In: Gressner A, Ramadori G, editors. Molecular and cell biology of liver fibrogenesis. Lancaster: Kluwer; 1992:176–80.
55. Miyazaki H, Van Eyken P, Roskams T, De Vos R, Desmet VJ. Transient expression of tenascin in experimentally induced cholestatic fibrosis in rat liver: an immunohistochemical study. J Hepatol. 1992:in press.
56. Rosen CB, Nagorney DM. Cholangiocarcinoma complicating primary sclerosing cholangitis. Semin Liver Dis. 1991;11:26–30.
57. Wee A, Ludwig J, Coffey RJ, LaRusso N, Wiesner R. Hepatobiliary carcinoma associated with primary sclerosing cholangitis and chronic ulcerative cholitis. Hum Pathol. 1985;16: 719–26.
58. Miros M, Kerlin P, Walker N, Lynch JH, Strong R. Predicting cholangiocarcinoma in patients with primary sclerosing cholangitis before transplantation. Gut. 1991;32:1369–73.

35
The immunogenetics of primary sclerosing cholangitis

R. W. CHAPMAN

INTRODUCTION

Primary sclerosing cholangitis (PSC) is a chronic cholestatic liver disease that is characterized by an obliterative inflammatory fibrosis of the biliary tract. This chronic inflammation frequently results in bile duct obliteration, biliary cirrhosis, hepatic failure and sometimes in cholangiocarcinoma[1].

The cause of PSC is unknown, but it is clear that any proposed aetiological factors must explain the close association with ulcerative colitis[2]. Approximately 5% of patients with total ulcerative colitis will develop PSC, and at least two-thirds of patients with PSC will have coexisting ulcerative colitis.

Recent studies have suggested that genetic and immunological factors are important in the pathogenesis of PSC[3]. Evidence for the importance of genetic factors was first provided by Quigley *et al.*, who reported on three families in whom two members developed ulcerative colitis and PSC[4]. Another report from Argentina has associated PSC in three siblings of one family[5]. The importance of immunological factors has been emphasized by the large number of recent reports that have shown humoral and cellular abnormalities in PSC. The cellular abnormalities include low values of circulating suppressor T cells in serum[6] and large increases in the numbers of both suppressor and helper T cells from the portal tracts of patients with PSC[7]. In addition an inhibition of leucocyte migration in response to biliary antigens[8], and aberrant expression of HLA DR antigens on biliary epithelium at early stages of the disease have been reported[9]. Humoral immune defects include increased levels of circulating immune complexes in blood[10], defective clearance of immune complexes[11], activation of the complement system[12], and circulating antibodies against neutrophil nuclei[13].

In the light of this evidence there has been increasing research into the immunogenetics, i.e. the study of inherited components of the immune system in relation to autoimmune liver disease in general and PSC in particular.

IMMUNOGENETIC BACKGROUND

Although immunogenetics is the study of all the inherited components of the immune response, in practice the majority of human immunogenetic research has involved the study of diseases in which particular HLA types are over-represented. HLA molecules are polymorphic cell surface heterodimeric glycoproteins which are essential for cell/cell recognition. The structure and functions of the HLA class I and HLA class II molecules are distinct. They are encoded on separate regions of the major histocompatibility complex (MHC) on the short arm of chromosome 6. The class I molecules are subdivided into HLA A, B and Cw, and consist of a peptide chain bound to β_2-microglobulin. They are found on the surface of all cells where they are responsible for self- and non-self by $CD8^+$ lymphocytes. The class II molecules consist of HLA DR, DQ and DP and consist of two chains – α and β – which are present on the surface of B lymphocytes, activated T lymphocytes and antigen-presenting cells. They have an important role in the initiation of the immune response to foreign antigen. Oligopeptides derived from the foreign antigen are processed in the antigen-presenting cell and then bound in a specialized binding groove in the external domain of the HLA class II molecule at the cell membrane. The next step is that the T cell receptor, in conjunction with the CD4 antigen on the helper T cell, recognizes and is stimulated by the oligopeptide fragment of the foreign antigen bound to the HLA class II molecule. The $CD4^+$ T lymphocyte will initiate humoral and cellular immunoresponses to the foreign antigen only if the HLA class II molecule is recognized by the T lymphocyte as self. An antigen-presenting cell from another individual with a different class II molecule will not produce an immune response. There are three methods in general use for the assignment of HLA class I and class II types.

1. *Serological HLA phenotyping*. In this technique, alloantisera containing antibodies to HLA molecules produce a cytotoxic effect on cells expressing the appropriate HLA molecule. This cytotoxicity is then assessed in a complement-dependent microcytotoxicity assay. The accuracy with which HLA types can be assigned using this method depends largely on the availability of alloantisera. In general this technique is suitable for the detection of polymorphisms of the HLA class I system, but the serological typing cannot detect much of the polymorphism known to exist among class II molecules.
2. *Restriction fragment polymorphism analysis of HLA class II alleles*. The polymorphism in the HLA class II molecular system is more easily detectable if the genes encoding HLA molecules are studied rather than the molecules themselves. Restriction length polymorphism (RFLP) analysis has been widely used to study the polymorphism of HLA class II molecules. DNA prepared from whole blood is digested by a restriction endonuclease. The choice of restriction enzyme is based on the distribution of informative restriction sites within the area of interest. The digestion of DNA produces fragments of varying lengths which are resolved using agarose electrophoresis. After transfer to nylon filters by

Southern blotting the restriction fragments are then revealed by means of a radiolabelled exon-specific probe followed by autoradiography. The pattern of restriction fragments corresponds to the HLA type of the individual. However, RFLP analysis cannot distinguish all alleles at a given locus since the polymorphic DNA sequences are not directly identified.

3. *Polymerase chain reaction and sequence specific oligonucleotide probing.* Polymorphism among HLA molecules is caused by differences in the amino acid sequences of the peptides. These can be deduced from the nucleotide sequence of the genes in the MHC. The genes of the MHC resemble immunoglobulin genes in that they contain variable and constant regions. MHC genes can be identified using oligonucleotide probes which are homologous with a variable region of a particular gene.

IMMUNOGENETIC STUDIES OF PRIMARY SCLEROSING CHOLANGITIS

In the early 1980s three immunogenetic studies were performed, although they were not recognized as such at the time! All three studies were based on serological phenotyping[14–16] a study of 25 patients with PSC from the Royal Free Hospital, a close association was found between the HLA B8 antigen and PSC[14]. HLA B8 was present in 60% of patients with PSC, with or without ulcerative colitis, compared with only 25% of 561 controls. HLA B12 was less frequent among patients at 8% than control with 30%. In a report from Oslo 20 patients with ulcerative colitis and hepatobiliary diseases were studied, of whom 16 had a firm diagnosis of PSC based on ERCP[15]. HLA B8 was present in 16 (80%) of the patients compared with 25% of controls. In addition, DR typing was performed and HLA DR3 was found significantly more frequently among patients (70%) as amongst controls (19%). These findings were confirmed in English patients with ulcerative colitis and PSC in Oxford, in whom B8 was found in 56% of 16 patients and DR3 in 75%[16].

HLA B8 and DR3 are in linkage disequilibrium and the HLA B8 DR3 haplotype is associated with a number of organ-specific autoimmune diseases such as lupoid chronic active hepatitis, type I diabetes mellitus, myasthenia gravis and thyrotoxicosis. The finding, therefore, of a markedly increased prevalence of HLA B8 and DR3 in PSC patients was strong suggestive evidence that immunological factors may be important in the pathogenesis, although at the time of the studies the possible mechanisms were not clear.

These results were confirmed and extended by a larger study performed in 1990 in 81 patients with PSC[17]. The results again showed a significant increase in the frequency of the antigens B8 and DR3 compared with controls, 53% versus 23% and 56% versus 21%, respectively. This was caused by a significant rise in the frequency of the HLA antigen A1 B8 DR3 haplotype; 40% versus 12% of controls. In contrast, a significant reduction was seen in the frequency of the antigens B44 and DR3, 12% versus 31% and 12% versus

34% respectively. When all the DR3-positive individuals were eliminated a significant association with DR2 was found: 25 (69%) of 36 remaining patients being DR2-positive compared with 27 (34%) of 79 DR3-negative controls. Interestingly, patients who were DR3-positive were first seen at a significantly younger age than those who were DR2-positive.

HLA A1 B8 DR3 and DR2 are equally distributed in PSC patients with and without ulcerative colitis. Moreover, these HLA antigens are not found in increased frequency in patients with ulcerative colitis[18]. These data suggest that HLA DR3, DR2, and ulcerative colitis are separate independent risk factors for the development of PSC.

Interest was heightened in the HLA associations in PSC by a report from Los Angeles[19] which studied the prevalence of the products of the recently discovered DR B3 and DR B4 genes, namely HLA DRw52a–c and DRw53. In a group of 29 patients with PSC undergoing liver transplantation all 29 were reported as having the HLA DRw52a antigen present, compared with only 35% of a control population[19]. Fifteen of these patients had a single common haplotype, namely HLA A1 B8 Cw7 DRw17 DQw2 DRw52a. DR7 DRw53 and DQw3 were significantly less frequent among patients than among controls. However, the study suffered from a number of shortcomings; firstly only a small number of patients were studied; secondly the patients studied were referred for liver transplantation, suggesting that they were suffering from endstage disease, perhaps introducing selection bias; and thirdly, and perhaps most importantly, serological typing was used to assign the patients to HLA DRw52a. Subsequently, a number of workers both in the USA and Europe have been unable to confirm the 100% association of HLA DRw52a with PSC[18,20,21]. The prevalence figures are shown to be anything from 45% to 65%. However, in a study from King's College Hospital in which HLA A, B, DQA and DQB genotypes were studied, DRw52a was the most strongly associated allele, although only found in 55% of the patients[22]. In this study survival was reduced amongst the DRw52a patients, which could account for the discrepancy between the findings originally reported and subsequent reports. However, this effect on survival is not clear-cut as a further study from Oxford and Birmingham has not confirmed these results (work in preparation).

There are several possible explanations why HLA DRw52a is not found in all patients with PSC, but only in approximately 55–65%. One possibility is that PSC is heterogeneous and that HLA DRw52a-positive and 52a-negative patients have distinct diseases which are not presently distinguishable by clinical means. However, this seems unlikely in view of the similarities with respect to age, sex ratio and associated ulcerative colitis in both the 52a-positive and 52a-negative patients with PSC. A second and more plausible explanation is that there is a second susceptibility allele in additiom to the allele which encodes 52a, namely DRB5*0101. This has been found in a recent study from King's College Hospital to be the most frequent allele amongst DRB3-0101 negative patients (DRB3*0101 encodes DR52a)[22]. The DRB5*0101 was found in 53% of patients who were 52a-negative. A role for DRB5-0101 would be consistent with the finding of a secondary association with HLA DR2 which was discussed earlier, since DRB5*0101, together with DRB1501, encodes the serological determinants of DR2.

Interestingly, both DRB3*0101 and DRB5*0101 encode a leucine residue at position 38 of the DR β-chain which is located in the floor of the peptide binding groove of the DR binding molecule. It is possible that amino acid substitutions at position 38 of DR-beta could affect the presentation of certain antigens to T cells, hence affecting the initiation of the immune response thought to be important in the aetiology of PSC. These data have led the King's group to hypothesize that the hydrophobicity of leucine at position 38 of DR-beta is the feature of the DR molecule which confirms susceptibility to PSC, and that alanine at this position in the molecule confirms protection against the development of PSC. That alanine affords protection is supported by the observed reduction in the frequency among the patients of DRB4*0101, the most frequent alanine 38 encoding allele. It would appear from the King's data that two DR-beta chains must have leucine at position 38 to produce a substantial relative risk and therefore substantial susceptibility.

However, only 28% of patients in the whole series of 71 patients were in this category. This suggests that, although immunogenetic predisposition is important, it is not essential in the development of PSC. This evidence would support the theory that if both DR-beta chains have a leucine residue at position 38, the environment in the peptide binding groove of the HLA molecule is particularly favourable for the initiation of the immune response leading to PSC. Conversely, if they both have alanine residues the environment is unfavourable. If a valine residue occupies position 38 in one or more DR molecules the position is intermediate. As the King's group themselves point out, although this hypothesis is attractive, a similar hypothesis for the protection from insulin-dependent diabetes mellitus has been tempered by the fact that genetic susceptibility to diabetes is a result of polymorphisms in at least three different chromosomes. The situation may be equally complex for PSC.

CONCLUSION

Current evidence suggests that PSC is an immunologically mediated disease. The factor or factors which trigger the immune process remain unknown. However, the presence of HLA DRw52a is the most strongly associated HLA antigen, being found in approximately 55–65% of patients with PSC. In patients who do not possess this antigen, HLA DR2 encoded by DRB5*0101 renders patients susceptible to the development of the disease. Both the alleles encoding for these HLA antigens encode a leucine residue at position 38 of the DR-beta molecule which may render patients susceptible to the disease. Conversely, DRB4*0101, which encodes DRw53, is less frequently found among patients with PSC, and encodes an alanine residue at this position, which may confer protection against the development of the disease. Ulcerative colitis would appear to be an independent risk factor. There is some suggestion that the presence of DRw52a may predispose to a more severe disease course, although this remains to be confirmed.

References

1. Wiesner RH, LaRusso NF. Clinicopathologic features of the syndrome of primary sclerosing cholangitis. Gastroenterology. 1980;79:200–6.
2. Chapman RW, Arborgh BA, Rhodes JM *et al.* Primary sclerosing cholangitis – a review of its clinical features, cholangiography and hepatic histology. Gut. 1980;21:870–7.
3. Chapman RW. Role of immune factors in the pathogenesis of primary sclerosing cholangitis. Semin Liver Dis. 1991;11:1–4.
4. Quigley EMM, LaRusso NF, Ludwig J *et al.* Familial occurrence of primary sclerosing cholangitis and ulcerative colitis. Gastroenterology. 1983;85:1160–5.
5. Jorge AD, Esley C, Ahumada J. Family incidence of primary sclerosing cholangitis associated with immunological diseases. Endoscopy. 1987;19:114–15.
6. Lindor KD, Wiesner RH, Katzman JA, LaRusso NF, Beaver SJ. Lymphocyte subsets in primary sclerosing cholangitis. Dig Dis Sci. 1987;32:720–5.
7. Whiteside TL, Lasky S, Si L, VanThiel DH. Immunologic analysis of mononuclear cells in liver tissues and blood of patients with primary sclerosing cholangitis. Hepatology. 1985;5:468–74.
8. McFarlane IG, Wojcicka BM, Tsantoulas DC *et al.* Leucocyte migration inhibition in response to biliary antigens in primary biliary cirrhosis, sclerosing cholangitis and other chronic liver diseases. Gastroenterology. 1979;76:1333–40.
9. Chapman RW, Kelly P, Heryet A *et al.* Expression of HLA = DR antigens on bile duct epithelium in primary sclerosing cholangitis. Gut. 1988;29:422–7.
10. Bodenheimer HCJ, LaRusso NF, Thayer WR Jr *et al.* Elevated circulating immune complexes in primary sclerosing cholangitis. Hepatology. 1983;3:150–4.
11. Minuk GY, Angus M, Brickman CM *et al.* Abnormal clearance of immune complexes from the circulation of patients with primary sclerosing cholangitis. Gastroenterology. 1985;88:166–70.
12. Senaldi G, Donaldson PT, Magrin S *et al.* Activation of the complement system in primary sclerosing cholangitis. Gastroenterology. 1989;97:1430–4.
13. Lo SK, Fleming KA, Chapman RW. Prevalence of anti-neutrophil antibody in primary sclerosing cholangitis and ulcerative colitis using an alkaline phosphatase technique. Gut. 1992;33:1370–5.
14. Chapman R, Vargiese Z, Gaul R *et al.* Association of primary sclerosing cholangitis with HLA-B8. Gut. 1983;24:38–41.
15. Schrumpf E, Fansa O, Forre O *et al.* HLA antigens and immunoregulatory T cells in ulcerative colitis associated with hepatobiliary disease. Scand J Gastroenterol. 1982;17: 187–91.
16. Shepherd HA, Selby WS, Chapman RW *et al.* Ulcerative colitis and liver dysfunction. Q J Med. 1983;52:503–13.
17. Donaldson PT, Farran JM, Wilkinson ML *et al.* Dual association of HLA DR2 and DR3 with primary sclerosing cholangitis. Hepatology. 1991;13:129–33.
18. Zetterquist H, Broome V, Einarsson K, Olerup O. HLA class II genes in primary sclerosing cholangitis and chronic inflammatory bowel disease: no HLA-DRw52a association in Swedish patients with sclerosing cholangitis. Gut. 1992;33:942–6.
19. Prochazka EJ, Terasaki PI, MinSik Park DVM *et al.* Association of primary sclerosing cholangitis with HLA-DRw52a. N Engl J Med. 1990;322:1842–4.
20. Mehal WZ, Wordsworth PB, Taylor CJ *et al.* Inability to attribute susceptibility to primary sclerosing cholangitis to specific aminoacid positions of the HLA-DRw52a allele. N Engl J Med. 1991;355–1252.
21. Munoz S, Westerberg S, Martin P *et al.* HLA-DRw52a: lack of universal association with primary sclerosing cholangitis. Gastroenterology. 1991;100:A778 (abstract).
22. Farrant JM, Doherty DG, Donaldson PT *et al.* Amino acid substitutions at position 38 of the DR B polypeptide confer susceptibility to and protection from primary sclerosing cholangitis. Hepatology. 1992;16:390–5.
23. Todd JA. Genetic control of autoimmunity in type I diabetes. Immunol Today. 1990;11: 122–9.

36
Antineutrophil cytoplasmic antibodies in primary sclerosing cholangitis and ulcerative colitis

A. VIDRICH and S. R. TARGAN

ANCA (ANTINEUTROPHIL CYTOPLASMIC ANTIBODIES)

Antibodies to cytoplasmic components of the neutrophil (and sometimes monocyte) are found in the sera of patients with certain chronic inflammatory conditions[1–5]. Davies and collaborators are credited with the first observation of ANCA (antineutrophil cytoplasmic antibodies). They found the antibodies when they examined a small population of patients with segmental necrotizing glomerulonephritis and systemic vasculitis[6]. By immunofluorescent microscopy, ANCA activity has been divided into two broad categories: cytoplasmic neutrophil staining (c-ANCA) and cytoplasmic staining with perinuclear highlighting (p-ANCA). These staining patterns are obtained with alcohol-fixed cytocentrifuged neutrophils. The use of a cytoplasmic staining pattern versus a perinuclear one to determine antigen localization should not be regarded as absolute since those patterns seem to be an artifact of alcohol fixation[7,9,15]. Nevertheless, this alcohol-induced localization can serve to differentially distinguish between two types of ANCA with unique antigens and different disease associations.

c-ANCA activity is most commonly found in patients with Wegener's granulomatosis[10] as first reported by Nölle *et al.* In that study a higher percentage (96%) of patients with active disease displayed c-ANCA activity, and that activity correlated with severity of disease. c-ANCA activity can also be found in polyarteritis nodosa, idiopathic crescentic glomerulonephritis and pulmonary-renal syndrome (ref. 1 and refs therein). However, c-ANCA is not found in non-Wegener's granulomatous pulmonary disease (i.e. tuberculosis). The c-ANCA antigen of Wegener's granulomatosis has been identified; it is a 29 kDa protein triplet of the azurophilic granules (primary lysosomes) also identified as proteinase 3[9,11,16–19]. Another c-ANCA identified recently is a 57 kDa cationic protein dubbed CAP57[1,20], also found in primary granules. While some patients express a single ANCA activity others will express more than one type[1].

Patients with systemic necrotizing vasculitis or idiopathic crescentic glomerulonephritis also display ANCA activity, but in these cases the immunofluorescent staining pattern is perinuclear in nature or p-ANCA[7]. Myeloperoxidase (MPO) of the primary granule[21] is the most common antigen recognized by this p-ANCA. Additional p-ANCAs identified to date include antibodies that recognize elastase (primary granule constituent) and lactoferrin, a component of secondary granules[22–24]. However these latter p-ANCAs are found with far less frequency than MPO-ANCA. Additionally, p-ANCA sera seem to display considerable heterogeneity in the number of reacting species recognized[1,25].

COMPARISONS OF p-ANCA OF ULCERATIVE COLITIS WITH ANCA OF WEGENER'S GRANULOMATOSIS AND OTHER VASCULITIDES

Antibodies to neutrophil cytoplasmic components have been identified in the sera of patients with inflammatory bowel disease (IBD)[26]. Initial studies showed that 68% of ulcerative colitis (UC) but only 20% of Crohn's disease (CD) sera showed a p-ANCA staining pattern, indicating that this activity could be used to differentiate between UC and CD[26]. Confirmation of these results and conclusion has come from a number of laboratories[27–32]. More important, the combination of a positive value in the fixed-neutrophil enzyme-linked immunosorbent assay (ELISA) and a perinuclear immunofluorescent staining pattern of alcohol-fixed neutrophils was shown to be highly specific (94%) for UC as compared to other colitides[33]. Other key features that distinguish UC p-ANCA from the ANCA of Wegener's granulomatosis and that of other vasculitides are: (1) neutrophil specificity with no staining of monocytes and (2) no correlation with extent of disease, disease activity or duration[26,33].

COMPARISONS OF PRIMARY SCLEROSING CHOLANGITIS ANCA AND UC p-ANCA

Sera of patients with primary sclerosing cholangitis (PSC) have been shown by R. Duerr and collaborators to contain ANCA activity similar to that found in the sera of patients with UC[34]. In that study a p-ANCA staining pattern was seen in 87% of 15 ELISA-positive UC sera, 79% of 42 ELISA-positive PSC sera and 73% of 11 ELISA-positive PSC without UC sera. The combination of a positive fixed-neutrophil ELISA and a perinuclear immunofluorescent staining pattern was 100% specific for PSC when compared to other chronic inflammatory liver diseases[34]. Similar to UC p-ANCA, PSC p-ANCA activity showed no correlation with disease duration. In addition, all 51 sera tested from PSC patients with and without UC were highly specific for neutrophils by immunofluorescence with no monocyte staining[34].

While all of the ANCA reactive antigens so far identified have been granule constituents, we and others have found no significant activity for anti-MPO, anti-elastase or anti-cathepsin G activity[26–32] in UC patient sera, nor any recognition of isolated primary granules[27]. In our laboratory, UC patient sera were assayed for binding to antigen-coated wells by ELISA and the antigen coating buffer used was varied to ensure optimal coating. No significant binding of UC p-ANCA sera to antigen-coated wells was obtained irrespective of the method of antigen coating. Increasing the concentration of antigen for coating to 10 μg/ml also resulted in no reaction. Similar to UC sera, PSC sera from patients with no histological evidence of UC and a p-ANCA immunofluorescent pattern were found not to react with authentic granule protein antigens[34].

The IgG subclass distribution of UC specific p-ANCA and PSC (non-UC) specific p-ANCA reactive IgG was examined in a preliminary study. It is well known that different effector functions can be ascribed to the IgG subclasses. Since similarities had been documented for the UC and PSC p-ANCA activity, it was of interest to determine whether these activities shared subclass specificity. A panel of p-ANCA-positive sera from patients with UC and PSC (non-UC) was examined in the fixed-neutrophil ELISA combined with a set of four mouse monoclonal antibodies specific for each human subclass to yield quantitative data for the distribution of autoantibody specificities. Distribution of the IgG subclasses in total serum of the UC and PSC patients, as well as normal control serum, was also determined. The distribution of IgG subclasses in control serum was as expected and previously reported[35]. No significant differences were seen in the IgG isotype distribution of total UC and PSC sera relative to normal sera. The isotype distribution of the UC p-ANCA reactive IgG also was not significantly different from that of normal serum. However, PSC p-ANCA activity was found to have a significant elevation of the IgG3 isotype with a concomitant reduction in IgG1 relative to total normal and PSC serum. While the precise meaning of this finding is unclear, it is the first significant difference found between UC and PSC p-ANCA positive sera. Predominance of one IgG subclass over another has been demonstrated for a variety of autoimmune diseases. In systemic lupus erythematosus the circulating double-stranded DNA antibodies are of IgG1, IgG2 and IgG3 isotypes[36], whereas in biliary cirrhosis the antimitochondrial antibodies are predominantly IgG3 and IgM[37]. Similarly, while IgG1 and IgG4 seemed to predominate in patients with 29-kDa ANCA and MPO ANCA, patients with Wegener's granulomatosis and renal involvement had higher levels of IgG3 subclass 29-kDa ANCA and MPO ANCA[38]. These data indicate that the same antigen is able to elicit variable isotype responses. Jayne *et al.*[39] have documented an enrichment of IgG3 for the ANCA activity in acute sera of systemic vasculitis. In time the ANCA activity switched from IgG3 to IgG2. The authors postulate that this switch is reflective of disease remission due to the diminished capacity of IgG2 to fix complement and bind to macrophages. Whether the persistence of an IgG1 and/or IgG3 response in UC and PSC p-ANCA is indicative of continued antigen presence needs to be determined. What factors may influence the seemingly differential IgG subclass response of UC p-ANCA versus PSC p-ANCA are unknown, but they may suggest some differences in underlying pathology, though not necessarily a different antigenic species.

To determine whether other similarities existed between the UC and PSC p-ANCA reactive antigen(s), we examined antigen stability by incubating neutrophils at 37 °C. Wells of microtitre plates were coated with a monolayer of neutrophils in Hanks' balanced salt solution. In one set (untreated), cells were allowed to attach for 30 min at room temperature, supernatant was removed, cells were air-dried and fixed with methanol as described[26]. In another set (treated), cells were first incubated at 37 °C for 5 h before processing as given above. Both neutrophil preparations were reacted with a panel of sera, positive for p-ANCA, from patients with PSC (without UC) and UC in the fixed-neutrophil ELISA at a serum dilution of 1:100 as described[26]. Both the UC and PSC ANCA reactive antigen(s) were unstable to the 37 °C treatment as described, and resulted in a lowered ELISA assay value as compared to that given by untreated control neutrophils (data not shown).

In order to identify the antigen(s) responsible for the UC p-ANCA pattern, we examined protein preparations of solubilized whole neutrophils by SDS-PAGE and Western blotting. When a panel of UC p-ANCA-positive sera was assayed a number of reactive bands were observed. However, the identical-sized bands were also recognized by a panel of normal control sera. Additionally, normal sera reacted with bands not obtained with the UC sera assayed. Analysing the neutrophil preparation by SDS-PAGE under non-denaturing conditions resulted in the same bands being recognized by UC p-ANCA-positive and normal patient sera (data not given). Varying the protein transfer time, or attempting to fractionate and solubilize neutrophils in a variety of ways, did not change the observation that both UC and normal patient sera react with similar-sized protein species. We concluded that the UC p-ANCA reactive antigen is not detectable by Western blotting.

Contrary to our findings, Klein and colleagues reported the identification, by Western blotting, of antigens responsible for the p-ANCA pattern found in PSC sera[40]. It is interesting to note that at least three of the five antigens reported by these authors to be PSC-specific are of the same molecular mass by SDS-PAGE as those we observed to be reactive with UC p-ANCA-positive and -negative (normal) control sera. As of this writing, Western blotting analysis has not yielded the identity of the UC p-ANCA antigen(s), and it is debatable whether this methodology has been successful in revealing the PSC p-ANCA antigen(s).

SUMMARY

The current data strongly support the thesis that the UC and PSC p-ANCA-reactive antigen(s) are similar and may be indicative of a common immunopathological mechanism. The following similarities have been observed: (1) both sera give a perinuclear immunofluorescent staining pattern with alcohol-fixed neutrophils, (2) there is no correlation with disease activity of either p-ANCA, (3) both PSC and UC p-ANCA are specific for neutrophils and (4) there is no reaction with any of the granule protein antigens implicated in other chronic inflammatory conditions. As of this writing, the UC p-ANCA antigen(s) cannot be identified by Western blotting, and it is doubtful that the PSC p-ANCA antigen(s) has yielded to such analysis. More recently we have adapted immunoprecipitation methodology to identify the UC p-ANCA-reactive antigens. We have been able to immunoprecipitate and resolve by SDS-PAGE antigens from whole neutrophil preparations that are recognized by UC p-ANCA-reactive sera but not by normal sera. While several bands are consistently resolved, the most frequently seen migrate with a molecular weight of 40–45 kDa and 32–36 kDa. Whether these same molecular species are recognized by PSC p-ANCA serum remains to be determined.

References

1. Jennette JC, Charles LA, Falk RJ. Antineutrophil cytoplasmic autoantibodies: disease associations, molecular biology, and pathophysiology. Int Rev Exp Pathol. 1991;32: 193–221.
2. Shanahan F, Landers C, Duerr R, Targan SR. Neutrophil autoantibodies as disease markers for ulcerative colitis. Immunol Res. 1991;10:479–84.
3. Nölle B, Specks U, Lüdemann J *et al.* Anticytoplasmic autoantibodies: their immunodiagnostic value in Wegener granulomatosis. Ann Intern Med. 1989;111:28–40.
4. Kallenberg CGM, Cohen Tervaert JW, van der Woude FJ *et al.* Autoimmunity to lysosomal enzymes: new clues to vasculitis and glomerulonephritis? Immunol Today. 1991;12(2): 61–4.
5. Falk RJ, Jennette JC. Wegener's granulomatosis, systemic vasculitis, and antineutrophil cytoplasmic autoantibodies. Annu Rev Med. 1991;42:459–69.
6. Davies DJ, Moran JE, Niall JF, Ryan GB. Segmental necrotising glomerulonephritis with antineutrophil antibody: possible arborvirus aetiology? Br Med J. 1982;285:606–10.
7. Falk RJ, Jennette JC. Anti-neutrophil cytoplasmic autoantibodies with specificity for myeloperoxidase in patients with systemic vasculitis and idiopathic necrotizing and crescentic glomerulonephritis. N Engl J Med. 1988;318:1651–7.
8. Lüdemann J, Utecht B, Gross WL. Detection and quantitation of anti-neutrophil cytoplasm antibodies in Wegener's granulomatosis by ELISA using affinity-purifed antigen. J Immunol Methods. 1988;114:167–74.
9. Goldschmeding R, van der Schoot CE, ten Bokkel Huinink D *et al.* Wegener's granulomatosis autoantibodies identify a novel diisopropylfluorophosphate-binding protein in the lysosomes of normal human neutrophils. J Clin Invest. 1989;84:1577–87.
10. Nölle B, Specks U, Lüdemann J *et al.* Anticytoplasmic autoantibodies: their immunodiagnostic value in Wegener granulomatosis. Ann Intern Med. 1989;111:28–40.
11. Niles JL, McCluskey RT, Ahmad MF, Arnaout MA. Wegener's granulomatosis autoantigen is a novel neutrophil serine proteinase. Blood. 1989;74(6):1888–93.
12. Hall JB, Wadham BMcN, Wood CJ *et al.* Vasculitis and glomerulonephritis: A subgroup with an antineutrophil cytoplasmic antibody. Aust NZ J Med. 1984;14:277–8.
13. van der Woude FJ, Rasmussen N, Lobatto S *et al.* Autoantibodies against neutrophils and monocytes: Tools for diagnosis and marker of disease activity in Wegener's granulomatosis. Lancet. 1985;i:425–9.
14. Falk RJ, Jennett JC. Anti-neutrophil cytoplasmic autoantibodies with specificity for myeloperoxidase in patients with systemic vasculitis and idiopathic necrotizing and crescentic glomerulonephritis. N Engl J Med. 1988;318:1651–7.
15. Pryzwansky KB, Martin LE, Spitznagel JK. Immunochemical localization of myeloperoxidase, lactoferrin, lysozyme, and neutral proteases in human monocytes and neutrophilic granulocytes. J Reticuloendothel Soc. 1978;24:295–310.
16. Lüdemann J, Utecht B, Gross WL. Antineutrophil cytoplasmic antibodies in Wegener's granulomatosis recognize an elastinolytic enzyme. J Exp Med. 1990;171:357–62.

17. Jennette JC, Hoidal JR, Falk RJ. Specificity of anti-neutrophil cytoplasmic autoantibodies for proteinase 3. Blood. 1990;75:2263–5.
18. Csernok E, Lüdemann J, Gross WL, Bainton DF. Ultrastructural localization of proteinase 3, the target antigen of anti-cytoplasmic antibodies circulating in Wegener's granulomatosis. Am J Pathol. 1990;137(5):1113–20.
19. Lüdemann J, Csernok E, Ulmer M *et al.* Anti-neutrophil cytoplasm antibodies in Wegener's granulomatosis: immunodiagnostic value, monoclonal antibodies and characterization of the target antigen. Neth J Med. 1990;36:157–62.
20. Ewert BH, Jennette JC, Falk RJ. The pathogenic role of antineutrophil cytoplasmic autoantibodies. Am J Kidney Dis. 1991;XVIII(2):188–95.
21. Falk FJ, Terrell RS, Charles L, Jennette JC. Anti-neutrophil cytoplasmic autoantibodies induce neutrophils to degranulate and produce oxygen radicals in vitro. Proc Natl Acad Sci USA. 1990;87:4115–19.
22. Goldschmeding R, Van der Schoot, Cohen Tervaert JW *et al.* Autoantibodies against myeloid lysosomal enzymes: a novel class of autoantibodies associated with vasculitic syndromes. Kidney Int. 1988;34:558–63.
23. Nässberger L, Johnsson H, Sjöhm AG. Circulating anti-elastase antibodies in systemic lupus erythematosus. Lancet. 1989;1:509.
24. Thompson RA, Lee SS. Antineutrophil cytoplasmic antibodies. Lancet. 1989;1:670.
25. Goldschmeding R, Cohen Tervaert JW, Gans ROB *et al.* Different immunological specificities and disease associations of c-ANCA and p-ANCA. Neth J Med. 1990;36:114–16.
26. Saxon A, Shanahan F, Landers C, Ganz T, Targan S. A subset of antineutrophil anticytoplasmic antibodies is associated with inflammatory bowel disease. J Allergy Clin Immunol. 1990;86:202–10.
27. Falk RJ, Sartor RB, Jones DA *et al.* Anti-neutrophil cytoplasmic autoantibodies (ANCA) in ulcerative colitis (UC). Clin Res. 1990;38:387 (abstract).
28. Rump JA, Scholmerich J, Gross V *et al.* A new type of perinuclear anti-neutrophil cytoplasmic antibody (p-ANCA) in active ulcerative colitis but not in Crohn's disease. Immunobiology. 1990;181:406–13.
29. Rustgi A, Podolsky D, McCluskey R, Niles J. Anti-neutrophilic antibodies in sera from patients with inflammatory bowel disease. Gastroenterology. 1991;100:612 (abstract).
30. Reumaux D, Colombel JF, Cortot A *et al.* Anti-neutrophil antibodies in sera from patients with inflammatory bowel disease. Gastroenterology. 1991;100:609 (abstract).
31. Hardarson S, LaBrecque DR, Mitros FA *et al.* Anti-neutrophil cytoplasmic antibody (ANCA) associated with ulcerative colitis and sclerosing cholangitis. Gastroenterology. 1991;100:585 (abstract).
32. Roth M, Rump JA, Gross WL *et al.* A new type of anti-neutrophil antibodies in sera from patients with ulcerative colitis but not Crohn's disease. Gastroenterology. 1991;100:244 (abstract).
33. Duerr RH, Targan SR, Landers CJ *et al.* Anti-neutrophil cytoplasmic antibodies in ulcerative colitis: comparison with other colitides/diarrheal illnesses. Gastroenterology. 1991;100: 1590–6.
34. Duerr RH, Targan SR, Landers CJ *et al.* Neutrophil cytoplasmic antibodies: a link between primary sclerosing cholangitis and ulcerative colitis. Gastroenterology. 1991;100:1385–91.
35. Klein F, Skvaril F, Vermeeren R *et al.* The quantification of human IgG subclasses in reference preparations. Clin Chim Acta. 1985;150:119–27.
36. Winkler TH, Henschel TA, Kalies I *et al.* Constant isotype pattern of anti dsDNA antibodies in patients with systemic lupus erythematosus. Clin. Exp. Immunol. 1988;72:434–9.
37. Surh CD, Cooper AE, Coppel RL *et al.* Predominance of IgG3 and IgM isotype anti-mitochondrial antibodies against recombinant fused mitochondrial peptide in patients with primary biliary cirrhosis. Hepatology. 1988;8:290–5.
38. Brouwer E, Cohen Tervaert JW, Horst G *et al.* Clin Exp Immunol. 1991;83:379–86.
39. Jayne DRW, Weetman AP, Lockwood CM. IgG subclass distribution of autoantibodies to neutrophil cytoplasmic antigens in systemic vasculitis. Clin Exp Immunol. 1991;84: 476–81.
40. Klein R, Eisenburg J, Weber P *et al.* Significance and specificity of antibodies to neutrophils detected by Western blotting for the serological diagnosis of primary sclerosing cholangitis. Hepatology. 1991;14:1147–52.

37
Animal models of sclerosing cholangitis: exploring mechanisms of hepatobiliary inflammation associated with intestinal injury

R. B. SARTOR and S. N. LICHTMAN

INTRODUCTION

Sclerosing cholangitis is an idiopathic inflammatory condition which leads to progressive destruction of intrahepatic and extrahepatic bile ducts. This disorder does not respond to conventional immunosuppressive therapy and currently accounts for the third leading cause of liver transplants in the United States. An interesting feature of sclerosing cholangitis is its relationship to inflammatory bowel disease (IBD). Approximately two-thirds of patients with sclerosing cholangitis have associated IBD, usually ulcerative colitis, although in some series in which evidence for intestinal inflammation is aggressively sought, nearly all sclerosing cholangitis patients have underlying colitis[1]. Conversely, a relatively small subset (2–6%) of IBD patients have clinically detected sclerosing cholangitis which is correlated with extent and location of intestinal inflammation. For example, ulcerative colitis patients with pancolitis have an 11-fold higher incidence of sclerosing cholangitis compared to patients with inflammation limited to the left colon. Crohn's disease patients with extensive colonic involvement have a much higher incidence of biliary inflammation than those patients with isolated ileitis[2]. These observations strongly suggest that intestinal inflammation is in some way linked to the pathogenesis of sclerosing cholangitis. This concept is further supported by the association of hepatobiliary inflammation with a variety of intestinal disorders, including ulcerative colitis, Crohn's disease, jejunoileal bypass for morbid obesity, Whipple's disease and coeliac disease. The common features of these diverse types of intestinal inflammatory conditions are enhanced mucosal permeability and overgrowth of anaerobic luminal bacteria.

Table 1 Potential mechanisms linking hepatobiliary inflammation with intestinal injury

1.	Shared aetiology
2.	Portal vein bacteraemia
3.	Mucosal absorption of phlogistic luminal products
4.	Portal vein transport of inflammatory mediators produced by the inflamed intestine

Table 2 Animal models of chronic hepatobiliary inflammation relevant to sclerosing cholangitis

1.	Intravenous injection of non-viable *E. coli*
2.	Chronic systemic administration of tumour necrosis factor
3.	Spontaneous colitis in cotton-topped tamarins
4.	Small intestinal bacterial overgrowth in genetically susceptible rats
5.	Indomethacin-induced enteritis in genetically susceptible rats

POTENTIAL MECHANISMS OF HUMAN HEPATOBILIARY INJURY

Several pathogenetic mechanisms could explain the association of intestinal and hepatobiliary inflammation (Table 1). Intestinal and hepatobiliary inflammation may share similar or identical aetiologies, such as infection, autoimmunity, dysregulation of the immune system or genetic predisposition. However, other factors must be involved since only a small minority of IBD patients develop clinically detectable hepatobiliary inflammation. Although portal vein bacteraemia occurs episodically in IBD, the lack of neutrophils in the periportal cellular infiltrate suggests alternative mechanisms of injury. A number of luminal constituents, including bacterial products, dietary antigens and bile acids, have well-documented proinflammatory effects which could induce hepatobiliary injury if they are absorbed across the deranged mucosal barrier of the inflamed intestine. Finally, distribution of proinflammatory soluble mediators, such as cytokines, arachidonic acid metabolites or reactive oxygen intermediates produced by the inflamed intestine, could damage the liver.

ANIMAL MODELS

These theories of pathogenesis can best be tested in animal models, but until recently no relevant chronic hepatobiliary models have been available (Table 2). Early attempts to produce inflammation with chronic portal vein infusions of viable *E. coli* were largely unsuccessful[3]. Lethal infection with *E. coli* produced periportal inflammation, Kupffer cell hyperplasia and increased alkaline phosphatase but sublethal doses had no apparent effect. More recently Kono *et al.*[4] repeatedly injected heat-killed non-pathogenic *E. coli* into the peripheral or portal veins of rabbits, which developed acute periportal and focal parenchymal inflammation. A chronic phase of granulomatous periportal inflammation with fibrosis, bile duct proliferation and Kupffer cell hyperplasia resolved 1 month after the last injection with residual periportal fibrosis. These results demonstrate the ability of non-viable bacterial products to induce protracted periportal inflammation, and suggest that bile duct proliferation is a result of the inflammatory process rather than biliary obstruction. This inflammatory response is probably mediated by cytokines which can also induce fibrosis. This concept is supported by the consequences of daily systemic injections of tumour necrosis factor (TNF-α) in rats[5]. After 8 days of TNF-α, rats developed hepatomegaly, bile duct proliferation, infiltration of portal tracts with mononuclear cells and focal parenchymal necrosis. Continuous interleukin-1 (IL-1) infusion for 1 week induced a slight elevation of transaminases, although the hepatic histology was not described[6]. In very preliminary observations it has been noted that hepatomegaly and periportal inflammation accompanies spontaneous colitis in the cotton-topped tamarin (B.F. Warren, verbal communication) and indomethacin-induced chronic enteritis in Lewis rats[7]. Collectively, these observations suggest that hepatobiliary inflammation can accompany chronic enterocolitis in experimental animals, and that chronic administration of bacterial products or cytokines can induce some of the histological features characteristic of sclerosing cholangitis.

The best-characterized experimental model of chronic hepatobiliary inflammation is that which occurs when genetically susceptible rat strains are exposed to small intestinal bacterial overgrowth[8]. Creation of a self-filling blind loop (SFBL) in the mid-jejunum induces a rapid proliferation of predominantly anaerobic bacteria, which are quite similar in profile to endogenous caecal flora. Female Lewis rats challenged with a SFBL develop hepatomegaly, splenomegaly, hepatobiliary inflammation, progressive increases in plasma AST values and a 50% mortality rate. Hepatobiliary injury begins approximately 2–3 weeks after creation of the SFBL. Periportal inflammation is the most remarkable histological finding, and consists of an influx of predominantly mononuclear cells with scattered neutrophils and evidence of biliary epithelial injury. This reaction is associated with bile duct proliferation, destruction and marked fibrosis (Fig. 1). Parenchymal injury, although less consistent, is manifested by focal chronic inflammation, hepatocellular dropout and Kupffer cell hyperplasia. The relevance of these lesions to sclerosing cholangitis is further documented by dilation, thickening and epithelial hyperplasia of the extrahepatic bile duct and cholangiographic abnormalities of intrahepatic and extrahepatic bile ducts[9] (Fig. 2).

MECHANISMS OF EXPERIMENTAL HEPATOBILIARY INFLAMMATION

We have begun to evaluate mechanisms of hepatobiliary injury associated with experimental small intestinal bacterial overgrowth (Table 3). Host genetic susceptibility is an important and unique feature of this model[8]. Inbred Lewis rats develop hepatobiliary inflammation 2–3 weeks after creation of the SFBL, and Wistar and Sprague-Dawley rats develop similar lesions within 8–12 weeks. However, inbred Buffalo and Fischer F344 rats fail to develop clinical, histological or biochemical evidence of hepatobiliary inflammation despite apparently identical luminal concentrations of bacteria and similar degrees of mucosal injury in the SFBL. Interestingly, Lewis and

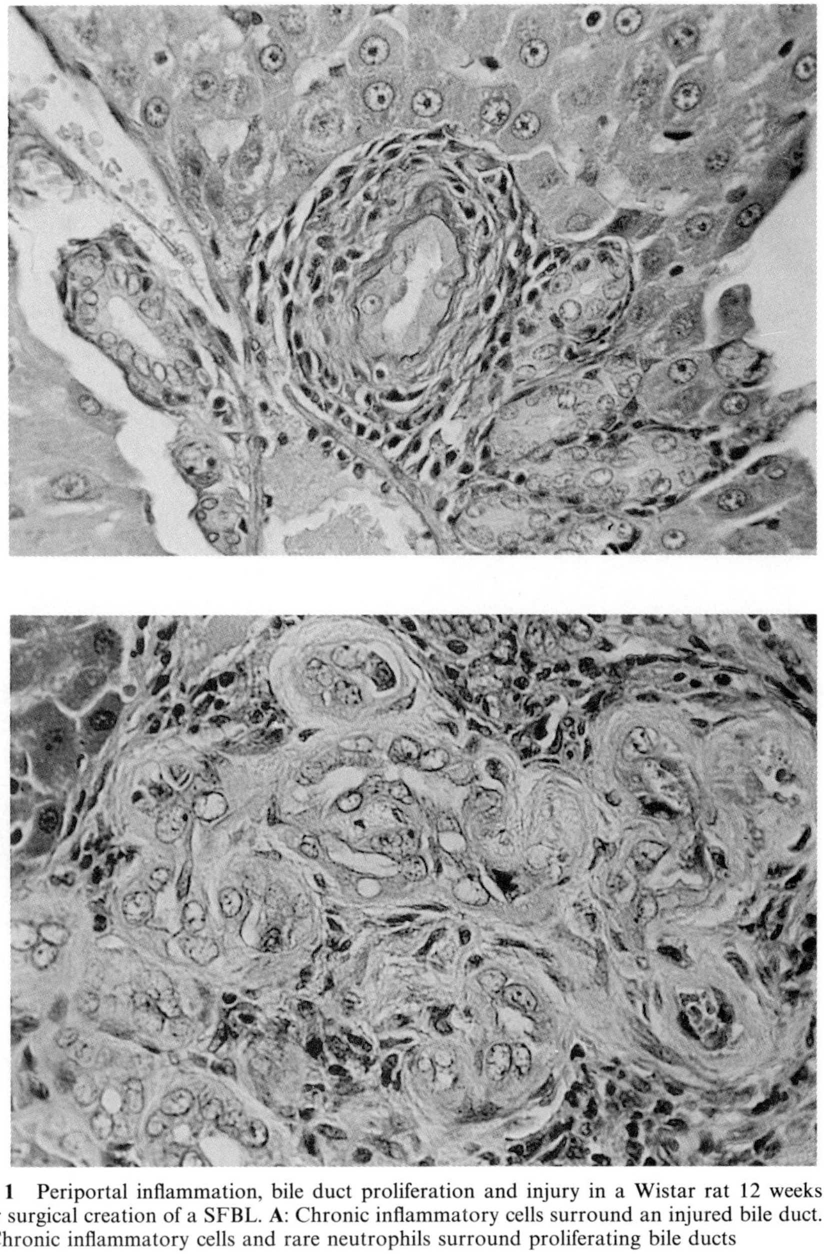

A

B

Fig. 1 Periportal inflammation, bile duct proliferation and injury in a Wistar rat 12 weeks after surgical creation of a SFBL. **A**: Chronic inflammatory cells surround an injured bile duct. **B**: Chronic inflammatory cells and rare neutrophils surround proliferating bile ducts

Fischer rats share identical MHC antigens, suggesting that the differential susceptibility to hepatobiliary inflammation is not a simple MHC-linked trait.

Proliferation of luminal anaerobic bacteria is an essential element in the

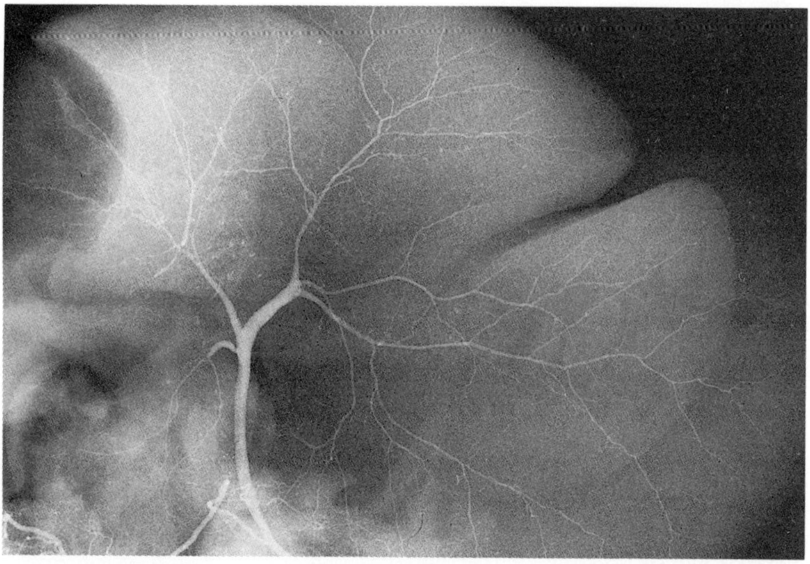

A

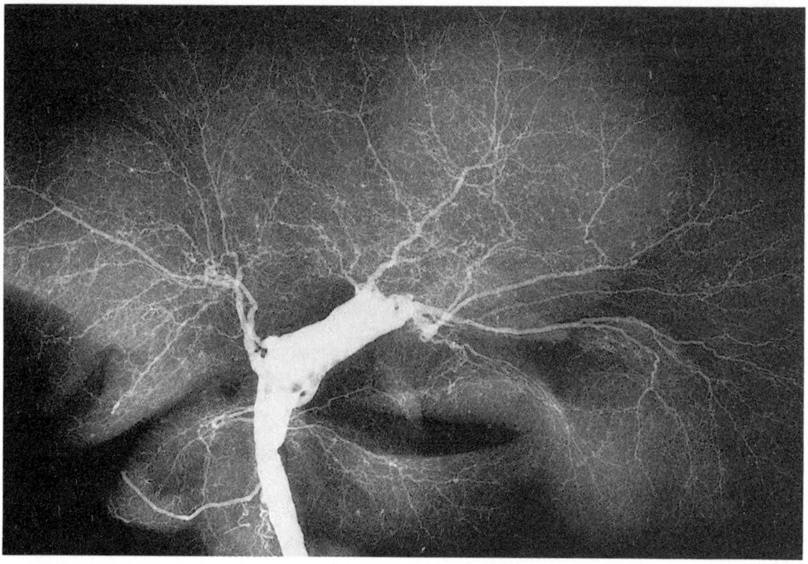

B

Fig. 2 Cholangiograms demonstrating (**A**) normal, smoothly tapering intrahepatic and extrahepatic bile ducts of a sham-operated rat and (**B**) a dilated extrahepatic duct with abruptly tapering and irregular intrahepatic ducts in a Lewis rat 4 weeks after SFBL surgery. Reprinted from ref. 9

Table 3 Pathogenesis of hepatobiliary inflammation associated with experimental small intestinal bacterial overgrowth

1.	Host genetic susceptibility
2.	Proliferation of luminal anaerobic bacteria (? *Bacteroides* spp.)
3.	Systemic absorption and biliary excretion of luminal peptidoglycan–polysaccharide polymers
4.	Cytokine (TNF-α) production (by Kupffer cells?)
5.	Inflammation, fibrosis, bile duct proliferation and injury

pathogenesis of this lesion[10]. Hepatobiliary inflammation is prevented and treated by metronidazole and tetracycline, but not by gentamicin or polymyxin-B. Interestingly, total anaerobic bacterial concentrations within the SFBL were diminished only slightly by chronic antibiotic therapy, but luminal *Bacteroides* spp. were eliminated by metronidazole and tetracycline. These data would suggest that only certain bacterial strains may be important in hepatobiliary inflammation and that *Bacteroides* spp. may be of particular relevance. This organism has previously been implicated as an important factor in vitamin B_{12} malabsorption and disaccharidase deficiency in the SFBL model[11], and has been suggested to have a role in the pathogenesis of Crohn's disease[12]. The rate of translocation of viable bacteria to mesenteric lymph nodes is no different in Lewis vs. Buffalo rats with SFBL (75–90%) and is not changed by metronidazole therapy. The liver, blood and peritoneal cavity of rats with hepatobiliary injury in this model are reproducibly sterile. Thus, bacterial infection of the liver or spread of viable bacteria to regional lymph nodes does not appear to produce the hepatic inflammation, suggesting that constituents or metabolites of the proliferating anaerobic bacteria within the lumen may be important.

Recent data convincingly implicate luminally derived peptidoglycan–polysaccharide (PG-PS) complexes in the pathogenesis of hepatobiliary injury associated with intestinal bacterial overgrowth. PG-PS is the primary structural component of nearly all bacteria, including enteric organisms. These polymers activate almost every limb of the inflammatory cascade and can produce acute and chronic inflammation after systemic or intestinal injection[12]. PG-PS from luminal bacteria is absorbed and systematically distributed in greater amounts after creation of a SFBL, as determined by increased plasma and luminal concentrations of anti-peptidoglycan IgG, IgM and IgA, and more directly by increased hepatic and serum levels of PG-PS injected into the SFBL[13]. PG-PS injected intravenously undergoes biliary excretion[14], suggesting a mechanism for injury that appears to be directed towards the bile duct in this model. Immune complex-mediated damage does not seem to be involved since plasma anti-peptidoglycan antibody concentrations do not correlate with the degree of hepatobiliary injury[13]. The most compelling evidence that PG-PS from an overgrowth of luminal bacteria causes hepatobiliary injury is prevention and treatment of the lesion by mutanolysin, an enzyme which specifically degrades PG-PS by splitting the β1-4 linkage of the polymer[15]. Mutanolysin has no antibiotic activity since it did not alter luminal concentrations of total bacteria or *Bacteroides* and had no apparent effect on mucosal injury. This drug apparently degrades absorbed PG-PS before the polymers can stimulate immune cells, as demonstrated by its prevention of elevated anti-peptidoglycan antibody and increased TFN-α plasma concentrations. Specificity for PG-PS in the pathogenesis of hepatobiliary injury in this model over other bacterial products such as endotoxin (lipopolysaccharide, LPS), is supported by the lack of efficacy of polymyxin-B, which binds and inactivates LPS[10] and failure of elevation of anti-lipid A antibodies[13]. However, PG-PS and LPS exert synergistic activities in activation of phagocytic cells, so an additive role for LPS and other proinflammatory bacterial products such as formylated oligopeptides (FMLP), which also undergo enterohepatic circulation[16], cannot be discounted. A primary role for PG-PS in chronic hepatobiliary inflammation associated with gut injury is supported by the fact that PG-PS injected either systemically or subserosally into the distal intestinal wall induces T lymphocyte-mediated chronic granulomatous hepatic inflammation with marked fibrosis in Lewis, but not Buffalo or Fischer inbred rats[17,18].

Evidence is now accumulating that cytokines, especially TNF-α, produced by Kupffer cells and recruited macrophages mediate hepatobiliary injury in this model. PG-PS, like LPS, stimulates TNF-α, IL-1 and transforming growth factor β (TGF-β) production by Kupffer cells and hepatic granuloma macrophages[19]. Plasma TNF-α is elevated in Lewis rats with experimental intestinal bacterial overgrowth; the increase in plasma TNF-α corresponds to the onset and progression of hepatobiliary injury[15]. Plasma TNF-α levels of rats treated with mutanolysin remain normal. Further documentation of a role for TNF-α produced by activated Kupffer cells is provided by the demonstration that pentoxifylline, which inhibits TNF-α production, and palmitate, which blocks phagocytosis by Kupffer cells, prevent hepatic injury in rats with experimental bacteria overgrowth[20]. Recent perfusion studies show that more TNF-α is released from livers of rats with SFBL than from those with sham operations, indicating that Kupffer cells are activated in this model[21]. Spontaneous and LPS-stimulated TNF-α production is increased in livers of rats with SFBL compared with control rats. Unexpectedly, in preliminary studies ursodeoxycholic acid, prednisone, methotrexate and cyclosporin A fails to prevent injury in this model[15].

CONCLUSIONS

Based on the observations in this model (Table 3) we propose that the following sequence of events is involved in the genesis of hepatobiliary inflammation that is associated with intestinal injury. A genetically susceptible host, which does not exhibit spontaneous hepatic injury, develops chronic, progressive hepatobiliary inflammation when continuously exposed to proinflammatory products of anaerobic bacteria which normally inhabit the distal intestine (Fig. 3). Increased mucosal permeability of the inflamed intestine leads to enhanced uptake of luminal PG-PS, LPS and FMLP into the portal vein, thus continuously stimulating Kupffer cells to secrete proinflammatory cytokines, stimulate fibrosis and induce bile duct proliferation and injury. Biliary excretion of PG-PS and FMLP may help localize

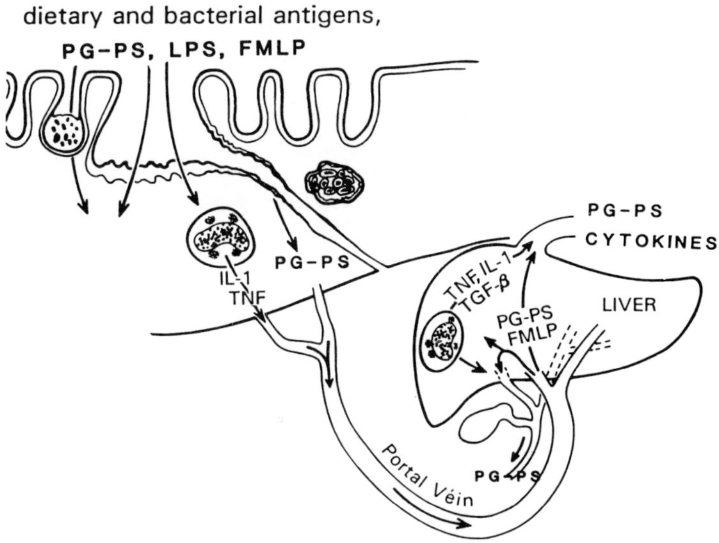

Fig. 3 Sequence of events leading to hepatobiliary inflammation associated with intestinal injury. Mucosal inflammation and ulceration leads to uptake of luminal bacterial products which are concentrated in the liver and bile. PG-PS and LPS activate Kupffer cells to secrete cytokines and inflammatory mediators. PG-PS and FMLP are excreted in the bile and cytokines and PG-PS are secreted into the systemic circulation

the inflammatory response to the bile duct. The mechanisms of genetic susceptibility in patients with sclerosing cholangitis remain to be determined, but preliminary evidence suggests that the Lewis rat has defective production of down-regulatory cytokines (for example, IL-1 receptor antagonist)[22]. The relatively low incidence of sclerosing cholangitis in ulcerative colitis patients suggests the gene(s) predisposing a person to hepatobiliary injury are independent from those associated with ulcerative colitis. Investigation of the genetic background of the subpopulation (approximately 20%) of patients who develop hepatic injury after jejunoileal bypass for obesity may help clarify the genetic susceptibility issue.

Identification of genetic and environmental factors in the Lewis rat model of hepatobiliary inflammation which develops as a consequence of experimental bacterial overgrowth will help focus investigation of the pathogenesis of human sclerosing cholangitis. Furthermore, these insights from the rat model suggest specific targets (i.e. TNF-α, PG-PS, luminal anaerobic bacteria, mucosal permeability changes) for pharmacological intervention in this debilitating and relentlessly progressive human disease.

Acknowledgements

The authors thank Shirley Willard for expert secretarial assistance. Original research supported by U.S. Public Health Service Grants RO1-DK-40249,

R29-DK-44233 and DK-34987 and the Crohn's and Colitis Foundation of America.

References

1. Aadland E, Schrumpf E, Fausa O *et al.* Primary sclerosing cholangitis: a long-term follow-up study. Scand J Gastroenterol. 1987;22:655–64.
2. Olsson R, Danielsson A, Jarnerot G *et al.* Prevalence of primary sclerosing cholangitis in patients with ulcerative colitis. Gastroenterology. 1991;100:1319–23.
3. Vinnik IE, Kern F, Struthers JE *et al.* Experimental chronic portal vein bacteremia. Proc Soc Exp Biol Med. 1964;15:311–14.
4. Kono K, Kunihiko O, Masao O *et al.* Experimental portal fibrosis produced by intraportal injection of killed nonpathogenic *Escherichia coli* in rabbits. Gastroenterology. 1990;98: 414–23.
5. Tracey KJ, Wei H, Manogue KR *et al.* Cachectin/tumor necrosis factor induces cachexia, anemia and inflammation. J Exp Med. 1988;167:1211–27.
6. Otterness IG, Golden HW, Brissette WH *et al.* Effects of continuously administered murine interleukin-1α: tolerance development and granuloma formation. Infect Immun. 1989;57:2742–50.
7. Sartor RB, Bender DE, Holt LC. Susceptibility of inbred rat strains to intestinal and extraintestinal inflammation induced by indomethacin. Gastroenterology. 1992;102:A690.
8. Lichtman SN, Sartor RB, Keku J, Schwab JH. Hepatic inflammation in rats with experimental small intestinal bacterial overgrowth. Gastroenterology. 1990;98:414–23.
9. Lichtman SN, Keku J, Schwab JH, Sartor RB. Biliary tract disease in rats with experimental small bowel bacterial overgrowth. Hepatology. 1991;13:766–72.
10. Lichtman SN, Keku J, Schwab JH, Sartor RB. Hepatic injury associated with small bowel bacterial overgrowth in rats is prevented by metronidazole and tetracycline. Gastroenterology. 1991;100:513–19.
11. Welkos SL, Toskes PP, Baer H, Smith GW. Importance of anaerobic bacteria in the cobalamin malabsorption of the experimental rat blind loop syndrome. Gastroenterology. 1981;80:313–20.
12. Sartor RB. Role of intestinal microflora in initiation and perpetuation of inflammatory bowel disease. Can J Gastroenterol. 1990;4:271–7.
13. Lichtman SN, Keku J, Schwab JH, Sartor RB. Evidence for peptidoglycan absorption in rats with experimental small bowel bacterial overgrowth. Infect Immun. 1991;59:555–62.
14. Lichtman SN, Sartor RB, Schwab JH. Elimination of peptidoglycan–polysaccharide in rat bile. Gastroenterology. 1988;94:A262 (abstract).
15. Lichtman SN, Okoruwa EE, Keku J *et al.* Degradation of endogenous bacterial cell wall polymers by the muralytic enzyme mutanolysin prevents hepatobiliary injury in genetically susceptible rats with experimental intestinal bacterial overgrowth. J Clin Invest. 1992: in press.
16. Hobson CH, Butt TJ, Ferry DM *et al.* Enterohepatic circulation of bacterial chemotactic peptide in rats with experimental colitis. Gastroenterology. 1988;94:1006–13.
17. Wahl SM, Allen JB, Dougherty S *et al.* T-lymphocyte-dependent evolution of bacterial cell wall induced hepatic granulomas. J Immunol. 1986;137:2199–209.
18. Sartor RB, Green KD, Anderle SK. Spontaneously reactivating granulomatous enterocolitis with extraintestinal inflammation induced by bacterial cell wall polymers in genetically susceptible rats. Gastroenterology. 1989;96:A442.
19. Manthey CL, Kossmann T, Allen JB *et al.* Role of Kupffer cells in developing streptococcal cell wall granulomas. Am J Pathol. 1992;140:1205–14.
20. Lichtman SN, Okoruwa NE, Currin RT, LeMasters JJ. Kupffer cells have a role in hepatic injury associated with small bowel bacterial overgrowth. Hepatology. 1991;14:168A (abstract).
21. Lichtman SM, Wang J, Currin R, Lemasters JJ. Peptidoglycan–polysaccharide (PG-PS) and endotoxin (LPS) induce less tumor necrosis factor (TNF) in susceptible strains of rats. Hepatology. 1992;16:164A (abstract).
22. McCall RD, Haskill JS, Sartor RB. Interleukin-1 and IL-1 receptor antagonist gene expression correlate with activity of inflammation in spontaneously relapsing enterocolitis in rats. Gastroenterology. 1991;100:A598 (abstract).

Section IX
Primary Biliary Cirrhosis

38
Primary biliary cirrhosis: definition and epidemiological features

S. SHERLOCK

DEFINITION

Primary biliary cirrhosis is a disease of unknown aetiology characterized by destruction of small intrahepatic bile ducts by a granulomatous reaction[1]. It predominantly affects females, is associated with cholestatic serum biochemical tests and a positive non-organ-specific serum antibody against the M2 component of the mitochondrial pyruvate dehydrogenase complex. Other diseases, largely autoimmune, may be associated. Main intrahepatic bile ducts are patent by cholangiography. These diagnostic points will now be discussed (Table 1).

Liver biopsy: a granulomatous hepatitis

The only hepatic lesion diagnostic of primary biliary cirrhosis is the injured septal or interlobular bile duct[2,3]. Such ducts are not often seen in needle

Table 1 Diagnosis of primary biliary cirrhosis at presentation

Symptomatic
1. Middle-aged woman with pruritus followed by slowly progressive jaundice
2. Liver palpable
3. Serum bilirubin about twice normal; serum alkaline phosphatase about 4 times normal; serum aspartate transaminase about twice normal; serum albumin normal
4. Serum mitochondrial antibody 1:40
5. Liver biopsy appearances compatible
6. ERCP (if diagnosis in doubt); normal intrahepatic bile ducts

Asymptomatic
1. Routine laboratory screen
2. Increased serum alkaline phosphatase
3. Positive serum mitochondrial antibody
4. Investigation of other disease, especially collagen or thyroid
5. Hepatomegaly

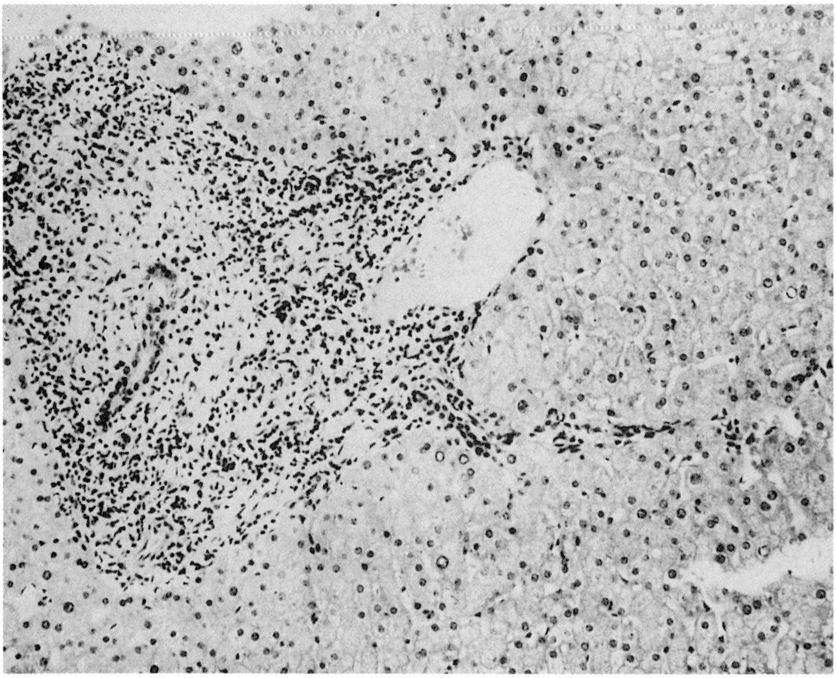

Fig. 1 Early primary biliary cirrhosis. The portal (zone 1) area is expanded by a cellular infiltrate and contains a damaged bile duct. Stained haematoxylin and eosin × 135

biopsy specimens, but are usually well represented in surgical biopsies (Fig. 1). Epithelial cells are swollen, irregular and more eosinophilic. The bile duct lumen is irregular and the basement membrane is disrupted. Surrounding the damaged duct is a cellular reaction which includes lymphocytes, plasma cells, eosinophils and histiocytes. Non-caseating granulomas commonly form, usually in zone 1.

Cytotoxic T cells can be seen infiltrating the bile duct epithelium, as are class 2 restricted T-4 lymphocytes. The final event is an attack by cytotoxic T cells on biliary epithelium. Suppressor T cells are reduced in number and function. Up-regulated display of HLA class 1 antigens and *de novo* expression of HLA class 2 antigens are compatible with immune-mediated duct destruction.

Later bile ducts disappear, and the sites are marked by aggregates of lymphoid cells; bile ductules begin to proliferate. Fibrosis progresses and ultimately an end-stage biliary cirrhosis is seen.

Diagnostic or compatible needle biopsy appearances are helpful in confirming the diagnosis, but liver biopsy is having a diminished role. A middle-aged woman with cholestatic biochemical tests and a strongly positive serum M2 test does not usually need a liver biopsy to confirm the diagnosis of primary biliary cirrhosis. Serial biopsies to follow progress are unnecessary unless the patient is part of a therapeutic clinical trial.

Sex and age

Ninety per cent of patients are female[2]. The cause for the prevalence in women is unknown. The patient is usually aged between 40 and 60 years, but can be as old as 80 years or as young as 20 years. The disease has a very long course, many years of which are asymptomatic[4]. In one series one-third of patients were diagnosed when asymptomatic[5]. The inclusion of such cases reduces the age at presentation.

Symptoms and serum biochemistry

The classical presentation is as insidious pruritus without jaundice, which follows a variable period later, usually within $2\frac{1}{2}$ years.

Widespread use of automated biochemical screening has resulted in an increasing number of patients being diagnosed when asymptomatic. Liver biopsy performed after finding a positive serum mitochondrial antibody during screening for autoimmune disease is almost always abnormal, and usually shows features consistent with primary biliary cirrhosis even if the patient is asymptomatic and the serum alkaline phosphatase is normal.

Patients with primary biliary cirrhosis can survive a very long time and remain asymptomatic even up to 20 years.

Serum biochemical tests usually show increased membrane-bound enzymes, serum alkaline phosphatase and γ-glutamyl transpeptidase. Cytosolic enzymes, alanine transferase and aspartate transaminase are only moderately increased. Serum IgM is usually increased, but the levels are not diagnostic. Serum cholesterol is variably elevated. Serum bilirubin levels rarely exceed 2 mg in asymptomatic patients. Total serum bile acids are increased.

In the early stages there is a striking elevation of high-density lipoproteins (HDL) with modest changes in apolipoprotein B-containing lipoproteins (VLDL and LDL). As the liver disease progresses HDL declines, with concomitant elevation of LDL to levels often greater than those encountered in patients suffering from familial hypercholesterolaemia. In one patient a serum cholesterol level exceeding 50 mmol/l was recorded, resulting in a hyperviscosity syndrome which necessitated plasma exchanges[7]. The elevation of LDL is largely due to the accumulation of an abnormal lipoprotein found in all forms of cholestasis (LpX).

Serum mitochondrial antibodies (anti-M2)

Virtually 100% of patients with primary biliary cirrhosis show circulating antibodies against mitochondrial components[8,9]. The antigens to which the antibodies are directed are localized in the inner mitochondrial membrane. The antigenic component specific for PBC serum is M2, a component of the pyruvate dehydrogenase complex of mitochondrial enzymes[10]. An ELISA has been developed against components of the M2 complex[11,12] and is 98% sensitive and 96% specific for the diagnosis of primary biliary cirrhosis. A further elegant refinement of the ELISA uses a recombinant dual-headed hybrid molecule and gives a sensitivity of 93%[13]. The diagnosis of primary biliary cirrhosis is unlikely in the absence of serum anti-M2. These specific sensitive tests may not be generally available and the routine serum antimitochondrial test is performed by indirect immunofluorescence on rat kidney substrate. This is a difficult technique and can give false-negative results in inexperienced laboratories. However, good comparisons have not been made between the ELISA and the immunofluorescence, and immunofluorescence continues to be the routine test in the clinic[14].

Endoscopic cholangiography

Visualization of the bile duct by endoscopic percutaneous cholangiography may be necessary in atypical patients. These include males and those with a negative serum mitochondrial antibody test, with inconclusive liver biopsy findings or with abdominal pain. Surgical exploration of the bile ducts is not necessary for diagnosis.

Associated diseases

Non-hepatic disorders are frequently associated with primary biliary cirrhosis[1]. These are frequently postulated autoimmune conditions. The collagenases, especially rheumatoid arthritis, dermatomyositis, mixed connective tissue disease and systemic lupus erythematosus, are particularly frequent. Primary biliary cirrhosis may be associated with scleroderma in 4% of patients and with the whole CREST syndrome. A sicca complex of dry eyes and mouth, with or without the arthritis completing Sjögren's syndrome, is found in about three-quarters of patients. Autoimmune thyroiditis is frequent, affecting about 20% of sufferers. Jejunal villus atrophy, resembling coeliac disease, has been associated.

Abnormal pulmonary gas transfer studies are associated with an abnormal chest X-ray showing nodules and interstitial fibrosis. Pulmonary interstitial giant cell granulomas have been described.

CT scanning shows 81% of patients with enlarged nodes in the gastrohepatic ligament and porta hepatis[15]. Enlarged paracardiac and mesenteric nodes are also seen.

DIFFERENTIAL DIAGNOSIS

Cholestatic drug reactions

These are excluded by the history and by the acute onset with rapidly deepening jaundice developing 4–6 weeks after the drug is started.

Table 2 Cholestatic sarcoidosis compared with primary biliary cirrhosis

	Sarcoidosis	*Primary biliary cirrhosis*
Sex	Equal	80% Female
Age	Young	Middle age
Pruritus	Yes	Yes
Jaundice	Yes	Yes
Respiratory complaints	Yes	No
Hepatosplenomegaly	Yes	Yes
Serum alkaline phosphatase	Raised	Raised
Hilar lymphadenopathy	Usual	Rare
Hepatic granulomas	Discrete	Poorly formed
	Clustered	Surrounded with mixed cells
Serum angiotensin-converting enzyme	Raised	Raised
Mitochondrial antibody	No	Yes (98%)
Kveim–Siltzbach test	Positive	Negative
Bronchoalveolar lavage		
Lymphocytosis	Present	Present
Activated macrophages	Present	Present

Primary sclerosing cholangitis

This may cause chronic cholestasis, more often in males than females. However, the serum anti-M2 is negative and, if necessary, endoscopic cholangiography shows the classical intrahepatic bile duct lesions.

Cholestatic sarcoidosis

This can cause real diagnostic difficulty. It may not be possible to exclude it on the basis of clinical features, serum biochemistry, serum angiotensin converting enzyme (SACE) or liver biopsy (Table 2)[16]. However, in sarcoidosis the serum mitochondrial antibody is negative.

Immune cholangiopathy

The patient shows features overlapping between primary biliary cirrhosis and autoimmune chronic active hepatitis[17–19]. These patients, usually women, present with cholestatic symptoms and biochemistry, and with liver biopsy histology resembling primary biliary cirrhosis[20]. However, the serum mitochondrial antibody (and the serum anti-M2) are negative while the serum antinuclear antibody (ANA) is usually strongly positive as is smooth muscle antibody (Table 3). The entity has been termed immune cholangitis[21]. The response to prenisolone therapy is rapid and beneficial[20,21]. This probably represents a variant of autoimmune chronic active hepatitis predominantly affecting bile ducts.

EPIDEMIOLOGY

Primary biliary cirrhosis has been reported from all parts of the world. Asians, Caucasians, Jews, Negroes and Orientals are all affected. There is

Table 3 Primary biliary cirrhosis compared with immune cholangiopathy

	Primary biliary cirrhosis	*Immune cholangiopathy*
Sex	Female	Female
Biochemistry	Cholestatic	Cholestatic
Liver biopsy		
Periportal infiltration	Present	Present
Bile duct lesions	Present	Present
Serum antibodies		
Mitochondrial	Present	Absent
Antinuclear	Absent	Present
Response to prednisolone	Fair	Good

great variability in the prevalence between different countries, and even between districts in the same country. It is extremely difficult to measure the geographical prevalence and death rates. Diagnosis is improving so that more asymptomatic patients are identified. Physician awareness, and particularly the presence of a newly arrived trained hepatologist in the community, changes the prevalence. The availability of such diagnostic tools as the mitochondrial antibody test varies from country to country. Primary biliary cirrhosis is believed to account for about 2% of patients dying from cirrhosis[22].

The International Association for the Study of the Liver have conducted a survey of 39 liver units in 19 countries covering 118 million persons. A total of 4300 cases were identified, giving a prevalence of 20–50 per million[23]. The prevalence per million was higher in countries such as Austria, Germany, Sweden and the United Kingdom, than in countries such as Argentina, South Africa and India. In northern Europe the prevalence was 100–150 per million compared with less than 5 per million for India and South Africa. The prevalence differs within one country. In Israel 28 patients were reported in Jews, but none in Arabs. From rural northern Sweden the mean annual incidence was 13.3 per million with point prevalence of 151 per million, which is the highest reported so far[24]. This was much higher than for southern Sweden where the value was 92 per million[25]. A wide survey of gastroenterologists in Ontario, Canada, revealed an incidence of 3.26 per million per year, with a prevalence of 22.39 per million[26]. There was no racial or geographical clustering. Some believe that the prevalence is higher in industrial than rural areas[5,27], but this was not confirmed by the Swedish study[24] or the Canadian one[26]. The disease seems to be increasing. In Newcastle-upon-Tyne, in the north of England, the prevalence rose from 18 per million in 1976 to 128.5 per million in 1987[5]. The disease seems to be increasing particularly rapidly in Japan, and especially in asymptomatic cases[28]. All these results may reflect better awareness of the disease and the more frequent recognition of the asymptomatic patient.

Genetic and environmental factors

There is family clustering, and primary biliary cirrhosis has been reported in sisters, twins, mothers and daughters[29,30]. In one study the familial incidence was 2.4%[5]. In a study in Sheffield, 200 relatives and spouse relatives of 45 patients showed a prevalence of M2 antibody in 7.6% of first-degree relatives compared with 7.2% in spouses and their relatives[23]. Environmental factors are also suggested by the development of the disease in a daughter, her mother and non-related close friend who nursed the daughter in her terminal illness[31]. Anti-M9 antibody (one of the family of mitochondrial antibodies) can occur in healthy controls exposed to primary biliary cirrhosis, i.e. relatives and laboratory workers[32]. From Victoria, Australia, it was found that the prevalence was 13 per million in Australian-born compared with 47 per million in north European-born persons[33].

In one study from Sheffield, primary biliary cirrhosis was associated with a particular water supply[34], and this study has been extended for a further 10 years and the original results confirmed[23].

Results for histocompatibility typing have given controversial results. Early work suggested that there was no association of primary biliary cirrhosis with any HLA, A, B or DR antigen[35–37]. In a white population from the United States, HLA DRw8 was associated with primary biliary cirrhosis[38] and an increased incidence of C4B2 reported from England[39]. A more recent study has included all three classes of HLA[40]. HLA class 1 antigen did not differ significantly from healthy controls. However, HLA class 2 antigen showed a highly significant increase of HLA DRw8 in patients with primary biliary cirrhosis compared with controls. C4A-QO, an HLA class III allele, is associated with many autoimmune diseases including autoimmune chronic active hepatitis and systemic lupus erythematosus. Genetic typing revealed an increased incidence for C4A-QO alleles. A highly significant proportion of PBC patients carried DRw8 and C4A-QO alleles. A mother and daughter and two sisters with primary biliary cirrhosis shared the major histocompatibility haplotype. Class 3 antigens are components of the complement system. This indicates a partial C4A deficiency in patients with primary biliary cirrhosis.

It is difficult to make a coherent story from all these genetic and environmental observations. They suggest a strong immunogenetic background for primary biliary cirrhosis which runs in families. Environmental factors cannot be ignored, and these presumably act on the genetically susceptible host.

References

1. Sherlock S, Dooley JC. Primary biliary cirrhosis. In: Diseases of the liver and biliary system, 9th edn. Oxford: Blackwell Scientific Publications; 1993;236–48.
2. Sherlock S, Scheuer PJ. The presentation and diagnosis of 100 patients with primary biliary cirrhosis. N Engl J Med. 1973;289:674–8.
3. Scheuer PJ. Primary biliary cirrhosis. Proc R Soc Med. 1967;60:1257–60.
4. Long RG, Scheuer PJ, Sherlock S. Presentation and course of asymptomatic primary biliary cirrhosis. Gastroenterology. 1977;72:1204–7.
5. Myszor M, James OFW. The epidemiology of primary biliary cirrhosis in north-east England: an increasingly common disease. Q J Med. 1990;75:377–85.
6. Mistry P, Seymour CA. Primary biliary cirrhosis – from Thomas Addison to the 1990s. Q J Med. 1992;82:185–96.

7. Rosenson RS, Baker AL, Chow MJ *et al.* Hyperviscosity syndrome in a hypercholesterolaemic patient with primary biliary cirrhosis. Gastroenterology. 1990;98:1351–7.
8. Walker JG, Doniach D, Roitt IM *et al.* Serological tests in the diagnosis of primary biliary cirrhosis. Lancet. 1965;1:827–31.
9. Munoz LE, Thomas HC, Scheuer PJ *et al.* Is mitochondrial antibody diagnostic of primary biliary cirrhosis? Gut. 1981;22:136–40.
10. Berg PA, Klein R, Lindenborn-Fotinos J. Antimitochondrial antibodies in primary biliary cirrhosis. J Hepatol. 1986;2:123–31.
11. Van de Water J, Cooper A, Surh CD *et al.* Detection of autoantibodies to recombinant mitochondrial proteins in patients with primary biliary cirrhosis. N Engl J Med. 1989;320:1377–80.
12. Heseltine L, Turner IB, Fussey SPM *et al.* Primary biliary cirrhosis: quantitation of autoantibodies to purified mitochondrial enzymes and correlation with disease progression. Gastroenterology. 1990;99:1786–92.
13. Leung PSC, Iwayama T, Prindiville T *et al.* Use of designer recombinant mitochondrial antigens in the diagnosis of primary biliary cirrhosis. Hepatology. 1992;15:367–72.
14. Bassendine MF, Yeaman SJ. Serological markers of primary biliary cirrhosis: diagnosis, prognosis and subsets. Hepatology. 1992;15:545–8.
15. Outwater E, Kaplan MM, Bankoff MS. Lymphadenopathy in primary biliary cirrhosis: CT observations. Radiology. 1989;171:731–3.
16. Sherlock S. The liver in sarcoidosis. Semin Resp Dis. 1992:in press.
17. Geubel AP, Baggenstoss AH, Summerskill WHJ. Responses to treatment can differentiate chronic active liver disease with cholangitic features from the primary biliary cirrhosis syndrome. Gastroenterology. 1976;71:444–9.
18. Okuno T, Seto Y, Okanque T, Takino T. Chronic active hepatitis with histological features of primary biliary cirrhosis. Dig Dis Sci. 1987;32:775–9.
19. Shouval D, Levij IS, Eliakim M. Chronic active hepatitis with cholestatic features. 1. A clinical and immunological study. Am J Gastroenterol. 1979;72:542–50.
20. Ben-Ari Z, Dhillon AP, Sherlock S. Autoimmune cholangiopathy? Part of the spectrum of autoimmune chronic active hepatitis. Hepatology. 1993: in press.
21. Brunner G, Klinge O. A cholangitis with antinuclear antibodies (immunocholangitis) resembling chronic non-suppurative destructive cholangitis. Dtsch Med. 1987;112:1454–8.
22. Hamlyn AN, Sherlock S. The epidemiology of primary biliary cirrhosis: a survey of mortality in England and Wales. Gut. 1974;15:473–9.
23. Triger DR. Epidemiology: is there an environmental contribution? Presented at the International Association for Study of the Liver, Brighton, England, 1992.
24. Danielsson A, Boqvist L, Uddenfeldt P *et al.* Epidemiology of primary biliary cirrhosis in a defined rural population in the northern part of Sweden. Hepatology. 1990;11:458–64.
25. Eriksson S, Lindgren S. The prevalence and clinical spectrum of primary biliary cirrhosis in a defined population. Scand J Gastroenterol. 1984;19:971–6.
26. Witt-Sullivan H, Heathcote J, Cauch K *et al.* The demography of primary biliary cirrhosis in Ontario, Canada. Hepatology. 1990;12:98–105.
27. Hamlyn AN, Macklon AF, James O. Primary biliary cirrhosis: geographical clustering and symptomatic onset seasonality. Gut. 1983;24:940–5.
28. Inoue K, Hirohara J, Nakano T *et al.* Prediction of prognosis in primary biliary cirrhosis: a study in Japan. Proceedings, International Association for the Study of the Liver, Brighton, 1992 (abstract).
29. Chohan MR. Primary biliary cirrhosis in twin sisters. Gut. 1973;14:213–16.
30. Tong MJ, Nies KM, Reynolds TB *et al.* Immunological studies in familial primary biliary cirrhosis. Gastroenterology. 1976;71:305–7.
31. Douglas JG, Finlayson NDC. Are increased individual susceptibility and environmental factors both necessary for the development of primary biliary cirrhosis? Br Med J. 1979;2:419–20.
32. Klein R, Berg PA. Demonstration of 'naturally occurring mitochondrial antibodies' in family members of patients with primary biliary cirrhosis. Hepatology. 1990;12:335–9.
33. Watson RGP, Goss B, Angus PW *et al.* Low prevalence of primary biliary cirrhosis (PBC) in Victoria, Australia. Proceedings, International Association for the Study of the Liver, Brighton, 1992 (abstract).

34. Triger DR. Primary biliary cirrhosis: an epidemiological study. Br Med J. 1980;281:772–5.
35. Hamlyn AN, Adams D, Sherlock S. Primary or secondary sicca complex? Investigation in primary biliary cirrhosis by histocompatibility testing. Br Med J. 1980;9:425–6.
36. Bassendine MF, Dewar PJ, James OFW. HLA-DR antigens in primary biliary cirrhosis: lack of association. Gut. 1985;26:625–8.
37. James SP, Jones EA, Schafer DF *et al.* Selective immunoglobulin A deficiency associated with primary biliary cirrhosis in a family with liver disease. Gastroenterology. 1986;90: 283–8.
38. Gores GJ, Moore SB, Fisher LD *et al.* Primary biliary cirrhosis: association with class II major histocompatibility complex antigens. Hepatology. 1987;7:889–92.
39. Briggs DC, Donaldson PT, Hayes P *et al.* A major histocompatibility complex class III allotype (C4B 2) associated with primary biliary cirrhosis (PBC). Tissue Antigens. 1987;29:141–5.
40. Manns MP, Bremm A, Schneider PM *et al.* HLA DRw8 and complement C4 deficiency as risk factors in primary biliary cirrhosis. Gastroenterology. 1991;101:1367–73.

39
Clinical relevance of different types of mitochondrial antibodies in primary biliary cirrhosis

P. A. BERG and R. KLEIN

INTRODUCTION

Primary biliary cirrhosis (PBC) is characterized by an inflammation of medium-sized bile ducts mediated by T cells. This immunological activity seems to determine the outcome of the disease. However, although there is no doubt that PBC can manifest itself as a rather progressive or a benign form[1,2], little is known about the natural course of the disease.

Recently we showed that the determination of different types of antimitochondrial antibodies is a reliable approach in differentiating between these two forms of PBC already at early stages[2]. Four AMA types (anti-M2, -M4, -M8, -M9) have been described[3], and retrospective studies clearly indicate that the association of complement fixing anti-M2/-M4 and -M8 antibodies especially heralds a rather progressive course[4–6].

In this chapter we will describe the different mitochondrial antigen–antibody systems and their application for the evaluation of prognosis of PBC in the early stages.

THE M2/ANTI-M2 SYSTEM

M2 could be released from inner membranes of beef heart mitochondria together with the enzyme ATPase by chloroform treatment ('ATPase-associated antigen', later named M2). Gel filtration and ion exchange chromatography lead to a separation of the ATPase enzyme from the M2 antigen[7,8]. However, using this 'ATPase fraction' in sensitive assays such as fluorometric or enzyme-linked immunoassay showed a high specificity for PBC, i.e. sera from patients with other hepatic and non-hepatic disorders did not react with this antigen[9–11]. Western blotting analysis revealed that this ATPase-associated M2 antigen consists of five antigenic determinants

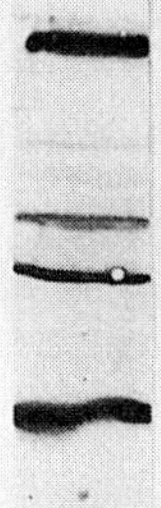

M2-determinants		identification of polypeptides	
- a	70 kD	I	E2-subunit of the pyruvate dehydrogenase complex (PDH) (dihydrolipoamid acetyltransferase)
- b	56 kD	II	protein X of PDH
- c	51 kD	III	E2-subunit of the branched chain 2-oxoacid dehydrogenase complex (branched chain acyltransferase)
		IV	E2-subunit of the 2-oxoglutarate dehydrogenase complex (succinyl transferase)
- d	45 kD	V	E1 alpha > subunit of the PDH complex
- e	36 kD	VI	E1 beta > subunit of the PDH complex

Fig. 1 Demonstration of the five major M2 determinants by Western blotting using the M2 fraction and their identification as the six polypeptides of the 2-oxoacid dehydrogenase complex

at 70 kDa (M2a), 56 kDa (M2b), 52 kDa (M2c), 45 kDa (M2d), and 36 kDa (M2e)[12]. These epitopes could be identified as subunits of the 2-oxoacid dehydrogenase complex of the inner mitochondrial membrane (Fig. 1)[13–16].

For the complement fixation test also this M2 fraction or the commercially available pyruvate dehydrogenase (PDH), the major component of the 2-oxoacid dehydrogenase complex, can be used. Highest titres are, however, obtained when these antigen fractions are applied to isopycnic sucrose density gradient centrifugation (100 000*g*, 24 h). The complement fixing M2-antigen bands at densities of 1.24–1.28 (Fig. 2). In contrast, cloned antigen fractions do not fix complement (unpublished observation).

The M2 antigen present in the ATPase fraction, as well as in the PDH, is protease-sensitive and can be destroyed by trypsin treatment (Figs 2 and 3).

THE M4/ANTI-M4 SYSTEM

Anti-M4 antibodies were initially detected when PBC sera were tested in the CFT against both the inner and outer mitochondrial membrane fractions derived from rat liver[4,17]. The M4 antigen can be further purified by subjecting a 100 000*g* supernatant from rat liver to ion exchange chromatography. The first peak contains M4[18]. In order to get an antigen fraction with high complement fixing activity, this 100 000*g* supernatant has to be layered onto isopycnic sucrose density gradients; the M4 antigen can be recovered at densities of 1.08–1.10 (Fig. 4)[19]. In contrast to M2 it is not destroyed by trypsin treatment (Figs 3 and 4).

Recently we showed that anti-M4 antibodies recognize epitopes which are associated with the sulphite oxidase, an enzyme of the mitochondrial intermembrane space[20]. This is a dimeric enzyme which consists of two subunits each of 55–60 kDa. Only PBC sera which were anti-M2 *and* anti-M4 positive reacted with this enzyme, and the anti-M4 antibody activity could be abolished by incubation of patients' sera with this enzyme. This commercially available enzyme can be used for the detection of anti-M4 in the ELISA but it shows only very weak complement fixing activity. M4-

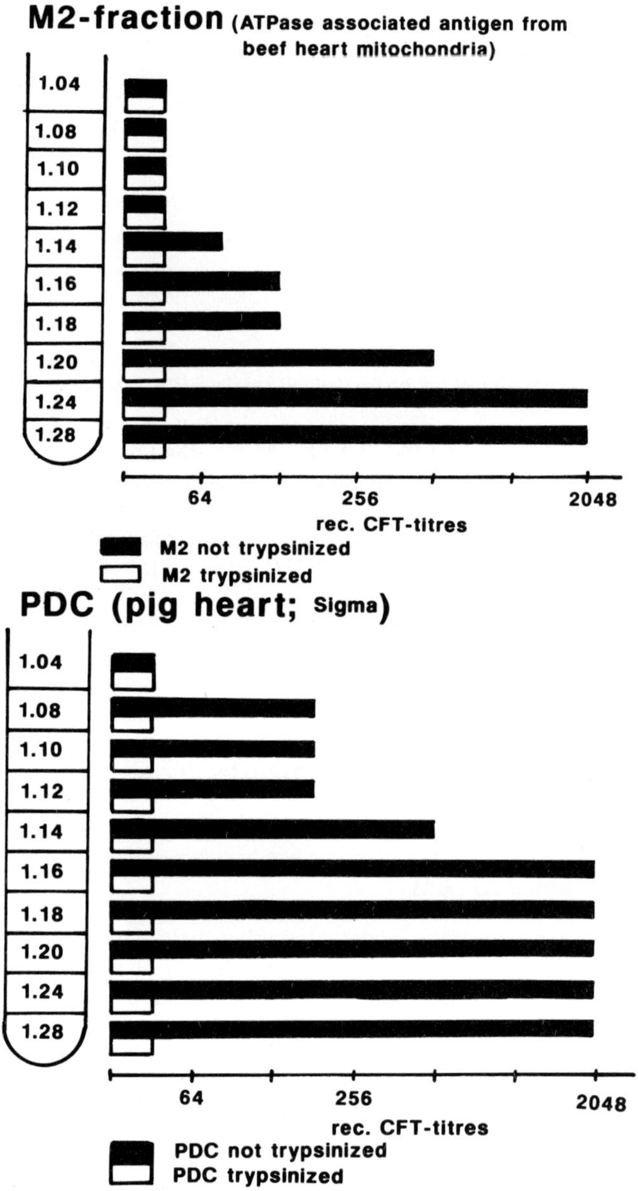

A

B

Fig. 2 Preparation of an M2 fraction with high complement-fixing activity subjecting either the ATPase-associated antigen fraction prepared from beef heart mitochondria (**A**) or the commercially available pyruvate dehydrogenase (PDC) from pig heart (Sigma, St Louis) (**B**) to isopycnic sucrose density gradient centrifugation (gradients 1.04–1.28). Testing the different gradients against a PBC serum with high anti-M2 titres in the complement fixation test (CFT), the M2 antigen was recovered in gradients 1.20–1.28 using the ATPase fraction (**A**) and 1.14–1.28 using the PDC (**B**). This reactivity was completely abolished when the antigen fractions were treated with trypsin

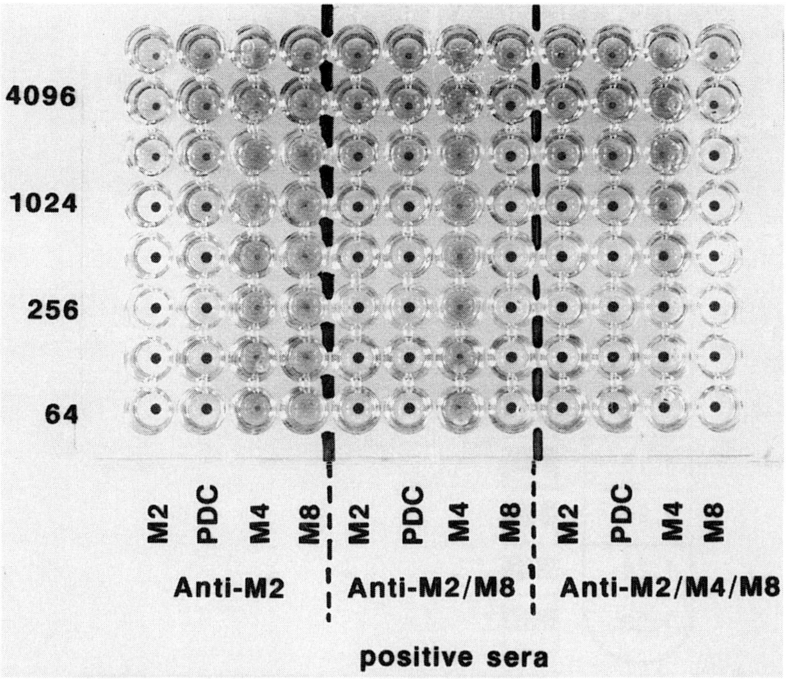

Fig. 3 Demonstration of anti-M2, -M4, and -M8 antibodies in the complement fixation test testing an anti-M2-positive/anti-M4- and -M8-negative serum, an anti-M2- and anti-M8 positive/anti-M4 negative serum and an anti-M2/-M4/-M8 positive serum against the M2 fraction, PDC, M4, and M8

specific determinants cannot be visualized in the Western blot using either the purified M4 fraction or the sulphite oxidase.

Anti-M4 antibodies were preferentially observed in sera from patients with active PBC, and in many instances these patients had histological features of chronic active hepatitis and showed an elevation of IgG and IgM globulins in parallel[4,19].

THE M8/ANTI-M8 SYSTEM

Evidence for a third complement-fixing AMA type came from the initial studies using an M2-negative antigen fraction obtained after sonication of human liver mitochondria. Subjecting this fraction to discontinuous sucrose density gradient centrifugation, M4 was again found at densities of 1.08–1.10 (see above) while the third complement-fixing antigen gathered at layers ranging from 1.14 to 1.18. This antigen was named M8[19].

Since it is difficult to get fresh human liver previously shown to contain high M8 activity, we tried to isolate M8 from mitochondria from animal tissue. It was found to be present in large amounts in pig kidney. The M8 antigen could be isolated from outer mitochondrial membranes or

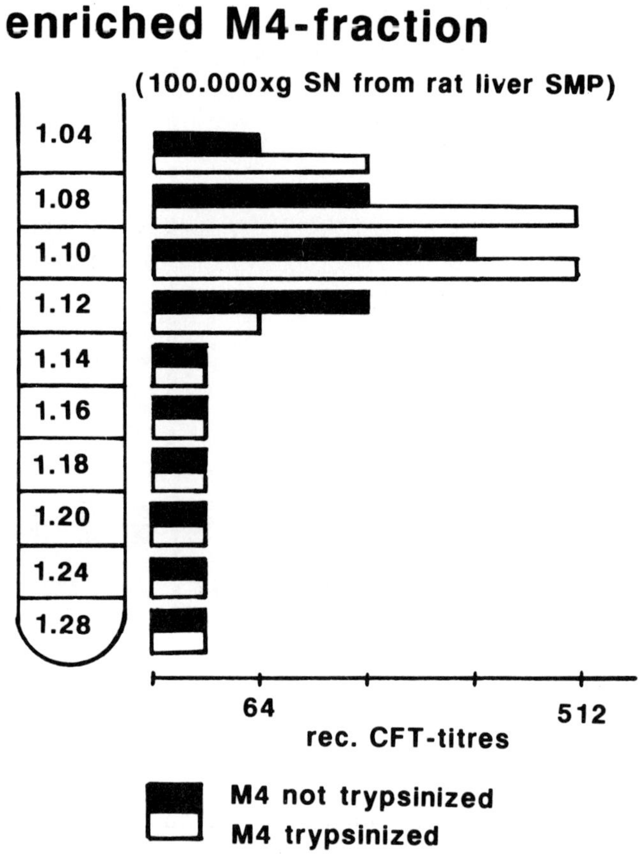

Fig. 4 Preparation of an M4 fraction with high complement-fixing activity subjecting an 100 000*g* supernatant (SN) from rat liver submitochondrial particles (SMP) to isopycnic sucrose density gradient centrifugation (gradients 1.04–1.28). Testing these gradients against a PBC serum with high anti-M2 and anti-M4 titres, the M4 antigen was recovered at densities of 1.04–1.12, and the reactivity was not abolished by trypsin treatment. No reaction was obtained with densities of 1.20–1.28, indicating that no M2 antigen was present in these antigen fractions

microsomes by Sepharose 6B gel filtration. It was found in the ascending part of the second peak, and this M8 fraction was devoid of M2 and M4 and could be used in ELISA and CFT[5].

In order to obtain high complement-fixing activity, sonicated pig kidney microsomes can also be applied to isopycnic sucrose density centrifugation; as with human liver mitochondria (see above), M8 again bands at 1.14–1.18 (Fig. 5).

Like M4, the M8 antigen does not react in the immunoblot, but in contrast to M4 it is destroyed by trypsin treatment (Figs 3 and 5). This antigen has not yet been identified.

The reaction of three marker sera showing only anti-M2, anti-M2 and anti-M8, and anti-M2,-M4,-M8 activity with the M2 fraction, PDC, and the

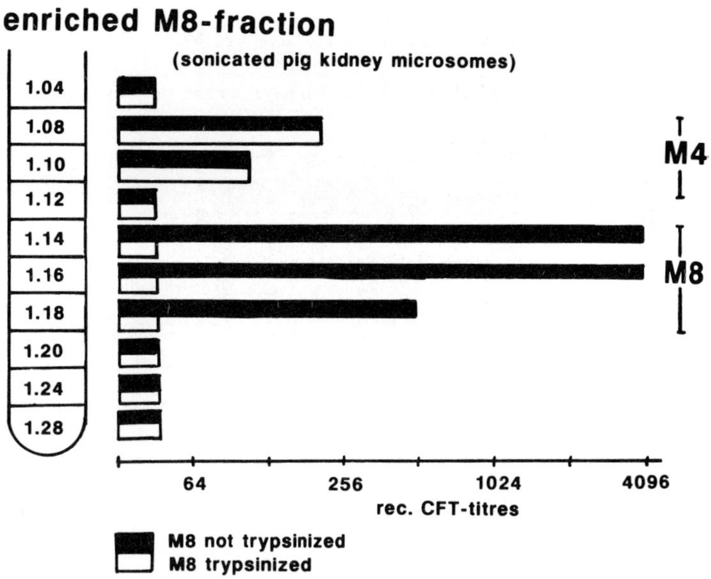

Fig. 5 Preparation of an M8 fraction with high complement-fixing activity subjecting sonicated pig kidney microsomes to isopycnic sucrose density gradient centrifugation (gradients 1.04–1.28). Testing these gradients against a PBC serum with high anti-M2/-M4/-M8 titres the M8 antigen was recovered at densities of 1.14–1.18, and this reactivity was abolished by trypsin treatment. Furthermore, the serum reacted with the trypsin-insensitive gradients 1.08–1.10, and this reaction was due to the presence of M4 in these fractions. No M2 activity could be detected, i.e. the serum did not react with gradients 1.20–1.28

M4 and M8 fractions in the complement fixation test (CFT) is shown in Fig. 6.

THE M9/ANTI-M9 SYSTEM

Anti-M9 antibodies were accidentally detected testing anti-M2-positive sera against trypsin-treated submitochondrial particles from rat liver which were devoid of M2[18]. The M9 antigen could be further purified by ion exchange chromatography using a 100 000*g* supernatant from rat liver SMP. The highest M9 activity was found in the peak eluted by 1 mol/l NaCl. This 'purified' M9 fraction revealed two determinants at molecular weights 98 and 59 kDa in Western blot. Anti-M9 antibodies cannot be detected by CFT.

Further studies indicated that M9 is associated with glycogen phosphorylase, a cytoplasmic enzyme which binds easily to mitochondrial membranes[21]. This enzyme is enriched in liver and skeletal muscle, and consists of subunits at 98 kDa. Although glycogen phosphorylase from skeletal muscle is commercially aailable, this enzyme fraction should not be used in the ELISA since it is not pure, and reacts with naturally occurring antibodies in sera from patients with infectious or chronic inflammatory diseases.

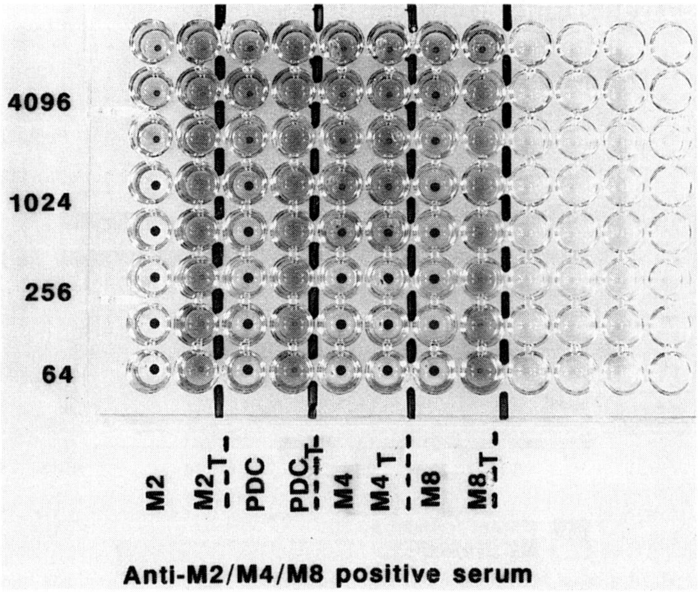

Fig. 6 Reactivity of an anti-M2/-M4/-M8-positive marker serum with M2, PDC, M4, and M8 before and after trypsin treatment (T) in the complement fixation test. Reciprocal CFT titres are given. The reaction with M2, PDC, and M8 became negative after trypsin treatment of these antigen fractions ($M2_T$, PDC_T, $M8_T$) while the M4 antigen was not destroyed by this procedure ($M4_T$)

THE FOUR AMA PROFILES IN PBC

From follow-up studies of PBC patients it emerged that anti-M2/anti-M9 antibodies were frequently found in patients with histological stages I/II while anti-M2-positive patients in advanced stages predominantly expressed anti-M4 and anti-M8[4,22]. We therefore defined four different AMA-profiles labelled A–D, based on different constellations of the four AMA types[6]:

A: only anti-M9-positive in the ELISA
B: anti-M9 and/or anti-M2-positive in the ELISA
C: anti-M2/-M4 and/or anti-M8-positive in the ELISA
D: anti-M2/-M4 and/or anti-M8-positive in ELISA *and* CFT.

The validity of the serological classification for the prediction of prognosis was analysed in three different groups of patients:

Group I: 76 PBC patients from the DRK hospital, Hamburg, all being in stage I/II at time of first diagnosis and followed continuously from 1970 to 1988 (median observation period 10 years); histology was analysed by only one pathologist (G. Klöppel, Brussels)[2].

Group II: 3000 patients collected from different hospitals mainly in Germany 1985–1992 (September); no follow-up, histology available in 1012 patients; in 519 of them the diagnosis of PBC could be histologically verified, in

Table 1 Frequency of the different PBC stages in relation to the AMA profiles in 519 patients

AMA profiles	*Number of patients*	*PBC stage (frequency, %)* I/II ($n = 353$)	III/IV ($n = 166$)
A	14	100	0
B	108	92	8
C	282	62	38
D	115	57	43

Table 2 Frequency of pathological IgG and bilirubin levels in relation to AMA profiles in 3000 PBC patients

		Pathological levels (frequency, %)	
AMA profiles	*Number of patients*	*IgG (> 2000 mg%)*	*Bilirubin (> 1.5 mg%)*
A	90	4	6
B	810	5	11
C	1530	24	31
D	570	32	32

the remaining 471 patients the histological diagnosis was ‘mixed form’, chronic active hepatitis, fatty liver disease, chronic hepatitis or cholangitis, and liver cirrhosis, and in 22 patients no pathological features were observed. Biochemical data were obtained at first presentation and before any therapy (unpublished data).

Group III: 29 PBC patients who had received a liver transplant (cooperative study with Professor Gips, Groningen, The Netherlands)[23].

Of the 76 group I patients, 44 had the profile A/B and 32 the profile C/D as early as in stage I/II. Only 3% of the 44 A/B patients progressed to stage III/IV within the observation period, in contrast to 70% of the 32 patients with profile C/D. Furthermore, survival time was shorter in patients of group C/D than of group A/B. Patients who had died of PBC, or who had received a liver transplant, all belonged to group C/D. AMA profiles remained unchanged during the whole observation period. Since anti-M4 and anti-M8 antibodies (profile C/D) can occur in the early stages of PBC, they are not a marker for advanced, but for progressive, PBC. In contrast, AMA or especially anti-M2 antibody titres did not correlate with prognosis as previously suggested by Heseltine *et al.*[24].

Of the 3000 group II patients 3% had profile A, 27% profile B, 51% profile C, and 19% profile D. Analysing these patients with respect to biochemical parameters it became evident that an elevation of IgG levels and bilirubin was preferentially found in patients with profile C/D (Table 1). Of the 519 patients with the histological diagnosis of PBC, 166 were in stage III/IV; 157 of these patients (95%) had the profile C/D (Table 2).

Following this concept that AMA profiles are prognostic indicators one has to postulate that PBC patients who had received liver transplant had AMA profiles with a bad prognosis before OLT. We, therefore, analysed sera from 29 PBC patients (group III) who were considered for OLT. Twenty-eight of these patients were anti-M2-positive, and one patient had only antibodies to 'nuclear dots' in the IFL on cell cultures. This antibody seems to occur preferentially in patients with progressive PBC (unpublished observation). Of the 28 anti-M2-positive patients 19 (68%) had profile D and seven (25%) had profile C but only two (7%) had profile B. One of these latter two patients also had antibodies to nuclei, smooth muscle antigens and actin, suggesting an overlap syndrome with autoimmune CAH; the other patient had antibodies to 'nuclear dots' in association with anti-M2.

These data again confirm the hypothesis that patients with profiles C/D especially develop late stages of PBC. It is, however, still unclear whether patients with profile A/B will never progress to cirrhosis, or whether the progression is very slow and extends our observation period which is currently about 20 years.

There are four major models for predicting survival for individual patients with PBC based on different risk variables[25–28]. Since these models are, however, based on variables which are indicators for advanced liver diseases (bilirubin, albumin, oedema, fibrosis, cirrhosis), the risk scores change during the course of PBC. They can therefore not differentiate at early stages between patients with high or low risk for disease progression, but they allow a rather accurate prediction of the appropriate timing of liver transplantation in patients prior to death.

In contrast, the AMA profiles are not primarily survival models, but they can help to define at early stages patients with good or bad prognosis, i.e. those in whom some years later OLT may become necessary. Furthermore, they may be helpful in analysing in more detail the efficacy of different therapeutic regimes in PBC.

Acknowledgements

This work was supported by the Deutsche Forschungsgemeinschaft, Bonn Bad Godesberg (Be 431/19).

References

1. Beswick DR, Klatskin G, Boyer JL. Asymptomatic primary biliary cirrhosis. A progress report on long-term follow-up and natural history. Gastroenterology. 1985;89:267–71.
2. Klein R, Klöppel G, Garbe W, Fintelmann V, Berg PA. Antimitochondrial antibody profiles determined at early stages of primary biliary cirrhosis differentiate between a benign and a progressive course of the disease. A retrospective analysis of 76 patients over 6–18 years. J Hepatol. 1991;12:21–7.
3. Berg PA, Klein R. Antimitochondrial antibodies in primary biliary cirrhosis and other disorders: definition and clinical relevance. Dig Dis. 1992;10:85–101.
4. Berg PA, Wiedmann KH, Sayers TJ, Klöppel G, Lindner H. Serological classification of chronic cholestatic liver diseases by the use of two different types of antimitochondrial antibodies. Lancet. 1980;2:1329–32.

5. Weber P, Brenner J, Stechemesser E, Klein R, Weckenmann U, Klöppel G, Kirchhof M, Fintelmann V, Berg PA. Characterization and clinical relevance of a new complement fixing antibody – anti-M8 – in patients with primary biliary cirrhosis. Hepatology. 1986;6:553–9.
6. Berg PA, Klein R. Clinical and prognostic relevance of different mitochondrial antibody profiles in primary biliary cirrhosis (PBC). Mol Aspects Med. 1985;8:235–47.
7. Sayers TJ, Leoutsakos A, Berg PA, Baum H. Antimitochondrial antibodies (AMA) in primary biliary cirrhosis. I. Separation of the PBC antigen activity from mitochondrial ATPase activity. J Bioenerg Biomemb. 1981;13:255–67.
8. Lindenborn-Fotinos J, Sayers TJ, Berg PA. Mitochondrial antibodies in primary biliary cirrhosis. VI. Association of the complement fixing antigen with a component of the mitochondrial F1–ATPase complex. Clin Exp Immunol. 1982;50:267–74.
9. Berg PA, Klein R, Lindenborn-Fotinos J, Klöppel G. ATPase-associated antigen (M2): marker antigen for serological diagnosis of primary biliary cirrhosis. Lancet. 1982;2: 1423–6.
10. Klein R, Lindenborn-Fotinos J, Berg PA. Use of ATPase-associated antigen (M2) for detection of antimitochondrial antibodies in primary biliary cirrhosis by fluorometric immunoassay. J Immunol Meth. 1983;64:227–38.
11. Berg PA, Klein R, Lindenborn-Fotinos J. Antimitochondrial antibodies in primary biliary cirrhosis. J Hepatol. 1986;2:123–31.
12. Lindenborn-Fotinos J, Baum H, Berg PA. Mitochondrial antibodies in primary biliary cirrhosis. Further characterization of the M2 antigen by immunoblotting revealing species and non-species specific determinants. Hepatology. 1985;5:763–9.
13. Gershwin ME, Mackay IR, Sturgess A, Coppel RL. Identification and specificity of a cDNA encoding the 70 kD mitochondrial antigen recognized in primary biliary cirrhosis. J Immunol. 1987;138:3525–31.
14. Yeaman SJ, Danner DJ, Mutimer DJ, Fussey SPM, James OFW, Bassendine MF. Primary biliary cirrhosis: identification of two major M2 mitochondrial autoantigens. Lancet. 1988;1:1067–70.
15. van de Water J, Surh CD, Leung PSC, Krams SM, Fregeau D, Davis P, Coppel R, Mackay IR, Gershwin ME. Molecular definitions, autoepitopes and enzymatic activities of the mitochondrial autoantigens of primary biliary cirrhosis. Semin Liver Dis. 1989;9:132–7.
16. Fussey SPM, Bassending MF, Fittes D, Turner IB, James OFW, Yeaman SJ. The E1alpha and beta subunits of the pyruvate dehydrogenase complex are M2′d′ and M2′e′ autoantigens in primary biliary cirrhosis. Clin Sci. 1989;77:365–8.
17. Berg PA, Baum H. The serology of primary biliary cirrhosis. Springer Semin Immunopathol. 1980;3:355–73.
18. Klein R, Berg PA. Characterization of a new mitochondrial antigen–antibody system (M9/anti-M9) in patients with anti-M2 positive and anti-M2 negative primary biliary cirrhosis. Clin Exp Immunol. 1988;74:68–74.
19. Berg PA, Weber P, Oehring J, Lindenborn-Fotinos J, Stechemesser E. Significance of different types of mitochondrial antibodies in primary biliary cirrhosis. In: Brunner H, Thaler H, editors. Hepatology: a festschrift for Hans Popper. New York: Raven Press; 1985:231–42.
20. Klein R, Berg PA. Anti-M4 antibodies in primary biliary cirrhosis react with sulfite oxidase, an enzyme of the mitochondrial intermembrane space. Clin Exp Immunol. 1991;84:445–8.
21. Klein R, Berg PA. Anti-M9 antibodies in sera from patients with primary biliary cirrhosis recognize an epitope of glycogen phosphorylase. Clin Exp Immunol. 1990;81:65–71.
22. Klein R, Klöppel G, Fischer R, Fintelmann V, Müting D, Berg PA. The antimitochondrial antibody anti-M9 – a marker for the diagnosis of early primary biliary cirrhosis (PBC). J Hepatol. 1988;6:299–306.
23. Klein R, Huizenga JR, Gips CH, Berg PA. Antimitochondrial antibody profiles in patients with primary biliary cirrhosis before orthotopic liver transplantation and titres of AMA-subtypes after transplantation. J. Hepatol. (in press).
24. Heseltine L, Turner IB, Fussey SPM, Kelly PJ, James OFW, Yeaman SJ, Bassendine MF. Primary biliary cirrhosis. Quantitation of autoantibodies to purified mitochondrial enzymes and correlation with disease progression. Gastroenterology. 1990;98:1786–92.
25. Shapiro JM, Smith H, Schaffner F. Serum bilirubin: a prognostic factor in primary biliary cirrhosis. Gut. 1979;20:137–40.

26. Roll J, Beswick JL, Barry D, Klatskin G. The prognostic importance of clinical and histologic features in asymptomatic and symptomatic primary biliary cirrhosis. N Engl J Med. 1983;308:1–7.
27. Christensen E, Neuberger J, Crowe J, Altman DG, Popper H, Portman B, Doniach D, Ranek L, Tygstrup N, Williams R. Beneficial effect of azathioprine and prediction of prognosis in primary biliary cirrhosis. Final results of an international trial. Gastroenterology. 1985;89:1084–91.
28. Dickson ER, Grambsch PM, Fleming TR, Fischer LD, Langworthy A. Prognosis in primary biliary cirrhosis: model for decision making. Hepatology. 1989;10:1–7.

40
Molecular basis of mitochondrial autoantigens associated with acyltransferases

M. F. BASSENDINE, J. M. PALMER, J. QUINN, D. E. J. JONES, A. G. DIAMOND, O. F. W. JAMES and S. J. YEAMAN

Antimitochondrial antibodies (AMA) were first described as serological markers of primary biliary cirrhosis (PBC) in 1965 by Walker *et al.* using immunofluorescence (IF) techniques[1]. They demonstrated antibodies that gave a characteristic pattern of fluorescence staining of composite tissue blocks in sera of virtually all patients with PBC[2]. This non-organ, non-species-specific staining was localized to the mitochondria by Berg, Doniach and Roitt in 1967[3]. Its usefulness as a serological test for PBC was documented by several investigators who reported detectable AMA by indirect IF in 84–99% of patients[4–6]. Furthermore the finding of AMA in serum by IF in a significant titre ($\geq$ 1:40) is strongly suggestive of PBC, even in the presence of a normal alkaline phosphatase and in the absence of any symptoms[7].

In view of the close association between AMA and PBC, much research has focused on identifying the mitochondrial autoantigen(s). The first advance came when Berg and colleagues showed that AMA in PBC sera reacted with a trypsin-sensitive antigen termed M2 on the inner mitochondrial membrane[8]. Subsequent characterization by Western immunoblotting showed that M2 consisted of several antigenic determinants with molecular masses of about 75–70, 56–50, 48–43 and 36 kDa, probably reflecting different antigen preparations, systems used in the SDS-PAGE and antibody detection techniques[9–12]. The dominant mitochondrial autoantigen was found to have a molecular mass of 70–75 kDa and to be present not only in a variety of mammalian organs (e.g. heart, liver, kidney) but also in different animals (e.g. rabbit, chicken, rat, frog, human) as well as yeast and bacteria. The identity of these non-organ, non-species-specific autoantigens remained elusive until 1988 when two groups independently showed that the major 70–75 kDa M2 antigen, that had been cloned by Gershwin and colleagues in 1987[13], was the E2 component of pyruvate dehydrogenase complex

(PDC)[14,15]. It rapidly became clear that the other M2 antigenic determinants visualized on immunoblotting were all polypeptide components of PDC or the other related 2-oxo acid dehydrogenase multienzyme complexes located in mammalian mitochondria within the inner membrane–matrix compartment[16].

THE 2-OXO ACID DEHYDROGENASE COMPLEXES

The 2-oxo acid dehydrogenase complexes (also called α-keto acid dehydrogenase complexes) are multienzyme systems which have been isolated from microbial and eukaryotic cells as functional units with molecular weights in the millions[17]. Three classes of multienzyme complexes that are involved in the oxidative decarboxylation of 2-oxo acids have been isolated in a highly purified state, one specific for pyruvate (PDC), a second specific for 2-oxoglutarate (2-oxoglutarate dehydrogenase complex, OGDC) and a third specific for the branched chain 2-oxo acids (branched-chain 2-oxo acid dehydrogenase complex, BCOADC). Each complex is composed of multiple copies of three enzymes: a substrate-specific decarboxylase-dehydrogenase (E1), a dihydrolipoamide acyltransferase (E2) specific for each type of complex and a dihydrolipoamide dehydrogenase (E3), a flavoprotein that is a common component of all three types of multienzyme complexes. The mammalian and yeast PDC also contain small amounts of protein X, which is apparently involved in high-affinity binding of E3[18].

Each of the three types of complex is organized about a core consisting of oligomeric E2, to which multiple copies of E1 and E3 are bound by non-covalent bonds. In the case of mammalian PDC there is a pentagonal dodecahedron core of 60 E2p subunits around which the E1p and E3 components are assembled: approximately 30 E1p tetramers ($\alpha_2\beta_2$) bind at the 30 edges and at least six E3 dimers on the 12 faces of the core[19]. In the case of mammalian OGDC and BCOADC the core consists of a cube with 24 E2 subunits arranged with octahedral symmetry. Research on the 2-oxo acid dehydrogenase complexes has concentrated mainly on the E2 component which not only has a central role in the structure and assembly of the multienzyme system, but also has a pivotal role in the catalytic activity of the complex.

Dihydrolipoamide acyltransferases

The E2 components (dihydrolipoamide acyltransferases) are specific for each complex but all possess a similar multidomain structure. The N-terminal region consists of one, two or three highly similar lipoyl domains arranged in tandem, each of about 80 amino acid residues; this is followed by another structurally distinct segment considered to be involved in the binding of the E3 component. Mammalian PDC is unique in containing the additional protein X which appears to play a major role in the binding of E3[20]. The C-terminal catalytic domain, in addition to containing the active site, binds

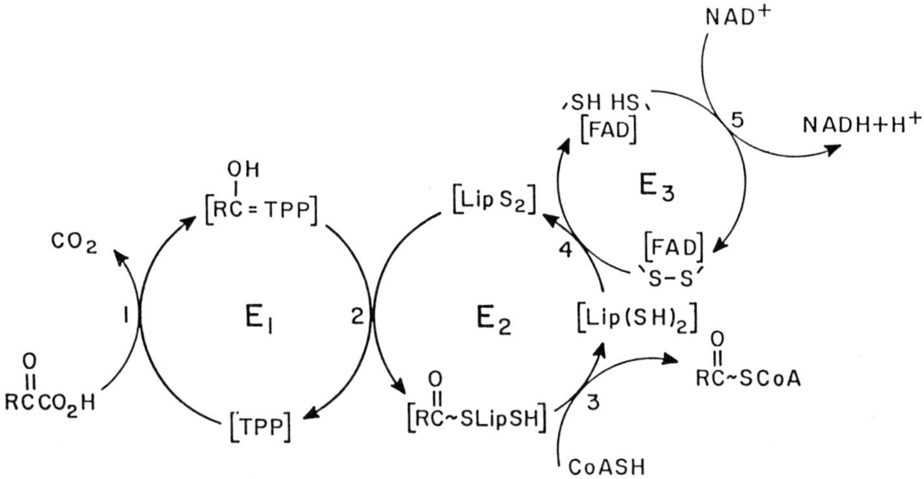

$$\mathrm{R\overset{O}{\overset{\|}{C}}CO_2H + CoASH + NAD^+ \rightarrow R\overset{O}{\overset{\|}{C}}{\sim}SCoA + CO_2 + NADH + H^+}$$

Fig. 1 Reaction mechanism for the oxidative decarboxylation of the 2-oxo acids by the 2-oxo acid dehydrogenase complexes. Reactions 1 and 2 are both catalysed by the E1 components of the respective complexes

to other E2 polypeptides to maintain the central core of the complex and is also thought to be responsible for the binding of E1. These independent domains are interconnected by flexible linker domains, characteristically rich in alanine and proline residues. The E2 component also has multiple roles in catalysis. In the case of PDC, its two lipoyl domains each contain a covalently-bound lipoyl cofactor which is reductively acetylated by E1p, the acetyl group then being transferred to CoA at the E2p active site. After acetyl transfer the reduced lipoamide is reoxidized by E3 to complete the catalytic cycle (Fig. 1).

The lipoyl domains of the dihydrolipoamide acyltransferases are of considerable interest. The lipoate residue of the domains is central to the activity of the complexes, providing a swinging arm that has sufficient rotational mobility to allow movement between the active sites of the three component enzymes[21]. However, surprisingly little is known concerning the enzymes responsible for the attachment and removal of this essential cofactor. The only information on the mammalian lipoylation system, to date, is its intra-mitochondrial localization[22]. The sequence surrounding the lipoate attachment site on several bacterial and mammalian complexes has been determined[23–25], and is highly conserved.

IDENTIFICATION OF M2 MITOCHONDRIAL AUTOANTIGENS

Following the identification of the major 70–75 kDa M2 antigen as the E2 component of PDC[14,15], it was apparent that the E2 components of

Table 1 Identification of M2 mitochondrial autoantigens

Identity of M2 antigen	*Apparent molecular weight* (kDa)	*Percentage PBC sera reacting to antigen on immunoblot*	*Reference*
E2 component of PDC	74	94	14,15
Protein X of PDC	52	94	27,30
E2 component of OGDC	50	89	26,27
E2 component of BCOADC	50	53	26,28
E1α subunit of PDC	41	41	32
E1β subunit of PDC	36	7	32

mammalian OGDC and BCOADC might also be autoantigens in view of their common domain structure and substantial degree of homology. This was confirmed by immunoblotting of PBC patients' sera against purified polypeptides[26,27] and recombinant human fetal liver BCOADC-E2[28]. In addition we reported that all PBC sera that reacted with PDC-E2 also reacted with protein X[14], which copurifies with it[29]. Furthermore, AMA reacting with PDC-E2 crossreact with protein X[30], but not with the E2 components of OGDC or BCOADC[31]. Subsequently PDC-E1α and β components have also been found to react with polypeptide-specific antibodies in a minority of PBC patients' sera[32] (Table 1).

Two recent reports suggested that alternative polypeptides may be major M2 autoantigens, but this has been refuted[33]. The finding of Frostell and colleagues[34], that a 75 kDa subunit of complex I of the respiratory chain is a major autoantigen can be explained by contamination of complex I with PDC. The report of Muno *et al.*[35] of the purification and N-terminal sequencing of a 36 kDa tryptic fragment of the major PBC-specific antigen, which did not show any identity with known sequences of PDC-E2[13,36] is not problematic once it is realized that the reported amino acid sequence corresponds to the N-terminal sequence of the intact PDC E1-β subunit[33]. Thus all the M2 antigens identified so far in PBC are components of the 2-oxo-acid dehydrogenase complexes. Recent work has also suggested that E3 also reacts with antibodies in PBC patients' sera[37]. We have, however, previously reported that the immunoreactive band with an apparent molecular weight of 55 kDa, that is sometimes visualized when PBC sera are immunoblotted against increasing amounts of PDC, is a proteolytic fragment of E2, not E3[31]. It is clear that confusion over the identity of autoantigens in PBC can easily arise if it is assumed that the major immunoreactive species in an immunoblot corresponds to the prominent polypeptide observed in that region on an SDS gel stained with Coomassie blue. In view of the sensitivity of the procedures employed in immunological analysis, it may be the case that a positive response is elicited by a minor immunogenic contaminant comigrating with a more abundant polypeptide. This may provide an explanation for the report that M9 antibodies in PBC patients' sera (which may be of prognostic relevance and associated with a benign course[38]) recognize an epitope of glycogen phosphorylase[39], an observation which we have been unable to substantiate[40]. Similarly we have been unable to observe any specific reactivity of PBC patients' sera with sulphite oxidase, the reported M4 autoantigen[41].

Crossreactivity of AMA with bacterial M2 antigens

Early immunoblotting experiments demonstrated that PBC sera react with prokaryotic antigens[9,42]. This observation was confirmed and extended using several Enterobacteriaceae as antigens[43], leading to the hypothesis that PBC may have a bacterial aetiology. We have suggested that the immunoreactivity observed with a variety of microorganisms is due to the highly conserved structure of the E2 polypeptides throughout evolution[44], and have confirmed that PBC sera react with *E. coli* PDC-E2 and OGDC-E2[45,46]. Stemerowicz and colleagues showed that PBC sera did not react with antigens from two archaebacteria[43], a finding which can be explained by the fact that archaebacteria do not contain PDC[47]. Although PBC sera contain antibodies capable of binding to both mammalian and bacterial PDC-E2 proteins, there is poor crossreactivity, indicating that distinct antibodies against these prokaryotic and eukaryotic antigens are present in PBC sera[31]. This is supported by evidence from Gershwin's laboratory[48]. Indeed, during the cloning of the mammalian autoantigen, the PBC sera used for screening the rat library were extensively preabsorbed with *E. coli* lysates[13]. In addition, antibody titre against mammalian PDC-E2 is approximately 100-fold higher than against bacterial PDC-E2[31] and PBC sera containing AMA to mammalian PDC-E1 subunits do not recognize *E. coli* PDC-E1[32]. Taken together these results argue against a bacterial origin for primary biliary cirrhosis.

MAPPING OF AUTOIMMUNIZING B-CELL EPITOPES

Following identification of E2p as the major M2 autoantigen, analysis of the main immunodominant region (MIR) on that polypeptide has been carried out using E2p from a variety of sources. Sub-cloning and expression of fragments of the rat E2p polypeptide localized the MIR to within the lipoyl domains[49]. By use of a series of overlapping synthetic peptides the MIR was further restricted to the region surrounding the site of lipoylation, with a synthetic peptide corresponding to that site being able to absorb out reactivity from PBC sera, albeit at high dilutions[49]. In a similar study, preparation of multiple recombinant fragments from the full-length human cDNA localized the MIR to the inner lipoyl domain[48]. A minimum of 93 amino acids were required for characteristic antibody binding. This suggests a conformational, non-linear epitope may be recognized.

In a separate practical approach, limited tryptic digestion of bovine heart E2p, which cleaves the polypeptide into two well-defined fragments[50], followed by immunoblotting, further indicated that the MIR was contained within the lipoyl domains of the protein[45].

The importance of the lipoyl domains was further supported by work using wild-type and mutant forms of E2p from *E. coli*. ELISA and immunoblotting studies against genetically restructured E2p polypeptides and isolated lipoyl domains indicated that the main immunogenic region lies within the lipoyl domains[46].

The localization of the MIR to the lipoyl domains prompted several investigations into the importance of the covalently attached lipoic acid co-factor in antibody recognition. A range of modified or non-modified *E. coli* lipoyl domains were tested for their ability to absorb out reactivity against *E. coli* E2p in an ELISA system. Only lipoylated domains or domains aberrantly substituted with octanoic acid were effective in pre-absorbing anti-E2p reactivity. In contrast, unlipoylated domains were apparently unrecognized. This demonstrated that PBC antibodies bind to a unique peptide-cofactor epitope within the domain[46].

A recent study has utilized an 18-residue synthetic peptide corresponding to the site of attachment of lipoic acid to the inner lipoyl domain of human E2p[51]. These workers found that only when this peptide contained a lipoate residue was it able to absorb out reactivity against E2p, or to be recognized itself in ELISA. This is in apparent contrast to the finding in ref. 49 that a non-lipoylated synthetic peptide can absorb out reactivity.

In order to further investigate the reactivity against E2p, and in particular the role of the lipoate cofactor, we have used recombinant human inner lipoyl domains with defined lipoate contents. When cDNA encoding the inner domain was expressed in *E. coli*, two forms of the domain were recovered, corresponding to unlipoylated and lipoylated forms[52]. These two forms were resolved by ion-exchange chromatography and used in both immunoblotting and in ELISA. It was found that PBC sera have both higher titre and affinity against the lipoylated than the non-lipoylated domains (Figure 2)[53].

To date, work with mammalian antigens has used either those of animal origin or else recombinant human protein expressed in *E. coli*. However, we have recently utilized native PDC and E2p purified from human heart to look at true autoantibody reactivity against human protein. Using both immunoblotting and ELISA, it was found that reactivity of AMA against human E2p was indistinguishable from that against bovine protein.

THE ROLE OF T CELLS

Immunohistochemical studies examining the nature of the extensive inflammatory cell infiltrate in the portal tracts of patients with PBC have found that the majority of the cells are lymphocytes with a higher proportion of T cells than B cells[54,55]. Conflicting results were initially obtained concerning the proportion of T-cell subsets in portal tracts, possibly due in part to variations in the histological stages of the liver biopsies examined[56–59]. More recent clonal analysis of liver-derived T cells in PBC has revealed activated $CD8^+$ are present and frequently predominate in the earlier precirrhotic stages of the disease[60,61]. Additionally bile duct epithelia in PBC have been shown to express large amounts of HLA class I and class II molecules[59,62,63]. These studies strongly suggest that T-cell-specific mechanisms are involved in the pathogenesis of damage to the biliary epithelial cells. Furthermore evidence has been presented showing that the T-cell population has a limited

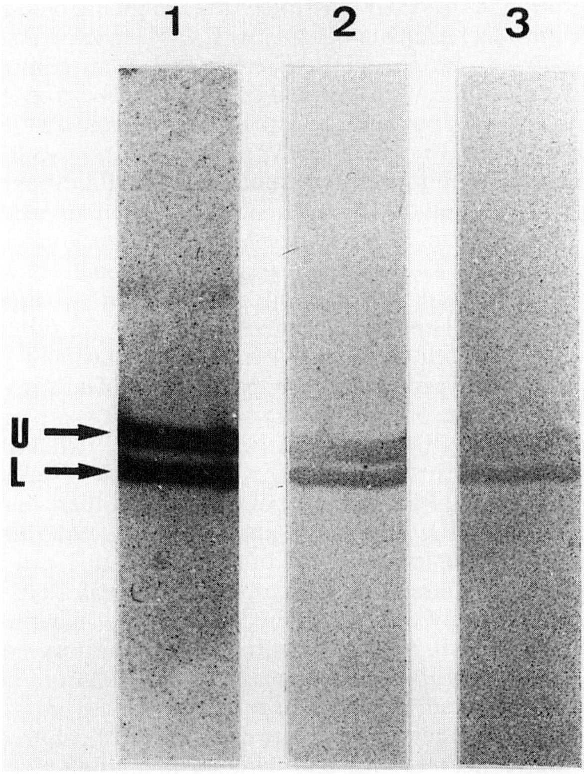

Fig. 2 Immunoblot illustrating differences in antibody binding to lipoylated and non-lipoylated PDC-E2 domain forms: lipoylated (L) and unlipoylated (U) domains (1 μg) were subjected to PAGE on 15% non-denaturing gels and stained with Coomassie brilliant blue (lane 1) or transferred to Fluorotrans membrane and immunoblotted against PBC serum in a dilution of 1:500 (lane 2) and 1:2000 (lane 3)

diversity[64,65], implying an oligoclonal T-cell response similar to that found in experimental autoimmune animal models[66].

There have, however, been only a limited number of studies examining the antigen specificity of the T-cell response in PBC. Preliminary studies examining the T-cell response to bovine PDC and PDC-E2 have been reported. Van de Water *et al.* showed that when PBC liver-derived lymphocytes were grown in bulk culture with interleukin-2 (IL-2) good growth was obtained[67]. When aliquots of the T-cell lines were re-cultured with antigen-presenting cells pulsed with bovine PDC-E2, IL-2 production occurred; this was taken as demonstrating an antigen-specific response. Limiting dilutional cloning of PDC-E2-responsive lines resulted in PDC-E2-restricted T-cell clones. When control liver was used, PDC-E2 specificity of derived T cells was not seen, leading to the conclusion that there are PDC-E2-specific T cells in the portal tract infiltrate in PBC but not in controls[67].

Lohr and colleagues have demonstrated that peripheral blood lymphocytes (PBL) from eight of 11 patients (72.7%) with PBC showed an HLA class II restricted response to bovine PDC, whereas PBL from controls did not[68]. In addition T-cell clones were isolated from diagnostic liver biopsies from two patients with PBC; nine clones reacted with bovine PDC presented by autologous B-cell lines. In contrast to Van de Water, no T-cell response was seen with bovine PDC-E2 (personal communication), although some of the clones with reactivity against the whole multienzyme complex recognized a crude preparation of human liver mitoplasts (i.e. mitochondria depleted of their outer membranes). These data suggest that autoreactive liver-infiltrating T cells in PBC recognize specific epitope(s) located on PDC which are different from the B-cell epitopes localized within the E2 subunit.

One problem with both these studies is that the PDC and PDC-E2 used in the proliferation assays is derived from beef heart, and is thus a xenoantigen. Unpublished work from our laboratory suggests that the peripheral blood T-cell response to beef PDC is not restricted to PBC patients but is found in some healthy normals. We have made PDC specific T-cell lines [$CD3^+$, $CD4^+$, $CD8^-$] from the PBL of these controls, tested these lines against the subunits E1, E2 and E3, and found that no one component enzyme is consistently immunodominant. In addition, when these T-cell lines that are restricted for beef PDC are tested for response to *human* PDC no reactivity is seen. This would imply that the original response was indeed xenogeneic in nature. In view of this, recent work from our laboratory has focused on assaying the response of PBLs to human PDC (derived from heart at organ allograft). PBLs from patients with primary biliary cirrhosis and controls (healthy normals and other chronic liver diseases) were cultured with *human* PDC at different concentrations and tritiated thymidine incorporation on day 6 assayed as a marker of proliferation. We have compared the PDC response to that seen to tetanus toxoid, a recall antigen presented by MHC class II positive cells. We have demonstrated a high incidence of proliferative responses (stimulation index > 2) to *human* PDC in PBC patients (23/29, 79%), that is largely absent in controls (4/26, 16%). In contrast the tetanus toxoid response is similar in both groups (PBC patients 20/29, 69%; controls 19/26, 73%). Our data suggest that the response to *human* PDC in patients with primary biliary cirrhosis is an antigen-specific phenomenon, and we are now further localizing the T-cell epitope by examining the proliferative response of PBLs and liver-derived T cells to the enzyme subunits of PDC, E1, E2 and E3. If limited T-cell receptor usage can be demonstrated, this could lead to the development of specific immunotherapy in primary biliary cirrhosis.

Acknowledgements

This work was supported by grants from the Wellcome Trust, the Medical Research Council and the Science and Engineering Research Council.

References

1. Walker JG, Doniach D, Roitt IM, Sherlock S. Serological tests in diagnosis of primary biliary cirrhosis. Lancet. 1965;1:827–31.
2. Doniach D, Roitt IM, Walker JG, Sherlock S. Tissue antibodies in primary biliary cirrhosis, active chronic (lupoid) hepatitis, cryptogenic cirrhosis and other liver diseases and their clinical implications. Clin Exp Immunol. 1966;1:237–62.
3. Berg PA, Doniach D, Roitt IM. Mitochondrial antibodies in primary biliary cirrhosis. Localisation of the antigen to mitochondrial membranes. J Exp Med. 1967;126:277–90.
4. Goudie RB, MacSween RNM, Goldberg DM. Serological and histological diagnosis of primary biliary cirrhosis. J Clin Pathol. 1966;19:527–38.
5. Klatskin G, Kantor FS. Mitochondrial antibody in primary biliary cirrhosis and other diseases. Ann Intern Med. 1972;77:533–41.
6. Munoz LE, Thomas HC, Scheuer PJ, Doniach D, Sherlock S. Is mitochondrial antibody diagnostic of primary biliary cirrhosis? Gut. 1981;22:136–40.
7. Mitchison HC, Bassendine MF, Hendrick A, Bennett MK, Bird G, Watson AJ, James OFW. Positive antimitochondrial antibody but normal alkaline phosphatase: is this primary biliary cirrhosis? Hepatology. 1986;6:1279–84.
8. Berg PA, Klein R, Lindenborn-Fotinos J, Kloppel W. ATPase-associated antigen (M2): marker antigen for serological diagnosis of primary biliary cirrhosis. Lancet. 1982;2: 1423–26.
9. Lindenborn-Fotinos J, Baum H, Berg PA. Mitochondrial antibodies in primary biliary cirrhosis: species and non-species specific determinants of M2 antigens. Hepatology. 1985;5:763–9.
10. Frazer IH, Mackay IR, Jordan TW, Whittingham S, Marzuki S. Reactivity of anti-mitochondrial autoantibodies in primary biliary cirrhosis: definition of two novel mitochondrial polypeptide autoantigens. J Immunol. 1985;135:1739–45.
11. Ishii H, Saifuku K, Namihisa T. Multiplicity of mitochondrial inner membrane antigens from beef heart reacting with antimitochondrial antibodies in sera of patients with primary biliary cirrhosis. Immunology Lett. 1985;9:325–30.
12. Mendel-Hartvig I, Nelson BD, Loof L, Totterman TH. Primary biliary cirrhosis: further biochemical and immunological characterisation of mitochondrial antigens. Clin Exp Immunol. 1985;62:371–9.
13. Gershwin ME, Mackay IR, Sturgess A, Coppel RL. Identification and specificity of a cDNA encoding the 70 kDa mitochondrial antigen recognised in primary biliary cirrhosis. J Immunol. 1987;138:3525–31.
14. Yeaman SJ, Fussey SPM, Danner DJ, James OFW, Mutimer DJ, Bassendine MF. Primary biliary cirrhosis: identification of two major M2 mitochondrial autoantigens. Lancet. 1988;1:1067–70.
15. Van de Water J, Fregeau D, Davis P, Ansari A, Danner D, Leung P, Coppel R, Gershwin ME. Autoantibodies of primary biliary cirrhosis recognise dihydrolipoamide acetyltransferase and inhibit enzyme function. J Immunol. 1988;141:2321–4.
16. Bassendine MF, Yeaman SJ. Primary biliary cirrhosis: nature of autoantigens. Springer Semin Immunopathol. 1990;12:73–83.
17. Reed LJ, Hackert ML. Structure–function relationships in dihydrolipoamide acyltransferases. J Biol Chem. 1990;265:8971–4.
18. Gopalakrishnan S, Rahmatullah M, Radke GA, Powers-Greenwood S, Roche TE. Role of protein X of the mammalian pyruvate dehydrogenase complex. Biochem Biophys Res Commun. 1989;160:715–21.
19. Barrra CR, Namihiri G, Hamilton L, Munk P, Eley MH, Linn TC, Reed LJ. α-Keto acid dehydrogenase complexes. Studies on the subunit structure of the pyruvate dehydrogenase complexes from bovine kidney and heart. Arch Biochem Biophys. 1972;148:343–58.
20. Neagle JC, Lindsay JG. Selective proteolysis of the protein-X subunit of the bovine heart pyruvate dehydrogenase complex – effects on dihydrolipoamide dehydrogenase (E3) affinity and enzymatic-properties of the complex. Biochem J. 1991;278:423–7.
21. Ambrose MC, Perham RN. Spin-label study of the mobility of enzyme-bound lipoic acid in the pyruvate dehydrogenase multienzyme complex of *Escherichia coli*. Biochem J. 1976;155:429–32.

22. Griffin TA, Wynn RM, Chuang DT. Expression and assembly of mature apotransacylase (E_{2b}) of bovine branched-chain α-keto acid dehydrogenase complex in *Escherichia coli*. J Biol Chem. 1990;265:12104–10.
23. Hale G, Perham RN. Amino acid sequence around lipoic acid residues in the pyruvate dehydrogenase multienzyme complex of *Escherichia coli*. Biochem J. 1980;187:905–8.
24. Bradford AP, Howell S, Aitken A, James LA, Yeaman SJ. Primary structure around the lipoate attachment site on the E2 component of bovine heart pyruvate dehydrogenase complex. Biochem J. 1987;245:919–22.
25. Hummel KB, Litwer S, Bradford AP, Aitken A, Danner DJ, Yeaman SJ. Nucleotide sequence of a cDNA for branched chain acyltransferase with analysis of the deduced protein sequence. J Biol Chem. 1988;263:6165–8.
26. Fussey SPM, Guest JR, James OFW, Bassendine MF, Yeaman SJ. Identification and analysis of the major M2 autoantigens in primary biliary cirrhosis. Proc Natl Acad Sci USA. 1988;85:8654–8.
27. Mutimer DJ, Fussey SPM, Yeaman SJ, Kelly PJ, James OFW, Bassendine MF. Frequency of IgG and IgM autoantibodies to four specific M2 mitochondrial autoantigens in primary biliary cirrhosis. Hepatology. 1989;10:403–7.
28. Surh CD, Danner AA, Coppel RC, Mackay IR, Dickson ER, Gershwin ME. Reactivity of primary biliary cirrhosis sera with a human fetal liver cDNA clone of branched-chain α-keto acid dehydrogenase dihydrolipoamide acyltransferase, the 52 kDa mitochondrial autoantigen. Hepatology. 1989;9:63–8.
29. De Marcucci O, Lindsay JG. Component X. An immunologically distinct polypeptide associated with mammalian pyruvate dehydrogenase multi-enzyme complex. Eur J Biochem. 1985;149:641–8.
30. Surh CD, Roche TE, Danner DJ, Ansari A, Coppel RL, Prindiville T, Dickson ER, Gershwin ME. Antimitochondrial autoantibodies in primary biliary cirrhosis recognise cross-reactive epitope(s) on protein X and dihydrolipoamide acetyltransferase of pyruvate dehydrogenase complex. Hepatology. 1989;10:127–33.
31. Fussey SPM, Lindsay JG, Fuller C, Perham RN, Dale S, James OFW, Bassendine MF, Yeaman SJ. Autoantibodies in primary biliary cirrhosis: analysis of reactivity against eukaryotic and prokaryotic 2-oxo acid dehydrogenase complexes. Hepatology. 1991;13: 467–74.
32. Fussey SPM, Bassendine MF, Fittes D, Turner IB, James OFW, Yeaman SJ. The E1α and β subunits of the pyruvate dehydrogenase complex are M2'd' and M2'e' autoantigens in primary biliary cirrhosis. Clin Sci. 1989;77:365–8.
33. Fussey SPM, West SM, Lindsay JG, Ragan CI, James OFW, Bassendine MF, Yeaman SJ. Clarification of the identity of the major M2 autoantigen in primary biliary cirrhosis. Clin Sci. 1991;80:451–5.
34. Frostell A, Mendel-Hartvig I, Nelson BD, Totterman TH, Bjorkland A, Ragan I. Evidence that the major primary biliary cirrhosis-specific mitochondrial autoantigen is a subunit of complex I of the respiratory chain. Scand J Immunol. 1988;28:157–65.
35. Muno D, Kominami E, Ishii H, Usui K, Saifuku K, Sakakibara Y, Namihisa T. Isolation of tryptic fragment of antigen from mitochondrial liver membrane proteins reacting with antimitochondrial antibody in sera of patients with primary biliary cirrhosis. Hepatology. 1990;11:16–23.
36. Coppel RL, McNeilage LJ, Surh CD, Van der Water J, Spithill IW, Whittingham S, Gershwin ME. Primary structure of the human M2 mitochondrial autoantigen of primary biliary cirrhosis: dihydrolipoamide acetyltransferase. Proc Natl Acad Sci USA. 1988;85: 7317–21.
37. Maeda T, Loveland BE, Rowley MJ, Mackay IR. Autoantibody against dihydrolipoamide dehydrogenase, the E3 subunit of the 2-oxoacid dehydrogenase complexes: significance for primary biliary cirrhosis. Hepatology. 1991;14:994–9.
38. Klein R, Kloppel G, Fischer R, Fintelmann V, Muting D, Berg PA. The antimitochondrial antibody anti-M9: a marker for the diagnosis of early primary biliary cirrhosis. J Hepatol. 1988;6:299–306.
39. Klein R, Berg PA. Anti-M9 antibodies in sera from patients with primary biliary cirrhosis recognise an epitope of glycogen phosphorylase. Clin Exp Immunol. 1990;81:65–71.
40. Palmer JM, Mitchison HC, James OFW, Yeaman SJ, Bassendine MF. Antimitochondrial

antibodies in primary biliary cirrhosis do not recognise glycogen phosphorylase identified as the 'M9' mitochondrial autoantigen. Hepatology. 1992;16:61A (abstract).

41. Klein R, Berg PA. Anti-M4 antibodies in primary biliary cirrhosis react with sulphite oxidase, an enzyme of the mitochondrial inter-membrane space. Clin Exp Immunol. 1991;84: 445–8.
42. Baum H, Palmer C. The PBC-specific antigen. Mol Aspects Med. 1985;8:201–34.
43. Stemerowicz R, Hopf U, Moller B, Wittenbrink C, Rodloff A, Reinhardt R, Freudenberg M, Galonos C. Are mitochondrial antibodies in primary biliary cirrhosis induced by R(rough)-mutants of enterobacteriaceae. Lancet. 1988;2:1166–9.
44. Yeaman SJ, Fussey SPM, Mutimer DJ, James OFW, Bassendine MF. M2 autoantigens in primary biliary cirrhosis. Lancet. 1989;1:103 (letter).
45. Fussey SPM, Bassendine MF, James OFW, Yeaman SJ. Characterisation of the reactivity of autoantibodies in primary biliary cirrhosis. FEBS Lett. 1989;246:49–53.
46. Fussey SPM, Ali ST, Guest JR, James OFW, Bassendine MF, Yeaman SJ. Reactivity of primary biliary cirrhosis sera with *Escherichia coli* dihydrolipoamide acetyltransferase (E2p): characterisation of the main immunogenic region. Proc Natl Acad Sci USA. 1990;87: 3987–91.
47. Kerscher L, Oesterhelt D. Pyruvate: ferridoxin oxidoreductase – new findings on an ancient enzyme. Trends Biochem Sci. 1982;7:371–4.
48. Surh CD, Coppel R, Gershwin ME. Structural requirement for autoreactivity on human pyruvate dehydrogenase-E2, the major autoantigen of primary biliary cirrhosis. J Immunol. 1990;144:3367–74.
49. Van de Water J, Gershwin ME, Leung P, Coppel R. The autoepitope of the 74 KD mitochondrial autoantigen of primary biliary cirrhosis corresponds to the functional site of dihydrolipoamide acetyltransferases. J Exp Med. 1988;167:1791–9.
50. Bleile DM, Hackert ML, Pettit FH, Reed LJ. Subunit structure of dihydrolipoyl transacetylase component of pyruvate dehydrogenase complex from bovine heart. J Biol Chem. 1981;256:514–19.
51. Tuaillon N, Andre C, Briand JP, Penner E, Muller S. A lipoyl synthetic octapeptide of dihydrolipoamide acetyltransferase specifically recognised by anti-M2 autoantibodies in primary biliary cirrhosis. J Immunol. 1992;148:445–50.
52. Quinn J, Diamond AG, Masters AK, Brookfield DE, Wallis NG, Yeaman SJ. Expression and lipoylation in *Escherichia coli* of the inner lipoyl domain of the E2 component of the human pyruvate dehydrogenase complex. Biochem J. 1993;289:81–5.
53. Quinn J, Diamond AG, Palmer JM, James OFW, Yeaman SJ. The role of lipoic acid in autoimmune recognition of dihydrolipoamide acetyltransferase (E2p), the major M2 autoantigen in primary biliary cirrhosis (PBC). Hepatology. 1992;16:62A (abstract).
54. Pape GR, Rieber EP, Eisenburg J, Hoffmann R, Balch CM, Paumgartner G, Reithmuller G. Involvement of the cytotoxic/suppressor T-cell subset in liver disease injury of patients with acute and chronic liver disease. Gastroenterology. 1983;85:657–62.
55. Van den Oord JJ, Fevery J, De Groote J, Desmet VJ. Immunohistochemical characterisation of inflammatory infiltrates in primary biliary cirrhosis. Liver. 1984;4:264–72.
56. Colucci G, Schaffner F, Paronetto F. In situ characterisation of the cell-surface antigens of the mononuclear cell infiltrate and bile duct epithelium in primary biliary cirrhosis. Clin Immunol Immunopathol. 1986;41:35–42.
57. Yamada G, Hyodo I, Tobe K, Mizuno M, Nishihara T, Kobayashi T, Nagashima H. Ultrastructural immunocytochemical analysis of lymphocytes infiltrating bile duct epithelia in primary biliary cirrhosis. Hepatology. 1986;3:385–91.
58. Shimizu M, Yuh K, Aoyama S, Ichihara I, Watanabe H, Shijo H, Okumura M. Immunohistochemical characterisation of inflammatory infiltrates at the site of bile duct injury in primary biliary cirrhosis. Liver. 1986;6:1–6.
59. Floreani A, Bennett MK, Mitchison HC, McLachlan SM, Bassendine MF, James OFW. Progression of autoimmune damage in primary biliary cirrhosis on immunohistochemical study. Autoimmunity. 1989;2:311–21.
60. Hoffman RM, Pape GR, Spengler U, Rieber EP, Eisenburg J, Dohrmann J, Paumgartner G, Reithmuller G. Clonal analysis of liver-derived T-cells of patients with primary biliary cirrhosis. Clin Exp Immunol. 1989;76:210–15.
61. Meuer SC, Moebius U, Manns M, Dienes HP, Ramadori G, Hess G, Hercend T, Meyer

zum Buschenfelde K-H. Clonal analysis of human T lymphocytes infiltrating the liver in chronic active hepatitis B and primary biliary cirrhosis. Eur J Immunol. 1988;18:1447–52.

62. Van den Oord JJ, Sciot R, Desmet VJ. Expression of MHC products by normal and abnormal bile duct epithelium. J Hepatol. 1987;3:310–17.
63. Spengler U, Paper GR, Hoffmann RM, Johnson JP, Eisenburg J, Paumgartner G, Riethemuller G. Differential expression of MHC Class II subregion products on bile duct epithelial cells and hepatocytes in patients with primary biliary cirrhosis. Hepatology. 1988;8:459–62.
64. Krams SM, Van de Water J, Coppel RC, Esquivel C, Roberts J, Ansari A, Gershwin ME. Analysis of hepatic T lymphocyte and immunoglobulin deposits in patients with primary biliary cirrhosis. Hepatology. 1990;12:306–13.
65. Moebius U, Manns M, Hess G, Kober G, Meyer zum Bushchenfelde K-H, Meuer SC. T-cell receptor gene rearrangements of T lymphocytes infiltrating the liver in chronic active hepatitis B and primary biliary cirrhosis (PBC): oligoclonality of PBC-derived T-cell clones. Eur J Immunol. 1990;20:889–96.
66. Zamvil S, Nelson P, Trotter J, Mitchell D, Knobler R, Fritz R, Steinman L. T-cell clones specific for myelin basic-protein induce chronic relapsing paralysis and demyelination. Nature. 1985;317:355–8.
67. Van de Water J, Ansari AA, Surh CD, Coppel R, Roche T, Donkovsky H, Kaplan M, Gershwin ME. Evidence for the targeting of 2-oxo-dehydrogenase enzymes in the T cell response of primary biliary cirrhosis. J Immunol. 1991;146:89–94.
68. Lohr H, Manns M, Fleischer B, Gerken G, Fussey S, Meyer zum Buschenfelde KH. Autoreactive liver-infiltrating T-cells in primary biliary cirrhosis. J Hepatol. 1992; 16(Suppl. 1):S60 (abstract).

41 T cell biology and cell surface expression of PDC-E2 in primary biliary cirrhosis

M. E. GERSHWIN, J. VAN DE WATER, P. S. C. LEUNG and R. COPPEL

INTRODUCTION

Primary biliary cirrhosis (PBC) results from autoimmune-mediated destruction of intrahepatic bile ducts with progressive inflammatory scarring followed by liver failure. The association of PBC with high-titre autoantibodies to mitochondrial antigens has long been recognized[1-3], and the possible significance discussed[4-6]. Characterization of the reactive antigens, designated as M2, was initially limited to a trypsin-sensitive moiety in the inner mitochondrial membrane, but further characterization proved slow[2,7]. In 1987 this situation was changed dramatically as a cDNA for the mitochondrial 74 kDa autoantigen of primary biliary cirrhosis was cloned and sequenced[8] by screening a rat liver cDNA library with sera from patients with PBC, and this led to the identification of the PBC autoantigen as the mitochondrial pyruvate dehydrogenase complex (PDC)[9-11]. Thereafter, a group of antigens associated with PDC, the OADC complex, were identified and characterized.

MOLECULAR STRUCTURE OF THE 2-OADC ENZYME ANTIGENS

The 2-OADC enzymes are functionally complex[12-15]. For PDC, the E1 subunit, α-decarboxylase, decarboxylates pyruvate releasing CO_2 and an acetyl group, the E2 subunit, dihydrolipoamide, effects the reductive transfer of the acetyl group by the lipoic acid cofactor to coenzyme A which enters the Krebs cycle; the E3 subunit reoxidizes lipoic acid with formation of reduced NAD (NADH). Since the E2 subunit carries the major antigenic reactivity of PDC, the 74 kDa antigen, it is appropriate to consider the molecular domains. The four structural/functional regions, from the

N-terminus, include the lipoyl binding domain(s), the alanine–proline-rich linker regions that confer flexibility on the molecule, a site at which there is binding of the other subunits E1 and E3 and, at the C terminus, the catalytic site at which transfer occurs of the acetyl group to coenzyme A. The structure of the lipoyl domains varies according to the source of the enzyme. *E. coli* PDC contains three lipoyl regions whereas mammalian PDC has two such regions, an outer and inner group, with the inner appearing more potent as an autoantigen than the outer. The other OADC enzymes have only one lipoyl binding region.

The overall structure of all three enzymes, PDC, OGDC and BCOADC, is similar in that each consists of multiple copies of three functionally equivalent subunit enzymes which have structural similarities but act on different substrates. PDC oxidatively decarboxylates pyruvate, OGDC decarboxylates α-oxoglutarate to form succinyl Co-A, and BCOADC catalyses the catabolism of the branched-chain amino acids, leucine, isoleucine and valine.

For each multienzyme complex the E2 component forms a symmetrical core around which the E1 and E3 components are arranged. For mammalian PDC there are some 60 E2 subunits and six protein X subunits, arranged in icosahedral symmetry[16]. The carboxyterminal inner domains self-associate to form a stable core to the complex. The attached lipoyl domains form freely rotating 'swinging arms' and support the sequential reactions at the well-separated active sites. The protrusion of the lipoyl sites and their mobility may account for their antigenicity[17,18]. In mammalian PDC, 20–30 copies of the $\alpha_2\beta_2$ tetramer which makes up the E1 component, and six copies of the E3 dimer, are associated with the complex. Thus, each of the 2-OADC complexes is very large, with a molecular mass of several million, and a diameter in solution of ~ 500 Å.

All of the subunits of these enzyme complexes are encoded by nuclear genes, and the polypeptides are separately imported from the cytoplasm into the mitochondrial matrix across two membranes for assembly on the inner membrane. During this process the appropriate cofactors must be inserted, and the proteins must fold and aggregate into the correctly assembled complexes. The process is energy-dependent, and involves proteolytic cleavage of the polypeptides[19]. Each of the precursor proteins is cleaved near the N-terminus during import. The size of the cleaved fragment varies in that the precursors of E1 subunits from mammalian PDC and OGDC have apparent molecular masses approximately 3 kDa greater than the mature polypeptides; the precursors of E2 from PDC and OGDC are approximately 8 kDa greater; and the precursor of E3 is approximately 1.5 kDa greater[20]. Neither the precursor polypeptide nor the mature protein is normally detected in the cytosol; however, in the presence of uncouplers to inhibit uptake and processing, precursors corresponding to the individual subunits may accumulate in the cytoplasm.

AUTOANTIBODIES TO MITOCHONDRIA

The anti-M2 mitochondrial autoantibodies in PBC have some notable features. First, the major reactivity appears to be with PDC, the 74 kDa antigen, since some 95% of sera are positive by immunoblotting. The frequency of reactivity against the E2 subunits of the other enzymes OGDC and BCOADC is lower, around 50–70%. In PBC there is usually reactivity against two, or even all three, of the 2-OADC enzymes, but serological crossreactivity is exceptional; the only crossreactivity observed among the M2 reactants is that between PDC and the protein X, which is a constituent of the same enzyme. Moreover, in keeping with this immunological specificity, the M2 antibodies are not crossreactive in enzyme inhibition assays[9,21,22], as described below. Second, there is more than one determinant on the M2 autoantigens. For PDC the E2 subunit contains a major site around the lipoyl binding region, other unmapped sites on the E1α and E1β subunits and a conformational site not identifiable by immunoblotting. Sites on the other 2-OADC enzymes are less well characterized, but the major reactivity can be confidently allocated to the single lipoyl binding domain of these enzymes. Third, there is a restriction to class and isotype of autoantibodies to the M2 antigens[18]. The M2 autoantibodies in PBC are not, as was formerly believed, predominantly IgM, but this isotype is nonetheless well represented, in contrast to antibodies in other autoimmune diseases which are predominantly IgG. Moreover, a low molecular type of IgM is present in PBC[23], and has anti-M2 reactivity. Among the IgG autoantibodies there is subclass restriction to IgG3 indicative of an influence of lymphokines from T cells that determine class-switching of antibody isotype. Fourth, M2 antibodies in PBC have very potent inhibitory effects on the catalytic function *in vitro* of the enzyme with which they react[9,21,22].

ENZYME INHIBITION

The inhibitory capacity of PBC sera is specific for each enzyme as judged by affinity purification of sera, giving a further indication that there are separate populations of antibodies reactive with each of the three 2-OADC enzymes. This is in a study based on the enzyme inhibitory capacity of PBC sera for PDC and OGDC[21]; 73/188 (39%) of PDC sera reacted with OGDC-E2 as judged by immunoblotting against purified OGDC, and the same PBC sera possessing OGDC-E2 reactivity specifically inhibited enzyme function of OGDC, whereas OGDC activity was not affected by PBC sera which contained autoantibodies to PDC-E2 and/or BCOADC-E2 but which lacked OGDC-E2 reactivity. Furthermore, affinity-purified PBC sera against OGDC-E2 inhibited only OGDC activity but did not alter the enzyme activity of either PDC or BCOADC, and OGDC-E2-specific affinity-purified antisera did not react by immunoblotting with any component enzymes of PDC or BCOADC[23]. Uibo *et al.*[24] likewise found that when PBC sera were affinity-purified on PDC-E2, the adsorbed preparation, in contrast to whole serum, reacted exclusively with PDC-E2 in serological and enzyme inhibition assays. The site on E1α with which autoantibodies react is unmapped; hence it is uncertain whether inhibition is due to specific interference with a functional sequence or to steric effects[21]. Although antibodies from patients with PBC strongly inhibit the mammalian enzymes, it is noteworthy that

Table 1 Enzyme subunits of the 2-oxoacid dehydrogenase complexes, and M2 mitochondrial autoantigens

Enzyme	*Molecular weight (kDa)*	*Frequency of antibody in PBC*	*M2 Antigen* a–e*
PDC-E1α pyruvate decarboxylase	41	41–66%	M2d
PDC-E1β pyruvate decarboxylase	36	2–7%	M2e
PDC-E2 acetyltransferase	74	95%	M2a
E3 lipoamide dehydrogenase†	55	38%	M2c
Protein X	52	95%	M2c
OGDC-E1 2-oxoglutarate decarboxylase	110	low	
OGDC-E2 succinyl transferase	48	39–88%	M2c
BCOADC-E1α acyl decarboxylase	46		
BCOADC-E1β acyl decarboxylase	38		
BCOADC-E2 acyl transferase	50	53–55%	M2c

*a–e nomenclature as cited by Berg and Klein[25]; M2b remains unidentified
†Lipoamide dehydrogenase, E3, is a common subunit to each enzyme complex; reactivity cited is at a low (1:100) serum dilution and occurs in PBC and some normal sera

such antibodies are almost totally non-inhibitory with purified bacterial PDC, despite the sera being reactive with both enzymes by immunoblotting. Table 1 summarizes the relationships that have been established between the various M2 antigens, the respective enzyme subunits and the prevalence of the reactivity in PBC patients.

Naturally occurring mitochondrial antibodies or 'NOMA' constitute reactivity to a large constellation of minor mitochondrial antigens reported from studies performing immunoblots using relatively concentrated (1:50) serum dilutions[26]. The molecular nature of the 'NOMAs' is not known. Klein and Berg have reported a relative deficiency of antibodies to these antigens among patients with PBC compared to their relatives, healthy controls and patients with a variety of infectious diseases. It was proposed that such a deficiency may predispose these individuals to the development of PBC by reason of a lack of naturally protective autoantibodies[26]. We specifically tested this hypothesis by immunoblotting for antibodies to the well-described oxo-acid dehydrogenase family of mitochondrial antigens (M2) using both dilute serum samples (1:1000) and concentrated (1:20) serum samples, with negative results. Our data suggest that NOMA may be a reactivity revealed by testing using low-dilution serum samples from normal volunteers, and that this reactivity is irrelevant to PBC. The significance of NOMA is still therefore a matter of debate.

EPITOPES

To finely map the major PDC-E2 epitope, a set of truncated constructs of PDC-E2 were generated by progressively creating cDNA restriction fragments at the amino and the carboxyl termini[27]. The cDNAs were subcloned and the resultant fusion proteins analysed by immunoblotting and ELISA using PBC sera at a 1:500 dilution. Of the N-terminal deletion constructs, the fusion protein that contained amino acid residues 128–227 from the N terminus of the mature protein was strongly reactive, whereas the fusion protein that contained residues 136–227 was less frequently and more weakly reactive. Thus, by immunoblotting, 23/26 sera reacted with the 128–227 protein, but only 14/26 PBC reacted with the 136–227 protein. Furthermore, although serum titres by blotting or ELISA against the 128–227 protein and the full-length fusion protein were similar for all of 10 sera analysed, the titres against the 136–227 fusion protein were 100-fold lower.

In previous work it was demonstrated that the immunodominant epitope of PDC-E2 was localized to the lipoic acid binding site[9]. Noting that human PDC-E2, in contrast to rat PDC-E2, has two lipoic acid binding sites, and by using a full-length human cDNA for PDC-E2 and preparation of multiple overlapping recombinant fusion proteins, we can specify that there are at least three autoepitopes present on human PDC-E2: the crossreactivity outer and inner lipoyl domains and a site surrounding the E1/E3 binding region. The dominant epitope is localized to the inner lipoyl region; the outer lipoyl region has only weak reactivity, and only 1/26 PBC sera reacted with the E1/E3 binding region. Strong evidence for a conformational autoepitope was obtained by Surh *et al.*[27] and Rowley *et al.*[28].

Studies of epitope mapping of PDC-E2 have primarily relied on whole sera. However, selective absorption studies using whole sera and a series of overlapping recombinant peptides of PDC-E2 have suggested that the epitope includes a large conformational component[27]. We have studied these issues by developing and characterizing five human monoclonal antibodies from a patient with PBC[29]. The monoclonal antibodies were produced by fusing regional hepatic lymph node B cells with the mouse human heterohybrid cell line F3B6. The five monoclonal antibodies that were generated included three IgG2a and two IgM antibodies. These antibodies were studied for antigen specificity against recombinant PDC-E2, recombinant BCOADC-E2, histone, dsDNA, IgG-Fc, collagen and a recombinant irrelevant liver-specific control, the F alloantigen. The antibodies were also used to probe blots of human, bovine, mouse and rat mitochondria. In addition, fine specificity was studied by selective ELISA and absorption against overlapping expressed fragments of PDC-E2. All five monoclonals were specific for PDC-2. Unlike polyreactive antisera they did not crossreact with protein X, suggesting that protein X contains an epitope distinct from that found on PDC-E2. Additionally, although all the three IgG2 monoclonals mapped within the inner lipoyl domain of PDC-E2, they recognized distinct specificities and different conformational epitopes[29].

T-CELL RESPONSES

The specificity of bile duct destruction in PBC, the presence of lymphoid infiltrates in the portal tracts, and the aberrant expression of HLA-DR molecules on biliary epithelium have suggested that intrahepatic biliary epithelial cells are the direct targets of an intense immune response[28–32]. Although the infiltrating T cells appear to be oligoclonal[32], there have been only limited reports on generating autoreactive cloned T cell lines[33]. In early lesions the $CD8^+$ T lymphocyte is the predominant cell type, but an increased tendency towards $CD4^+$ cells is noted in advanced stages, but whether (and if so, how) these actually cause the damage is uncertain. Activated T cells may produce lymphokines which act locally to recruit non-specific T cells to the sites of inflammation. It is, therefore, particularly appropriate to note that T cell cloned lines derived from liver biopsies of patients with PBC produced IL-2 specifically when stimulated with PDC-E2 or BCOADC-E2, but not ovalbumin, PPD or BGG[33]. The availability of such T cell lines will provide a valuable tool to address the basic issues of clonality, T cell repertoire and epitope mapping.

CELL SURFACE EXPRESSION OF M2 AUTOANTIGENS

There are some studies suggesting that autoantigens relevant to PBC may be present on the surface of hepatocytes or biliary epithelium. Earlier, studies[34] reported that PBC sera reacted with the surface of teased-out hepatocytes, and intact hepatoma cells, and that reactivity was abolished by prior absorption of sera with mitochondria. Others[35] detected reactivity of PBC sera with guinea-pig hepatocytes, and with 67 and 50 kDa components of isolated rat hepatocellular plasma membranes.

We have examined antigen distribution in liver tissue from PBC patients by use of a mouse monoclonal antibody which reacted with the inner lipoyl domain of PDC-E2 similar to PBC sera. A distinct and intense reactivity with the bile ducts of patients with PBC was demonstrated when the mAb was used at a 1:100 dilution of culture supernatant[33]. In these studies, bile ducts of liver tissue from normals, patients with chronic active hepatitis and progressing sclerosing cholangitis gave a mitochondrial pattern of reactivity, but detectable only at a dilution of antibody of 1:2. In similar studies using purified rabbit antibodies there was very strong staining with antibody to E2 in the biliary epithelium, and in a subset of macrophages in the portal lymph nodes. By contrast, staining with antibodies to E1 and E3 produced characteristic mitochondrial reactivity but in both PBC and control tissue[35,36].

Therefore, sera from patients with primary biliary cirrhosis (PBC) clearly react with enzymes of the 2-oxo-dehydrogenase pathways, particularly PDC-E2. These enzymes are present in all nucleated cells, yet autoimmune damage is confined to biliary epithelial cells. Using a panel of eight mouse monoclonal antibodies and a human combinatorial antibody specific for PDC-E2, we examined, by confocal microscopy sections of liver from patients with PBC, progressive sclerosing cholangitis (PSC) and hepatocarcinoma. The monoclonal antibodies gave typical mitochondrial immunofluorescence on biliary epithelium and on hepatocytes from patients with either PBC, PSC or hepatocarcinoma. However, one of eight mouse monoclonal antibodies (C355.1) and the human combinatorial antibody reacted with great intensity and specificity with the luminal surface of biliary epithelium from patients with PBC. Simultaneous examination of these sections with an anti-isotype reagent for human IgA revealed high IgA staining at the luminal surface of biliary epithelial cells in patients with PBC. IgG and IgA antibodies to PDC-E2 were detected in the bile of patients with PBC but not normal controls. We believe these data may be interpreted as indicating that PDC-E2 or a crossreactive protein is expressed at high levels at the luminal surface of biliary epithelial cells in PBC.

EPIDEMIOLOGICAL AND FAMILIAL CONSIDERATION

There are various other possibilities which could determine surface expression of autoantigenic proteins including M2. One is the assembly process of the 2-OADC enzymes (M2 antigens) which are encoded in the nucleus, synthesized in the cytoplasm, and from there transferred via a leader sequence to the mitochondria, to their correct location for assembly of the complex on the inner mitochondrial membrane or matrix. Any mechanism which interfered with this process could lead to an accumulation of the protein in the leader sequence of the cytoplasm and cell surface expression. Alternatively, the occurrence of a somatic mutation on the gene for PDC-E2 could disrupt the process, and lead to cell surface expression.

Using immunoblotting, ELISA, and enzyme inhibition with both purified mitochondrial proteins and recombinant autoantigens, family members and spouses of patients with PBC have been studied in our laboratory for the presence of antimitochondrial antibodies[39]. This study included 27 index patients with PBC, 15 spouses, and 48 first- and second-degree relatives. Overall, seven relatives (11%) were positive for autoantibodies by indirect immunofluorescence against mouse liver and stomach sections. The pattern strictly conformed to that of AMA in only one of these seven people, a sibling with mild pruritus and a liver biopsy diagnostic of PBC despite a normal serum alkaline phosphatase. Inhibition of enzyme activity of PDC was seen at a serum dilution of 1:500 in this sibling. In addition, the mother of a patient of PBC had a history of sarcoidosis and was positive by immunoblotting for antibodies to PDC-E2 and protein X. All other relatives were negative for all of the assays. More importantly, in the healthy relatives, antibodies to the 2-OADC enzymes were absent, as were the recently proposed family of 'naturally occurring mitochondrial antibodies'[26]. We also note that by history one brother died of PBC, a father died of an unknown liver disease and one sister is reported to have PBC but was unavailable for testing. Further, there were a number of relatives with other autoimmune diseases, including the sicca complex, thyroiditis and rheumatoid arthritis. These data reinforce a (weak) genetic predisposition to PBC, and a general predisposition to autoimmunity; they also reinforce the disease-specific nature of AMA when tested for purified or recombinant autoantigens.

Primary biliary cirrhosis (PBC) is described among various ethnic and racial populations, but the incidence and prevalence varies quite widely, from the highest among northern European populations to lower in Japan and vanishingly low in certain other parts of Asia[40–44]. Moreover, even among populations derived from northern European sources there is a striking difference in prevalence, e.g. between that reported for northern England

and Canada. Also, it is our undocumented impression tha the Australian prevalence is closer to that of Canada than that of northern Europe. There has hitherto not been a detailed immunological profile of antimitochondrial antibodies (AMA) according to geographical region. We have used recombinant or purified preparations from the 2-OADC enzymes (PDC-E2, BCOADC-E2, OGDC, protein X and PDC-E1α) to compare the reactivity of sera from either Japanese or American–Caucasian patients with PBC[45]. The clear regional differences in the incidence of PBC were accompanied by interesting differences in the pattern of AMA immunoreactivity among North American Caucasians and Japanese patients with PBC. In particular, only 65% of Japanese patients reacted by ELISA with PDC-E2 compared with more than 95% of the North American group and, moreover, the level of enzyme-inhibitory antibodies to PDC was lower in the Japanese. Our findings prompt the need for characterization of specific susceptibility genes and environmental factors in various parts of the world to clarify the aetiology of PBC, noting that the clinical manifestations of the disease appear similar between geographical regions. It is clear that the different regional frequencies in PBC and the subtle differences in serological reactivity point to yet-to-be-determined genetic and environmental determinants of this disease. Surprisingly, detailed data on the prevalence of PBC throughout the world accumulated from independent studies over a period of 3–10 years are still rather limited, being available only for western European countries and, more recently, Canada and Japan. Available data for annual incidence include 128/million population for Sweden[40], 128.5/million for England[41], 23/million for several western European countries[42], and 23/million for Canada[43], all in contrast to Japan, wherein the annual incidence is only 5.16/million[44]. The disease is predominantly female in all populations surveyed. None of these demographic studies have taken advantage of modern serological assays using cloned mitochondrial autoantigens in the screening process, and the numbers reported reflect only those with clinical disease. In other words there are no comparative interpopulation data on asymptomatic PBC or on asymptomatic subjects.

References

1. Mackay IR. Primary biliary cirrhosis showing high titre of autoantibody: report of a case. N Engl J Med. 1958;258:185–7.
2. Berg PA, Doniach D, Roitt IM. Mitochondrial antibodies in primary biliary cirrhosis. I. Localization of the antigen to mitochondrial membranes. J Exp Med. 1967;126:277–90.
3. Walker JG, Doniach D, Roitt IM, Sherlock S. Serological tests in the diagnosis of primary biliary cirrhosis. Lancet. 1965;1:827–9.
4. Kaplan MM. Primary biliary cirrhosis. N Engl J Med. 1987;316:521–8.
5. Gershwin ME, Coppel RL, Mackay IR. Primary biliary cirrhosis and mitochondrial autoantigens – insights from molecular biology. Hepatology. 1988;8:147–51.
6. Gershwin ME, Mackay IR. Primary biliary cirrhosis: paradigm or paradox for autoimmunity. Gastroenterology. 1991;100:822–33.
7. Mendel-Hartvig I, Nelson BD, Loof L, Totterman TH. Primary biliary cirrhosis: further biochemical and immunological characterisation of mitochondrial antigens. Clin Exp Immunol. 1985;62:371–9.

8. Gershwin ME, Mackay IR, Sturgess A, Coppel RL. Identification and specificity of a cDNA encoding the 70 kD mitochondrial antigen recognized in primary biliary cirrhosis. J Immunol. 1987;138:3525–31.
9. Van de Water J, Fregeau D, Davis P, Ansari A, Danner D, Leung P, Coppel R, Gershwin ME. Autoantibodies of primary biliary cirrhosis recognize dihydrolipoamide acetyltransferase and inhibit enzyme function. J Immunol. 1988;141:2321–4.
10. Coppel RL, McNeilage LJ, Surh CD, Van de Water J, Spithill TW, Whittingham S, Gershwin ME. Primary structure of the human M2 mitochondrial autoantigen of primary biliary cirrhosis: dihydrolipoamide acetyltransferase. Proc Natl Acad Sci USA. 1988;85: 7317–21.
11. Fussey SPM, Guest JR, James OFW, Yeaman SJ. Identification and analysis of the major M2 autoantigens in primary biliary cirrhosis. Proc Natl Acad Sci USA. 1988;85:8654–8.
12. Mackay IR, Gershwin ME. Molecular basis of mitochondrial autoreactivity in primary biliary cirrhosis. Immunol Today. 1989;10:315.
13. Yeaman SJ. The mammalian 2-oxoacid dehydrogenases: a complex family. Trends Biochem Sci. 1986;11:293–6.
14. Roche TE, Lawlis VB. Structure and regulation of α-ketoglutarate dehydrogenase of bovine kidney. Ann NY Acad Sci. 1982;378:236.
15. Patel MS, Roche TE. Molecular biology and biochemistry of pyruvate dehydrogenase complexes. FASEB J. 1990;4:3224–33.
16. Perham RN, Packman LC. 2-Oxo acid dehydrogenase multienzyme complexes: domains, dynamics, and design. Ann NY Acad Sci. 1989;573:1–20.
17. Surh CD, Roche TE, Danner DJ, Ansari A, Coppel RL, Prindiville T, Dickson ER, Gershwin ME. Antimitochondrial autoantibodies in primary biliary cirrhosis recognize cross-reactive epitope(s) on protein X and dihydrolipoamide acetyltransferase of pyruvate dehydrogenase complex. Hepatology. 1989;10:127–33.
18. Surh CD, Cooper AE, Coppel RL, Leung P, Ahmed A, Dickson R, Gershwin ME. The predominance of IgG3 and IgM isotype antimitochondrial antibodies against recombinant fused mitochondrial polypeptide in patients with PBC. Hepatology. 1988;8:290–5.
19. Roise D, Schatz G. Mitochondrial presequences. J Biol Chem. 1988;263:4509–11.
20. De Marcucci OGL, Gibb GM, Dick J, Lindsay JG. Biosynthesis, import and processing of precursor polypeptides of mammalian pyruvate dehydrogenase complex. Biochem J. 1988;251:817–23.
21. Fregeau DR, Roche TE, Davis PA, Coppel R, Gershwin ME. Primary biliary cirrhosis. Inhibition of pyruvate dehydrogenase complex activity by autoantibodies specific for E1α, a non-lipoic acid containing mitochondrial enzyme. J Immunol. 1990;144:1671–6.
22. Fregeau DR, Prindiville T, Coppel RL, Kaplan M, Dickson ER, Gershwin ME. Inhibition of α-ketoglutarate dehydrogenase activity by a distinct population of autoantibodies recognizing dihydrolipoamide succinyltransferase in primary biliary cirrhosis. Hepatology. 1990;11:975–81.
23. Harris R, Beckman I, Roberts-Thomson PJ. Low molecular weight IgM detection using immunoblotting. J Immunol Methods. 1986;88:97.
24. Uibo R, Mackay IR, Rowley M, Humphries P, Armstrong J McD, McNeilage J. Inhibition of enzyme function by human autoantibodies to an autoantigen pyruvate dehydrogenase E2: different epitope for spontaneous human and induced rabbit autoantibodies. Clin Exp Immunol. 1990;80:19–24.
25. Berg PA, Klein R. Heterogeneity of antimitochondrial antibodies. Semin Liver Dis. 1989;9:103–16.
26. Klein R, Berg PA. Demonstration of naturally occurring mitochondrial antibodies in family members of patients with primary biliary cirrhosis. Hepatology. 1990;12:335–41.
27. Surh CD, Coppel R, Gershwin ME. Structural requirement for autoreactivity in human pyruvate dehydrogenase-E2, the major autoantigen of primary biliary cirrhosis. J Immunol. 1990;144:3367–74.
28. Rowley MJ, McNeilage LJ, Armstrong JMcD, Mackay IR. Inhibitory autoantibody to a conformational epitope of the pyruvate dehydrogenase complex, the major autoantigen in primary biliary cirrhosis. Clin Immunol Immunopathol. 1991;60:356–70.
29. Leung PSC, Krams S, Munoz S, Surh CP, Ansari A, Kenny T, Robbins DL, Fung J, Starzl TE, Maddrey W, Coppel RL, Gershwin ME. Characterization and epitope mapping of

human monoclonal antibodies to PDC-E2, the immunodominant autoantigen of primary biliary cirrhosis. J Autoimmunity. 1992;5:703–18.
30. Ballardini G, Bianelli GB, Doniach D, Mirakiam R, Pisi E, Botazzo GF. Aberrant expression of HLA-DR antigens on bile duct epithelium in primary biliary cirrhosis, relevance to pathogenesis. Lancet. 1984;2:1009–11.
31. Yamada G, Hyodo I, Tobe K, Mizuno M, Nishihara T, Kobayashi T, Nagashima H. Ultrastructural immunocytochemical analysis of lymphocytes infiltrating bile duct epithelia in primary biliary cirrhosis. Hepatology. 1986;3:385–91.
32. Moebius U, Manns M, Hess G, Kober G, Zum Buschenfelde KHM, Meuer SC. T-cell receptor gene rearrangements of lymphocytes-T infiltrating the liver in chronic active hepatitis B and primary biliary cirrhosis (PBC): oligoclonality of PBC-derived T cell clones. Eur J Immunol. 1990;20:889–93.
33. Van de Water J, Ansari AA, Surh CD, Coppel R, Roche T, Bonkovsky H, Kaplan M, Gershwin ME. Evidence for the targeting by 2-oxo-dehydrogenase enzymes in the T cell response of primary biliary cirrhosis. J Immunol. 1991;146:89–94.
34. Ghadiminejad I, Baum H. Evidence for the cell-surface localization of antigens cross-reacting with 'mitochondrial antibodies' of primary biliary cirrhosis. Hepatology. 1987;7: 743–50.
35. Sundin U, Sundqvist KG. Plasma membrane association of primary biliary cirrhosis mitochondrial marker antigen M2. Clin Exp Immunol. 1991;83:407–12.
36. Krams SM, Van de Water J, Coppel RL, Esquivel C, Roberts J, Ansari A, Gershwin ME. Analysis of hepatic T lymphocyte and immunoglobulin deposits in patients with primary biliary cirrhosis. Hepatology. 1991;12:306–13.
37. Joplin R, Lindsay JG, Johnson GD, Strain A, Neuberger J. Membrane dihydrolipoamide acetyltransferase (E2) on human biliary epithelial cells in primary biliary cirrhosis. Lancet. 1992;339:93–4.
38. Joplin R, Lindsay JG, Hubscher SG, Johnson GD, Shaw JC, Strain AJ, Neuberger JM. Distribution of dihydrolipoamide acetyltransferase (E2) in the liver and portal lymph nodes of patients with primary biliary cirrhosis: an immunohistochemical study. Hepatology. 1991;14:442–7.
39. Cladwell SH, Leung PSC, Spivey JR, Prindiville T, De Medina M, Saicheur T, Rowley M, Reddy KR, Coppel R, Jeffers LJ, Mackay IR, Schiff ER, Gershwin ME. Antimitochondrial antibodies in kindreds of patients with primary biliary cirrhosis: Antimitochondrial antibodies are unique to clinical disease and are absent in asymptomatic family members. Hepatology. 1992;16:899–905.
40. Lofgren J, Jarnerot G, Danielsson D, Hemdal I. Incidence and prevalence of primary biliary cirrhosis in a defined population in Sweden. Scand J Gastroenterol. 1985;20:647–50.
41. Myszor M, James OF. The epidemiology of primary biliary cirrhosis in north-east England: an increasingly common disease? Q J Med. 1990;75:377–85.
42. Triger DR, Berg PA, Roder J. Epidemiology of primary biliary cirrhosis. Liver. 1984;4: 195–200.
43. Witt-Sullivan H, Heathcote J, Cauch K, Blendis L, Chent C, Katz A, Milner R, Pappas SC, Rankin J, Wanless IR. The demography of primary biliary cirrhosis in Ontario, Canada. Hepatology. 1990;12:98–105.
44. Yasutoshi M. Annual of Hepatitis Research Committee of Japan (in Japanese) 1989:8–10.
45. Iwayama T, Leung PSC, Rowley M, Munoz S, Nishioka M, Nakagawa T, Dickson ER, Coppel RL, Mackay IR, Gershwin ME. Comparative immunoreactive profiles of Japanese and American patients with primary biliary cirrhosis against mitochondrial autoantigens. Int Arch Allergy Immunol. 1992;99:28–33.

42
Immunogenetic influences in primary biliary cirrhosis

P. T. DONALDSON, D. G. DOHERTY, J. A. UNDERHILL and R. WILLIAMS

The exact pathogenesis of primary biliary cirrhosis (PBC) is unclear. However, several features including raised serum IgM levels[1], abnormalities of the cellular immune response including *in-vitro* cytotoxicity to hepatocytes[2], sensitization to bile duct- and liver-specific antigens[3,4], bile duct disruption by mononuclear cells[5], defective suppressor T cell function[6,7], circulating immune complexes and accelerated complement turnover[8], the association with autoantibodies to nuclear and mitochondrial antigens[9-12], and in particular, increased HLA class II expression on bile duct epithelium[13,14], suggest an immune pathogenesis. More recently demonstration of expression of the E2 antigen on cultured bile duct epithelial cells may have identified one potential target autoantigen[15]. Taken together these observations support the concept that PBC is an autoimmune disease. However, unlike two other autoimmune liver diseases, autoimmune hepatitis (AIH) and primary sclerosing cholangitis (PSC), PBC is not associated with an over-representation of the HLA A1-B8-DR3 haplotype[16], nor are there secondary associations with HLA DR4 or DR2 as reported in AIH and PSC[17,18]. The story of immunogenetic associations in PBC is considerably more complex, and requires an understanding of the genetic structure of the short arm of chromosome 6[19].

The HLA region on the short arm of chromosome 6 (Fig. 1) spans approximately 4000 kilobases. This short piece of DNA represents the most studied genetic system in the human genome and the most polymorphic. For the sake of convenience we can consider the region in three parts: class I, class II and class III. These definitions are based on the structure and function of the gene products encoded by the three regions.

The HLA class I region encodes the HLA A, B, Cw, E, F G and H antigens. The products of the HLA A, B and Cw loci are known to be important in transplant rejection and antigen presentation. Each locus represents a single gene, with a single polypeptide product. The HLA A, B and Cw antigens are expressed as cell surface glycoproteins on all nucleated

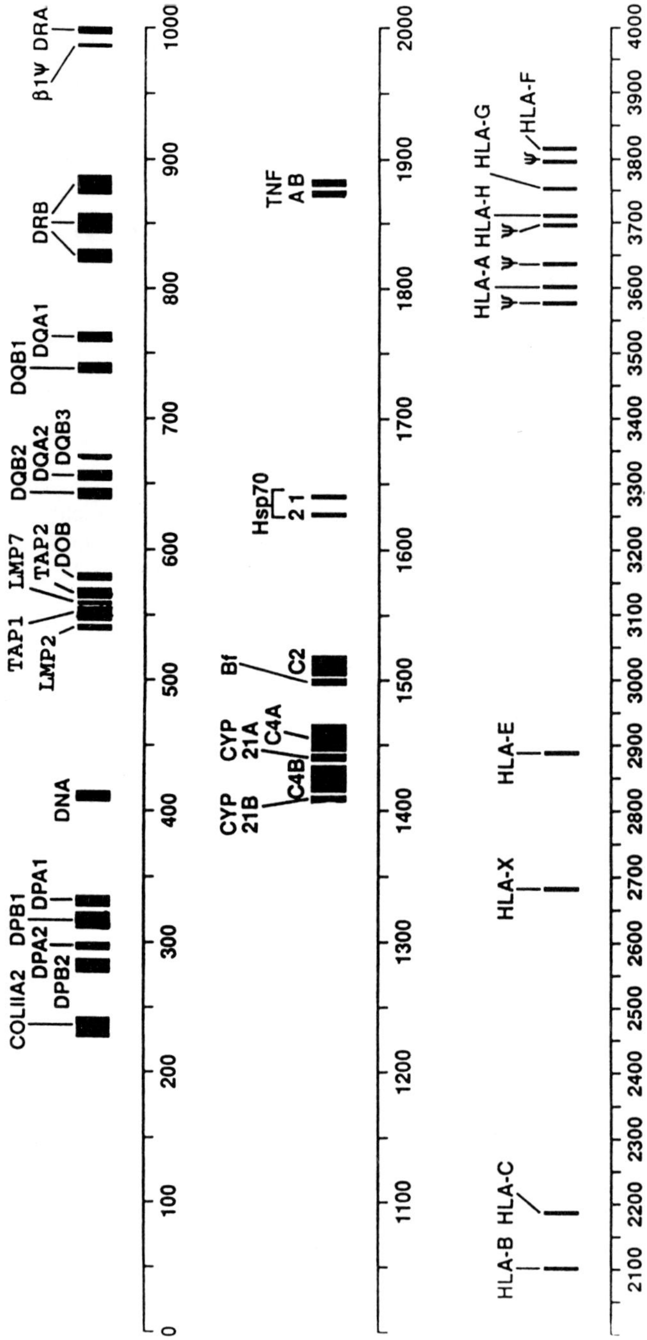

Fig. 1 Genetic map of the short arm of chromosome 6 (see ref. 19). ψ indicates pseudogenes

cells. They consist of a single α-chain of 45 kDa with three domains and a short transmembrane section. The α-chain is non-covalently associated with a β_2-microglobulin molecule. The β_2-microglobulin molecule or β-chain is encoded on chromosome 15 and is not polymorphic. In the expressed form as an α/β heterodimer the two membrane distal domains of the α-chain form a groove. X-ray crystallographic studies[20] of purified HLA class I proteins show the groove as a complex structure, with two α-helices, one from each domain – representing the walls and a series of eight criss-crossing β pleated sheets – which form the floor. The products of the HLA A, B and Cw loci are all highly polymorphic. Recent DNA sequencing studies have demonstrated that the majority of that polymorphism is encoded by nucleotides representing amino acid positions in the wall and floor of the groove[21].

To date at least 30 genes in the class II regions are recognized, including genes involved in peptide cleavage (low molecular weight proteases, LMP2, LMP7) and peptide transport (peptide transporter genes TAP1 and TAP-2)[22–24]. This review is concerned with the classical HLA class II genes, i.e. those which encode the HLA DR, DQ and DP antigens. Other class II loci include DO, DN and what appear to be ancestral HLA class II genes DMA and DMB. The function of these other HLA class II genes is currently not known.

The organization of the class II genes (Fig. 2) is considerably more complex than that of the HLA A, B and Cw genes. There are striking similarities and important differences between class I and class II. As with the class I antigens, each HLA D antigen is expressed as an α/β heterodimer, but for the HLA D antigens both the α-chain and β-chain are encoded (by an A gene and a B gene) on chromosome 6. Unlike HLA class I, where the β-chain (β_2-microglobulin) is invariable for the HLA D antigens both the α-chain and the β-chain may be polymorphic. In practical terms the DRA gene is invariable, but the DRB, DQA, DQB, DPA and DPB genes are all polymorphic. In addition there are usually two expressed DR genes in each haplotype. Thus whilst there is a single essentially monomorphic DRA gene there are five different polymorphic DRB genes. Of these DRB1 encodes the classical serological variants DR1–DR18; DRB2 is a pseudogene (with no expressed product); DRB3 encodes three variants of DR52: DR52a, DR52b, and DR52c; DRB4 encodes DR53 and the product of DRB5 encodes the recently named DR51 specificity. There is such linkage disequilibrium within haplotypes that nearly all those with DRB1 types DR3, DR5 or DR6 carry the DRB3 gene, those with DRB1 types DR4, DR7 or DR9 carry DRB4, DRB1 types DR2 carry DRB5, whilst those with the DRB1 type DR8 are exceptional, having only one expressed DRB allele (Fig. 2). As with the class I genes, the products of the class II genes are cell surface glycoproteins, but unlike HLA A, B and Cw antigens these antigens are expressed on a restricted number of cell types including cells involved in antigen presentation (B lymphocytes, macrophages – including tissue macrophages, e.g. Kupffer cells, activated T cells, etc.), and also (albeit weakly) on endothelial and epithelial cells[25]. After immune stimulation there are local increases in class II expression. The predicted structure of the class II glycoproteins is very similar to that of their class I cousins; however, with class II molecules the

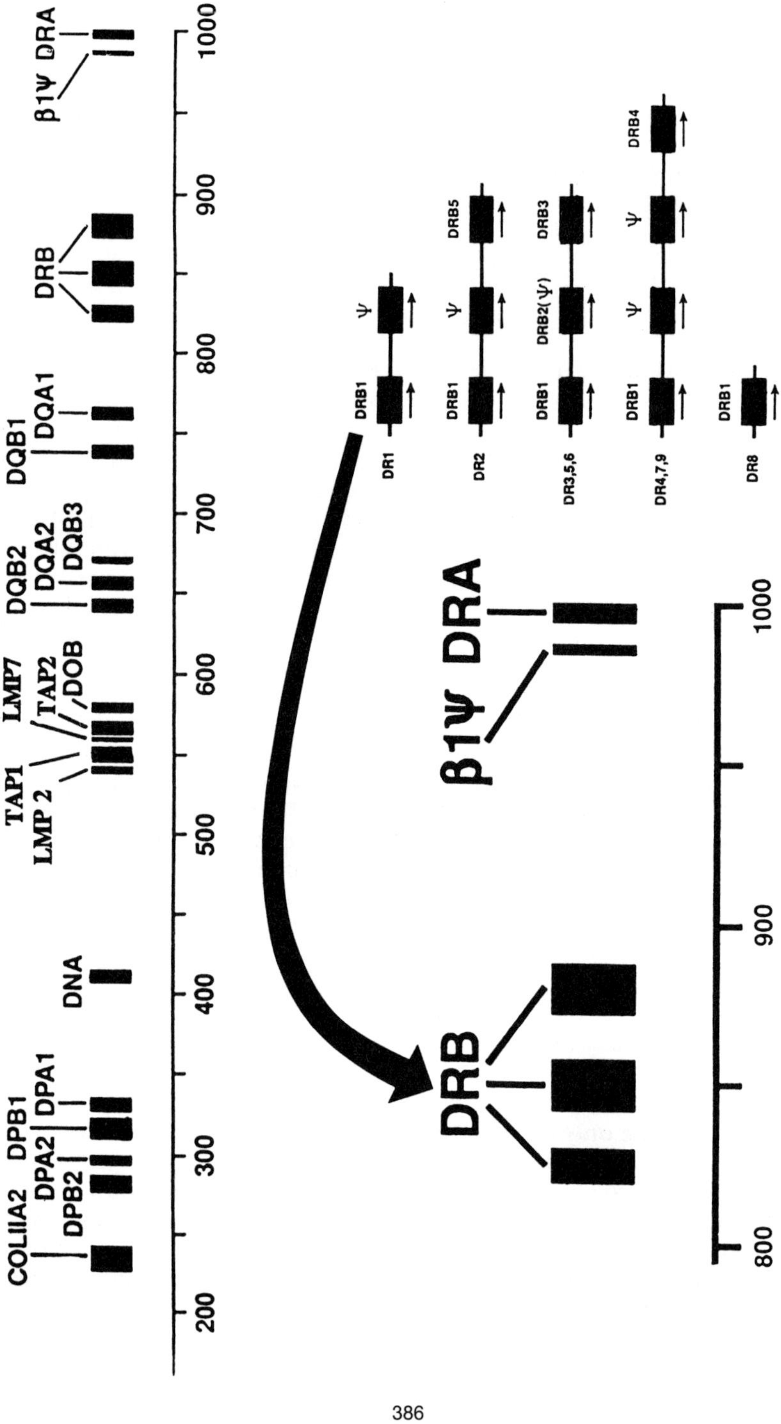

Fig. 2 Genetic complexity of the HLA DRB sub-region

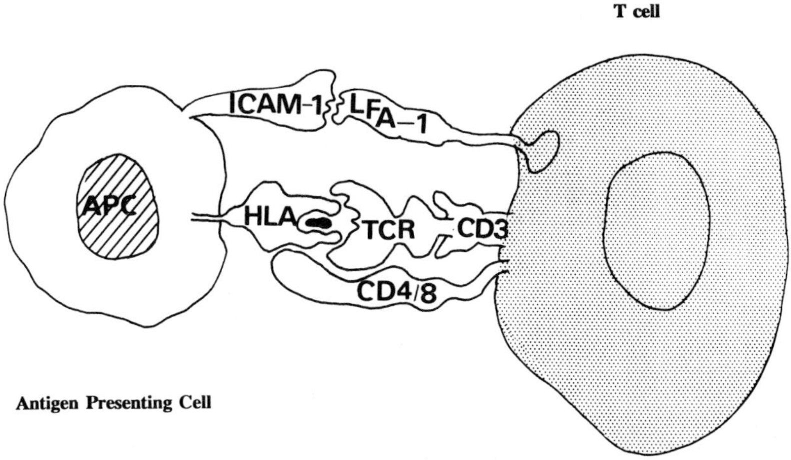

Fig. 3 Simplified view of antigen presentation. Antigen (peptide) is presented in the HLA binding groove to the T cell receptor of a T cell. HLA class I and class II molecules have separate binding sites for CD8 and CD4 respectively. Adhesion molecules bind ligands forming bridges between the cells, thereby adding further stability to the coupling process

antigen-binding groove is formed from the membrane distal domain of the α-chain and the membrane distal domain of the β-chain. As with the HLA class I DNA sequences class II DNA sequencing reveals that the majority of the encoded polymorphism maps within the groove[26].

The term HLA class III is a misnomer, since the products of this region are not cell surface glycoproteins – or human leucocyte antigens. The genes in this region encode a collection of immunologically active serum and plasma proteins. This includes the genes for the classical complement pathway components C4A, C4B and C2 and the alternative pathway equivalent Bf (factor B or properdin factor), tumour necrosis factor α and β (TNF), two steroid cytochrome P450 21-hydroxylase enzymes (CYP21A and CYP21B) and also genes for the heat shock protein – hsp70.

Although the MHC genes were first described in 1936[27], the importance of MHC products in antigen presentation was not realized for several decades. It is now generally accepted that MHC molecules, or HLA molecules in humans, present fragments of antigen in the form of peptides to T cells (Fig. 3). HLA class I molecules present peptides which are derived from proteins that are produced endogenously in the cell. During antigen processing antigens are degraded in the cytosol and the peptides derived are transported to the endoplasmic reticulum, where further degradation may take place. In the endoplasmic reticulum peptides bind to, and take part in the assembly of, class I molecules; finally the whole peptide–HLA class I complex is transported to the cell surface and displayed on the plasma membrane[28,29]. Recent work suggests that for class I molecules a restricted repertoire of peptides are bound, requiring specific amino acids at specific anchor sites within the antigen binding groove. By requiring specific motifs for each allele the number and variety of peptides bound by a given class I molecule is restricted[30]. Though peptides of varying lengths may be bound

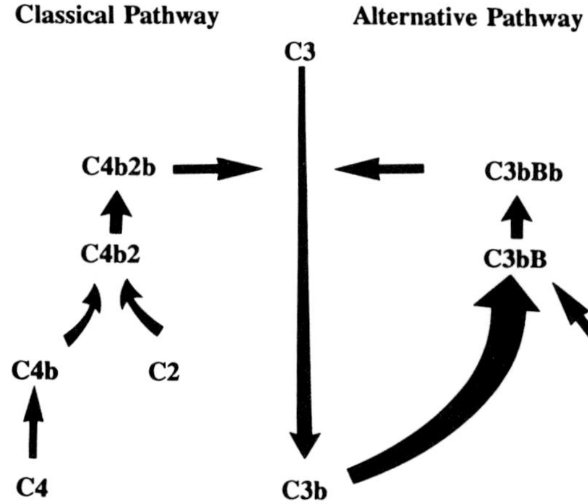

Fig. 4 Alternative and classical complement pathways illustrating the role of the HLA class II complement proteins C4 (both C4A and C4B), C2 and Bf

in the groove, trimming by proteolytic enzymes reduces the peptide which is displayed for presentation to the T cells to eight or nine amino acids long. Once trimmed to a short length the peptide–HLA class I complex is very stable.

HLA class II molecules are primarily involved in the presentation of peptides derived from extracellular fluids. Antigens are taken into the cell by endocytosis or phagocytosis. Inside the cell the endocytic vesicle fuses with an acidic lysosome, where the antigen is proteolytically digested. At the same time HLA class II molecules are synthesized in the endoplasmic reticulum, budded to the transgolgi and fuse with the acidic lysosome. At low pH the invariant chain which is non-covalently bound with the class II molecule is replaced by the antigenic peptide. The whole HLA–class II antigen complex is then transported to the cell surface where it is displayed on the cell membrane[31].

It is of some interest that the function of the HLA region encoded complement proteins is C4A and B, and C2 is in the conversion of C3 to C3b in the classical activation pathway, whilst the other HLA-encoded complement protein Bf is involved in exactly the same process in the alternative activation pathway (Fig. 4). This critical transformation C3 to C3b is common to both complement pathways, though the classical pathway is essentially antibody dependent and the alternative pathway is not. No other complement alleles are known to map to the short arm of chromosome 6. In fact the remaining complement proteins appear to be randomly scattered throughout the human genome.

The high female preponderance in PBC, and the occasional report of the disease within families, suggests that there is at least one genetic element to disease susceptibility. Interest in the autoimmune hypothesis for PBC was sufficient to warrant investigation of other potential genetic susceptibility factors. The early 1970s saw an explosion of interest in the relationship between HLA and disease[32]. At that time most autoimmune diseases were

Table 1 History of HLA class I in PBC

Principal author	*Year*	*Country*	*Reference*
Galbraith	1974	UK	28
Ercilla	1979	Spain	31
Hamlyn	1980	UK	29
Miyamori	1983	Japan	33
Bassendine	1985	UK	30
Donaldson		UK	*
Gores	1987	USA	34
Manns	1991	Germany	41

*Unpublished data (n = 110)

found to be associated with the antigens A1 and B8. PBC was an exception; the first study of HLA and PBC from the King's group[33] which included two UK populations: 45 patients from southeast England and 28 from southwest Scotland, the frequencies of A1 were 44% and 29% compared with 22% and 31% for controls (respectively). The authors found no correlation with autoantibodies to nuclear factor and mitochondrial antigen. These data were a striking contrast to data on AIH presented in the same paper. These findings were later confirmed by two other UK studies[34,35]. To date there is general agreement on this point. No fewer than eight studies, from six centres (Table 1) have confirmed the lack of an HLA class I association in PBC.

HLA class II associations were first reported in 1979 in 21 white Caucasian PBC patients from Spain[36]. In that study 12/21 (57.1%) had DR3 compared to 11/74 (14.8%) unrelated controls. These data appear to contradict earlier reports suggesting the lack of an association with HLA B8 in PBC, since in northern Europe 90% of DR3-positive individuals have B8[37]. The authors suggested that in Spain the linkage disequilibrium between DR3 and B8 was weaker. To add to the confusion DR2 was associated with PBC in Japanese[38]. In light of the data from Spain this seemed plausible since, in Japan, DR3 is almost absent and DR2 is most often associated with autoimmune diseases. However, both of these studies were based on very small patient groups and have a high risk of statistical error. In addition the arguments about linkage disequilibrium are the subject of debate, since delta values derived from small numbers of controls are very inaccurate.

In 1985, data from a study of 75 UK patients[35] suggested that there is no DR association with PBC. Our own unpublished data on over 100 patients confirmed these observations. However, a study of 114 patients from the Mayo Clinic[39] described an increase in the frequency of DR8 in patients with PBC, 30.1% of patients were DR8-positive compared to 4.7% of 171 controls. In addition the frequency of DR5 was lower in patients, 9.8% compared to 25.2% in controls. The apparent differences between this study, that of Bassendine and our own series (unpublished) are simple to explain. In our own series DR8 was not tested, due to the lack of well-defined monospecific sera. A similar explanation can be made for the Bassendine study – a later review by the authors suggests that the sera used for the definition of DR8 were poor[40]. However, unlike Gores, neither UK series demonstrated a negative association with DR5; this may also be due to problems with monospecific antisera. The antigens DR5 and DR8 crossreact, the majority of antisera against DR5 react with DR8 and vice-versa; thus if DR8 was not assigned, the serotyping pattern would suggest DR5 as the next most logical antigen. Additional problems may arise from sera which react with combinations of DR6, DR5 and DR8.

This sort of variation is typical of HLA disease association studies in the 1970s and 1980s. With the introduction of molecular DNA-based techniques in the late 1980s HLA typing has become more precise. One method in particular has been widely applied for HLA DR typing – restriction fragment length polymorphism (RFLP) analysis[41]. RFLP analysis of more than 4000 DNA samples from renal transplant recipients and donors reveals that up to 25% HLA DR assignments based on classical serology may be incorrect[42]. Although the introduction of better cell separation techniques and more well-defined typing sera has led to a global improvement in serological tissue typing, there are still severe limitations on the use of serology for disease studies. Our own experience reveals that the accuracy of serological DR typing for a given antigen may vary from 70.4% for DR8 to 98% for DR3[43]. The degree of accuracy reflects the availability of well-defined monospecific antisera and not the competence of the operator.

RFLP typing is ideal for the assignment of DR8. Using a standard one enzyme protocol with 10 μg of genomic DNA[41], DR8 can be assigned with nearing 100% accuracy as a single 8.66 kB Taq 1 band. Two studies, both from the UK, have now used RFLP typing to investigate HLA DR associations in PBC. The data are remarkably similar. In our own series DR8 (as determined by the 8.66 kb Taq 1 band) was present in 11% of 159 northern European white patients compared to 4% of 162 racially matched controls[44]. In the second study DR8 was present in 10% of 80 patients compared to 4.6% of 363 controls[45]. These associations are significant despite the fact that the majority of patients (approximately 90%) do not have the susceptibility allele. However, DR5 was not associated with susceptibility to, or protection from, PBC in either of these studies. Furthermore the frequency of DR8 is considerably lower than that reported by Gores *et al.* It has been suggested that this may reflect differences in the genetic background of northern European whites compared to North American whites. There may be an historical precedent for this view (Julia Bodmer, personal communication). However, a more recent study, based on serological assignment of DR8 in 25 patients from Germany, reported 36% of patients with DR8 (versus 3.6% of controls)[46]. Since such large differences in HLA antigen frequencies between UK and German populations cannot be explained by racial variation, a more likely explanation is that DNA-based techniques are more precise in defining DR8.

It would be incorrect to give the impression that all the differences between studies are due to technical imperfections. One study from Sweden[47] recently reported a strong association with DR7 in PBC. In this case we cannot question the accuracy of the DR typing, since RFLP analysis was used. All of the patients in the above study were from Malmo, Sweden, and it is possible that such a homogeneous population may have a different HLA association. However, this report is an exception. Even in Japanese, where there are considerable genetic differences compared to a northern European population, DR8 is raised in PBC. As with series from Europe and the USA, the values quoted vary between studies depending on whether serology or DNA-based techniques are used. In one report, based on serotyping, 78.6% of patients were DR8-positive[48], in another report, based on DNA typing, only 36.8% had DR8[49].

Despite the variations, in the majority of PBC populations tested DR8 is raised. However, in Europeans the association accounts for a minority of patients. The data may be an indication that the 'susceptibility allele' lies some distance from the HLA DR genes. Candidate alleles include the closely linked DQ loci and DP loci, or alternatively susceptibility to PBC may be determined by genes within the HLA class III region. A recent study from our own institute investigated DQB polymorphisms by polymerase chain reaction amplification and allele- or sequence-specific oligonucleotide probing[44]. One allele, DQB1*0402, was more frequent in patients compared to controls, being present in 11% of 89 patients and in 4% of 181 controls. Though this difference was not significant, all nine patients had DR8. Since these two antigens are in linkage disequilibrium and the greatest relative risk associated with the presence of both antigens (RR = 5.4) it was assumed that the haplotype DR8–DQB1*0401 is primarily associated with PBC. In Japanese the DR8 haplotype associated with PBC may be different, since Seki reported DQ3 in 79.4% of 38 patients[49]. Furthermore the same study investigated the HLA DPB locus; 84.8% of patients were DPB1*0501-positive compared to 55% of controls. The authors suggest that DPB1*0501 may be the primary susceptibility allele in PBC. These observations await confirmation in other series.

The class III complement genes, in particular C4A and C4B, have attracted considerable attention in relation to autoimmune disease. In PBC a catalogue of complement abnormalities has been recorded. Observations in the early 1980s that C4A null alleles were raised in systemic lupus erythematosus[50] and in children with AIH[51] – were encouragement to investigate class III alleles and in particular C4 in PBC. However, in the first report of C4 allotypes in PBC, null alleles for C4A and C4B (C4AQ0 and C4BQ0) were not increased, as the authors expected[52]. This is a marked contrast to AIH and many other autoimmune diseases. Instead there was a significant increase in the frequency of the C4B 2 allotype, 15/33 (45%) of patients were C4B 2-positive compared to 53/307 (17%) controls. In addition there was an increased frequency of the C4A 4 allotype, which was present in 21% of patients compared to 6% of controls. These two C4 alleles are in linkage disequilibrium and the authors suggest that the primary association is with C4B 2. A number of other diseases have been associated with the C4B 2 allotype including multiple sclerosis[53], juvenile rheumatoid arthritis[54] and Alzheimer's disease[55]. At the 9th international histocompatibility workshop, C4B 2 was not found to be in linkage with DR8[32]. Therefore these two associations may be independent, possibly defining two subsets of the disease, although studies to date have failed to relate either DR8 or C4B 2 to particular clinical or immune features of PBC. A second study of class III in PBC from Germany on 25 patients[46] failed to confirm the association with C4B 2, though this allotype was present in 8/25 (32%) of patients and 23/176 (15.4%) controls. Similarly the frequency of the C4A 4 allotype was higher in patients, though not significant (24% versus 12%). In contrast to the study of Briggs, Manns observed a two-fold difference in the frequency of C4AQ0 between patients and controls (72% versus 34.5%). The effect of C4AQ0, in terms of disease susceptibility, was even more striking when combined with DR8 (RR = 183.75). The most difficult aspect of this report is that DR8 and C4AQ0 are thought to be in negative linkage disequilibrium in caucasoid populations. Both studies can be criticized for the small number of patients studied and, though interesting, these data should be considered as preliminary observations. A third study of the class III region has demonstrated an association with a specific TNF-α restriction fragment[56], though it remains to be seen whether this has any functional significance.

The relationship between these immunogenetic alleles and PBC is speculative. The association with DR8 may be a marker for a stronger association with a distant locus on the short arm of chromosome 6. The most likely HLA D locus would be DP; alternatively there may be associations with other non-classical class II genes – such as the protease or transporter genes. All of these associations imply a role for the class II gene in the pathogenesis of the disease, through antigen presentation or processing. It is interesting to note that AIH and PSC, both of which are thought to be autoimmune liver diseases, have been recently associated with specific amino acid substitutions located within the antigen-binding groove of the HLA DR molecule[57] (D. Doherty unpublished observation, 1992; Fig. 5). We may speculate on the functional significance of these changes. It is possible that these substitutions may be sufficient to alter significantly the binding of a putative autoantigen, thus changing the balance in favour of an autoimmune reaction. However autoreactivity will occur only if potentially autoreactive clones have been able to survive the process of clonal deletion during T cell development and maturation in the thymus. Thus most healthy individuals have one or more HLA alleles which have been associated with susceptibility to disease. The associated susceptibility allele is a risk factor for disease, but alone is insufficient to lead to disease. In addition, in both AIH and PSC there is considerable evidence that the HLA alleles may not only determine susceptibility to, and protection from, but also the severity of, disease[17,18,57]. Such an explanation for the DR8 association with PBC is possible though, as stated above, to date there has been no correlation between HLA DR or DQ and clinical or immune features of the disease[34].

Associations between PBC and complement alleles are easier to explain. Clearly there are abnormalities in complement metabolism in PBC, though whether these are secondary to the disease is unknown. Inherited deficiencies in complement are reported. Such disorders are usually dramatic with high mortality, though not associated with PBC. Partial complement deficiencies may be possible where one allele is defective, though under normal circumstances the maternal alleles will make up for deficiencies in paternal complement allele function and vice-versa. Therefore in practice those with one null or defective allele do not have deficiencies in circulating complement

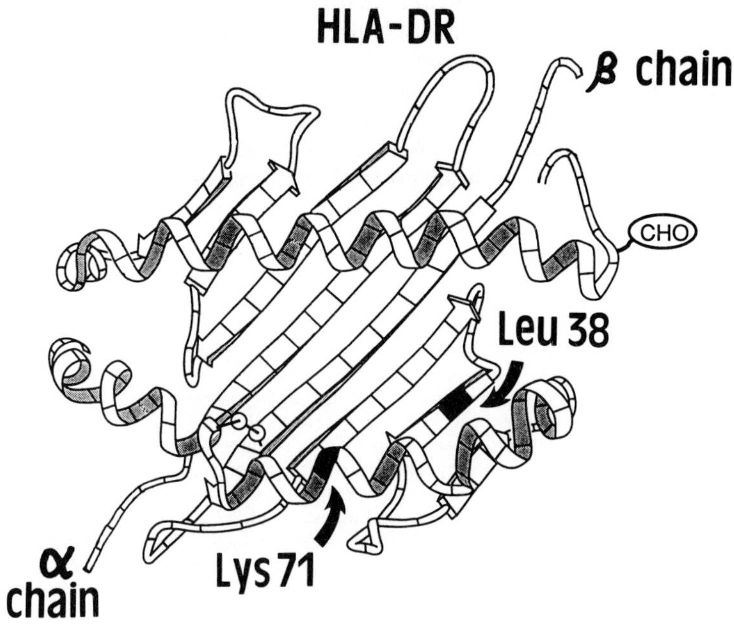

Fig. 5 Predicted structure of the first domains of the HLA DR molecule (see ref. 65) showing amino acid positions which are currently thought to encode susceptibility to AIH and PSC (ref. 52 and D. Doherty, personal communication, 1992)

levels. There may, however, be circumstances in which complement deficiencies can be engineered by infection or immune stimulation. The C4A and C4B alleles are known to have different affinities for polypeptides and carbohydrate substrates. In hydralazine-induced systemic lupus erythematosus C4 null alleles have been reported, though most patients are heterozygous null carriers. The most common second allele in these patients has a high affinity for hydralazine[58]. Thus a functional deficiency may arise through interaction of the drug with the one functional C4 allele.

Finally it would be incorrect to give the view that immunogenetics is entirely the study of HLA and the short arm of chromosome 6. Other immune active polypeptides are known to be polymorphic, in particular the other members of the immunoglobulin supergene family: the T cell receptor and immunoglobulin genes. Although both T cell receptor and Ig genes undergo somatic mutation and recombination to achieve functional diversity, there are a number of well-characterized polymorphisms of germline genes[59,60]. As with HLA associations there has been considerable interest in the relationship between these genes and disease susceptibility. Many studies seeking associations between autoimmune diseases and specific immunoglobulin allotypes have been performed[60]. These allotypes are genetically determined polymorphisms in the constant region genes of the IgG and IgM heavy and light chains. Most notably the IgG1 subclass (g-1-

m) allotypes 'a' and 'x' are associated with AIH[61], and similar studies suggest interaction of HLA and Gm in susceptibility to Grave's disease[62]. A number of T cell receptor germline polymorphisms have recently attracted attention in diabetes[63]. These RFLP-defined variants of the $V\beta$ and $C\beta$ genes are thought to increase susceptibility to diabetes. Preliminary data suggest that similar associations are found in AIH (K. Manabe, unpublished observations, 1991). To date there have been no similar investigations of these genes in PBC.

References

1. Fiezi T. Immunoglobulins in chronic liver disease. Gut. 1968;9:193–8.
2. Veirling JM, Nelson DL, Strober W, Bundy BM, Jones EA. *In vitro* cell-mediated cytotoxicity in primary biliary cirrhosis and chronic hepatitis; dysfunction of spontaneous cell-mediated cytotoxicity in primary biliary cirrhosis. J Clin Invest. 1977;60:1116.
3. McFarlane IG, Wojcicka BM, Tsantoulas DC, Portmann B, Eddleston ALWF, Williams R. Leucoctye migration inhibition response to biliary antigens in primary biliary cirrhosis, sclerosing cholangitis and other chronic liver disease. Gastroenterology. 1979;76:1333.
4. Tsantoulas D, Perperas A, Portmann B, Eddleston ALWF, Williams R. Antibodies to a human liver membrane lipoprotein (LSP) in primary biliary cirrhosis. Gut. 1980;21:557.
5. Schaffner F, Popper H. Clinical pathological relations in primary biliary cirrhosis. In: Popper H, Schaffner F, editors. Progress in liver disease, vol. VII. New York: Grune & Stratton; 1982:529.
6. Zetterman RK, Woltjen JA. Suppressor cell activity in primary biliary cirrhosis. Dig Dis Sci. 1980;25:104.
7. Nouri-Aria KT, Hegarty JE, Neuberger J, Eddleston ALWF, Williams R. *In vitro* studies on the mechanisms of increased serum IgM levels in primary biliary cirrhosis. Clin Exp Immunol. 1985;61:297–304.
8. Wands JR, Dienstag JL, Bahn AK, Feller ER, Isselbacher KJ. Circulating immune complexes and complement activation in primary biliary cirrhosis. N Engl J Med. 1978;298:233–7.
9. Walker JG, Doniach D, Roitt IM. Serological tests in the diagnosis of primary biliary cirrhosis. Lancet. 1965;1:827–31.
10. Doniach D, Riott IM, Walker JG, Sherlock S. Tissue antibodies in primary biliary cirrhosis, active chronic (lupoid) hepatitis, cryptogenic cirrhosis and other liver diseases and their clinical implication. Clin Exp Immunol. 1966;1:237–62.
11. Berg PA, Doniach D, Roitt IM. Mitochondrial antibodies in primary biliary cirrhosis. Localisation of the antigen to mitochondrial membranes. J Exp Med. 1967;126:277–99.
12. Mackay IR, Gershwin ME. Molecular basis of mitochondrial autoreactivity in primary biliary cirrhosis. Immunol Today. 1989;10:315–18.
13. Ballardini G, Mirakian R, Bianchi FB, Pisi E, Doniach D, Bottazzo GF. Aberrant expression of HLA-DR antigens on bile duct epithelium in primary biliary cirrhosis: relevance to pathogenesis. Lancet. 1984;2:1009–13.
14. Nakanuma Y, Naoko K. Expression of HLA DR antigens on interlobular bile ducts in primary biliary cirrhosis. Hum Pathol. 1991;22:431–6.
15. Joplin R, Lindsay JG, Johnson GD, Strain A, Neuberger J. Membrane dihydroloamide acetyltransferase E2 on human biliary epithelial cells in primary biliary cirrhosis. Lancet. 1992;339:93–4.
16. Mackay IR, Tait BD. HLA associations with autoimmune-type chronic active hepatitis: Identification of B8-DRw3 haplotype by family studies. Gastroenterology. 1980;79:95–8.
17. Donaldson PT, Doherty DG, Hayllar KM, McFarlane IG, Johnson PJ, Williams R. Susceptibility to autoimmune chronic active hepatitis: Human leucocyte antigens DR4 and A1-B8-DR3 are independent risk factors. Hepatology. 1991;13:701–6.
18. Donaldson PT, Farrant JM, Wilkinson ML, Hayllar KM, Portmann BC, Williams R. Dual association of HLA DR2 and DR3 with primary sclerosing cholangitis. Hepatology. 1991;13:129–33.

19. Trowsdale J, Campbell RD. Complexity in the major histocompatibility complex. Eur J Immunogenet. 1992;19:45–55.
20. Bjorkman PJ, Saper MA, Samraoui B, Bennett WS, Strominger JL, Wiley DC. Structure of the human class I histocompatibility antigen, HLA-A2. Nature. 1987;329:506–12.
21. Zemmour J, Parham P. HLA class I nucleotide sequences, 1991. Immunogenetics. 1991;33:310–20.
22. Spies T, Bresnahan M, Bahram S, Arnold D, Blanck R, Mellins E, Pious P, DeMars R. A gene in the human major histocompatibility complex class II region controlling the class I antigen presentation pathway. Nature. 1990;348:744–7.
23. Glynne R, Powis SH, Beck S, Kelly A, Kerr L-A, Trowsdale J. A proteosome-related gene between the two ABC transporter loci in the class II region of the human MHC. Nature. 1991;353:357–60.
24. Kelly A, Powis SH, Glynne R, Radley E, Beck S, Trowsdale J. Second proteosome-related gene in the human MHC class II region. Nature. 1991;353:667–8.
25. Daar AS, Fuggle SV, Fabre JW, Ting A, Morris PJ. The detailed distribution of MHC class II antigens in normal human organs. Transplantation. 1984;38:293–6.
26. Marsh SGE, Bodmer JG. HLA class II nucleotide sequences, 1991. Hum Immunol. 1991;31:207.
27. Gorer PA. Genetic and antigenic basis of tumour transplantion. J Pathol Bacteriol. 1937;44:691–7.
28. Monaco JJ. A molecular model of MHC class I restricted antigen processing. Immunol Today. 1992;13:173–9.
29. Elliot T, Townsend A, Cerundolo V. Naturally processed peptides. Nature. 1990;348: 195–7.
30. Rotschke O, Falk K. Naturally-occurring peptide antigens derived from the MHC class-I restricted processing pathway. Immunol Today. 1991;12:447–55.
31. Neejfes JJ, Ploegh HL. Intracellular transport of MHC class II molecules. Immunol Today. 1992;13:179–84.
32. Tiwari JL, Terasaki PI. HLA and disease associations. 1st edn. New York: Springer Verlag; 1985.
33. Galbraith RM, Eddleston ALWF, Smith MG, Williams R, McSween RNM, Watkinson G, Dick H, Kennedy LA, Batchelor JR. Histocompatibility antigens in active chronic hepatitis and primary biliary cirrhosis. Br Med J. 1974;3:604–5.
34. Hamlyn AN, Adams D, Sherlock S. Primary or secondary sicca complex? Investigation in primary biliary cirrhosis by histocompatibility testing. Br Med J. 1980;281:425–6.
35. Bassendine MF, Dewar PJ, James OFW. HLA DR antigens in primary biliary cirrhosis; lack of association. Gut. 1985;26:625–8.
36. Ercilla G, Pares A, Arriga F, Brugera M, Castillo R, Rodes J, Vives J. Primary biliary cirrhosis associated with HLA DR3. Tissue Antigens. 1979;14:449–52.
37. Baur MP, Neugebauer M, Albert ED. Reference table of two-locus haplotype frequencies for all MHC marker loci. In Albert ED, Bauer MP, Mayr WR, editors. Histocompatibility testing. New York: Springer Verlag; 1984:667–755.
38. Miyamori H, Kato Y, Koboyashi K, Hattoi N. HLA antigens in Japanese patients with primary biliary cirrhosis and autoimmune chronic active hepatitis. Digestion. 1983;26: 213–17.
39. Gores GJ, Moore SB, Fisher LD, Powell FC, Dickson ER. Primary biliary cirrhosis: association with class II major histocompatibility complex antigens. Hepatology. 1987;7: 889–92.
40. James OFW, Myszor M. Epidemiology and genetics of primary biliary cirrhosis. Prog Liver Dis. 1990;9:523–36.
41. Bidwell JL, Bidwell EA, Savage DA, Middleton D, Klouda PT, Bradley BA. A DNA RFLP typing system that positively identifies serologically well defined and ill defined HLA DR and DQ alleles including DRw10. Transplantation. 1988;45:640–6.
42. Opelz G, Mytilineos J, Scherer S, Dunckley H, Trejaut J, Chapman J, Middleton D, Savage D, Fischer O, Bignon JD, Bensa JC, Albert E, Noreen H. Survival of DNA HLA DR typed and matched cadaver kidney transplants. Lancet. 1991;338:461–3.
43. Doherty DG, Donaldson PT. HLA DRB and DQB typing by a combination of serology, RFLP and PCR SSO probing. Eur J Immunogenet. 1991;18:111–24.

44. Underhill J, Donaldson P, Bray G, Doherty D, Portmann B, Williams R. Susceptibility to primary biliary cirrhosis is associated with the HLA-DR8-DQB1*0402 haplotype. Hepatology. 1992;16:1404–8.
45. Gregory W, Mehal W, Daly AK, Dunn AN, Cavanagh G, Chapman R, Idle J, James OFW, Bassendine MF. Analysis of major histocompatibility complex class II genotype in primary biliary cirrhosis using RFLP and PCR. Hepatology. 1992:in press (abstract).
46. Manns MP, Bremm A, Schneider PM, Notghi A, Gerken G, Prager-Eerbele M, Stradmann-Bellinghausen B, Meyer zum Buschenfelde KH, Ritner C. HLA DRw8 and complement C4 deficiency as risk factors in primary biliary cirrhosis. Gastroenterology. 1991;101:1367–73.
47. Lindgren S, Kockum I, Lernmark A, Sundkvist G, Wassmuth R, Eriksson S. HLA DR gene polymorphisms in primary biliary cirrhosis. J Hepatol. 1991;13(suppl 2):165 (abstract).
48. Maeda T, Onoshi S, Saibara T, Iwasaki S, Yamamoto J. HLA DR8 and primary biliary cirrhosis. Gastroenterology. 1992;103:1118–19.
49. Seki T, Kiyosawa K, Ohta M, Sodeyama, T, Tahaka E, Yoshizawa K, Yabu T, Furuta K, Usuda S, Furuta S, Mizuki N, Ando LA, Inoko H. HLA typing using PCR in PBC. Acta Hepatol Jpn. 1992;33 (suppl. 1): 164 (abstract).
50. Fielder AHL, Walport MJ, Batchelor JR, Rynes RI, Black CM, Dodi IA, Hughes GRV. Family study of the major histocompatibility complex in patients with systemic lupus erythematosus: importance of null alleles of C4A and C4B in determining disease susceptibility. Br Med J. 1983;286:425–8.
51. Vergani D, Wells L, Larcher VF, Nasaruddin BA, Davies ET, Mieli-Vergani G, Mowat AP. Genetically determined low C4: a predisposing factor to autoimmune chronic active hepatitis. Lancet. 1985;2:294–8.
52. Briggs DC, Donaldson PT, Hayes P, Welsh KI, Williams R. A major histocompatibility complex Class III allotype C4B2 associated with primary biliary cirrhosis. Tissue Antigens. 1987;29:141–5.
53. Schroder R, Zander H, Andreas A, Mauff G. Multiple sclerosis: immunogenetic analysis of sib-pair double family cases. II. Studies on the association of multiple sclerosis with C2, C4, BF, C3, C6 and GLO polymorphisms. Immunobiology. 1983;164:160–70.
54. Hall PJ, Burman S, Laurent MR, Briggs DC, Venning HE, Leak AM, Bedford PA, Ansell BM. Genetic susceptibility to early onset articular juvenile arthritis: a study of HLA and complement marker in 159 British patients. Ann Rheum Dis. 1986;45:464–74.
55. Nerl CW, Mayeux R, O'Niell GJ. Complement C4 allotypes in Alzheimer's disease. Lancet. 1982;2:1343.
56. Fugger L, Morling N, Ryder LP, Platz P, Georgson J, Jackobson BK, Svejgaard A, Dalhoff K, Ranek L. Nco I RFLP of tumour necrosis factor alpha region in primary biliary cirrhosis in healthy Danes. Scand J Immunol. 1989;30:185–9.
57. Farrant JM, Doherty DG, Donaldson PT, Vaughan RW, Hayllar KM, Welsh KI, Eddleston ALWF, Williams R. Amino acid substitutions at position 38 of the DRβ polypeptide confer susceptibility and protection from primary sclerosing cholangitis. Hepatology. 1992;16: 390–5.
58. Speirs C, Fielder AHL, Chapel H, Davey NJ, Batchelor JR. Complement system protein C4 and susceptibility to hydralazine-induced systemic lupus erythematosus. Lancet. 1989;1:922–4.
59. Niven MJ, Caffrey C, Moore RH, Sachs JA, Mohan V, Festenstein H. T-cell receptor β-subunit gene polymorphism and autoimmune disease. Human Immunol. 1990;27:360–7.
60. Propert DN. Detection of immunoglobulin polymorphisms. In: Simons MJ, Tait BD, editors. Detection of immune-associated genetic markers of human disease. (Practical methods in clinical immunology 7). New York: Churchill Livingstone; 1984:65–81.
61. Whittingham S, Mathews JD, Schanfield MS, Tait BD, Mackay IR. Interaction of HLA and gm in autoimmune chronic active hepatitis. Clin Exp Immunol. 1980;43:80–6.
62. Uno H, Sasazuki T, Tamai H, Matsumoto H. Two major genes, linked to HLA and Gm, control susceptibility to Graves' disease. Nature. 1981;292:768–70.
63. Hibberd ML, Millward BA, Wong FS, Demaine AG. T-cell receptor constant chain polymorphisms and susceptibility to type I diabetes. Diabet Med. 1992;9:929–33.
64. Brown JH, Jardetzky T, Saper MA, Samraoui B, Bjorkman PJ, Wiley DC. A hypothetical model of the foreign antigen binding site of class II histocompatibility molecules. Nature. 1988;332:845–50.

43
Nuclear autoantibodies in primary biliary cirrhosis

I. R. MACKAY, M. J. ROWLEY and S. F. WHITTINGHAM

INTRODUCTION

Primary biliary cirrhosis (PBC) is a paradoxical organ-specific autoimmune disease[1]. The lesions are mostly limited to intrahepatic biliary ductules yet the demonstrable autoantigens are non-tissue-specific. The most characteristic reactivity, known as anti-M2, is with the enzymes of the 2-oxo-acid dehydrogenase complexes (OADC) in mitochondria and, in particular, with the E2 subunit of the pyruvate dehydrogenase complex (PDC-E2)[1]. The characterization of this reactivity, and mapping of an immunodominant epitope to the lipoyl domain of PDC-E2, have been significant advances, and have overshadowed the occurrence in PBC of other serological reactivities. These include autoantibodies to nuclear autoantigens (discussed in this chapter), smooth muscle autoantigens seen particularly in the overlap syndrome of PBC with autoimmune hepatitis[2] and thyroid autoantigens[3,4].

There are three major sets of nuclear autoantigens that are part of the serological profile of PBC: centromeric antigen(s), the Sp-100 antigen and nuclear lamins. The importance of these antinuclear responses in PBC is threefold (Fig. 1). First, the autoantibodies are directed to particular nuclear

1. Non-random: to discrete nuclear subsets — **centromere**, **Sp-100**, **lamins**

2. Syndrome associated: centromere antibodies with scleroderma–CRST

3. Non-crossreactivity: mitochondrial and nuclear antibodies

Fig. 1 Nuclear antibodies in PBC – likely relevance

1. Centromere
1970 : CRST association
1980 : anti-centromere

2. Speckled-dot (Sp-100)
1984 : immunofluorescence
1987 : immunoblotting: MW 100 kDa
1990 : cDNA for Sp-100

3. Nuclear membrane – lamins
1985 : immunofluorescence
1988 : immunoblotting: various MWs
1990 : nuclear pore glycoprotein

Fig. 2 Nuclear autoantigens in PBC – background

constituents, since the more usual antinuclear reactivities, e.g. anti-dsDNA, anti-histone, anti-Ro, as seen for example in systemic lupus erythematosus, are seldom observed[2]. Second, the reactivity to centromeric antigens is matched by the clinical association with PBC of the corresponding clinical syndrome, peripheral scleroderma-CRST, as described below. Third, the populations of autoantibodies to mitochondrial and nuclear autoantigens are independent and non-crossreactive, as would be suspected from non-homology in cloned and sequenced mitochondrial and centromeric or Sp-100 proteins. We here present data from affinity chromatographic partition of sera with antimitochondrial and antinuclear reactivities.

HISTORICAL BACKGROUND AND OVERVIEW

The development of knowledge on reactions to nuclear autoantigens in PBC is summarized in Fig. 2.

Primary biliary cirrhosis–scleroderma–anticentromere

A PBC–scleroderma overlap was reported initially as a clinical association by Reynolds *et al.*[5,6] and Murray-Lyon *et al.*[7]. Both groups concurred that although previous instances of chronic liver disease and scleroderma had been recorded, the co-occurrence specifically of PBC with calcinosis–Raynaud phenomena–sclerodactyly–telangiectasia (CRST) could be regarded as a newly recognized syndrome. Early indications of the frequency of CRST in PBC were given as 6% (11 of 188 cases)[8] and 3% (3 of 100 cases)[9]. There were subsequent reports of higher frequencies, 17% (14 of 83 cases)[10], and 18% (20 of 110 cases)[11], and lower frequencies, 2%[12] although the latter showed that 12% of the cases of PBC had centromere antibody.

In 1980, centromere autoantibody identified by immunofluorescence was recognized as a characteristic accompaniment of CRST-type scleroderma, by Moroi *et al.*[13] and Fritzler *et al.*[14]. Thereafter assessments were made in cases of PBC of the frequency of both scleroderma and centromeric antibody. The initial studies showed the expected association between PBC and centromere antibody, but the clinical accompaniment differed. Thus in the 110 consecutive patients with PBC reported by Bernstein *et al.*[11], scleroderma (CRST-type) was diagnosed clinically in 20 (18.2%) yet centromeric antibody was detected only in 10 (9.1%). Other reports indicate that in PBC centromeric antibody could exist without clinical evidence of scleroderma, or may even precede the onset of the clinical syndrome. Makinen *et al.*[15] reported a 29% incidence of centromeric antibody in PBC (14 of 48 cases), with 5 of the 14 cases lacking any clinical evidence of CRST-scleroderma.

There is less comment on the frequency of PBC ascertained among case-series of scleroderma (systemic sclerosis). There are a number of case reports on the coexistence of scleroderma and PBC[16] but these were not ascertained through systematic surveys of scleroderma cases. Fregeau *et al.*[16] analysed serum samples from 250 patients with scleroderma from three referral sources. Of these, 141 had CRST-type disease, 101 had diffuse cutaneous disease and 8 unclassified disease. There were 19 sera (7.6%) with anti-M2 reactivity and 15 were from cases of CRST syndrome. Of these 19 cases with anti-M2, only 3 had PBC (which developed after the occurrence of scleroderma), 1 had chronic active hepatitis and 3 had abnormal liver function tests, giving an aggregate frequency of liver disease of 2.8%. McHugh *et al.*[17] analysed patients with scleroderma (systemic sclerosis) attending a connective tissue disease clinic. There were 72 cases studied and, whereas none had clinical evidence of liver disease, 8 (11%) had IgG and/or IgM antibody to M-2, specifically to pyruvate dehydrogenase complex, by ELISA.

Primary biliary cirrhosis and anti-Sp-100

A second antinuclear reactivity in PBC was described in 1984 by Bernstein *et al.*[18], using immunofluorescence which gave a characteristic pattern of speckled dots not associated with nucleoli or condensed chromatin. This autoantibody was found by Szostecki *et al.*[19] in 1987 to react by immunoblotting with a nuclear protein with an electrophoretic mobility of 100 kDa, and hence was called Sp- (for speckled) 100. Fusconi *et al.*[20] reported two bands of immunoblotting, 78–92 and 96–100 kDa. Unlike what pertains for centromeric antibody, there is no clear-cut clinical subset of PBC that accompanies Sp-100. An association of Sp-100 with lacrimal dysfunction was suspected[19], and the occurrence occasionally in PBC of anti-Sp-100 in the absence of anti-M2 raised the suggestion that anti-Sp-100 could mark a particular type of PBC[21], but this has not been substantiated. The reported frequency of the Sp-100 autoantibody in PBC has varied; the antibody specified as PBC 95K was present in 44% (22 of 50)[22], and that specified as multiple nuclear dot (MND) ANA in about 15%[20].

Szostecki *et al.*[21] derived a partial cDNA and an expressed fusion protein that had Sp-100 reactivity, so allowing for large-scale screening by ELISA for anti-Sp-100 in various autoimmune diseases. Their results based on 525 disease sera showed a high degree of specificity of anti-Sp-100 for PBC. Among 184 cases of PBC there were 50 (27.2%) positive by ELISA, with no cases positive among 70 cases with other chronic hepatobiliary inflammatory diseases. Among the 271 cases of rheumatoid diseases tested, anti-Sp-100 was detected by ELISA in 7 of 97 (7.2%) cases of primary systemic sclerosis and 2 of 102 (1.9%) of cases of SLE.

Primary biliary cirrhosis and antibodies to nuclear membrane components

The third antinuclear reactivity in PBC, initially characterized by immunofluorescence as nuclear membrane staining, is anti-lamin. The first report, by Ruffatti *et al.*[23], described an antinuclear antibody specific for the nuclear membrane with an incidence in PBC of 28.5% (18 of 63 cases). This antinuclear membrane antibody (ANMA) was usually present to a higher titre than anti-M2, and reacted with a linear or ring-like staining of the limiting membrane of the nucleus. It had high specificity, since it was rarely detected in control sera, but there were no accompanying clinical associations that distinguished ANMA-positive cases of PBC. Curiously, ANMA was present as the only autoantibody in the serum of a woman with PBC whose sister, also with PBC, had only anti-M2[23]. The prevalence of perinuclear antibody in two subsequent PBC case series was 52%[24] and 29%[25].

The nuclear envelope comprises a double membrane, pore complexes and the nuclear lamina, that include three major proteins of 74, 68 and 60 kDa, called A, B and C lamins[26,27]. Although ring-like staining of the nucleus initially was specified as anti-DNA, it is now attributable also to autoantibodies to proteins of the nuclear lamina (lamins), and to a major glycoprotein of the nuclear pore complex[28]. By immunoblotting, sera containing anti-lamins react with proteins of molecular weights of 74, 68 and 60 kDa, corresponding to lamins A, B, C. These are members of the cytoskeletal protein family, since there is a close sequence similarity between lamin proteins and intermediate filaments[29,30]. Hence autoantibodies to lamins can be expected as markers of various autoimmune liver diseases, including PBC, as well as appearing also in miscellaneous other diseases. Initially Lassoued *et al.*[31] found that of 50 sera with a ring-like nuclear fluorescence, 11 contained anti-lamins and 8 of these were from cases of chronic liver disease. Wesierska-Gadek *et al.*[32] described anti-lamins by immunofluorescence in 15 sera, of which 3 were from patients with PBC and 12 from patients with lupoid hepatitis.

Lassoued *et al.*[25] studied 150 sera from patients with PBC of which 43 displayed a perinuclear ring-like staining by immunofluorescence. Studies by immunoblotting showed that of these 43, there were 40 that reacted with a 200 kDa nuclear envelope protein; sera from 2 reacted with both lamins A and C, and 1 serum was negative by immunoblotting. The previously described 200 kDa antigen[33] was subsequently identified as gp210 which is an integral membrane protein believed to be involved in the formation of nuclear pores and the anchorage of pore complex constituents to the nuclear membrane[34]. In contrast to autoantibodies to lamins, autoantibody to the 200 kDa nuclear pore glycoprotein appears to be highly specific for PBC, since it is not detectable in other autoimmune diseases[25].

METHODS

The purpose of the studies to be described was to test for crossreactivity using preparations of PBC serum that had anti-M2 activity together with a nuclear reactivity, anti-centromere or anti-Sp-100, after affinity purification of serum on recombinant PDC-E2.

Sera

The sera tested were from two patients with PBC diagnosed with classical clinical and histological features[36]. Each serum, 'a' and 'b', gave the pattern of cytoplasmic immunofluorescence characteristic of antimitochondrial reactivity. In addition, each serum contained a specific antinuclear reactivity: serum 'a' contained anti-centromere antibodies that reacted against CENP A and CENP B, and serum 'b' contained antibodies to Sp-100.

Analysis of antibodies by immunofluorescence

Antinuclear antibodies and antimitochondrial antibodies were tested by immunofluorescence on HEp-2 cells (Kaalestadt) by standard techniques. Sera were screened initially at 1/40 and titrated in four-fold dilutions. Fractions from the affinity column were tested undiluted. The reactivities by immunofluorescence are shown in Fig. 3.

Analysis of antibodies by ELISA

Antibodies to the pyruvate dehydrogenase complex were measured by ELISA as described previously[37]. The antigen used was a human glutathione-*S*-transferase recombinant PDC-E2 protein purified by affinity chromatography from lysates of *E. coli* transformed with the plasmid expression vector pGEX containing a cDNA insert of 1350 base pairs encoding the human PDC-E2 autoantigen[38]. Polystyrene microtitre plates were coated with 50 μl of antigen, 10 μg/ml, and incubated overnight at 4°C with 50 μl of antibody. Antibody binding was detected using peroxidase-conjugated anti-human IgG (Silenus, Hawthorn, Victoria, Australia), and 0.5 mg/ml 2,2′-azinobis(3-ethylbenzathiazoline sulphonic acid) (ABTS) in 0.1 mol/l citrate–phosphate buffer pH 4 as substrate.

Analysis of antibodies by immunoblotting

Immunoblot detection of mitochondrial antibodies to the 2-OADC antigens was carried out as previously described[37]. Extracts of bovine heart mitochon-

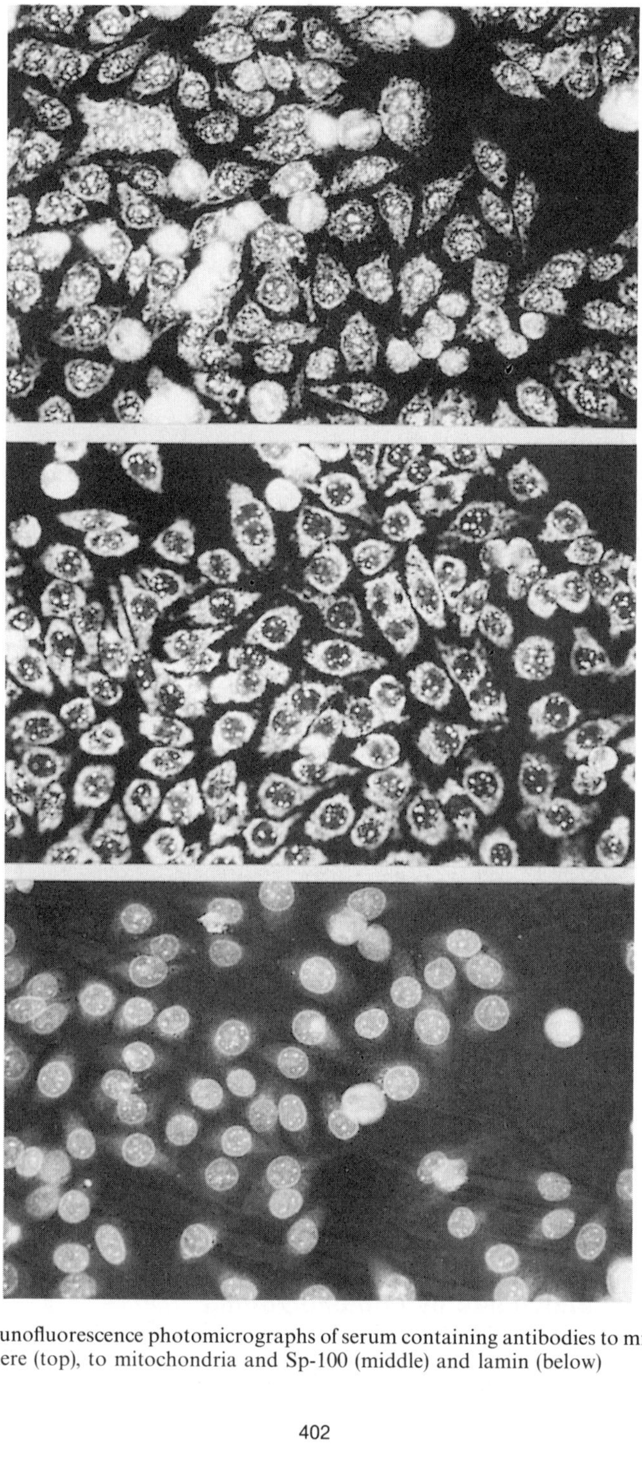

Fig. 3 Immunofluorescence photomicrographs of serum containing antibodies to mitochondria and centromere (top), to mitochondria and Sp-100 (middle) and lamin (below)

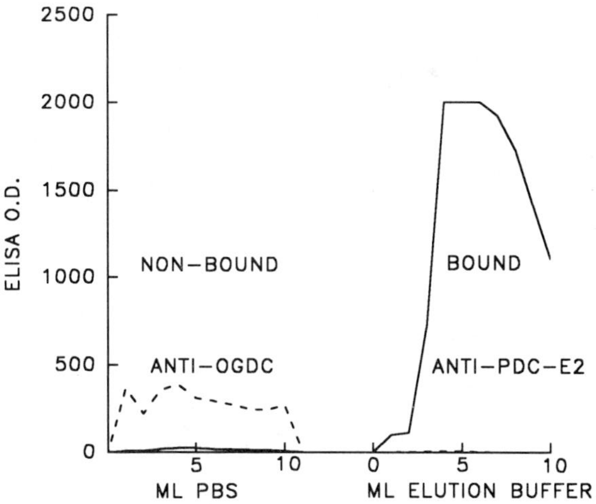

Fig. 4 Antibody profile from serum 'b' fractionated on an affinity column. The non-bound peak contained antibody eluted with PBS that did not bind to PDC-E2, and the bound peak contained antibody that did bind to PDC-E2. Fractions were diluted 1:400 and were tested by ELISA on recombinant PDC-E2 (solid line) and on OGDC (dotted line). Antibody that reacted with PDC-E2 was not detected in the non-bound peak after separation

dria were separated under reducing conditions on 10% or 12.5% resolving gels and proteins were electrotransferred to nitrocellulose. Sera were tested at 1:1000 dilution. Peroxidase-coupled affinity-purified anti-human IgG (Silenus) was used as a second antibody, and 4-chloro-naphthol solution (Sigma) as peroxidase substrate.

Affinity separation of antibody populations in serum

Antibody populations were purified using Sepharose CL-4B affinity columns coupled with recombinant PDC-E2[37]; 50 μl of serum was diluted 1:10 in phosphate buffered salin (PBS), and applied to the column. Non-bound protein was eluted with PBS and the first 10 ml was collected in 1 ml fractions, representing the non-bound (NB) peak. After extensive washing, the antibodies bound to the column were eluted using 0.58% acetic acid in 0.15 mol/l NaCl, pH 3.0, as 10 fractions of 0.5 ml representing the bound (B) peak.

Each of the 10 fractions from the two peaks from the column was tested for antibodies to recombinant PDC-E2 by ELISA at a dilution of 1:400.

RESULTS

Separation of each serum on the affinity column gave two fractions (Fig. 4). Antibodies that reacted with PDC-E2, the 74 kDa antigen, by immunoblotting, bound to the column, and were eluted at low pH. Antibodies that were

Table 1 Reactivities of affinity-purified fractions of PBC sera that contained an anti-mitochondrial and antinuclear reactivity

Serum	*Fraction*	*ELISA titre (PDC-E2)*	*Immunofluorescence*	
			Anti-M2	*Other*
'a'	Whole serum	10 000	+ + + +	anti-centromere
	NB	—	—	anti-centromere
	B	1 600	+ + +	—
'b'	Whole serum	1 000 000	+ + + +	anti-Sp-100
	NB[a]	—	+ +[b]	anti-Sp-100
	B	250 000	+ + + +	—

[a]After two absorptions with PDC-E2 (see Fig. 4)
[b]Serum 'b' contained antibodies by immunoblotting that reacted with branched chain OADC-E2 (55 kDa), and oxoglutaric DC-E2 (48 kDa) as well as with PDC-E2 (74 kDa); these additional anti-M2 reactivities were not removed by PDC-E2 affinity purification, and hence the non-bound fractions from serum 'b' also showed antimitochondrial antibodies by immunofluorescence

unreactive with PDC-E2, and all other serum proteins, were washed through the column with PBS.

Affinity separation of anti-PDC-E2 and anti-centromere

For serum 'a', after separation on the column, the bound fractions contained antibodies to PDC-E2 by ELISA, but there were no detectable antibodies to PDC-E2 in the non-bound peak (Fig. 4). Moreover, the antibody that bound to the column showed by immunofluorescence strong antimitochondrial reactivity, but no nuclear reactivity. By contrast, the protein that did not bind to the column gave clear anti-centromere reactivity, but no antimitochondrial reactivity (Table 1).

Affinity separation of anti-PDC-E2 and anti-Sp-100

For serum 'b', after separation on the column, the bound fractions, but not the unbound fractions, contained antibodies to PDC-E2 by ELISA. The antibody that bound to the column showed by immunofluorescence strong antimitochondrial reactivity but no nuclear reactivity. The fractions that did not bind to the column gave the pattern of nuclear dots characteristic of reactivity with Sp-100 (Table 1). A montage with results of affinity purification on PDC-E2 (this study) and on recombinant Sp-100 (from Szostecki *et al.*[21]) is shown in Fig. 5.

DISCUSSION

The classification of autoimmune diseases into 'organ-specific' and 'multi-system' has practical utility. However, there are in limbo a group of paradoxical autoimmune diseases, notably PBC, Sjögren's syndrome and

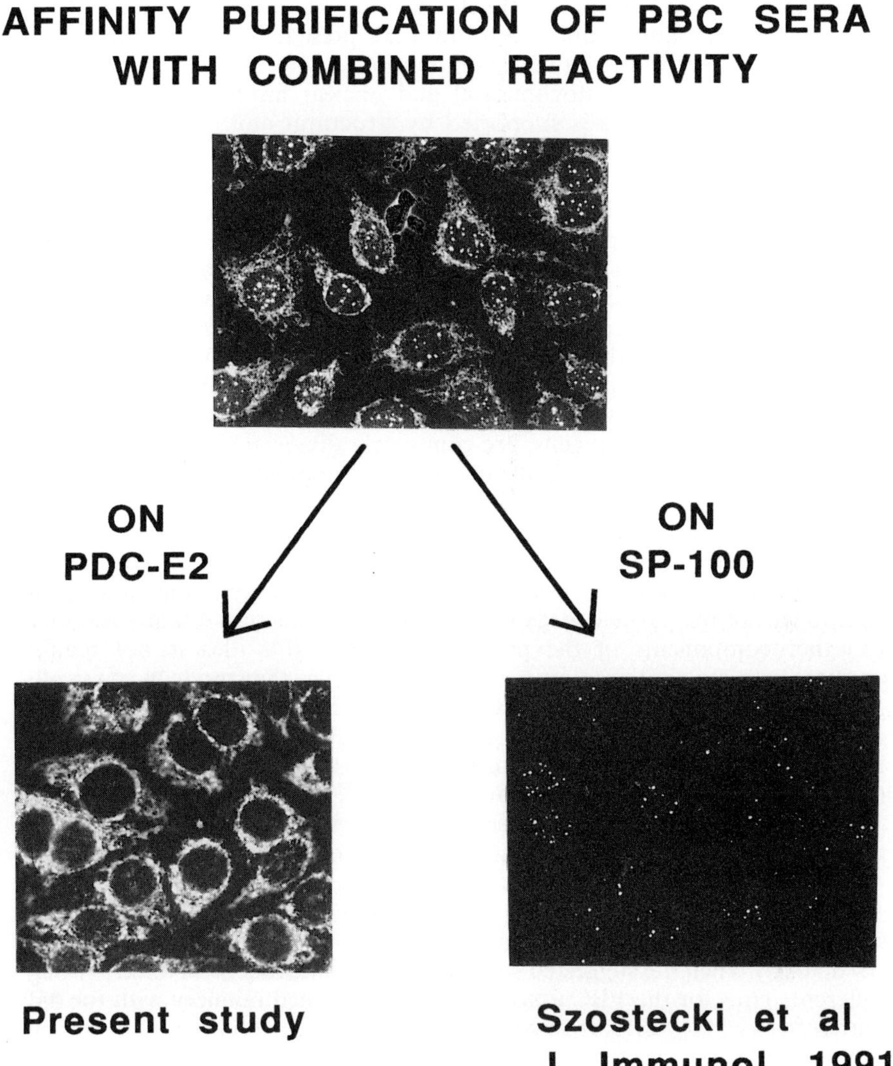

Fig. 5 Montage illustrating reactivity by immunofluorescence of PBC sera with autoantibodies to mitochondria and Sp-100 before (top), and after affinity purification either on recombinant PDC-E2 or recombinant Sp-100. The affinity purified fractions had monospecific reactivity with mitochondria (bottom left) or Sp-100 (bottom right). (Data and illustrations for Sp-100 kindly provided by Dr. Carin Szostecki)

polymyositis among others, in which an organ-specific focus is accompanied by 'multisystem'-type autoantibodies to non-organ-specific antigens. This paradox, which in the case of PBC is amplified by coexisting sets of 'multisystem'type autoantibodies to antigens present in tissues throughout the body, has received less than due attention.

The likelihood that mitochondrial and nuclear antibodies in PBC are independent populations is supported by structural molecular evidence. A cloned cDNA has been derived for the major mitochondrial reactant in PBC, PDC-E2[1], and also for two of the three major nuclear reactants, the centromeric antigen CENP[39] and the Sp-100[21] antigen. The deduced amino acid sequences of these proteins lack any sites of homology, and this negates the likelihood of crossreactivity although, since epitopes for antibodies including autoantibodies are often conformational structures, there could still be homology on a conformational rather than a sequential basis. However, the data on the lack of crossreactivity of autoantibodies in PBC, in previous and the present studies using affinity purification procedures, appear conclusive. Thus reactivities to mitochondrial PDC-E2, and either centromere or Sp-100 antigens, are completely dissociated.

The existence of independent autoantibody populations, in multisystem autoimmune disease in general and PBC in particular, raises interesting questions. Tan *et al.*[40] combined the concepts of an antigen-driven response and an autoimmunogenic capacity of an entire subcellular particle, to account for a diversity of antibody specificities. Possibly reactivity to one 'dominant' component of the particle leads to recruitment of the autoimmune response to other components of the particle. However, this idea is not readily applicable to reactivities to autoantigenic molecules that reside in physically separate compartments of the cell. As another possible explanation for multiple autoimmune specificities, new reactivities could arise through idiotypic network interactions as recently proposed for autoantibody profiles ('parallel sets') in SLE in mice[41] and humans[42].

The availability of a structural sequence for an autoantigenic protein from a cDNA allows for an examination for homology, i.e. mimicry with other proteins including those of microorganisms, to explain an immune response to the self-protein. However, the existence of independent sets of autoantibodies puts some strain on simple versions of the mimicry hypothesis, particularly when the suggested sources of the mimicking proteins are widely different. Thus for the PBC autoantigens, the claimed mimicry with the M2 autoantigens involves corresponding enzymes of bacterial species. On the other hand, the suggested mimicries for the nuclear Sp-100 include two sets of proteins of quite different provenance, one set being the transcriptional regulatory proteins encoded in the 3′-long terminal repeat region of certain viruses, and the transactivator E1A protein of human adenovirus 5, and the other included in the amino acid sequence 76–116 of MHC class 1 molecules of humans and various animals[21]. The existence was postulated of a (retro)virus in PBC patients 'expressing a transcription factor to which antibodies are produced which crossreact with the Sp-100 host protein'[21]. How this might be aligned with the coexistence of mitochondrial antibodies to PDC-E2 is problematical.

It is our preference in autoimmune disease to nominate host proteins themselves as the immunogens as well as the reactants. This concept requires that the immune repertoire would include a capacity on the part of T and B cells to recognize critical (auto)epitopes on particular intracellular molecules, with the assumption that such T and B cells would not have undergone deletion in the thymus (T cells) or the bone marrow (B cells). However, these autoantigenic epitopes would seldom be engaged, by reason of their intracellular location and the existence of a peripheral tolerogenic process(es). Exceptionally, however, in states in which there is release of tissue proteins in the course of inflammatory damage, together with disruption of peripheral tolerance by reason, say, of excessive helper influences (IL-2, etc.), a potential would exist for various anti-self reactivities to develop. As evidence for a genetic contribution to a defect of tolerance, there are reports on the occurrence in excess of autoantibodies of varying specificities in relatives of patients with autoimmune diseases including PBC[36].

Finally we are still far from understanding what provides the major tissue focus for spontaneously occurring autoimmune diseases in humans. Experimentally, the focus for expression of autoimmune disease is provided either by incorporating a tissue-specific autoantigen within a potent adjuvant, or directing a potential 'autoantigen' to a particular tissue by transgenic technology. However, it is uncertain to what degree such procedures represent true models for autoimmunity in humans. Perhaps the tissue focus is provided initially by what would otherwise be an irrelevant episode of cellular injury but, in genetically predisposed individuals, there occurs *in situ* an uncontrolled immune response to those autoantigens for which there has been an escape from deletional and/or peripheral tolerance. In addition, autoimmune responses may require an increase in cell-surface expression of intracellular autoantigens for which there is evidence in PBC[43], but again the existence of multiple reactive intracellular autoantigens challenges this interpretation. Thus the questions posed by the coexisting mitochondrial and nuclear reactivity in PBC are clearly fundamental to the complete understanding of autoimmunity in general.

References

1. Gershwin ME, Mackay IR. Primary biliary cirrhosis: paradigm or paradox for autoimmunity. Gastroenterology. 1990;100:822–33.
2. Berg PA, Klein R. Autoantibody patterns in primary biliary cirrhosis. In: Krawitt EL, Wiesner RH, editors. Autoimmune liver diseases. New York, Raven Press; 1991:123–42.
3. Crowe JP, Christensen E, Butler J. Primary biliary cirrhosis: the prevalence of hypothyroidism and its relation to thyroid antibodies and sicca syndrome. Gastroenterology. 1980;78:1437–41.
4. Elta GH, Sepersky RA, Bodberg MJ, Connors CM, Miller KB, Kaplan MM. Increased incidence of hypothyroidism in primary biliary cirrhosis. Dig Dis Sci. 1983;28:971–5.
5. Reynolds TB, Denison EK, Frankel HD, Liebermann FL, Peter RL. New syndrome combination of primary biliary cirrhosis, scleroderma, and hereditary hemorrhagic telangiectasia. Gastroenterology. 1970;58:290 (abstract).
6. Reynolds TB, Denison EK, Frankl HD, Lieberman FL, Peters RL. Primary biliary cirrhosis with scleroderma, Raynaud's phenomenon and telangiectasia. Am J Med. 1971;50:302–12.
7. Murray-Lyon IM, Thompson RPH, Ansell ID, Williams R. Scleroderma and primary biliary cirrhosis. Br Med J. 1970;3:258–9.

8. Klatskin G, Kantor FS. Mitochondrial antibody in primary biliary cirrhosis and other diseases. Ann Intern Med. 1972;77:533–41.
9. Sherlock S, Scheuer PJ. The presentation and diagnosis of 100 patients with primary biliary cirrhosis. N Engl J Med. 1973;289:674–8.
10. Clark AK, Galbraith RM, Hamilton EBD, Williams R. Rheumatic disorders in primary biliary cirrhosis. Ann Rheum Dis. 1978;37:42–7.
11. Bernstein RM, Callender ME, Neuberger JM *et al.* Anticentromere antibody in primary biliary cirrhosis. Ann Rheum Dis. 1982;41:612–14.
12. Powell FC, Schroeter AL, Dickson ER. Primary biliary cirrhosis and the CREST syndrome: a report of 22 cases. Q J Med. 1987;62:75–82.
13. Moroi Y, Peebles C, Fritzler MJ *et al.* Autoantibody to centromere (kinetochore) in scleroderma sera. Proc Natl Acad Sci USA. 1980;77:1627–31.
15. Makinen D, Fritzler M, David P, Sherlock S. Anticentromere antibodies in primary biliary cirrhosis. Arthritis Rheum. 1983;26:914–17.
16. Fregeau D, Leung PSC, Coppel RL *et al.* Autoantibodies to mitochondria in systemic sclerosis: frequency and characterization using recombinant cloned autoantigen. Arthritis Rheum. 1988;31:386–92.
17. McHugh NJ, James IE, Fairburn K, Maddison PJ. Antibodies to mitochondrial and centromere antigens in primary biliary cirrhosis and systemic sclerosis. Clin Exp Immunol. 1990;81:244–9.
18. Bernstein RM, Neuberger JM, Bunn CC *et al.* Diversity of autoantibodies in primary biliary cirrhosis and chronic active hepatitis. Clin Exp Immunol. 1984;55:553–60.
19. Szoztecki C, Krippner H, Penner E, Bautz FA. Autoimmune sera recognize a 100 kDa nuclear protein antigen (SP-100). Clin Exp Immunol. 1987;68:108–16.
20. Fusconi M, Cassani F, Govoni M *et al.* Anti-nuclear antibodies of primary biliary cirrhosis recognize 78-92 kD and 96-100 kD proteins of nuclear bodies. Clin Exp Immunol. 1991;83:291–7.
21. Szostecki C, Guldner HH, Netter HJ, Will H. Isolation and characterization of cDNA encoding a human nuclear antigen predominantly recognized by autoantibodies from patients with primary biliary cirrhosis. J Immunol. 1990;145:4338–47.
22. Evans J, Reuben A, Craft J. (1991) PBC 95K, A 95-kilodalton nuclear autoantigen in primary biliary cirrhosis. Arthritis Rheum. 1991;34:731–6.
23. Ruffatti A, Arslan P, Floreani A *et al.* Nuclear membrane-staining antinuclear antibody in patients with primary biliary cirrhosis. J Clin Immunol. 1985;5:357–61.
24. Lozano F, Pares A, Borche L *et al.* Autoantibodies against nuclear envelope-associated proteins in primary biliary cirrhosis. Hepatology. 1988;8:930–8.
25. Lassoued K, Brenard R, Degos F *et al.* Antinuclear antibodies directed to a 200-kilodalton polypeptide of the nuclear envelope in primary biliary cirrhosis. A clinical and immunological study of a series of 150 patients with primary biliary cirrhosis. Gastroenterology. 1990;99: 181–6.
26. Newport JW, Forbes DJ. The nucleus: structure, function, and dynamics. Ann Rev Biochem. 1987;56:335–65.
27. Gerace L, Burke B. Functional organization of the nuclear envelope. Ann Rev Cell Biol. 1988;4:335–74.
28. Senecal J-L, Raymond Y. Autoantibodies to DNA, lamins, and pore complex proteins produce distinct peripheral fluorescent antinuclear antibody patterns on the HEp-2 substrate. Arthritis Rheum. 1991;34:249–51.
29. Raymond Y, Gagnon R. Lamin B shares a number of distinct epitopes with lamins A and C and with intermediate filament proteins. Biochemistry. 1988;27:2590–7.
30. Tan EM. Autoantibodies to nuclear lamins. Ann Intern Med. 1988;108:897–8.
31. Lassoued K, Guilly M-N, Danon F *et al.* Antinuclear autoantibodies specific for lamins. Characterization and clinical significance. Ann Intern Med. 1988;108:829–33.
32. Wesierska-Gadek J, Penner E, Hitchman E, Sauermann G. Antibodies to nuclear lamins in autoimmune liver disease. Clin Immunol Immunopathol. 1988;49:107–15.
33. Lassoued K, Guilly MN, Andre C *et al.* Autoantibodies to 200 kD polypeptide(s) of the nuclear envelope: a new serologic marker of primary biliary cirrhosis. Clin Exp Immunol. 1988;74:283–8.
34. Courvalin J-C, Lassoued K, Bartnik E *et al.* The 210 kD nuclear envelope polypeptide

recognized by human autoantibodies in primary biliary cirrhosis. J Clin Invest. 1990;86: 279–88.

35. Senecal J-L, Raymond Y. Autoantibodies to DNA, lamins and pore proteins produce distinct peripheral fluorescent antinuclear antibody patterns on the HEp-2 substrate. Arthritis Rheum. 1991;34:249–51.
36. Mackay IR. Autoimmune diseases of the liver: chronic active hepatitis and primary biliary cirrhosis. In: Rose NR, Mackay IR, editors. The autoimmune diseases. Orlando: Academic Press, 1985:291–337.
37. Rowley MJ, McNeilage LJ, Armstrong JMcD, Mackay IR. Inhibitory autoantibody to a conformational epitope of the pyruvate dehydrogenase complex, the major autoantigen in primary biliary cirrhosis. Clin Immunol Immunopathol. 1991;60:356–70.
38. Coppel RL, McNeilage LJ, Suhr CD *et al.* Primary structure of the human M2 mitochondrial autoantigen of primary biliary cirrhosis: Dihydrolipoamide acetyltransferase. Proc Natl Acad Sci USA. 1988;85:7317–21.
39. Earnshaw WC, Sullivan KF, Macklin PS *et al.* Molecular cloning of a cDNA for CENP-B, the major human centromere autoantigen. J Cell Biol. 1987;104:817–29.
40. Tan EM, Chan EKL, Sullivan KF, Rubin RL. Antinuclear antibodies (ANAs): diagnostically specific immune markers and clues towards the understanding of autoimmunity. Clin Immunol Immunopathol. 1988;47:121–41.
41. Migliorini P, Ardman B, Kaburaki J, Schwartz RS. Parallel sets of autoantibodies in MRL-*lpr*/*lpr* mice. An anti-DNA, anti-SmRNP, anti-gp70 network. J Exp Med. 1987;165:483–99.
42. Talal N, Garry RF, Schur PH *et al.* A conserved idiotype and antibodies to retroviral proteins in systemic lupus erythematosus. J Clin Invest. 1990;85:1866–71.
43. Joplin R, Lindsay JG, Hubscher SG *et al.* Distribution of dihydrolipoamide acetyltransferase (E2) in the liver and portal lymph nodes of patient with primary biliary cirrhosis: an immunohistological study. Hepatology. 1991;14:442–7.

44
Animal models of primary biliary cirrhosis

D. L. THIELE and F. H. WILLIAMS

INTRODUCTION

A variety of approaches have been taken towards establishing animal models of primary biliary cirrhosis (PBC). A number of investigators have attempted to reproduce PBC-like disease in animals by generating immune responses to bile duct cell membrane antigens or more recently to recombinant mitochondrial antigens[1–3]. While there has been at least one report of PBC-like bile duct lesions following immunization of rabbits with antigenic preparations from bovine gallbladder mucous membranes[1], no apparent follow-up information regarding the reproducibility or utility of this model in exploring mechanisms of PBC has appeared in the literature. More recently, following the characterization and cloning of cDNA encoding the mitochondrial antigens recognized by the characteristic antimitochondrial antibodies present in human PBC, multiple animal species have been immunized with these antigens[3]. While antimitochondrial antibodies were readily produced, histological evidence of PBC-like non-suppurative cholangitis was not observed[3]. Of interest, transfer of peripheral blood lymphocytes from humans with PBC to severe combined immunodeficient (SCID) mice has been associated with production of both antimitochondrial antibodies and bile duct lesions typical of PBC[4]. However, similar, albeit less severe, biliary lesions were noted in SCID mouse recipients of normal human peripheral blood lymphocytes, suggesting that xenogeneic graft versus host disease (GVHD) might have contributed to generation of the cellular characteristics of PBC present in these mice[4].

The histological similarity of hepatic GVHD and PBC has been noted frequently[5–12]. Of interest, not only is hepatic GVHD characterized by histological features of non-suppurative cholangitis such as lymphocytic infiltration of bile duct epithelia, segmental necrosis of biliary epithelial cells and destruction of interlobular ducts that are typical of the pathological lesions of PBC[5–12], but both diseases are associated in some cases with similar salivary gland and scleroderma-like skin lesions[5,6,8]. For these

Table 1 MHC and non-MHC alleles of mouse strains used in the current studies

Strains	*Alleles at H-2 region*				*Non-MHC differences relative to B6?*
	K	*I-A*	*I-E*	*D*	
C57BL/6J (B6)	b	b	—	b	No
bm1 × B6 F1	bm1/b	b	—	b	No
B6 × bm12 F1	b	bm12/b	—	b	No
bm1 × bm12 F1	bm1/b	bm12/b	—	b	No
Balb.B × B6 F1	b	b	—	b	Yes
Balb.B × bm12 F1	b	bm12/b	—	b	Yes

reasons GVHD has been proposed as a useful model for examining immune mechanisms responsible for generating PBC-like non-suppurative cholangitis[8]. Our laboratory has utilized a murine model of GVHD to explore the role of different T effector mechanisms in generation of various aspects of GVHD[13–17]. As part of these studies we have examined the role of MHC encoded and multiple non-MHC encoded antigenic differences in eliciting immune responses leading to destructive non-suppurative cholangitis, and have sought to determine the role of individual T effector cell populations in mediating such pathological changes.

MATERIALS AND METHODS

Mice

C57BL/6J (B6) and B6.C-H-2^{bm1} (bm1) mice were purchased from the Jackson Laboratory, Bar Harbor, ME, and B6.C-H-2^{bm12} (bm12), and Balb.B mice were obtained from Dr James Forman, University of Texas Southwestern Medical Centre at Dallas, Dallas, TX. B6 × bm12 F1, bm1 × B6 F1, bm1 × bm12 F1, Balb.B × bm12 F1 and Balb.B × B6 F1 mice were produced in our animal colony. The MHC and non-MHC differences of the recipient strains relative to the donor B6 mice are shown in Table 1.

Reagents

Anti-Thy1.2 (HO-13-4), anti-L3T4 (GK1.5, 2B6), anti-Lyt2 (3.155) and anti-Lyt2.2 (HO-2.2) were culture supernatants or ascitic fluid produced from hybridoma cells obtained from the American Type Culture Collection, Rockville, MD (HO-13-4, GK1.5, 3.155, HO-2.2,18–21) or from Dr Ethan Shevach (2B6,22). L-Leucyl-L-leucine methyl ester (Leu–Leu–OMe) was synthesized from leucyl–leucine (Sigma Chemical Co., St Louis, MO) as previously described[23].

Cell preparation

Suspensions of bone marrow cells (BMC) and spleen cells (SpC) were prepared as previously detailed[14,16]. To remove Thy1$^+$, CD4$^+$ or CD8$^+$ cells, BMC or SpC were suspended at a concentration of 40×10^6 in HBSS supplemented with 25 mmol/l Hepes, 10^{-4} mol/l 2-mercaptoethanol and 0.3% bovine serum albumin (Sigma). Appropriate concentrations of anti-Thy 1.2 (HO-13-4), anti-CD4 (GK1.5, 2B6) or anti-CD8 (HO-2.2,3.155) mAb were added and the cells were incubated at 4°C for 30 min. Rabbit C (1:8 Pel Freez, Rogers, AR) previously absorbed with mouse spleen cells was added, and the cell suspension was incubated at 37°C for 50 min. The cells were then filtered through sterile nylon mesh and washed with HBSS. For removal of Leu–Leu–OMe sensitive CTL and natural killer (NK) cells[17], BMC or SpC were suspended in pH 7.4 phosphate buffered saline and incubated for 15 min at room temperature with 250 μmol/l Leu–Leu–OMe. Cells were then washed with a 4-fold excess volume of HBSS. BMC were treated with anti-Thy 1.2 and C and Leu–Leu–OMe such that the bone marrow provided a source of T and NK depleted stem cells.

Transplantation

In all experiments, 6–10-week-old male B6 mice were used as a source of donor cells. Groups of three to 10 male recipient mice (age 6–10 weeks) were maintained on acidified (pH 2), antibiotic (neomycin, 100 mg/l and polymyxin B, 10 mg/ml) water for 2–3 days prior to transplantation and 10 days after transplantation. On the day of transplantation all recipient mice were irradiated (600 cGy) and then infused intravenously via the lateral tail vein with 5×10^6 anti-Thy1 + C and Leu–Leu–OMe treated BMC and varying numbers of B6 SpC or cells.

Histology

At 2–8 weeks after transplantation the mice were sacrificed. A portion of the liver was removed, fixed in 10% phosphate buffered formalin, embedded in paraffin and four or five μm sections were stained with haematoxylin and eosin and Masson's trichrome stain. Twenty portal tracts in each liver were examined by light microscopy in a blinded fashion, and the extent of mononuclear cell infiltrate in each portal tract was graded semi-quantitatively (0–4+). For each mouse, a weighted inflammation score was determined from the formula: weighted inflammation score = Σ inflammation scores of individual portal tracts/total number of tracts examined. In addition, each portal tract was scored for the presence or absence of lymphocytic invasion or destruction of the bile duct wall. Lymphocytic invasion of the bile duct was defined as the presence of one or more lymphocytes between adjoining bile duct epithelial cells. Destructive bile duct lesions were defined as either a loss of continuity of the bile duct wall or frank obliteration of the duct. Results are represented as the mean of values obtained from examination of

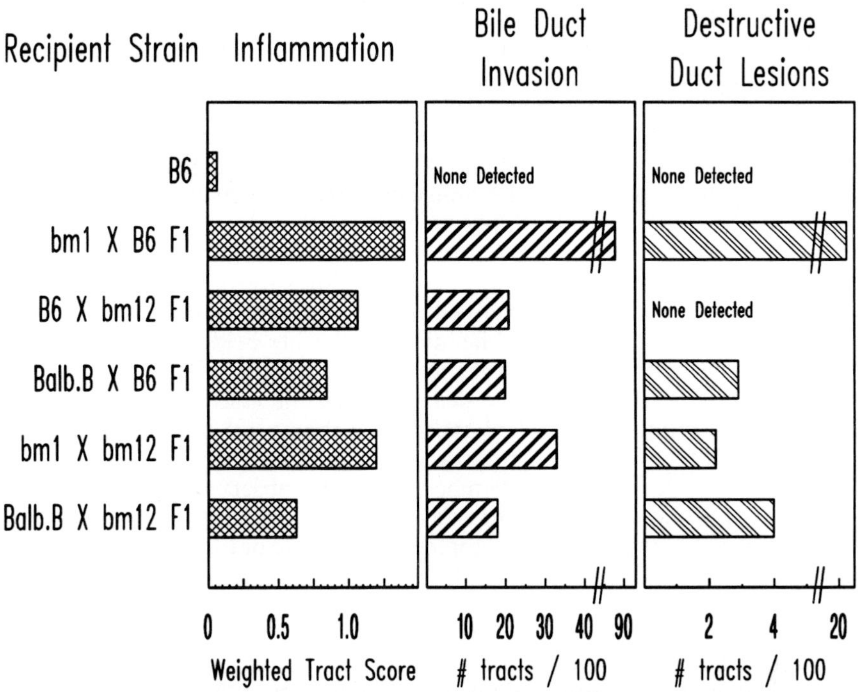

Fig. 1 Non-suppurative cholangitis develops after transfer of B6 donor cells to class I MHC disparate, class II MHC disparate or multiple non-MHC encoded antigen disparate F1 recipients. Results are given for histological evaluation of livers sacrificed 3 weeks after transfer of 5×10^6 T and NK-depleted B6 bone marrow and 10^7 B6 spleen cells

60–200 portal tracts in livers from three to 10 animals included in each experimental group.

RESULTS

In initial studies, livers from recipients of 10^7 control B6 SpC and 5×10^6 T and NK depleted B6 BMC were examined 14–21 days after transplantation for evidence of non-suppurative cholangitis. Irradiated B6 recipients of syngeneic B6 SpC and BMC were found to have minimal portal tract inflammation (see Fig. 1). In contrast, non-suppurative cholangitis was seen following transfer of B6 donor SpC to irradiated class I MHC disparate, class II MHC disparate, or multiple non-MHC disparate F1 recipient mice. To facilitate comparison of severity of GVHD lesions in different strain combinations, 20 portal tracts within liver sections from each of multiple animals in each experimental group were semi-quantitatively graded in a blinded fashion for extent of mononuclear cell infiltrate, and a weighted inflammation score was calculated as detailed in the methods section. In addition, each portal tract was evaluated for evidence of lymphocytic invasion of the bile duct wall and for destruction or degeneration of bile duct epithelium. As summarized in Fig. 1, in all allogeneic strain combinations examined, the weighted inflammation score was significantly higher than that seen in the syngeneic controls. Moreover, in addition to portal tract inflammation, frank lymphocytic invasion of the bile duct wall was observed in all F1 recipients of B6 donor cells. A very high percentage of portal tracts of livers of B6 → bm1 × B6 F1 mice displayed evidence of invasive or destructive bile duct lesions, while such lesions were observed less frequently in portal tracts of Balb.B × B6 F1, Balb.B × bm12 F1 and bm1 × bm12 F1 recipient mice. Of note, while portal tracts within livers of B6 × bm12 F1 recipients of B6 donor SpC contained readily apparent periportal infiltrates and lymphocytic invasion of bile duct walls, no evidence of bile duct epithelium cell destruction or degeneration was noted.

Multiple previous studies have demonstrated the essential role of donor T cells in generating GVHD[24–26] and during the course of previous studies of murine GVHD elicited in response to class I + II MHC and multiple non-MHC encoded antigen differences we have observed that pan-T cell depletion of donor inocula with anti-Thy1 + C or anti-CD4 and anti-CD8 + C treatment prevents development of hepatic or other organ manifestations of GVHD[16]. Concurrent with the studies detailed in Fig. 1, additional F1 recipient mice were infused with varying numbers of B6 donor SpC depleted of Leu–Leu–OMe sensitive CTL[14] or of $CD4^+$ or $CD8^+$ T cells, and liver pathology was evaluated at varying time points after transplantation. As detailed in Figs 2 and 3, depletion of Leu–Leu–OMe sensitive donor CTL resulted in a significant reduction in class I MHC disparate, bm1 × B6 F1 recipients (Fig. 2) or multiple non-MHC disparate Balb.B × B6 F1 mice (Fig. 3) examined 21 days after transplantation. The lesions produced by Leu–Leu–OMe resistant effector cells in bm1 × B6 F1 recipients were self-limited in that minimal infiltration or bile duct invasion was seen 42 days after transplantation. As infusion of 10^7 control B6 donor cells into bm1 × B6 F1 recipients resulted in 100% mortality by day 24, the temporal course of non-suppurative cholangitis induced by control donor cells could not be evaluated.

In contrast to the course of GVHD in B6 → bm1 × B6 F1 mice, when Balb.B × B6 F1 recipients of 10^7 Leu–Leu–OMe treated B6 spleen cells were examined at later times after transplantation, delayed onset of non-suppurative cholangitis was observed. Thus, as detailed in Fig. 4, by day 40 the extent of portal tract inflammatory infiltrates in these mice had evolved to a level approximately equal to that seen at day 21 in animals receiving control spleen cells. The frequency of destructive duct lesions observed at day 40 in livers of Balb.B × B6 F1 recipients of Leu–Leu–OMe treated B6 donor cells actually exceeded that seen at any time point in recipients of control donor cells. Thus Leu–Leu–OMe treated donor cells were found to generate a delayed cholangitic response that was as extensive as that observed at earlier time points following transfer of control cells. In additional studies it was noted that when the B6 donor spleen cell inoculum was increased to 3×10^7 cells per recipient Balb.B × B6 F1 mouse, biliary lesions induced by Leu–Leu–OMe resistant donor cells were apparent at earlier time points.

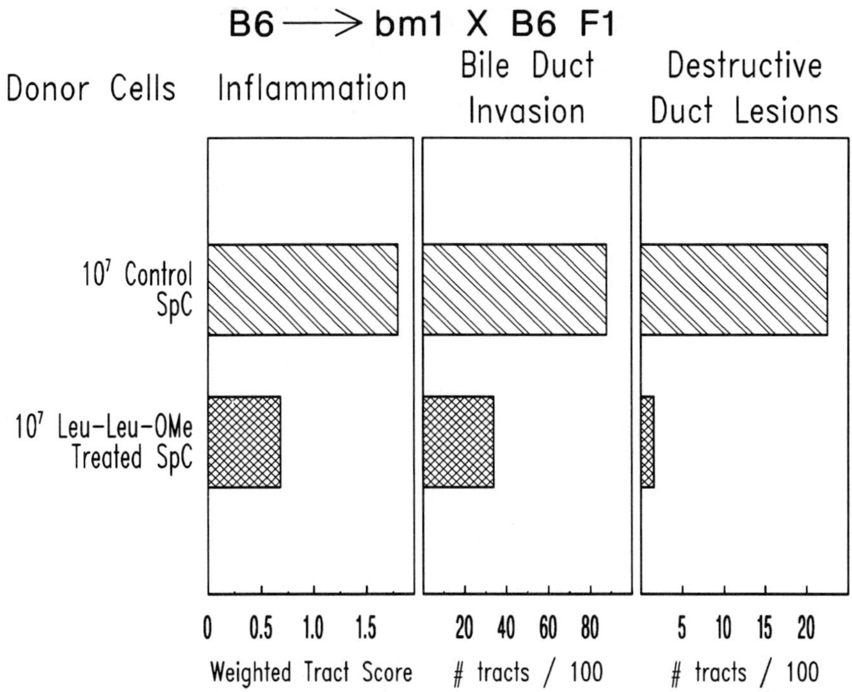

Fig. 2 Depletion of Leu–Leu–OMe sensitive cytotoxic donor lymphocytes significantly decreases the severity of non-suppurative cholangitis generated in class I MHC disparate bm1 × B6 F1 recipients

As detailed in Fig. 5, treatment of B6 spleen cells with anti-CD4 + C resulted in a marked reduction in the weighted inflammation score and the level of bile duct invasion or destruction. However, anti-CD8 + C did not decrease the degree of biliary disease. In fact, as demonstrated by the data detailed in Fig. 5, treatment of the B6 donor SpC with anti-CD8 + C or both anti-CD8 + C and Leu–Leu–OMe resulted in increased severity of lesions in the biliary tracts of Balb.B × B6 F1 recipient mice. Thus transfer of Leu–Leu–OMe resistant, $CD4^+$ donor T cells alone was sufficient to generate the full histological spectrum of non-suppurative cholangitis in this strain combination. In additional studies (data not shown), transfer of Leu–Leu–OMe treated, $CD8^-$ B6 donor T cells was found to be sufficient to generate destructive cholangitis in class I + II MHC disparate bm1 × bm12 F1 mice.

DISCUSSION

The present studies were designed to examine directly the role of different classes of alloantigens and different effector T cell subsets in the evolution of non-suppurative cholangitis. The results indicate that periportal mononuclear cell infiltrates and lymphocytic bile duct infiltration and/or destruction

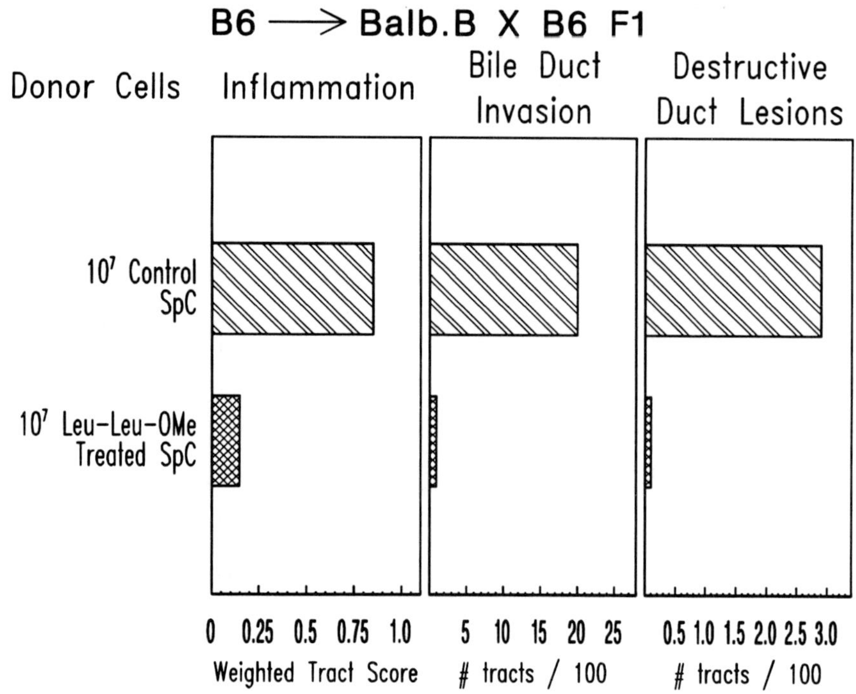

Fig. 3 Depletion of Leu–Leu–OMe sensitive cytotoxic donor lymphocytes significantly decreases the severity of non-suppurative cholangitis generated in multiple non-MHC encoded antigen disparate Balb.B × B6 F1 recipients

typical of the histological lesions previously reported during the course of GVHD, liver allograft rejection or primary biliary cirrhosis can be generated during GVH reactions directed at multiple non-MHC encoded or discrete class I MHC or class II MHC differences. However, lesions associated with frank destruction of the bile duct wall were seen only in strain combinations in which class I MHC or multiple non-MHC encoded allogeneic differences were present. In class II MHC only disparate, B6 × bm12 F1 recipients of B6 donor cells, extensive periportal and bile duct wall lymphocytic infiltrates were noted, but in over 400 bile ducts examined in B6 → B6 × bm12 F1 mice in the course of these studies, frank disruption of bile duct walls was not observed. GVHD directed at class I MHC differences has been shown to be mediated by $CD8^+$ donor T cells while GVHD elicited in response to class II MHC differences has been shown to be mediated by $CD4^+$ T cells[26]. As the present studies demonstrated that transfer of Leu–Leu–OMe sensitive donor CTL was required to elicit the high frequency of destructive duct lesions observed in GVHD directed at class I MHC differences, the absence of such lesions in B6 → B6 × bm12 F1 mice probably relates in part to diminished frequency of cytotoxic effector cells among the $CD4^+$ T cells previously shown to mediate GVHD in this class II MHC disparate strain combination.

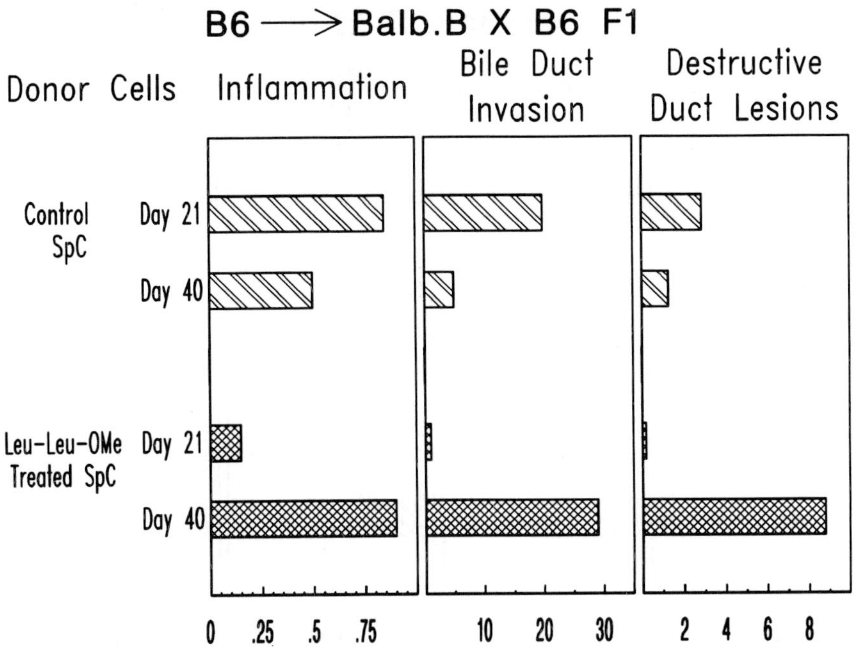

Fig. 4 Time course of non-suppurative cholangitis in Balb.B × B6 F1 recipients of control or Leu–Leu–OMe treated B6 donor cells

However, the total absence of destructive duct lesions in B6 → B6 × bm12 F1 mice does not appear to relate to an absolute inability of $CD4^+$ effector T cells to mediate destructive cholangitis. Thus, in both class I + II MHC disparate bm1 × bm12 F1 and multiple non-MHC antigen disparate Balb.B × B6 F1 recipients of $CD8^+$T cell depleted, $CD4^+$ T cell enriched donor cell populations, destructive cholangitis developed. Leu–Leu–OMe treatment of donor cells also did not prevent generation of destructive cholangitis in the B6 → Balb.B × B6 F1 strain combination, although such treatment delayed the onset of destructive cholangitis generated by smaller numbers of donor cells. Treatment of human or murine lymphoid cells with this agent has been shown to deplete dipeptidyl peptidase I enriched precursors of both $CD4^+$ and $CD8^+$ CTL[14,27–29]. In class I + II MHC and multiple non-MHC disparate murine bone marrow transplant models, Leu–Leu–OMe treatment of donor cells has been shown to be very effective in preventing *in vivo* donor anti-host CTL generation and lethal GVHD[14,15,30]. Thus, the present findings suggest that $CD4^+$ T helper cell responses alone are sufficient to generate destructive cholangitis in the multiple non-MHC antigen disparate B6 → Balb.B × B6 F1 and the class I + II MHC disparate B6 → bm1 × bm12 F1 strain combinations. $CD4^+$ T cells classically respond to antigenic peptides presented in the context of class II MHC molecules[31]. The results of the present studies therefore suggest that peptide fragments of class I MHC or non-MHC encoded alloantigens presented by self class II MHC molecules (I–A^b in the present studies) expressed on the surface of

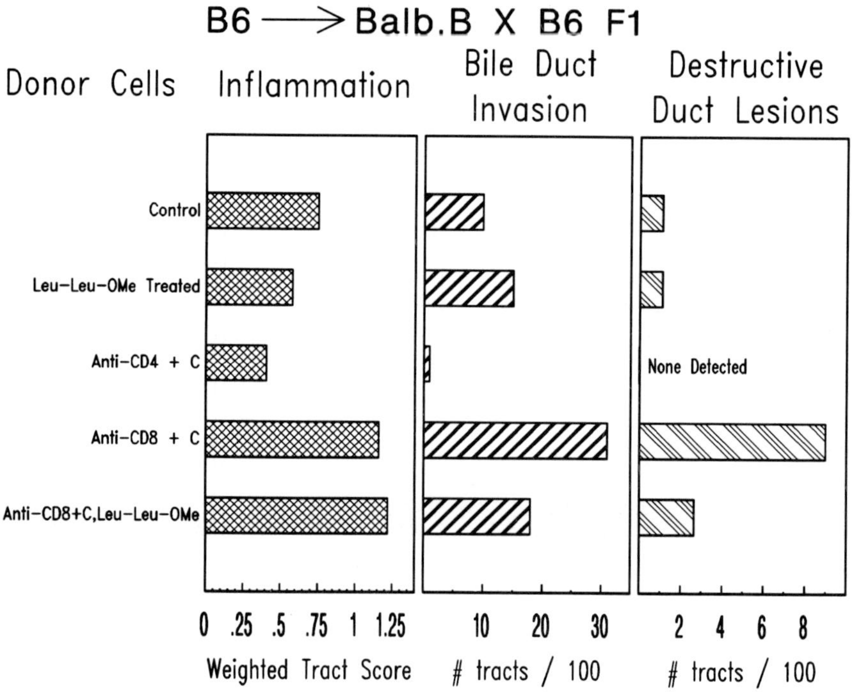

Fig. 5 Transfer of Leu–Leu–OMe resistant, CD8$^-$ B6 donor T cells is sufficient to generate destructive cholangitis in Balb.B × B6 F1 mice

bile duct epithelial cells might be responsible for eliciting immune responses leading to the lesions of non-suppurative cholangitis in bm1 × bm12 F1 or Balb.B × B6 F1 recipients of B6 CD4$^+$ donor T cells.

A variety of previous findings also suggest that class II MHC restricted CD4$^+$ T cells play a major role in development of destructive non-suppurative cholangitis during GVHD or liver allograft rejection. Such observations have included the observed expression of class II MHC antigens on the surface of normally class II MHC antigen negative biliary epithelial cells in temporal association with development of non-suppurative cholangitis and a predominance of CD4$^+$ T cells in cholangitic lesions present in a variety of GVHD or liver transplant models[32–36]. Aberrant expression of class II MHC antigens has also been noted on bile duct epithelial cells during the course of PBC[37,38]. However as allogeneic class II MHC molecules expressing self or allogeneic peptides can also directly elicit CD4$^+$ T cell responses[26], the presence of lymphocytic bile duct infiltration, but not frank bile duct destruction, in the class II MHC disparate B6 → B6 × bm12 F1 strain combination employed in these studies is notable. These results suggest that the profile of CD4$^+$ T cytokine or other effector mechanisms elicited in direct response to major class II histocompatibility differences may be quite different from that elicited in response to peptide fragments of other classes of alloantigens presented in the context of self class II MHC.

In contrast to the results of the present studies, Saitoh *et al.*[36,39] have reported the development of non-suppurative cholangitis during GVHD in the class II MHC disparate B6 → B6 × bm12 F1 strain combination, but not in B6 → bm1 × B6 F1 or B6 → bm1 × bm12 F1 mice. In such studies, host bone marrow-derived cells were not depleted by pretransplant irradiation. In addition, high levels of autoantibody formation and circulating immune complexes were also documented[39]. Such autoantibody formation during murine GVHD has been observed only in the course of GVH reactions produced in non-irradiated mice in which mixed chimerism persists for prolonged time intervals and appears to be related to a donor $CD4^+$ T cytokine response that drives autoantibody production by host-derived B cells[40]. Preparative irradiation that ablates or greatly reduces host marrow-derived cell lineages and/or the concomitant presence of strong donor $CD8^+$ T cell responses directed at host class I MHC differences has been observed to prevent GVHD-related immune complex-mediated disease and instead lead to different patterns of T cytokine response and more aggressive GVHD with respect to both end-organ damage and survival[40]. In contrast to the studies of Saitoh *et al.*, in which recipients were not irradiated, the present studies utilized a preparative irradiation regimen that has been demonstrated previously to enhance GVH responses elicited by donor T cells and favour establishment of complete chimerism[14,16]. Thus, apparent discrepancies between the results of the studies of Saitoh *et al.* and the present studies may relate to the presence of host-derived B cell autoantibody responses and a relative paucity of donor anti-host cytotoxic T cell responses in the model employed by Saitoh *et al.*

A number of findings in the present studies clearly suggest that T cytotoxic responses play an important and in some cases a principal role in generating destructive bile duct lesions. In the class I MHC disparate B6 → bm1 × B6 F1 strain combination, Leu–Leu–OMe treatment of donor cells significantly decreased periductular and intraductular lymphocytic infiltration and reduced the incidence of destructive bile duct lesions by approximately 90%. Previous studies have noted that *in-vitro* B6 anti-bm1 T cell responses, as well as B6 anti-bm1 GVHD or skin graft rejection responses, appear to be mediated largely by $CD8^+$ responder T cells capable of both T cytokine and T cytotoxic responses[41]. In additional studies (data not shown), we have found that bm1 × B6 F1 recipients of $CD8^+$ T cell-depleted B6 donor cells develop scant liver or other end-organ evidence of GVHD. Thus the results of prior and current studies suggest that Leu–Leu–OMe sensitive $CD8^+$ cytotoxic T cell responses are primarily responsible for the extensive destructive bile duct lesions present in B6 → bm1 × B6 F1 GVHD mice. In Balb.B × B6 F1 recipients of lower numbers of B6 donor cells, Leu–Leu–OMe treatment of donor cells also was associated with dramatic reduction in frequency of destructive cholangitis observed 21 days after transplantation. These findings therefore suggest a major role for Leu–Leu–OMe sensitive cytotoxic T cells in mediating acute destruction of bile duct epithelial cells expressing non-MHC encoded antigenic differences. The complete absence of destructive bile duct lesions in Balb.B × B6 F1 recipients of donor cell inocula depleted of $CD4^+$ T cells raises the possibility that Leu–Leu–OMe sensitive $CD4^+$ cytotoxic T cells may be responsible for acute destructive bile duct lesions in this strain combination, although such findings are also consistent with a requirement for $CD4^+$ T helper cells in generating donor anti-host $CD8^+$ cytotoxic T cell responses.

One of the characteristics of the non-suppurative cholangitis lesions noted in the present and previous studies of hepatic GVHD pathology is the often focal nature of the lesions. Thus portal tracts with extensive lymphocytic infiltration are often found in relatively close proximity to portal tracts with little or no histological abnormality. In the strain combinations in which CTL were found to play a major role in generation of destructive duct lesions in the current studies, such lesions were not infrequently observed in portal tracts with relatively sparse lymphocytic infiltrates. This dichotomy between degree of inflammatory infiltration and presence of apparently immunologically mediated bile duct destruction has also been noted in previous studies of human hepatic GVHD or allograft rejection[6,42]. In contrast, in GVHD mediated by CTL depleted, $CD4^+$ T helper cell-enriched B6 donor cells in bm1 × bm12 F1 or Balb.B × B6 F1 recipient mice, destructive duct lesions were invariably associated with marked periductular lymphocytic infiltrates. In addition, we and other investigators[36,39] have noted the presence of non-caseating epithelioid granulomas in murine GVHD lesions generated by $CD4^+$ T helper cell responses.

The results of these studies demonstrate that generation of destructive non-suppurative cholangitis cannot be simply attributed to either a single immune effector mechanism or to responses directed at a single class of histocompatibility antigens. However, while either cytotoxic T cell or non-cytotoxic T cell effector mechanisms appear capable of mediating destructive cholangitis in livers of mice expressing both class I and class II MHC or multiple non-MHC encoded antigen differences, the GVHD histology generated by $CD4^+$ T helper cell-mediated mechanisms appears to bear the greatest similarity to pathological abnormalities noted during the course of human PBC.

Abbreviations

bm1, B6.C-H-2^{bm1}; bm12, B6.C-H-2^{bm12}; B6, C57BL/6J; BMC, bone marrow cells; BMTx, bone marrow transplantation; CTL, cytotoxic T lymphocyte; GVHD, graft-versus-host disease; Leu–Leu–OMe, leucyl–leucine methyl ester; NK, natural killer cell; SpC, spleen cell.

Acknowledgements

This work was supported by National Institutes of Health grant AI24639.

References

1. Kawai K, Kitagawa H, Highashimori T, Matsui T, Fujiyama S, Monna T, Yamamoto S, Morisawa S. Experimental chronic non-suppurative destructive cholangitis in rabbits

following immunization with bile duct antigen. Gastroenterol Jpn. 1980;15:337–45.
2. Kochar DK, Gupta KD, Jatkar PR, Vyas UK. Primary biliary cirrhosis like lesions following experimental autoimmunization. Ind J Pathol Microbiol. 1982;25:173–4.
3. Krams SM, Surh CD, Coppel RL, Ansari A, Ruebner B, Gershwin ME. Immunization of experimental animals with dihydrolipoamide acetyltransferase, as a purified recombinant polypeptide, generates mitochondrial antibodies but not primary biliary cirrhosis. Hepatology. 1989;9:411–16.
4. Krams SM, Dorshkind K, Gershwin ME. Generation of biliary lesions after transfer of human lymphocytes into severe combined immunodeficient (SCID) mice. J Exp Med. 1989;170:1919–30.
5. Thomas ED, Storb R, Clift RA, Fefer A, Johnson FL, Neiman PE, Lerner KG, Glucksberg H, Buckner CD. Bone-marrow transplantation (second of two parts). N Engl J Med. 1975;202:895–902.
6. Shulman HM, Sullivan KM, Weiden PL, McDonald GB, Striker GE, Sale GE, Hackman R, Tsoi T-S, Storb R, Thomas ED. Chronic graft-versus-host syndrome in man. A long-term clinicopathologic study of 20 Seattle patients. Am J Med. 1980;69:204–17.
7. Vierling JM, Fennel RH Jr. Histopathology of early and late human hepatic allograft rejection: Evidence of progressive destruction of interlobular bile ducts. Hepatology. 1985;5:1076–82.
8. Sherlock S. The syndrome of disappearing intrahepatic bile ducts. Lancet. 1987;2:493–6.
9. Vierling JM, Ruderman WB. Hepatic lesions in murine chronic graft-versus-host disease to minor histocompatibility antigens. A reproducible model of nonsuppurative destructive cholangitis. Transplantation. 1989;48:717–18.
10. Shulman HM, Sharma P, Amos D, Fenster LF, McDonald GB. A coded histologic study of hepatic graft-versus-host disease after human bone marrow transplantation. Hepatology. 1988;8:463–70.
11. Knapp AB, Crawford JM, Rappeport JM, Gollan JL. Cirrhosis as a consequence of graft-versus-host disease. Gastroenterology. 1987;92:513–19.
12. Stechschulte DJ, Jr, Fishback JI, Emami A, Bhatia P. Secondary biliary cirrhosis as a consequence of graft-versus-host disease. Gastroenterology. 1990;98:223–35.
13. Charley M, Thiele DL, Bennett M, Lipsky PE. Prevention of lethal murine graft versus host disease by treatment of donor cells with L-leucyl-L-leucine methyl ester. J Clin Invest. 1986;78:1415–20.
14. Thiele DL, Charley MR, Calomeni A, Lipsky PE. Lethal graft-versus-host disease across major histocompatibility barriers: Requirement for leucyl-leucine methyl ester sensitive cytotoxic T cells. J Immunol. 1987;138:51–7.
15. Thiele DL, Bryde SE, Lipsky PE. Lethal graft-vs-host disease induced by a class II MHC antigen only disparity is not mediated by cytotoxic T cells. J Immunol. 1988;141:3377–82.
16. Thiele DL, Eigenbrodt ML, Bryde SE, Eigenbrodt EH, Lipsky PE. Intestinal graft-versus-host disease is mediated by donor T cells distinct from classic cytotoxic T lymphocytes. J Clin Invest. 1989;84:1947–56.
17. Thiele DL, Lipsky PE. The impact of major histocompatibility complex (MHC) and non-MHC antigenic differences on graft-versus-host disease mediated by helper T cells. In: Transactions of the Association of American Physicians, Vol. CII, pp. 59–67.
18. Marshak-Rothstein A, Fink P, Gridley T, Raulet DH, Bevan MJ, Gefter ML. Properties and applications of monoclonal antibodies directed against determinants of the Thy-1 locus. J Immunol. 1979;122:2491–7.
19. Dialynas DP, Wilde DB, Marrack P, Pierres A, Wall KA, Havran W, Otten G, Loken MR, Pierres M, Kappler J, Fitch FW. Characterization of the murine antigenic determinant, designated L3T4a, recognized by monoclonal antibody GK1.5: expression of L3T4a by functional T cell clones appears to correlate primarily with class II MHC antigen-reactivity. Immunol Rev. 1983;74:29–56.
20. Sarmiento M, Glasebrook AL, Fitch AFW. IgG or IgM monoclonal antibodies reactive with different determinants of the molecular complex bearing Lyt2 antigen block T cell-mediated cytolysis in the absence of complement. J Immunol. 1990;125:2665–72.
21. Raulet DH, Gottlieb PD, Bevan MJ. Fractionation of lymphocyte populations with monoclonal antibodies specific for Lyt-2.2 and Lyt-3.1. J Immunol. 1980;125:1136–43.
22. Wassmer P, Chan C, Loegdberg L, Shevach EM. Role of the L3T4-antigen in T cell

activation. II. Inhibition of T cell activation by monoclonal anti-L3T4 antibodies in the absence of accessory cells. J Immunol. 1985;135:2237–42.
23. Thiele DL, Lipsky PE. Regulation of cellular function by products of lysosomal enzyme activity: Elimination of human natural killer cells by a peptide methyl ester generated from L-leucine methyl ester by monocytes or polymorphonuclear leukocytes. Proc Natl Acad Sci USA. 1985;82:2468–72.
24. Korngold R, Sprent J. Lethal graft-versus-host disease after bone marrow transplantation across minor histocompatibility barriers in mice. Prevention by removing mature T cells from marrow. J Exp Med. 1978;148:1687–98.
25. Martin PJ, Hansen JA, Buckner CD, Sanders JE, Deeg HJ, Stewart P, Appelbaum FR, Clift R, Fefer A, Witherspoon RP, Kennedy MS, Sullivan KM, Flournoy N, Storb R, Thomas ED. Effects of *in vitro* depletion of T cells in HLA-identical allogeneic marrow grafts. Blood. 1985;66:664–72.
26. Korngold R, Sprent J. Surface markers of T cells causing lethal graft-vs-host disease to class I vs class II H-2 differences. J Immunol. 1985;135:3004–10.
27. Thiele DL, Lipsky PE. The immunosuppressive activity of L-leucyl-L-leucine methyl ester: selective ablation of cytotoxic lymphocytes and monocytes. J Immunol. 1986;136:1038–48.
28. Thiele DL, Lipsky PE. Mechanism of L-leucyl-L-leucine methyl ester-mediated killing of cytotoxic lymphocytes: dependence on a lysosomal thiol protease dipeptidyl peptidase I, that is enriched in these cells. Proc Natl Acad Sci USA. 1990;87:83–7.
29. Thiele DL, Lipsky PE. The action of leucyl-leucine methyl ester on cyotoxic lymphocytes requires uptake by a novel dipeptide-specific facilitated transport system and dipeptidyl peptidase I-mediated conversion to membranolytic products. J Exp Med. 1990;172:183–94.
30. Thiele DL, Geissler GH, Williams FH, Lipskey PE. The role of leucyl-leucine methyl ester-sensitive cytotoxic cells in skin allograft rejection. Transplantation. 1992;53:1334–40.
31. Brown JH, Jardetzky T, Saper MA, Samraoui B, Bjorkman PJ, Wiley DC. A hypothetical model of the foreign antigen binding site of class II histocompatibility molecules. Nature. 1988;332:845–50.
32. Suitters AJ, Lampert IA. Class II antigen induction in the liver of rats with graft-versus-host disease. Transplantation. 1984;38:194–6.
33. Demetris AJ, Lasky S, van Thiel DH, Starzl TE, Whiteside T. Induction of DR/IA antigens in human liver allografts. An immunocytochemical and clinicopathologic analysis of twenty failed grafts. Transplantation. 1985;40:504–9.
34. Steinhoff G, Wonigeit K, Ringe B, Lauchart W, Kemnitz J, Pichlmayr R. Modified patterns of major histocompatibility complex-antigen expression in human liver grafts during rejection. Transplant Proc. 1987;XIX:2466–9.
35. Hubscher SG, Adams DH, Elias E. Changes in the expression of major histocompatibility complex class II antigens in liver allograft rejection. J Pathol. 1990;162:165–71.
36. Saitoh T, Fujiwara M, Asakura H. L3T4+ T cells induce hepatic lesions resembling primary biliary cirrhosis in mice with graft-versus-host reactions due to major histocompatibility complex class II disparity. Clin Immunol Immunopathol. 1991;59:449–61.
37. Ballardini G, Mirakian R, Bianchi FB. Aberrant expression of HLA-DR antigens on bile duct epithelium in primary biliary cirrhosis: Relevance to pathogenesis. Lancet. 1984;2: 1009–13.
38. Kaplan MM. Primary biliary cirrhosis. Adv Intern Med.1987;32:359–78.
39. Saitoh T, Fujiwara M, Nomoto M, Makino M, Watanabe H, Ishihara K, Kamimura T, Ichida F. Hepatic lesions induced by graft-versus-host reaction across MHC class II antigens: an implication for animal models of primary biliary cirrhosis. Clin Immunol Immunopathol. 1988;49:166–72.
40. Via CS, Shearer GM. T-cell interaction in autoimmunity: insights from a murine model of graft-versus-host disease. Immunol Today. 1988;9:207–13.
41. Sprent J, Schaefer M, Lo D, Korngold R. Properties of purified T cell subsets. II. In vivo responses to class I vs. class II H-2 differences. J Exp Med. 1986;163:998–1011.
42. Wiesner RH, Ludwig J, van Hoek B, Krom RAF. Current concepts in cell-mediated hepatic allograft rejection leading to ductopenia and liver failure. Hepatology. 1991;14:721–9.

45
Disturbed lymphokine production in patients with primary biliary cirrhosis: a functional defect of T lymphocytes?

G. R. PAPE, G. MESSER, U. SPENGLER, M.-C. JUNG and E. H. WEISS

Primary biliary cirrhosis (PBC) is believed to be an autoimmune disease. It is initially characterized by an immunoinflammatory destruction of small to medium-sized bile ducts that result in, and is compounded by, progressive liver fibrosis and cirrhosis. PBC is a systemic disease with numerous immunological abnormalities. Although substantial progress has been made in the identification of the antigens recognized by the disease-specific antimitochondrial antibodies (AMA), the pathogenesis of the disease remains a matter of hypotheses[1-5].

Lymphocytes, particularly T cells, which are the histological hallmark of the early stages of PBC, become an issue of increasing interest in this disease. In addition to the phenotypic identification of the liver tissue-infiltrating lymphocytes, recently available immunological tools offer new prospects for the functional analysis of these cells.

Lymphokine production represents an essential function of activated T lymphocytes. Cytokines (lymphokines) are soluble transmitters which function as an interactive communication network to coordinate the immune response in the development of inflammation and specific immunity. Cytokines are often produced only transiently and at picomolar concentrations in order that the response be limited to a discrete local radius. Recent investigations suggest that local lymphokine production may be necessary for the induction of autoreactive T lymphocytes[6]. Thus, a dysregulated synthesis of cytokines or reception of their signals could contribute to the development of autoimmunity.

Recently, we became interested in the function of T lymphocytes in PBC, particularly in their production of cytokines upon activation, for several reasons:

1. The localization of the tumour necrosis factor (TNF) genes in tandem within the major histocompatibility complex (MHC) on the short arm of chromosome 6[7-10] has raised the suspicion that the TNF loci might play a role in the notable association between HLA and various autoimmune diseases. For example in a mouse model for SLE (systemic lupus erythematosus) nephritis, both a decreased TNF-α production, and a RFLP (restriction fragment length polymorphism) have been correlated with the development of the disease[11]. However, in this disease the linkage of the decreased TNF-α production with a mutation in the TNF-α locus has been questioned, since the presumptive autoimmune TNF-α allele has been found in many mouse strains[12].
2. The aberrant expression of molecules of the MHC class II antigens on biliary epithelial cells may play an important role in the pathogenesis of PBC[13,14]. Pujol-Borrel *et al.* showed that the lymphokine TNF-β in concert with interferon-γ (IFN-γ) could stimulate an aberrant expression of MHC class II antigens on human epithelial (pancreatic) cells[15]. Thus, the analysis of local lymphokine production in liver tissue of patients with PBC may be an important issue to understand the mechanisms involved in bile duct damage.
3. Fugger *et al.* have reported a Nco I RFLP of the TNF region with significant association to patients with PBC[16].

We investigated lymphokine secretion *in vitro* by mitogen-stimulated T lymphocytes from liver biopsies and from peripheral blood of patients with PBC and for comparison of patients with various liver diseases (Fig. 1).

T cell lines were established either from liver tissue or from the peripheral blood. They were left for 10 days without adding fresh feeder cells before the stimulation experiments. Lymphokine production was induced by addition of PHA (for details see legend to Fig. 1). Control experiments without PHA were always run in parallel to check for inadvertent activation of T cells by the medium.

A diminished synthesis of TNF-β, TNF-α and IFN-γ was found both in T cell lines from liver tissue and from peripheral blood. The reduction was most prominent in TNF-β in early histological stages of PBC. The synthesis of this lymphokine was analysed in more detail at the molecular level. In the context of our findings the disturbed TNF-β production in PBC was associated with reduced mRNA levels of this cytokine, when analysed in parallel with the secretion profiles of activated peripheral blood mononuclear cells (PBMC)[17].

Since a RFLP has been characterized in the TNF region[16,18-21], we localized this RFLP by chromosomal restriction mapping and sequence analysis in the first intron at position +210 from the transcriptional start site of the TNF-β gene. Amplification of the corresponding alleles by polymerase chain reaction (PCR) and sequence analysis showed that the presence of the Nco I restriction site (allele TNFB*1) is associated with a variant amino acid at position 26 (aa 26, Asn), coding for asparagine, whereas the TNFB*2 allele, lacking the Nco I site, codes for threonine (thr)[22]. Interestingly, a reduced level of TNF-β production upon stimulation with

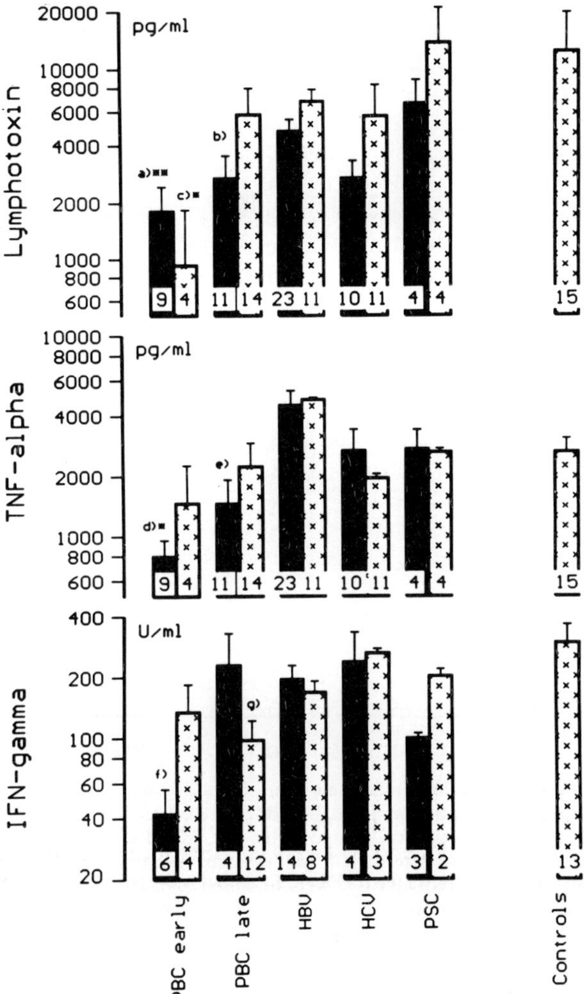

Fig. 1 Lymphotoxin (TNF-β), tumour necrosis factor alpha (TNF-α) and interferon-γ (IFN-γ) production of stimulated T-cell lines in patients with inflammatory liver diseases. *Ordinate*: Lymphotoxin (pg/ml), TNF-α (pg/ml) and IFN-γ (U/ml) in supernatants of PHA-stimulated T-cell lines derived from liver tissue (■) and peripheral blood (☒). Supernatants (1 ml/well) were removed from 2×10^6 T cells on day 3 after the addition of 2 μg PHA (Sigma, Germany) and frozen at $-70\,^{\circ}C$ until analysis by ELISA. *Abscissa*: Patients with early and late PBC (histological stage I and II versus stage III and IV, see text), with chronic hepatitis B (HBV), with chronic hepatitis C (HCV), with primary sclerosing cholangitis (PSC) and healthy controls were tested. For ethical reasons T-cell lines from healthy controls were established only from peripheral blood. The number of T-cell lines tested is given in the figure. Results of the Kruskal–Wallis test are indicated by * for $p < 0.05$ and ** for $p < 0.01$. Differences between groups were evaluated by the Mann–Whitney test as (a) early PBC versus chronic HBV: $p = 0.0160$, versus PSC: $p = 0.0308$; (b) late PBC versus chronic HBV: $p = 0.0489$, versus PSC: $p = 0.0265$; (c) early PBC versus controls: $p = 0.0051$, versus chronic HBV: $p = 0.009$; (d) early PBC versus chronic HBV: $p = 0.0053$, versus chronic HCV: $p = 0.0549$; versus PSC: $p = 0.0055$; (e) late PBC versus chronic HBV: $p = 0.0489$; (f) early PBC versus chronic HBV: $p = 0.0065$, versus PSC: $p = 0.0065$; (g) late PBC versus controls: $p = 0.0462$

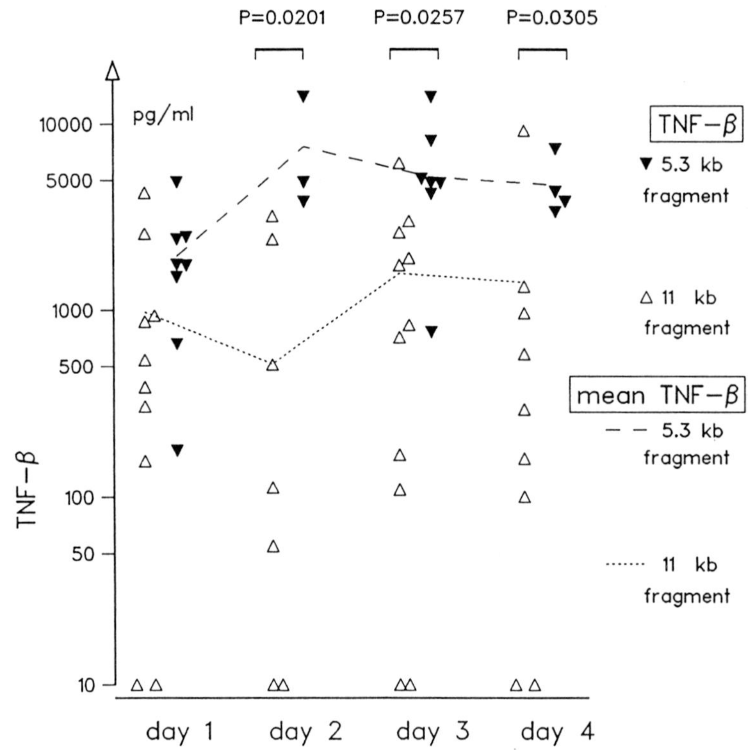

Fig. 2 Stimulation of PBMC of individuals either homozygous for the allele TNFB*1 (5.3 kb fragment; filled arrow heads) or the allele TNFB*2 (11 kb fragment; open arrow heads) with 2 μg PHA. TNF-β protein levels were assayed after 1, 2, 3, and 4 days after activation and are shown in pg/ml; p values were determined by the Mann–Whitney test. Significant differences between the alleles TNFB*1 and TNFB*2 were observed after 2 ($p = 0.02$), 3 ($p = 0.0257$), and 4 days ($p = 0.0305$) of stimulation

Table 1A Frequency of the TNFB alleles in 179 healthy randomly collected individuals. The numbers of observed genotypes represent results obtained in the random controls group. Expected values are calculated according to the Hardy–Weinberg equilibrium for the distribution of the TNFB*1 and TNFB*2 alleles, and present no significant deviation

	Observed	*Expected*
TNFB*1	20 (11.2%)	19.5 (10.8%)
TNFB*1/2	78 (43.6%)	78.8 (44%)
TNFB*2	81 (45.2%)	80.4 (44.9%)

PHA *in vitro* was observed for PBMC of donors, homozygous for TNFB*2 after 2, 3, and 4 days (Fig. 2).

Fugger *et al.* (1989) reported a significantly elevated occurrence of the RFLP pattern corresponding to TNFB*1 in 22 patients with PBC[16], which

Table 1B Distribution of the TNFB phenotypes in 60 patients with PBC (primary biliary cirrhosis) in comparison to 179 healthy individuals. The phenotype is given in numbers and as calculated percentage (in parentheses); the gene frequencies of TNFB*1 and TNFB*2 are depicted below. Relative risk for PBC in the TNFB*2 group (RR = 1.16) is calculated by Haldane's formula

	*TNFB*1*	*TNFB*1/TNFB*2*	*TNFB*2*
PBC ($n = 60$)	6 (10%) 0.3	24 (40%)	30 (50%) 0.7
Controls ($n = 179$)	20 (11.2%) 0.33	78 (43.6%)	81 (45.2%) 0.67

RR = 1.16; chi-square = 0.4

might be linked to a higher TNF-β response. We have tested whether a certain allele of the TNF-β gene is associated with the disease PBC in our collective of patients which might be directly responsible for the low TNF-β production. A large panel of 60 PBC patients was analysed[23].

The amplification of a 740 bp exon 1/intron 3 carrying fragment of the human TNF-β gene was performed from genomic DNA by the use of the PCR (Fig. 3). DNA oligonucleotide primers were chosen such that the Nco I restriction site was in excentric position and Nco I restriction of the TNFB*1 amplification product resulted in two fragments of 185 bp and 555 bp in length (Fig. 3b and c).

In addition, the TNFB allele frequencies of 179 healthy, randomly selected individuals of the Munich area were studied for the normal frequency of the TNFB alleles. Table 1 gives the observed gene frequencies: 0.33 for the TNFB*1 allele and 0.67 for TNFB*2 and 0.3 and 0.7 in PBC patients, respectively. No difference in the frequency of TNFB*1 phenotypes in patients with PBC was found (10%) in comparison to controls (11.2%). Heterozygosity was decreased (40%) and the TNFB*2 phenotype was slightly increased in patients (50%) compared to controls (43.6% and 45.2%, respectively). In summary, no significant deviation from the expectations, according to Hardy-Weinberg equilibrium, was found when comparing PBC patients with the control collective or with the female subgroup. These results suggest that the reduced TNF-β response of PBC patients is not linked to a particular TNF-β allele. Furthermore, our results do not confirm the observation of Fugger *et al.* in a smaller collective of patients[16].

To investigate whether a correlation with certain HLA haplotypes could be found, we have analysed HLA class I and class II antigens by standard NIH complement-dependent microcytotoxicity assays in patients which were available for typing (PBC, $n = 29$ and control, $n = 44$). The distribution of HLA alleles in PBC patients did not differ strongly from gene frequencies in the control group, and was similar to those obtained by the population analysis of Baur *et al.*[24]. Taken together a similar increase of certain HLA-class I antigens has been observed, as previously reported by Prochazka *et al.*[25].

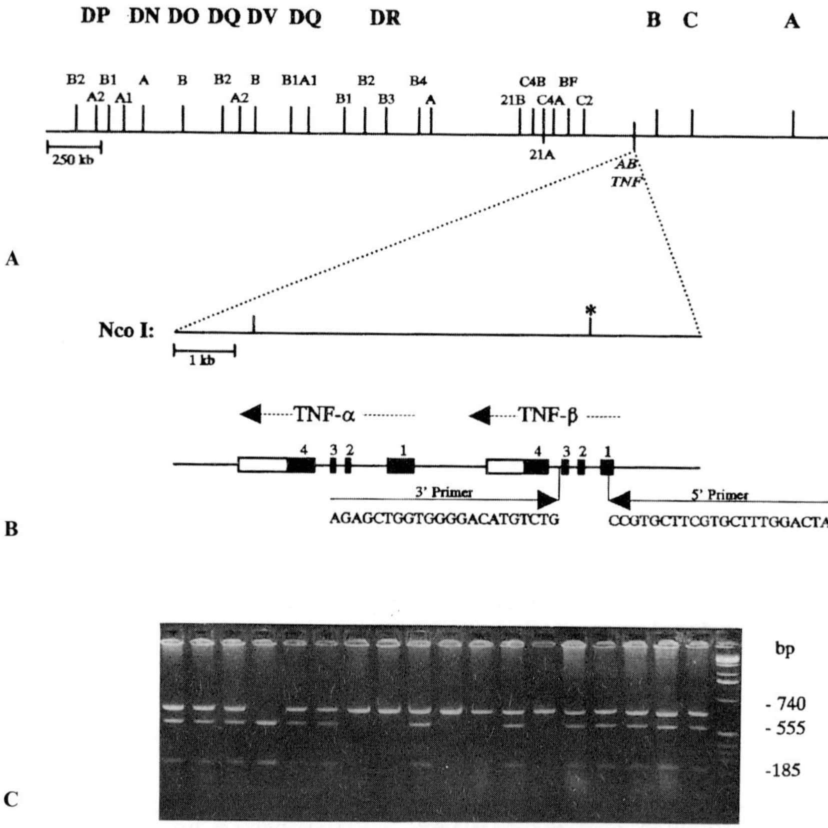

Fig. 3 **A**: Map of the MHC complex on the short arm p of chromosome 6. TNFA and TNFB were mapped by pulsed field gel electrophoresis and chromosomal walking experiments[22]. At least 19 novel genes were detected within the HLA class III region[26] between HLA-B and centromeric HLA-DR. **B**: Strategy for PCR-typing of the Nco I RFLP of the human TNF-β gene. The genomic structure of the linked human TNF-β and TNF-α genes is shown in A. Exons are indicated as black boxes with the numbers above. The position and sequence of the oligonucleotide primers used for PCR-amplification of genomic DNA resulting in a 740 bp fragment, are depicted underneath. The asterisk indicates the Nco I restriction site present in the first intron of the TNFB*1 allele. **C**: The result of the Nco I restricted products obtained from 18 different PBC patients. The 1 kb molecular weight marker (BRL, Karlsruhe) was co-electrophoresed in the last lane on the right. The sizes of the fragments after Nco I restriction are given on the right side (740 bp for the TNFB*2 allele; 555 bp and 185 bp for the TNFB*1 allele). Patient 4 from the left is homozygous for the TNFB*1 allele

DISCUSSION

A strong association with the HLA haplotype HLA-B8 and HLA-DR3 has been described to be common to multiple autoimmune diseases[24]. Furthermore, the linkage of the allele TNFB*1 with the B8-DR3 haplotype[19,21,26,27] has raised the suspicion that variations of the TNF genes might be related to individual disease susceptibilities, perhaps as a cofactor in the promotion of chronic inflammation. This hypothesis explains the

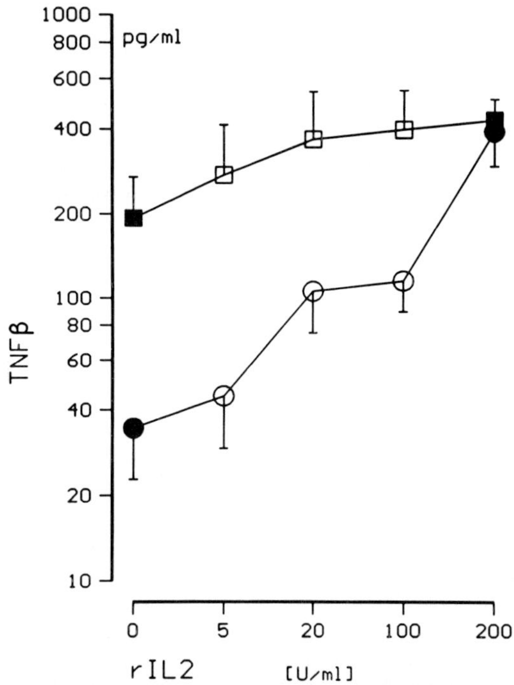

Fig. 4 Stimulation of TNF-β (lymphotoxin) production of PBMC by recombinant interleukin-2 (IL-2). TNF-β (pg/ml) produced by 2 × 10^6 PBMC of patients with PBC (open circles, $n = 7$; black circles, $n = 15$) and healthy controls (open squares, $n = 4$; black squares, $n = 7$) during PHA stimulation after addition of recombinant IL-2

enthusiastic manner in which the TNF-β RFLP was examined in several autoimmune diseases with an immunogenetic background. Initially the diallelic Nco I RFLP was studied only in small collectives of patients with primary biliary cirrhosis[16], diabetes mellitus (IDDM[19,27]), Grave's disease[28], systemic lupus erythematosus (SLE), pauciarticular juvenile rheumatoid arthritis (P-JRA), rheumatoid arthritis (RA), and primary Sjögren's syndrome (pSS)[20]. Later testing in larger collectives of patients with PBC[23], myasthenia gravis[26], multiple sclerosis, optic neuritis[29], ankylosing spondylitis[30], Hashimoto's thyroiditis[31], and spontaneous abortions[32] demonstrated that no increase in the frequency of one TNFB allele was found when compared to HLA-matched controls. A higher number of heterozygotes among patients with IDDM was observed[19,27], and in SLE the allele TNFB*1 was significantly increased in the patients (RR = 1.96; $p = 0.002$)[33]. This supports the concept that the linkage disequilibrium of certain HLA haplotypes (e.g. HLA-A1, -B8, -DR3, DQw2) and TNF is responsible for the increased occurrence of TNFB*1. The same conclusion has been drawn for patients with PM-Scl-antibody positive systemic sclerosis[34] (Messer *et al.*, unpublished observation).

In conclusion, no association can be found between PBC and the Nco I RFLP of the TNF-β gene. RFLP typing in various autoimmune diseases thus far reflects a pattern of allelic distribution in linkage with the corresponding HLA haplotypes found. Although the gene frequencies differ between the control groups, this might be due to the immunogenetic background and the composition of HLA haplotypes therein. In certain groups of patients with significant positive associations to HLA-B8, -DR3, like IDDM, myasthenia gravis and PM-Scl-positive systemic sclerosis patients, the TNFB*1 allele frequencies obtained are so far only significantly increased, when compared to non-matched controls for HLA[19]. In context with PBC, the data presented here argue against a predominant involvement of a particular TNF-β allele in the pathogenesis of PBC.

A detailed investigation of the production of lymphokines of mitogen-stimulated T cells from liver tissue and peripheral blood from patients with PBC showed a reduced production of TNF-β, TNF-α, and IFN-γ compared to healthy controls and patients with acute (data not shown) and chronic hepatitis B, chronic hepatitis non-A–non-B/C, primary sclerosing cholangitis, and healthy controls. Impaired lymphokine production was detected irrespective of the dose of mitogen. It was correlated neither to cholestasis nor to inter-individual alterations in the phenotypic composition of T-cell preparations. Disturbed lymphokine production was a persistent phenomenon when T-cell lines were tested after longer periods of tissue culture (up to 6 weeks tested). Lymphokine production was particularly low in patients with early stages of disease (stage I and II). This was also true for TNF-β and TNF-α production of PBMC (TNF-β/TNF-α in pg/ml in PBC stage I and II ($n = 28$): $280 \pm 172/333 \pm 105$, in PBC stage III and IV ($n = 18$): $1542 \pm 503/4864 \pm 2934$; in chronic hepatitis B ($n = 41$): $2391 \pm 764/2310 \pm 393$; in chronic hepatitis non-A–non-B/C ($n = 16$): $3791 \pm 1729/3461 \pm 1819$; in primary sclerosing cholangitis ($n = 10$): $1451 \pm 636/2338 \pm 1256$; and in healthy controls ($n = 28$): $1729 \pm 613/1127 \pm 512$. The differences of TNF-β and TNF-α production between patients in early stages of PBC and patients with various inflammatory liver diseases were statistically significant.

As demonstrated in Fig. 4, TNF-β production upon stimulation was modulated by interleukin 2 (IL-2). Addition of high amounts of recombinant IL-2 (200 U/ml) to T cells of PBC patients resulted in an increased production of TNF-β. Likewise addition of anti-IL-2 antibodies reduced TNF-β production of T cells (data not shown).

Interestingly, the observation of a superinduction of the TNF-β response *in vitro* by addition of recombinant IL-2 (Fig. 4), and the subsequent response of previously non- or low-responding PBMC of PBC patients suggests a role for regulatory mechanisms in T lymphocytes causing this immune phenomenon. This leads us to propose a certain stage of anergy as an explanation for the reduced production of TNF-β mRNA and protein and IL-2[35] in patients with PBC. Due to results reported recently, this might be caused by a reduced activation of the *cis*-activating nuclear factor AP-1 (activator protein-1)[36], binding to elements in the IL-2 and TNF-β gene in parallel[22,37] upon activation. A reduced or defective signalling via AP-1 might be involved in the observed reduction of transcription of TNF-β and IL-2 genes[17], resulting in a reduced protein production[17,35].

Our data demonstrate a functional impairment of T lymphocytes in patients with PBC. This functional impairment is demonstrated by reduced lymphokine production[17].

The disturbed lymphokine production was observed both in T cell lines derived from peripheral blood and from liver tissue. Several groups, including our own, have characterized T cell lines from liver tissue in PBC demonstrating that, at least phenotypically, liver-derived T cell lines correspond to portal lymphocellular infiltrates[38–40]. Provided that these T cells reflect the functional stage of tissue-infiltrating T lymphocytes, these data indicate that cell activation and lymphokine secretion may be impaired in T cells at the site of tissue damage. The reduced functional capacity of T cells was evident in early stages (stage I and II) and was not statistically significant in late stages (stage III and IV) of PBC. Reduced lymphokine production was also detected at the level of mRNA, e.g. low amounts of TNF-β mRNA corresponded with reduced TNF-β secretion.

The interpretation of the results is difficult. Current evidence indicates that T cells require costimulatory signals for activation in addition to triggering of the T cell receptor complex (TCR). It has been speculated that aberrant expression of several distinct molecules of MHC class II antigens on biliary epithelial cells in PBC may qualify these cells for antigen presentation and triggering of the TCR complex (TCR). Aberrant expression of MHC class II molecules is prominent in the early stages of PBC, whereas in the late stages bile ducts are destroyed and replaced by fibrotic tissue. However, since these non-professional antigen-presenting cells lack costimulatory activity, it is an intriguing speculation that in PBC one reason for the unresponsiveness of T lymphocytes with regard to production of certain lymphokines might be the result of prior contact with parenchymal cells aberrantly expressing MHC class II molecules.

However, different interpretations are possible, and further elucidation of the functional capacity of liver tissue-infiltrating T cells has to await, e.g., lymphokine analysis *in situ* by *in situ* hybridization or by *in situ* PCR, as well as a detailed study of activating nuclear factors binding to the respective lymphokine gene *cis*-activating elements[36]. Reduced production of TNF-α, TNF-β, and IFN-γ has been reported in a variety of human autoimmune diseases which are characterized by aberrant MHC class II expression[41–46].

While the role of cytokines and their interrelationship in immunologically determined inflammatory responses, including PBC, is very complex, the failure of production of some lymphokines may lead to inappropriate or ineffective antigen processing, presentation and elimination by B and T cell responses, or to inappropriate activation of T cells, resulting in failure to resolve the inflammatory process.

Acknowledgements

This work has been supported by grants from the Wilhelm Sander Stiftung (Grant No. 83.015.4 Pa) and the Deutsche Forschungsgemeinschaft (SFB 217).

References

1. Thomas HC, Epstein O. Pathogenetic mechanisms in primary biliary cirrhosis. Springer Semin Immunopathol. 1980;3:375–84.
2. Kaplan MM. Primary biliary cirrhosis. N Engl J Med. 1987;9:521–8.
3. Ludwig J. New concepts in biliary cirrhosis. Springer Semin Liver Dis. 1987;7:293–301.
4. Gershwin ME, Mackay IR. Primary biliary cirrhosis: current knowledge, perspectives, future directions. Springer Semin Liver Dis. 1989;9:149–57.
5. Pape GR, Spengler U, Hoffmann RM, Jung MC. Pathogenesis of primary biliary cirrhosis: new aspects for a role of T-lymphocytes. In: Krawitt EL, Wiesner RH, editors. Autoimmune liver disease. New York: Raven Press; 1991:43–62.
6. Sarvetnick N, Liggitt D, Pitts SL, Hansen SE, Stewart A. Insulin-dependent diabetes induced in transgenic mice by ectopic expression of class II MHC and interferon-gamma. Cell. 1988;52:773–82.
7. Dunham I, Sargent CA, Trowsdale J, Campbell RD. Molecular mapping of the human major histocompatibility complex by pulsed-field gel electrophoresis. Proc Natl Acad Sci USA. 1987;84:7237–41.
8. Carroll MC, Katzman P, Alicot EM, Koller BH, Geraghty DE, Orr HT, Strominger JL, Spies T. Linkage map of the human major histocompatibility complex including the tumor necrosis factor genes. Proc Natl Acad Sci USA. 1987;84:8535–9.
9. Inoko H, Trowsdale J. Linkage of TNF genes to the HLA-B locus. Nucl Acids Res. 1987;15:9857–62.
10. Ragoussis J, Blömer K, Weiss EH, Ziegler A. Localisation of the genes for tumor necrosis factor and lymphotoxin between the HLA class I and class III regions by field inversion gel electrophoresis. Immunogenetics. 1988;27:66–9.
11. Jacob CO, McDevitt HO. Tumor necrosis factor-α in murine autoimmune 'lupus' nephritis. Nature. 1988;331:356–8.
12. Richter G, Quin Z, Diamantstein T, Blankenstein T. Analysis of restriction fragment polymorphism in lymphokine genes of normal and autoimmune mice. J Exp Med. 1989;170:1439–43.
13. Ballardini G, Mirakian R, Bianchi FB, Pisi E, Donaich D, Botazzo GF. Aberrant expression of HLA-DR antigens on bile duct epithelium in primary biliary cirrhosis: relevance to pathogenesis. Lancet. 1984;II:1009–13.
14. Spengler U, Pape GR, Hoffmann RM, Johnson JP, Eisenburg J, Paumgartner G, Riethmüller G. Differential expression of MHC class II subregion products on bile duct epithelial cells and hepatocytes in patients with primary biliary cirrhosis. Hepatology. 1988;8:459–62.
15. Pujol-Borrel R, Todd I, Doshi M, Botazzo GF, Sutton R, Gray D, Adolf GR, Feldmann M. HLA class II induction in human islet cells by interferon-gamma plus tumor necrosis factor or lymphotoxin. Nature. 1987;362:304–6.
16. Fugger L, Morling N, Ryder LP, Platz P, Georgsen J, Jakobsen BK, Svejgaard A, Dalhoff K, Ranek L. NcoI restriction fragment length polymorphism (RFLP) of the tumor necrosis factor (TNF-α) region in primary biliary cirrhosis and in healthy Danes. Scand J Immunol. 1989;30:185–9.
17. Spengler U, Möller A, Jung MC, Messer G, Zachoval R, Hoffmann RM, Eisenburg J, Paumgartner G, Riethmüller G, Weiss EH, Pape GR. T lymphocytes from patients with primary biliary cirrhosis produce reduced amounts of lymphotoxin, tumor necrosis factor and interferon gamma upon mitogen stimulation. J Hepatol. 1992;15:129–35.
18. Nedospasov SA, Shakov AN, Turetskaya RL, Mett VA, Azizov MM, Georgiev GP, Korobko VG, Dobrynin VN, Filipov SA, Bystrov NS, Boldyreva EF, Chuvpilo SA, Chumakov SM, Shingarova LN, Ovchinnikov YA. Tandem arrangement of genes coding for tumor necrosis factor (TNF-α) and lymphotoxin (TNF–β) in the human genome. Cold Spring Harbor Symp Quant Biol. 1986;51:611–24.
19. Badenhoop K, Schwarz G, Trowsdale J, Lewis V, Gale EAM, Botazzo GF. TNF-α gene polymorphisms in type 1 (insulin-dependent) diabetes mellitus. Diabetologia. 1989;32: 445–8
20. Fugger L, Morling N, Ryder LP, Georgsen J, Jakobsen BK, Svejgaard A, Andersen V, Oxholm P, Karup Pedersen F, Friis J, Halberg P. NcoI restriction fragment length

polymorphism (RFLP) of the tumor necrosis factor (TNF-α) region in four autoimmune diseases. Tissue Antigens. 1989;34:17–22.

21. Dawkins RL, Leaver A, Cameron PU, Martin E, Kay PH, Christiansen FT. Some disease-associated ancestral haplotypes carry a polymorphism of TNF. Human Immunol. 1989;26:91–7.
22. Messer G, Spengler U, Jung MC, Honold G, Pape GR, Riethmüller G, Weiss EH. Polymorphic structure of the TNF locus: a NcoI polymorphism in the first intron of the human TNF-β gene correlates with a variant amino acid in position 26 and a reduced level of TNF-β production. J Exp Med. 1991;173:209–19.
23. Messer G, Spengler U, Jung MC, Honold G, Eisenburg J, Scholz S, Albert ED, Pape GR, Riethmüller G, Weiss EH. Allelic variation in the TNF-β gene does not explain the low TNF-β response in patients with primary biliary cirrhosis. Scand J Immunol. 1991;34: 735–40.
24. Albert ED, Baur MP, Mayr WR. Histocompatibility testing. New York, Berlin, Heidelberg, Tokyo: Springer-Verlag; 1984.
25. Prochazka EJ, Terasaki PI, Park MS, Goldstein LI, Busuttil RW. Association of primary sclerosing cholangitis with HLA-DRw52a. N Engl J Med. 1990;25:1842–4.
26. Degli-Esposti MA, Andreas A, Christiansen FT, Schalke B, Albert E, Dawkins RL. An approach to the localization of the susceptibility genes for generalized myasthenia gravis by mapping recombinant ancestral haplotypes. Immunogenetics. 1992;35:355–64.
27. Pociot F, Mölvig J, Wogensen L, Worsaae H, Dalboge H, Baek, Nerup J. A tumour necrosis factor beta gene polymorphism in relation to monokine secretion and insulin-dependent diabetes mellitus. Scand J Immunol. 1991;33:37–49.
28. Badenhoop K, Schwarz G, Schleusener H, Weetman AP, Recks S, Peters H, Botazzo GF, Usadel KH. Tumor necrosis factor beta gene polymorphisms in Graves' disease. J Clin Endocrinol Metab. 1992;74:287–91.
29. Fugger L, Morling N, Sandberg-Wollheim M, Ryder LP, Svejgaard A. Tumor necrosis factor alpha gene polymorphism in multiple sclerosis and optic neuritis. J Neuroimmunol. 1990;27:85–8.
30. Verjans GM, van der Linden SM, van Eys GJJM, de Waal LP, Kijlstra A. Restriction fragment length polymorphism of the tumor necrosis factor (TNF) region in patients with ankylosing spondylitis. Arthritis Rheum. 1991;34:486–9.
31. Badenhoop K, Schwarz G, Walfish PG, Drummond V, Usadel KH, Botazzo GF. Susceptibility to thyroid autoimmune disease: Molecular analysis of HLA-D region genes identifies new markers for goitrous Hashimoto's thyroiditis. J Clin Endocrinol Metab. 1990;71:1131–7.
32. Laitinen T, Lokki ML, Tulppala M, Ylikorkala O, Koskimies S. Tumour necrosis factor B gene polymorphism in relation to complotype in couples with spontaneous abortions and in control families. Scand J Immunol. 1992;35:131–5.
33. Bettinotti MP, Hartung K, Deicher HRG, Messer G, Keller E, Weiss EH, Albert DA. Polymorphism of the tumour necrosis factor beta gene in systemic lupus erythematosus. TNFB-MHC haplotypes. Immunogenetics. 1992;37:449–54.
34. Genth E, Mierau R, Genetzky P, Mühlen C von, Kaufmann S, Wilmowsky H von, Meurer M, Krieg T, Pollmann HJ, Hartl PW. Immunogenetic associations of scleroderma-related antinuclear antibodies. Arthritis Rheum. 1990;33:657–65.
35. Saxena S, Nouri-Aria KT, Anderson MG. Interleukin 2 activity in chronic liver disease and the effect of in vitro α-interferon. Clin Exp Immunol. 1986;63:541–8.
36. Kang SM, Beverly B, Tran AC, Brorson K, Schwartz RH, Lenardo MJ. Transactivation by AP-1 is a molecular target of T cell clonal anergy. Science. 1992;257:1134–8.
37. Serfling E, Bathelmäs I, Pfeuffer B, Schenk S, Zarius S, Swoboda R, Mercurio F, Karin M. Ubiquitous and lymphocyte-specific factors are involved in the induction of the mouse interleukin 2 gene in T lymphocytes. EMBO J. 1989;8:465–73.
38. Hoffmann RM, Pape GR, Spengler U, Rieber EP, Eisenburg J, Döhrmann J, Paumgartner G, Riethmüller G. Clonal analysis of liver derived T cells of patients with primary biliary cirrhosis. Clin Exp Immunol. 1989;76:210–15.
39. Meuer SC, Moebius U, Manns MM, Dienes HP, Ramadori G, Hess G, Hercend T, Meyer zum Büschenfelde K-H. Clonal analysis of human T lymphocytes infiltrating the liver in chronic active hepatitis B and primary biliary cirrhosis. Eur J Immunol. 1988;18:1447–52.

40. Krams SM, Van de Water J, Coppel RL, Esquivel C, Roberts J, Ansari A, Gershwin ME. Analysis of hepatic T lymphocyte and immunoglobulin deposits in patients with primary biliary cirrhosis. Hepatology. 1990;12:306–13.
41. Stolzenberg T, Binz H, Fontana A, Felder M, Wagenhaeuser FJ. Impaired mitogen-induced interferon-gamma production in rheumatoid arthritis. Scand J Immunol. 1988;27:73–81.
42. Ziegler EJ. Tumor necrosis factor in humans. N Engl J Med. 1988;318:1533–5.
43. Franchimont P, Reuter A, Gysen P, Bernier J, Vrindts-Gevaert Y. Tumor necrosing factor α: Un mediateur de la fonction macrophagique. Actions biologiques et dosage radioimmunologique. Med Hyg. 1987;45:2160–8.
44. Sachs JA, Whichelow CE, Hitman GA, Niven M, Thode H, Meager A. The effect of HLA and insulin-dependent diabetes mellitus on the secretion levels of tumour necrosis factors alpha and beta and gamma interferon. Scand J Immunol. 1990;32:703–8.
45. Satoh J, Seino H, Abo T, Tanaka S, Shintani S, Ohta S, Tamura K, Sawait T, Nobunaga T, Oteki T. Recombinant tumor necrosis factor alpha suppresses autoimmune diabetes in NOD mice. J Clin Invest. 1989;84:1345–8.
46. Jacob CO, Aiso S, Michie SA, McDevitt HO, Acha-Orbea H. Prevention of diabetes in non obese diabetic mice by tumor necrosis factor (TNF): Similarities between TNF-alpha and interleukin 1. Proc Natl Acad Sci USA. 1990;87:968–72.

46
Antigen expression and presentation on bile duct epithelium

J. NEUBERGER, R. AYRES, A. STRAIN and R. JOPLIN

INTRODUCTION

Although extrahepatic organs are also affected in primary biliary cirrhosis (PBC), it is the liver that bears the brunt of the disease, and hepatic disease is the commonest cause of morbidity and mortality in such patients. Within the liver, morphological studies suggest that it is the middle-sized intrahepatic bile ducts that are the targets. Although immunosuppressive drugs, to date, have been shown to have very little effect on the natural history of the disease, the association with complement activation and, on histology, the presence of lymphoid aggregates, granulomas, and immunoglobulin deposition in and around the bile ducts, has led to the concept that immune mechanisms are responsible for the progressive bile duct damage characteristic of the disease. The involvement of immune mechanisms in the pathogenesis and progression of the disease is further supported by the large number of humoral and cellular immunological abnormalities which have been well characterized and reported in a number of reviews. In this chapter we will concentrate on antigen presentation and expression on bile duct epithelium.

ANTIGEN EXPRESSION IN TISSUE

The MHC antigens

Since Ballardini's original description of increased expression of MHC class II antigens by biliary epithelial cells in PBC[1], there has been an increasing interest in the pattern of MHC expression in both normal and diseased liver. In the normal liver, class I antigens can be seen to be expressed on biliary epithelial cells and sinusoidal cells but not on hepatocytes (Table 1)[2]. Class II antigens are expressed on sinusoidal cells only. In patients with PBC there is increased expression of MHC antigens on both biliary epithelial cells and periportal hepatocytes[3,4]. As might be anticipated, these findings are not

Table 1 MHC expression in liver

	Sinusoidal cells	*BEC*	*Hepatocytes*
Normal			
Class I	+	+	−
Class II	+	−	−
PBC			
Class I	+	+	+
Class II	+	+	±
Cholestasis			
Class I	+	+	+
Class II	+	+	±

Table 2 Mean intensity scoring of ICAM-1 in normal and diseased liver[16]

			Bile ducts		
	Hepatocytes	*Endothelium*	*Ductule*	*Lobular*	*Medium*
Normal liver	0.6	1.0	n.a.	0.3	0.9
PBC	2.3	0.96	2.9	2.9	0.05
PSC	1.8	1.0	2.6	2.7	0
Cirrhosis	1.5	0.5	0.4	0.1	0.04

n.a. = Not applicable

specific to PBC, and similar observations have been made in other conditions where there is presumed immune-mediated damage to the liver, such as liver allograft rejection, chronic active hepatitis and sclerosing cholangitis[5–7] (Table 2).

It must, however, be questioned whether the enhanced expression of MHC antigens on the biliary epithelial cells is a consequence of the cholestasis or may be more central to the pathogenesis of the disease[8]. This question has been partly resolved by studies by Calmus and others, who have examined the appearance of membrane MHC expression in patients and in animals with cholestasis[8,9].

In rats after bile duct ligation a substantial increase in the number of hepatocytes expressing class I antigen was observed. In contrast, no increased expression of class II antigens was seen on the hepatocytes, biliary epithelial cells or endothelial cells. Pretreatment of rats with immunosuppressive agents such as corticosteroids and cyclosporin had no effect in reducing this increased hepatocyte class I expression[4]. In contrast, ursodeoxycholic acid treatment was associated with a reduction in class I antigen expression. Patients with PBC treated with ursodeoxycholic acid were also found to have a reduction in class I MHC expression on hepatocytes, but no change in class II expression by biliary epithelial cells was observed. The significance of these observations is uncertain since in PBC, target damage is manifest primarily on the biliary epithelial cells rather than the hepatocytes[10]. More recent studies[11] have provided additional support that class II expression may not be implicated in disease. Balb/C mice were given interleukin-2 (IL-

2) intraperitoneally daily for 35 days. In the liver there was strong luminal expression of MHC class I antigens on the biliary epithelial cells which were surrounded by T cells (mainly CD3, L3T4 and IL-2 positive). Half were positive for asialo-GM1 and one-third were interferon-α positive. There was no evidence of bile duct damage and no autoantibodies were found serologically. Thus aberrant class II expression may be a secondary phenomenon, and not necessarily associated in the pathogenesis of bile duct damage.

Blood group antigens

A further group of antigens present on the surface of biliary epithelial cells is the blood group antigens. In normal liver, ABH antigens are expressed on septal ducts while Lewis antigens are present on ducts and ductules of all sizes[12,13]. These observations add further evidence for the phenotypic heterogeneity between biliary epithelial cells in different regions of the biliary tree. In diseases such as primary sclerosing cholangitis (PSC), there may be inappropriate expression of A and B antigens compared with normal controls and other disease groups (including PBC)[14]. However, in PBC, PSC and in the presence of extrahepatic bile duct obstruction, there is increased biliary expression of Lewis blood group antigens compared with normal liver and with alcoholic liver disease. Reasons for these differences are not clear and require further elucidation.

Adhesion molecules

It is now recognized that interaction between immune cells and target cells is a complex reaction involving participation of many different molecules. Among these are the intercellular adhesion molecules (ICAM) of which three subgroups have been identified (ICAM-1, ICAM-2 and ICAM-3). Although it is thought that ICAM-2 is not inducible, ICAM-1 does appear inducible[15]. The membrane expression of ICAM-1 in PBC liver was studied using a three-step immuno-alkaline phosphatase method[16]. Sections were stained with a mouse monoclonal antibody recognizing ICAM-1. Sections were examined and the staining intensity graded in a semi-quantitative scale (0–3). This technique has been validated using confocal laser microscopy[17]. In normal liver (Table 2) there was some staining of endothelium, some hepatocyte staining and very little staining observed on lobular or medium-sized bile ducts. In contrast, in sections from patients with primary biliary cirrhosis there was no increase in endothelial ICAM-1 expression but significant increase of ICAM-1 expression both on the lobular bile ducts and the ductules. This pattern is similar to that observed in sections from patients with PSC, but contrasts with that seen in sections of livers from patients with cirrhosis due to other causes where no increased expression of ICAM-1 on bile ducts was observed. It was of interest that in PBC the middle-sized bile ducts were negative even in the presence of active inflammation. The

Table 3 Intensity of E2 staining in liver[19] (mean score)

		Bile ducts		
	Hepatocytes	*Ductules*	*Interlobular*	*Septal*
Normal liver	0.83	n.a.	1.75	1.75
PBC	2.01	2.86	2.86	2.67

hepatocellular staining by anti-ICAM-1 was predominantly periseptal in distribution. This appearance is possibly related to the fibrosis. Very similar results are observed in patients with acute or chronic liver allograft rejection[17]. However, not all authors have been able to reproduce these results[18].

E2 expression

The close association between PBC and antimitochondrial antibodies is well recognized. The characterization of E2 is described in other chapters. Using a similar technique to that for ICAM-1, the intensity and pattern of distribution of E2 in liver tissue was studied and assessed semi-quantitatively. Antibodies to E3 and E2 were raised in rabbits by Dr Gordon Lindsay (University of Glasgow) using methods described in detail elsewhere[19]. The results of the staining of E2 are shown in Table 3. The pattern of staining of E2 did not parallel the reported distribution of mitochondria in the liver. In both normal and PBC liver, E2 staining was greater in biliary epithelial cells than in hepatocytes (Fig. 1). Furthermore in PBC there was greater staining of E2 in the septal and interlobular bile ducts compared with normal liver. By contrast, staining with antibodies to E3 produced uniform intensity and distribution of staining in both normal and PBC liver (Fig. 2). This apparent dissociation between the distribution of E2 and of mitochondria is further supported by additional studies[20] where the distribution of E2 was compared with that of a marker for mitochondrial inner membranes. While the mitochondrial marker was seen in greater intensity in hepatocytes compared with biliary epithelial cells, E2 was found in up to 30 times greater concentration in bile duct cells compared with hepatocytes.

We were also able to study lymph nodes from patients with PBC, PSC and normal subjects. Up to 25% of the sinus macrophages from the portal lymph nodes from patients with PBC stained intensely with anti-E2. These lymph nodes were taken from patient's liver removed at the time of transplantation (Fig. 3).

In contrast, no such staining of macrophages by anti-E2 in portal nodes of patients with PSC was seen. Because we were unable to find portal lymph nodes in normal liver adequate for study, as a control, iliac nodes from normal subjects were used. In these lymph nodes, the macrophages in normal subjects were no more intensely stained than other cell types (Table 4).

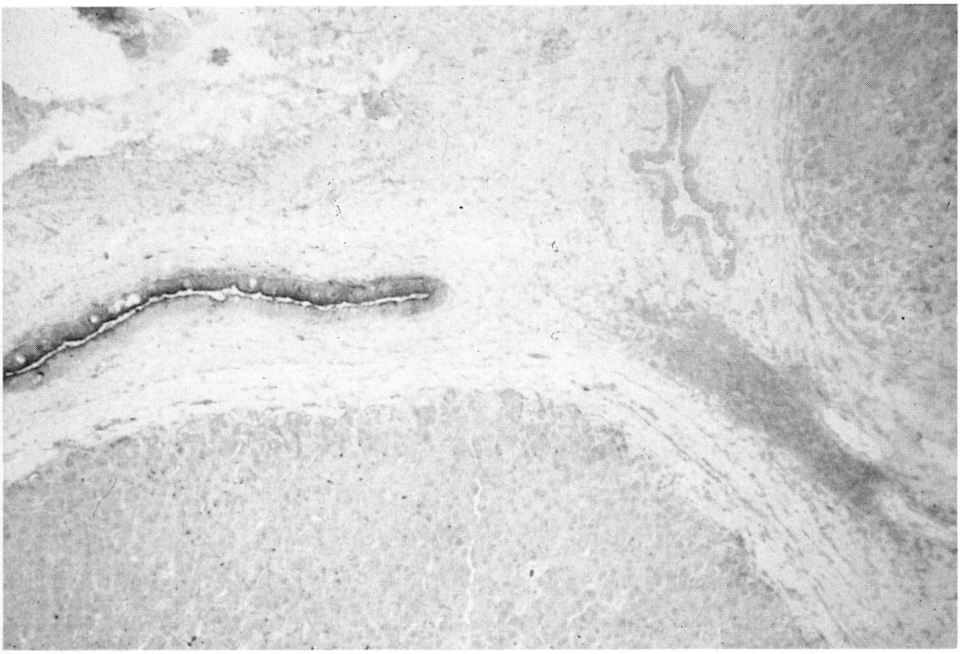

Fig. 1 Histological section of a liver from a patient with PBC, stained with anti-E2 showing intense staining of one bile duct with little staining of hepatocytes

ANTIGEN EXPRESSION ON ISOLATED BECs

The results obtained from staining of liver tissue give some idea of the pattern of distribution of the various antigens examined, but cannot actively define the location of the antigen stained. In order to investigate further the pattern of distribution of these antigens, techniques for isolation and maintenance in tissue culture of biliary epithelial cells isolated from normal and PBC livers were developed[21,22]. The method, described in detail elsewhere, involves collagenase digestion, differential density centrifugation and immuno-isolation using an antibody which, in the liver, is specific for biliary epithelial cells. Cells can be maintained in tissue culture for up to 6–12 weeks without loss of the phenotypic or morphological characteristics of biliary epithelial cells.

Distribution of E2

Distribution of E2 on biliary epithelial cells isolated both from normal and PBC livers was studied using these isolated cells in order to determine whether E2 was present on the membrane of these cells[23].

No membrane staining for E2 was seen on cells either freshly isolated or cells that had been in culture for up to 3 days. In contrast, the BECs isolated

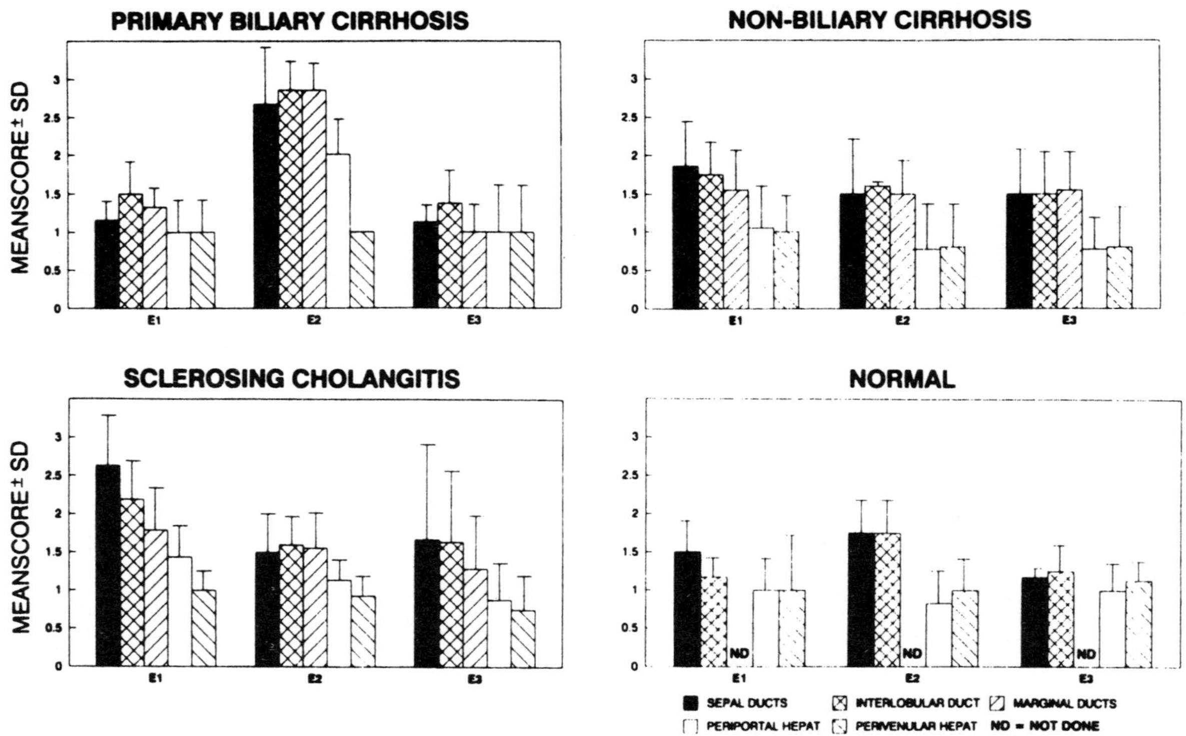

Fig. 2 Intensity of E1, E2 and E3 staining of different cell types in livers from patients with normal liver, PBC, PSC and other causes of cirrhosis

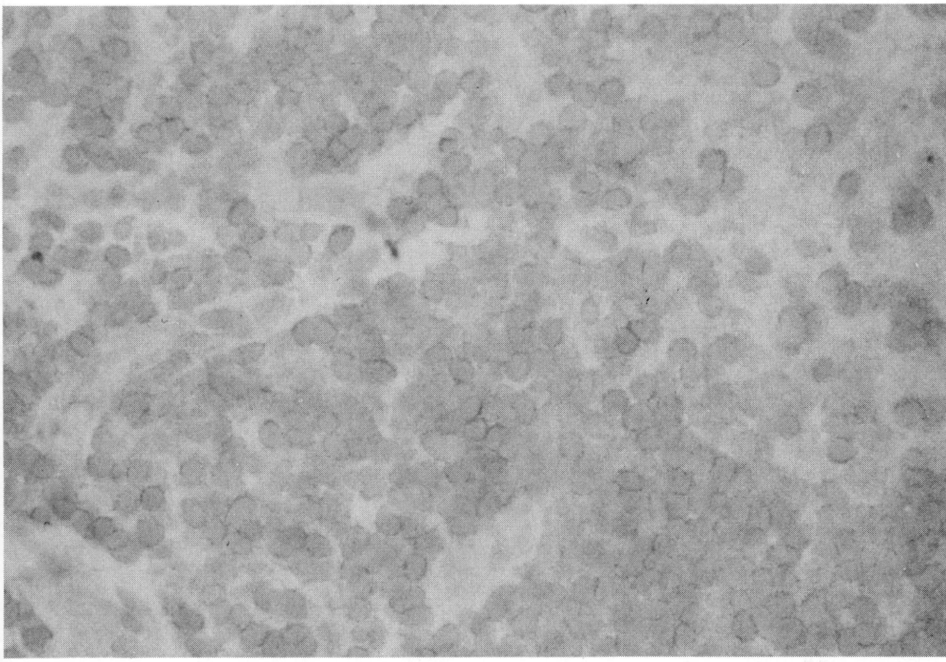

Fig. 3 Portal lymph node from patients with PBC stained with anti-E2 showing sinus macrophages in PBC node strongly reacting

Table 4 Intensity of E2 staining in lymph nodes[19]

	Vessels	*Macrophages*	*Lymphocytes*
Normal iliac node	2.00	1.17	1.00
PBC portal node	1.88	2.75	1.13

from patients with PBC showed an increasing proportion of colonies staining for E2 on the membrane (Fig. 4).

Thus by 7–10 days after isolation the immuno-isolated colonies showed positive membrane staining for E2. In contrast, of the seven normal livers used, only one preparation showed staining for E2 – this was observed only 3 days after isolation. The pattern of E2 staining was similar to that observed for the membrane antigen, HEA125, present on all colonies of both normal and PBC-derived epithelial cells.

Isolated biliary epithelial cells were studied in further experiments. Cells were isolated and incubated with anti-E2, fixed and then further incubated with a labelled second antibody. Confocal laser microscopy clearly showed a pattern of membrane distribution of E2 similar to that observed for the membrane protein HEA125. Epithelial cells from normal subjects showed no such distribution. In contrast, when the cells were fixed prior to staining with anti-E2, thus allowing antibodies access to intracellular proteins, both

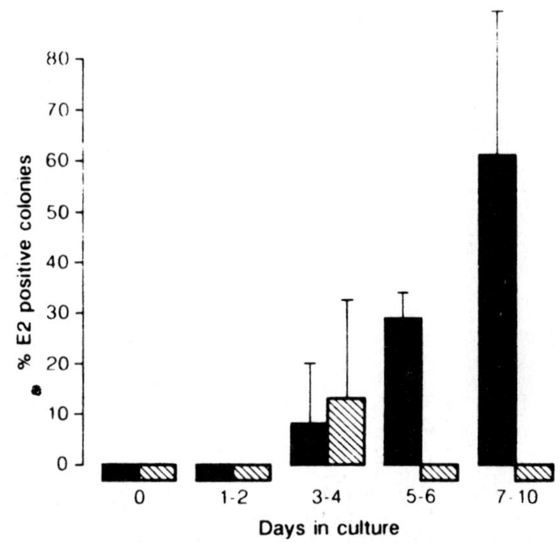

–Biliary epithelial cell E2 antibody staining.

■ PBC; ▨ normal.

Fig. 4 Percentage of colonies of isolated biliary epithelial cells from isolated normal and PBC livers staining for E2 (Courtesy of *Lancet*)

PBC and normal BECs showed an intracellular distribution of E2, which was similar in the two groups examined. A limited number of studies have been performed with BECs isolated from patients with primary sclerosing cholangitis; the behaviour of E2 in these patients closely resembled those of normal subjects (unpublished data). To date we have not observed membrane distribution of E2 in any group other than PBC (Fig. 5).

Thus, these studies strongly suggest that E2 is present on the membrane of biliary epithelial cells isolated from patients with PBC but not normal subjects. It remains to be confirmed whether this membrane expression is that of the whole of E2 or of a sub-unit. The possibility of crossreaction cannot be excluded, although immunoblotting studies have failed to provide any evidence of this.

MHC expression by isolated biliary epithelial cells

Using these biliary epithelial cells in culture it was possible to examine the effect of various pro-inflammatory cytokines on membrane expression of HLA class I, class II and ICAM-1[24]. Cells between 6 and 9 days in culture were stimulated *in vitro* with either tumour necrosis factor, interferon-γ or interleukin-1 for 24 hours. In some experiments the cells were simultaneously incubated with methylprednisolone (2.6×10^{-7} mol/l). The stimulated cells were then examined using monoclonal antibodies and the antibodies detected using an alkaline phosphatase (APAAP) technique. Because these cells were in colonies and were not confluent, staining was scored semi-quantitatively

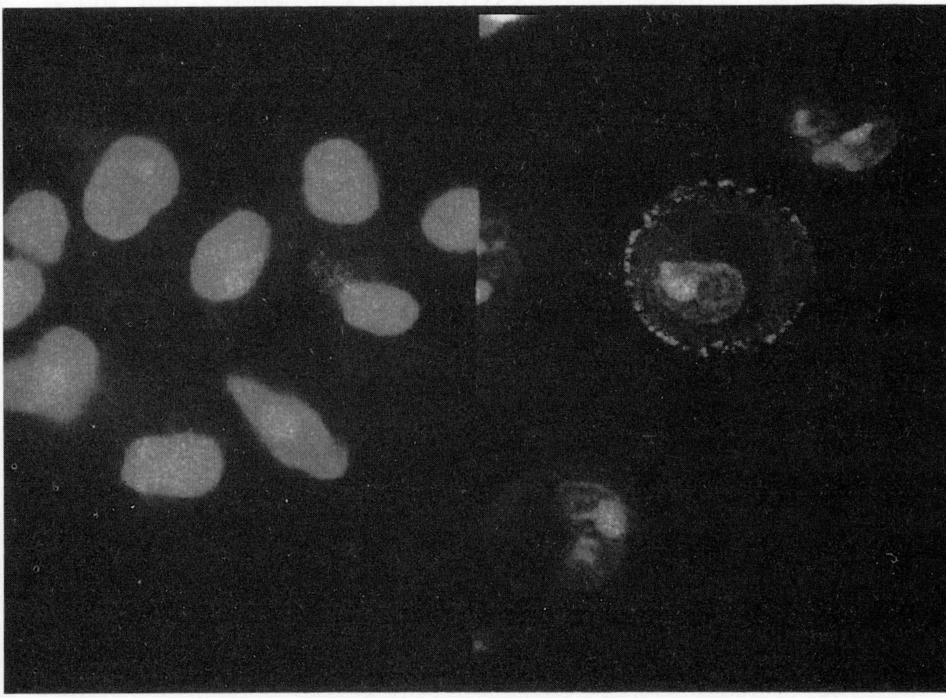

Fig. 5 Isolated biliary epithelial cells from control (left) and (right) PBC livers stained with anti-E2 (green); the red counterstain is propidium iodide

Table 5 Intensity of staining of various antigens induced by stimulation with pro-inflammatory cytokines on BECs from PBC and normal liver[24]

Antigen	*Control*	*TNF (500 units/ml)*	*IFN (500 units/ml)*	*IL-1 (5 units/ml)*	*Normal*
ICAM-1	2.5	1.85*	1.85*	1.73*	0.93**
HLA class I	0.83	0.26	0.27	1.02*	0.64
HLA class II	0.83	1.0	1.1*	1.3*	0.58**

*$p < 0.01$ compared with control PBC livers; **$p < 0.05$ PBC control compared normal control

by three independent observers. This approach was validated elsewhere using vascular endothelial cells[20]. Scores were calculated from the mean of each set of triplicates and the results are shown in Table 5. ICAM-1 was increased by TNF, interleukin-1 and interferon-γ. Co-culture with corticosteroids had no effect on the amount of ICAM-1 observed. HLA class I was found to be significantly increased after incubation only with interleukin-1. Incubation with tumour necrosis factor had no effect on the amount of HLA class II, whereas preincubation with both interferon and interleukin-1 significantly increased the amount of HLA class II in these cells. Comparison of BECs isolated from normal and PBC liver showed that 'normal' BECs had, when unstimulated, significantly less ICAM-1 and HLA class II than PBC BECs. This mirrors the situation found *in vivo* (see above).

These results must be regarded as preliminary findings only. More objective methods of assessing the degree of antigen membrane expression require the use of confluent layers of cells.

Preliminary studies of the effect of tauro-ursodeoxycholic acid, ursodeoxycholic and tauro-ursochenodeoxycholic acid have failed to provide any evidence that these bile salts will affect the expression of ICAM-1, HLA class I or II antigen expression.

ANTIGEN PRESENTATION

The results outlined above have suggested that both HLA products and E2 may be abnormally expressed on biliary epithelial cells from patients with primary biliary cirrhosis. This raises the possibility that these biliary epithelial cells are able to present E2 to the immune system, thus resulting both in the appearance in serum of mitochondrial antibodies and of bile duct damage. In order to assess this possibility we used a proliferation assay based on the response of HLA class II restricted T cell clones to specific antigens in order to assess the ability of biliary epithelial cells to present antigen. BECs were grown to 80% confluence using standard techniques and then γ-irradiated. HLA-DR identical clones were established in tissue culture by Dr Hill Gaston, Department of Rheumatology, Queen Elizabeth Hospital. Peripheral blood lymphocytes were obtained from HLA-DR matched volunteers and γ-irradiated. Biliary epithelial cells, T cell clones, and peripheral blood mononuclear cells were established in co-culture in various combinations and stimulated with antigens, either PPD, P1 or phytohaemagglutinin plus interleukin-2. Preliminary results so far obtained failed to provide any evidence that biliary epithelial cells *in vitro* can be shown to present antigen resulting in proliferation of the T cell. There may be many reasons for the inability to demonstrate antigen presentation by biliary epithelial cells.

Clearly there are other potential systems which can be used to assess this possibility. However, it must be emphasized that studies on the distribution of E2 in lymph nodes show that a significant proportion of the sinus macrophages from PBC are very heavily stained with E2. The ability of macrophages to present antigen is well recognized, and it may be that biliary epithelial cells are able either not at all or only weakly to present antigen, and that presentation of E2 to the immune system occurs not in the liver but in the draining lymph nodes.

CONCLUSIONS

Biliary epithelial cells, the presumed target of immune-mediated damage in primary biliary cirrhosis, have aberrant expression of class II antigens and E2 on the membrane. The expression of MHC class II antigens on the membrane may be a consequence of locally released cytokines. However, the presence of E2 on the membrane of biliary epithelial cells from patients with primary biliary cirrhosis provides a possible link between the appearance of antimitochondrial antibodies and the generation of bile duct damage.

However, there are still very many questions to be answered. For example, it has not yet been shown whether E2 is co-expressed with MHC class II antigens. The nature of the E2 recognized by AMA on BECs is unclear; the mechanism whereby there is apparent membrane expression of E2 also requires further investigation. Furthermore the discordant appearance of E2 and E3 in biliary epithelial cells and hepatocytes requires further examination. Whether biliary epithelial cells can present antigen *in vivo* is uncertain. Our *in-vitro* studies have failed to provide any evidence of this.

The demonstration of E2 in the macrophages of the lymph nodes shown in the liver raises alternative possibilities for E2 presentation to the immune system. Approaches using isolated biliary epithelial cells may contribute to the understanding of this enigmatic disease.

References

1. Ballardini G, Mirakian R, Bianchi FB *et al.* Aberrant expression of HLA-DR antigens on bile duct epithelium in primary biliary cirrhosis. Lancet. 1984;2:1009–13.
2. Franco A, Barnaba V, Natali P *et al.* Expression of class I and class II major histocompatibility complex antigens on human hepatocytes. Hepatology. 1988;8:449–54.
3. Van Den Ord J, Selot R, Desmet V. Expression of MHC products by normal and abnormal bile duct epithelium. J Hepatol. 1986;3:310–17.
4. Calmus Y, Gane P, Rouger P, Poupon R. Hepatic expression of class I and class II major histocompatibility complex molecules in primary biliary cirrhosis. Hepatology. 1990;11: 12–15.
5. Chapman RW, Kelly P, Heryet A *et al.* Expression of HLA-DR antigens on bile duct epithelium in primary sclerosing cholangitis. Gut. 1988;29:422–7.
6. Steinhoff G, Wonigeit K, Pichlmayer R. Analysis of sequential changes in major histocompatibility complex expression in human liver grafts after transplantation. Transplantation. 1988;45:394–401.
7. So S, Platt J, Ascher N, Snover D. Increased expression of class I major histocompatibility complex expression in human liver grafts after transplantation. Transplantation. 1987;43: 79–85.
8. Calmus Y, Arvieux C, Gane P *et al.* Cholestasis induces major histocompatibility complex class I expression in hepatocytes. Hepatology. 1992;102:1371–7.
9. Innes G, Nagafuchi Y, Fuller B, Hobbs K. Increased expression of major histocompatibility antigens in the liver as a result of cholestasis. Transplantation. 1988;45:749–51.
10. Lindor K. What is the role of major histocompatibility complex expression in cholestasis? Gastroenterology. 1992;102:1429–30.
11. Himeno H, Saibara T, Onishi S *et al.* Administration of Interleukin-2 induces major histocompatibility complex class II antigens on the biliary epithelial cells, possibly through endogenous interferon production. Hepatology. 1992;16:409–17.
12. Okado Y, Sinnon K, Showsuke M *et al.* Blood group antigens in the intrahepatic biliary tree. I. Distribution in normal liver. J Hepatol. 1988;6:63–70.
13. Nakanuma Y, Sasaki M. Expression of blood group related antigens in the intrahepatic biliary tree and hepatocytes in normal liver and various hepatobiliary diseases. Hepatology. 1989;10:174–8.
14. Bloom S, Herryat A, Fleming K, Chapman RW. Inappropriate expression of blood group antigens on the biliary epithelium in PSC. Hepatology. 1990;12:841 (abstract).
15. Dustin M, Rothlein R, Bhan A *et al.* Induction by IL-1 and interferon, tissue distribution, biochemistry and function of natural adherence molecule (ICAM-1). J Immunol. 1986;137:245–51.

16. Adams D, Hubscher S, Shaw J *et al.* Increased expression of intercellular adhesion molecule-1 (ICAM-1) on bile duct in primary biliary cirrhosis and primary sclerosing cholangitis. Hepatology. 1991;14:426–31.
17. Adams D, Hubscher S, Shaw J *et al.* Intercellular adhesion molecule-1 on liver allografts during rejection. Lancet. 1989;2:1122–5.
18. Hultcrantz R, Broome U, Scheynius A. Lack of ICAM-1 expression in bile ducts from patients with PBC and PSC. Hepatology. 1991;14:63A.
19. Joplin R, Lindsay JG, Hubscher S *et al.* Distribution of dihydrolipoamide acetyltransferase in the liver and periportal lymph nodes of patients with primary biliary cirrhosis. Hepatology. 1991;14:442–7.
20. Joplin R, Johnson G, Lindsay JG *et al.* Distribution of dihydrolipoamide acetyltransferase (E2) in PBC does not correspond to that of the mitochondrial marker MCA151A. J Hepatol. 1992;16:A17.
21. Joplin R, Strain A, Neuberger J. Immunoisolation and culture of biliary epithelial cells from normal human liver. In vitro Cell Dev Biol. 1989;25:1189–92.
22. Joplin R, Strain A, Neuberger J. Biliary epithelial cells from the liver of patients with PBC: isolation, characterisation and short term culture. J Pathol. 1990;162:255–60.
23. Joplin R, Lindsay JG, Johnson G *et al.* Membrane dihydrolipoamide acetyltransferase (E2) on human biliary epithelial cells in primary biliary cirrhosis. Lancet. 1992;339:93–4.
24. Ayres RCS, Neuberger J, Shaw J, Adams D. *In vitro* induction of ICAM-1 and MHC antigens in human biliary epithelial cells by pre-inflammatory cytokines. Hepatology. 1991;14:97A.

47
Can enterobacterial antigens induce a primary biliary cirrhosis?

U. HOPF and R. STEMEROWICZ

THE IMMUNOPATHOLOGY OF PBC

In its precirrhotic phase primary biliary cirrhosis (PBC) might be more accurately designed chronic destructive non-suppurative cholangitis. It represents a syndrome with intrahepatic and extrahepatic manifestations and is often associated with inflammatory activity in secretory organs, including the salivary glands, the tear glands and the pancreas, which may constitute arthritis or other rheumatic and autoimmune diseases[1–3]. The syndrome of PBC bears some resemblance to chronic graft versus host disease[4–6].

PBC demonstrates a number of characteristics which suggest an immunological mechanism of disease. The presence of antimitochondrial antibodies (AMA) is a characteristic serological finding in PBC[7–10]. AMA which are specific for PBC react with species-unspecific antigens from the inner mitochondrial membrane and demonstrate three chief bands at approximately 40, 50 and 70–75 kDa in the immunoblot when incubated with mitochondria from beef heart or swine kidney[11–15]. These three mitochondrial target antigens of PBC-specific AMA have been associated with the 'M2 complex'[16]. They were identified as components of pyruvate dehydrogenase (PDH) and related enzymes[17–20]. The antibodies reacting with the PDH complex recognize the lipoyl-containing region of the polypeptide[21–23].

Additional immunological and serological characteristics of PBC include elevated serum IgM levels, circulating immune complexes[24,25], and activation of the complement system[26]. Antinuclear antibodies including anti-DNA antibodies are present in some cases. So-called mixed forms of PBC and autoimmune chronic active hepatitis may involve liver membrane antibodies (LMA), antibodies against actin and other subcellular structures[27].

Histological studies on livers from patients with PBC demonstrate inflammatory activity around the small intrahepatic bile ducts as well as destruction and proliferation of the ducts[28]. The inflammatory infiltrate is composed primarily of T cells[29]. Granulomas are common. The target of immunological attack is apparently the epithelium of the small bile ducts, which expresses

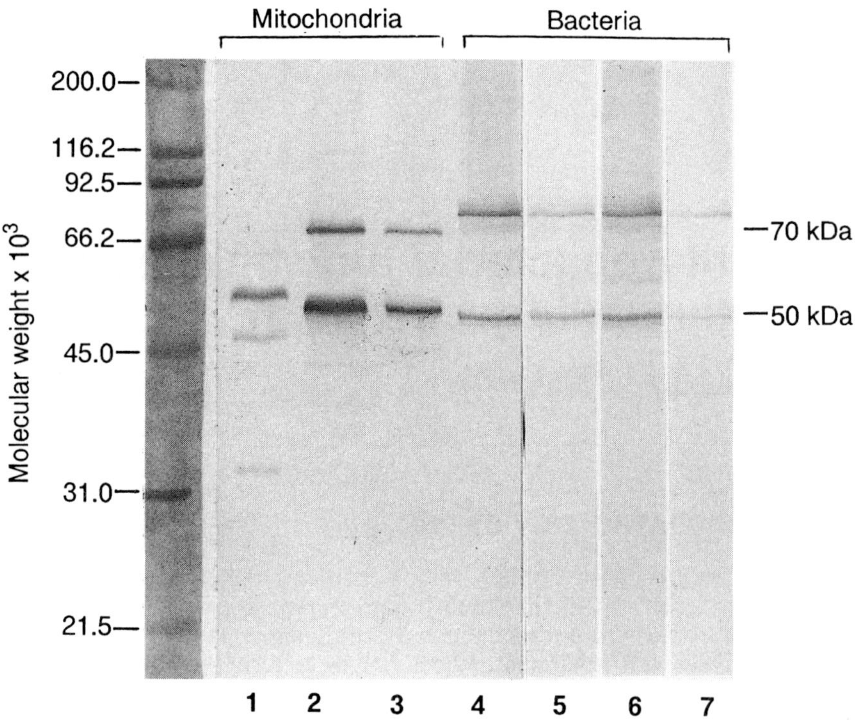

Fig. 1 Immunoblots of a representative serum sample from a patient with PBC tested against mitochondria and Enterobacteriaceae as antigens after separation by SDS-PAGE. (1) Mitochondria from rat liver. (2) Mitochondria from beef heart. (3) Mitochondria from swine kidney. (4) *E. coli* wild form. (5) *E. coli* R-form. (6) *Salmonella abortus equi.* (7) *Acinetobacter calcoaceticus*

histocompatibility antigens in a particular fashion[30] and PDH complex in their cytoplasm (see Chapter 46).

RELATIONSHIP BETWEEN PBC-SPECIFIC AMA AND ENTEROBACTERIACEAE

The AMA which appear in PBC represent a specific phenomenon which may be used for diagnosis of the disease, although the origin and significance of these antibodies have yet to be elucidated. It seems unlikely that they are involved in the pathogenesis of the disease. We believe that AMA and, ultimately, PBC are induced by exposure to enterobacterial antigens. Recent data supporting this hypothesis will be presented here. In the immunoblot PBC-specific antibodies recognize enterobacterial proteins which correspond to mitochondrial target proteins in molecular weight at 50 and 70–80 kDa[31,32] (Fig. 1). Absorption studies suggest partial identity between AMA-reactive mitochondrial and bacterial proteins. Our investigations have shown that all Gram-negative bacteria tested contain these proteins (Table

Table 1 Polypeptide antigens of various Gram-negative bacteria reacting in immunoblot studies with AMA-positive sera from patients with PBC

Bacterial strains	*LPS-form*	*Recognized polypeptides (kDa)*	
Escherichia coli 06;K2:H1	S	75–80	52
Escherichia coli H9	R	75–80	52
Salmonella typhimurium	S	70–85	50
Salmonella enteritidis	S	70–85	50
Salmonella abortus equi	S	70–85	50
Salmonella minnesota R60	Ra	75	
Salmonella minnesota R343	Rb	(75)	50
Salmonella minnesota R5	Rc	75	(50)
Salmonella minnesota R7	Rd1	75	50
Salmonella minnesota R595	Re	75	50
Klebsiella pneumoniae	S	80–85	50
Bacteroides fragilis	S	60	50
Acinetobacter calcaceticus	S	80–90	55; 40
Enterobacter cloacae	S		52
Neisseria meningitidis	S	70–75	47
*Halobacterium merismortui**	–	–	–
*Sulfolobus acidocaldarius**	–	–	–

*Archebacteria
Data from ref. 31

1), and the reaction is evident with whole bacteria and with enterobacterial plasma membranes as antigens (Fig. 2). Earlier biochemical studies have demonstrated dihydrolipoyl dehydrogenase in membranes of bacteria[33–36].

The expression of common antigenic epitopes between Gram-negative bacteria and mitochondria is compatible with endosymbiotic theory[37]. Since the structure and metabolism of aerobic bacteria and mitochondria are similar, it is possible to conclude that mitochondria derive phylogenetically from bacteria as a result of the integration of bacteria in amoeboid cells. This interesting hypothesis has gained support from analyses of RNA from ribosomes and mitochondria[38] and from our data showing common antigenic epitopes of membrane proteins. According to the endosymbiotic hypothesis the inner mitochondrial membrane represents the outer bacterial membrane, and this interpretation is compatible with the reactivity of PBC-specific AMA.

On the basis of these observations it was our intention to induce experimental PBC-specific AMA with Enterobacteriaceae. In order to test this possibility we immunized rabbits with a spectrum of available wild forms of *E. coli* and *Salmonella minnesota* as well as rough forms of *Salmonella*. Two animals inoculated with *Salmonella minnesota* R-mutants (R5 and R345) demonstrated AMA similar to those found in PBC[31,32] as shown by immunoblot with mitochondria (Fig. 3) or purified mammalian PDH (Fig. 4) as antigens. None of the rabbits immunized with enterobacterial wild forms developed AMA.

The fact that some enterobacterial R-mutants cause experimental animals to produce AMA equivalent to that found in PBC raises important questions about the specific characteristics of these R-mutants. Their most important characteristic is a defect in the lipopolysaccharide (LPS) molecule. This

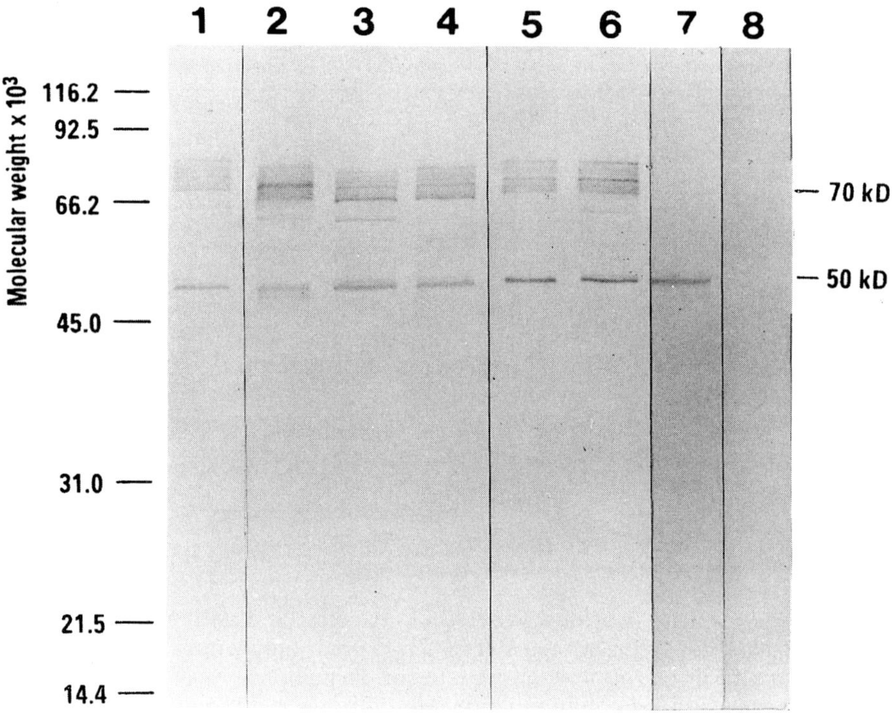

Fig. 2 Immunoblots with a representative PBC serum and *E. coli* subfractions as antigens. (1) *E. coli* 06 K2:H1 (whole bacterium). (2) Plasma membrane preparation of *E. coli* K1:H7. (3) External plasma membrane of *E. coli* K1:H7. (4) Plasma membranes from *E. coli* 0 114:H4. (5) Plasma membranes from *E. coli* 0 114:K9. (6) Ribosomes. (7) 30 S ribosomal subunit. (8) 50 S ribosomal subunit. (Antigen preparations were furnished by Dr L. Beutin of the Robert-Koch Institut, Berlin)

involves the absence of *O*-polysaccharide and an incomplete core polysaccharide[39,40]. This alters the membrane characteristics of the bacteria, since absence of the *O*-polysaccharide – which represents a strong antigen – leads to expression of other superficial antigens. The surface of R-mutants is more lipophilic and less readily water-soluble than that of S-forms[39–42].

CIRCULATING IMMUNE COMPLEXES (CIC) IN PBC

Increased levels of CIC are found in patients with PBC regardless of the stage of disease[43,44]. Dissociation of the complexes liberates antigens which have been characterized as biliary[43] and mitochondrial components[44].

We recently performed a study to identify antigens in CIC associated with PBC[45]. CIC were precipitated with polyethylene glycol, separated by SDS-PAGE, and transferred to nitrocellulose. Subsequent immunoblot studies were performed with AMA-positive sera from patients with PBC and with AMA-positive experimental antisera against *Salmonella minnesota* R5. Both

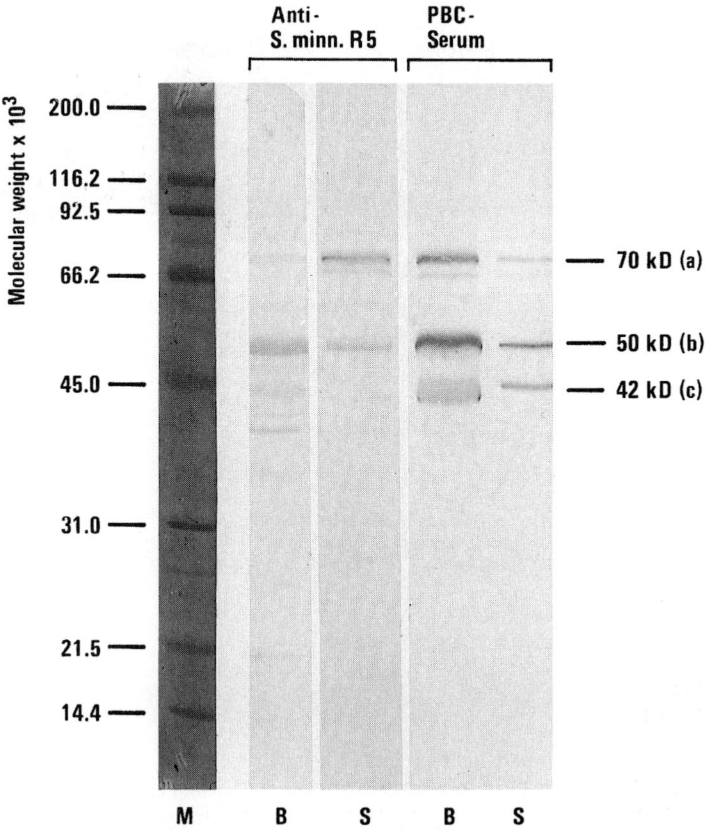

Fig. 3 Immunoblots with an experimental rabbit serum induced against *Salmonella minnesota* R5 and a representative PBC serum tested against mitochondria from beef heart (B) and swine kidney (S) as antigens

sera demonstrated bands at 50 kDa. We conclude that the 50 kDa protein is an enterobacterial component which may be identical to the biliary antigen described by Amoroso *et al.*[43] and with the mitochondrial antigen reported by Penner *et al.*[44].

DEMONSTRATION OF ENTEROBACTERIAL R-FORMS IN PATIENTS WITH PBC

The observation that certain R-mutants of *Salmonella minnesota* express immunogenic PBC-specific antigens led us to search for R-forms of Enterobacteriaceae in the faeces of patients with PBC and other liver diseases. All stool samples from patients with PBC contained R-forms of *E. coli* which comprised up to 50% of all aerobic Gram-negative bacteria in the samples[46]. Demonstration of R-forms from *E. coli* was much less common in patients with other liver diseases and in healthy controls.

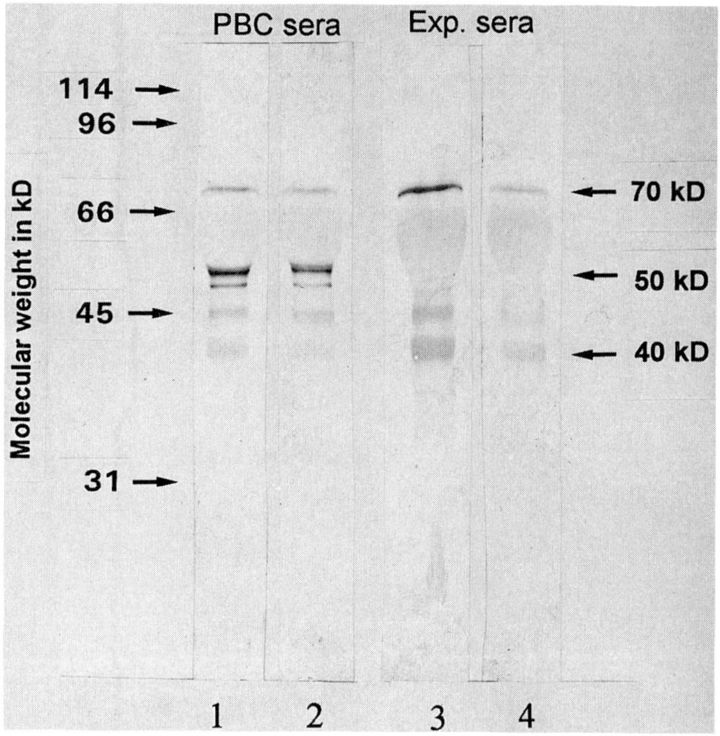

Fig. 4 Immunoblot of PBC sera (lanes 1 and 2) and experimental anti-sera against *Salmonella minnesota* R5 (lanes 3 and 4) with purified mammalian pyruvate dehydrogenase (Sigma Chemicals) as antigen

Patients with PBC commonly suffer urinary tract infections with Gram-negative bacteria[47,48]. Burroughs and co-workers recently documented a high proportion of R-forms in these cases[49,50]. There was also an association between urinary tract infection and circulating AMA against M2 complex in a group of patients without PBC. Additional studies will be necessary to demonstrate whether R-forms are present in the intestinal flora of these patients, and follow-up examinations will show whether this group is at increased risk of developing PBC. The close relationship between the presence of enterobacterial R-forms in the gut and urinary tract, and demonstration of PBC-specific AMA, suggests the possibility that AMA may be induced by Enterobacteriaceae.

LIPID A IN LIVER TISSUE OF PATIENTS WITH PBC

Enterobacterial antigens reach the liver from the gut, and LPS has been documented in the portal circulation of individuals without disease of the liver or the gut[51–53]. However, the concentration of LPS in portal blood is

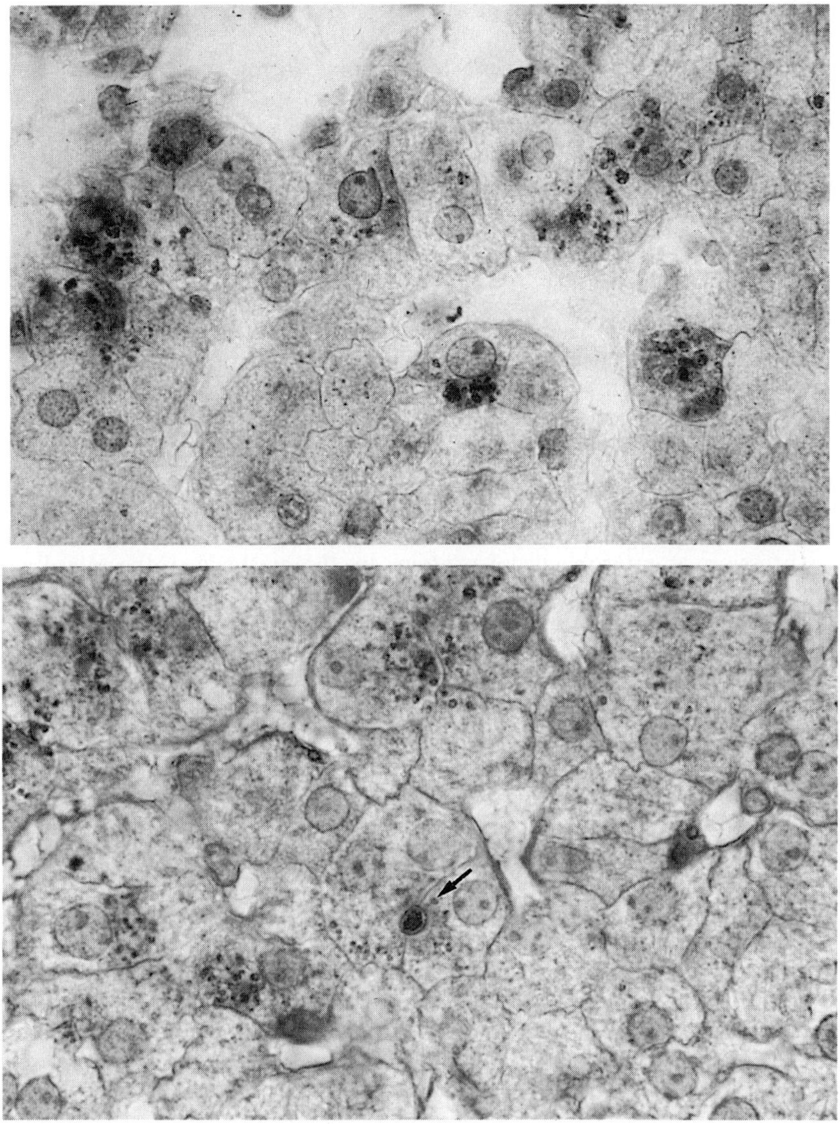

Fig. 5 Immunohistochemical demonstration (APAAP technique) of lipid A in liver tissue from a patient with PBC. Lipid A is visible as a coarse granular pattern in the cytoplasm of hepatocytes (upper part) and bile canaliculi (lower part, arrow) (× 324)

low and hepatic clearance of LPS is high, with the result that it was not possible to demonstrate LPS in human liver tissue. Recent studies using monoclonal antibodies have succeeded in demonstrating the presence of lipid A in liver tissue of patients with PBC[46]. Lipid A was found in the cytoplasm of hepatocytes and in bile canaliculi (Fig. 5).

Early experimental studies have shown different clearance patterns for lipid A and LPS from R- and S-forms in the liver[41,42,54]. The latter are taken up primarily by RES, while LPS from R-forms and free lipid A pass directly into hepatic cells and are excreted as metabolites with the bile. Therefore demonstration of lipid A in the hepatocytes in patients with PBC supports the hypothesis that the lipid A is derived from enterobacterial R-forms.

A HYPOTHESIS ON THE AETIOLOGY OF PBC

We assume that Enterobacteriaceae with altered plasma membrane characteristics represent the causative agent in PBC. Surface alterations are found in R-mutants, but the presence of plasmids or bacteriophages is another possibility. These questions require further clarification.

Our hypothesis is based on the assumption that enterobacterial plasma membrane proteins form complexes with LPS or lipid A and interact with the immune system in the gut and the spleen. The enterobacterial structures are taken up by the liver, metabolized, and excreted with the bile, resulting in expression of enterobacterial proteins by the epithelia of the bile ducts. Enterobacterial antigens in bile might bind to epithelium or metabolic components of the proteins might be expressed on the epithelia. Sensitized T cells originating from the lymphoid tissue of the gut would then attack enterobacterial antigens present on the epithelial surface of bile ducts.

Although AMA appear to have no role in the pathogenesis of PBC, it is possible that AMA-reactive proteins – epitopes of the PDH complex – are relevant target antigens. It is conceivable that other enterobacterial membrane antigens not associated with the PDH complex cause PBC, since PBC-specific AMA are not demonstrable in some individuals without PBC, and since AMA are not present in all patients with PBC.

AMA-reactive proteins have been phylogenetically preserved and there is natural immune tolerance to them. A number of factors are required to disturb immune tolerance and to increase immunity. LPS and lipid A fulfil these requirements and explain other immunological characteristics of PBC such as increased serum IgM levels, complement activation, and expression of histocompatibility antigens. Lipid A is the biologically active component of the LPS molecule and it induces reactions typical of endotoxin, e.g. adjuvant effect, mitogenicity with stimulation of IgM production, complement activation, and induction of endogenous mediators such as tumour necrosis factor (TNF) and interferon-γ[39,55–59]. In this way cells are stimulated to express MHC antigens. Lipid A itself is a weak antigen; therefore antibodies against lipid A are found at low titres, if at all, in patients with chronic liver disease[60,61]. The exception is alcoholic liver cirrhosis, in which ascension of flora in the small intestine is known[62].

The hypothesis presented above implies a number of open questions, the most important of which concerns characterization of the epithelial target antigens in bile ducts recognized by T lymphocytes in PBC. Are the target antigens components of the PDH complex and/or other polypeptides? Are the target antigens of autologous or microbiological origin? If the antigens were to prove identical to structures in enterobacterial membranes, then this would constitute significant evidence supporting the hypothesis. The genetic aspect of the disease remains to be considered. The preponderance of females among patients with PBC and the association of the disease with HLA-DRw3[63] and HLA DRw8[64] suggest a genetic disposition. This interpretation has been used to explain the fact that AMA are demonstrated more often than would otherwise be expected in the relatives of patients with PBC[65,66]. However, epidemiological factors may be implicated in this phenomenon.

References

1. James O, Macklon AF, Watson AJ. Primary biliary cirrhosis: a revised clinical spectrum. Lancet. 1981;1:1278–81.
2. Culp KS, Fleming CR, Duffy J. Autoimmune associations in primary biliary cirrhosis. Mayo Clin Proc. 1982;57:365–70.
3. Kaplan MM. Primary biliary cirrhosis. N Engl J Med. 1987;316:521–8.
4. Bernau D, Gisselbrecht C, Deveregie A, Feldmann G, Gluckmann E, Marty M, Boiron M. Histological and ultrastructural appearance of the liver during graft-versus-host disease complicating bone marrow transplantation. Transplantation. 1980;29:236–44.
5. Epstein O, Thomas HC, Sherlock S. Primary biliary cirrhosis: a dry gland syndrome with features of chronic graft-versus-host disease. Lancet. 1980;1:1164–8.
6. Siegert W, Stemerowicz R, Hopf U. Antimitochondrial antibodies in patients with chronic graft-versus-host disease. Bone Marrow Transplant. 1992;10:221–7.
7. Walker JG, Doniach D, Roitt IM, Sherlock S. Serological tests in the diagnosis of primary biliary cirrhosis. Lancet. 1965;i:827–31.
8. Berg PA, Doniach D, Roitt IM, Cooper HM. Mitochondrial antibodies in primary biliary cirrhosis. IV. Significance of the membrane structure for the complement fixing antigen. Immunology. 1969;17:281–7.
9. Sherlock S, Scheuer PJ. The presentation and diagnosis of 100 patients with primary biliary cirrhosis. N Engl J Med. 1973;289:674–8.
10. Kaplan MM, Gandolfo JV, Quaroni EG. An enzyme-linked immunosorbent assay (ELISA) for detecting antimitochondrial antibody. Hepatology. 1984;4:727–30.
11. Lindenborn-Fotinos J, Baum H, Berg PA. Mitochondrial antibodies in primary biliary cirrhosis: species and nonspecies specific determinants of M2 antigen. Hepatology. 1985;5:763–9.
12. Mendel-Hartvig I, Nelson BD, Lööf L, Tötterman TH. Primary biliary cirrhosis: further biochemical and immunological characterization of mitochondrial antigens. Clin Exp Immunol. 1985;62:371–9.
13. Baum H, Palmer C. The PBC-specific antigen. Mol Aspects Med. 1985;8:201–34.
14. Frazer IH, Mackay IR, Jordan TW, Whittingham S, Marzuki S. Reactivity of anti-mitochondrial autoantibodies in primary biliary cirrhosis; definition of two novel mito-chondrial peptide autoantigens. J Immunol. 1985;135:1739–45.
15. Ishii H, Saifuku K, Namihisa T. Reactivities and clinical relevance of antimitochondrial antibodies to four mitochondrial inner membrane proteins in sera of patients with primary biliary cirrhosis. Hepatology. 1987;7:134–6.
16. Berg PA, Klein R, Lindenborn-Fotions J, Klöppel G. ATP-ase associated antigen (M2): marker antigen for serological diagnosis of primary biliary cirrhosis. Lancet. 1982;2: 1423–6.
17. Yeaman SJ, Fussy SPM, Dannon DJ, James OFW, Martinez DJ, Bassendine MF. Primary biliary cirrhosis: identification of two major M2 mitochondrial autoantigens. Lancet. 1988;1:1067–70.
18. Fussey SPM, Guest JR, James OFW, Bassendine MF, Yeaman S. Identification and analysis of the two major M2 autoantigens in primary biliary cirrhosis. Proc Natl Acad Sci USA. 1988;85:8654–8.

19. Gershwin ME, Mackay IR, Sturgess A, Coppel RL. Identification and specificity of a cDNA encoding the 70 kD mitochondrial antigen recognized in primary biliary cirrhosis. J Immunol. 1987;138:3525–31.
20. Suhr CK, Danner DD, Ahmed A, Coppel RL, Mackay IR, Dickson ER, Gershwin ME. Reactivity of primary biliary cirrhosis sera with a human fetal liver cDNA clone of branched-chain α-keto acid dehydrogenase dihydrolipamide acetyltransferase, the 52 kD mitochondrial autoantigen. Hepatology. 1989;9:63–8.
21. Surh SD *et al.* Antimitochondrial autoantibodies in primary biliary cirrhosis recognize cross-reactive epitope(s) on protein X and dihydrolipoamide acetyltransferase of pyruvate dehydrogenase complex. Hepatology. 1989;10:127–33.
22. Fussey SPM, Ali ST, Guest JR, James OFW, Bassendine MF, Yeaman SJ. Reactivity of primary biliary cirrhosis sera with Escherichia coli dihydrolipoamide acetyltransferase (E2p): Characterization of the main immunogenic region. Proc Natl Acad Sci USA. 1990;87:3987–91.
23. Fussey SPM, Lindsay JG, Fuller C, Perham RN, Dale S, James OFW, Bassendine MF. Autoantiodies in primary biliary cirrhosis: analysis of reactivity against eukaryotic and prokaryotic 2-oxo acid dehydrogenase complexes. Hepatology. 1991;13:467–74.
24. Fakunle YM, Aranguibel F, DeVilliers D, Thomas HC, Sherlock S. Monomeric (7S) IgM in chronic liver disease. Clin Exp Immunol. 1979;38:204–10.
25. Thomas HC, DeVilliers D, Potter BJ, Hodgson H, Jain S, Jewell DP, Sherlock S. Immune complexes in acute and chronic liver diseases. Clin Exp Immunol. 1978;31:150–7.
26. Lindgren S, Laurell AB, Eriksson S. Complement compounds and activation in primary biliary cirrhosis. Hepatology. 1984;4:9–14.
27. Hopf U, Möller B, Lobeck H, Klein R, Berg PA. Immunserologische Differenzierung chronisch-cholestatischer Leberentzündungen. Dtsch Med Wochenschr. 1985;110:1924–9.
28. Scheuer PJ. Primary biliary cirrhosis: liver biopsy interpretation, 3rd edn. London: Baillière Tindall; 1980;47–56.
29. Van den Oord JJ, Fevery J, DeGroote D, Desmet VJ. Immunohistochemical characterization of inflammatory infiltrates in primary biliary cirrhosis. Liver. 1984;4:264–74.
30. Ballardini G, Mirakian R, Bianchi FB, Pisi E, Doniach D, Bottazzo GF. Aberrant expression of HLA-DR antigens on bile duct epithelium in primary biliary cirrhosis: relevance to pathogenesis. Lancet. 1984;2:1009–13.
31. Stemerowicz R, Hopf U, Möller B, Wittenbrink C, Rodloff A, Reinhardt R, Freudenberg M, Galanos C. Are mitochondrial antibodies in primary biliary cirrhosis induced by R(rough)-mutants of Enterobacteriaceae? Lancet. 1988;2:1166–70.
32. Hopf U, Stemerowicz R, Möller B, Rodloff A, Reinhardt R, Freudenberg M, Galanos C. Wird die primäre biliäre Zirrhose (PBC) durch enterobakterielle Antigene induziert? Neuere Daten und hypothetische Aspekte. In: Thaler H, ed. Gastroenterologie aus immunologischer Sicht. Thieme-Verlag, Stuttgart; 1989:149–55.
33. Owen P *et al.* Identification of antigen 19/27 as dihydrolipoyl dehydrogenase and its probable involvement in ubiquinone-mediated NADH-dependent transport phenomena in vesicles of *Escherichia coli.* FEBS Microbiol Lett. 1980;7:345–8.
34. Kerscher L, Oesterholt D. Pyruvate ferredoxin oxidoreductase – new findings on an ancient enzyme. Trends Biochem Sci. 1982;7:371–4.
35. Danson MJ *et al.* Dihydrolipoamide dehydrogenase from holophilic archaebacteria. Biochem J. 1984;218:811–18.
36. Danson MJ *et al.* Dihydrolipoamide dehydrogenase from *Trypanosoma brucei.* Characterization and cellular location. Biochem J. 1987;243:661–5.
37. Margulis L. Origin of eukaryotic cells. New Haven: Yale University Press; 1970.
38. Künzel H, Köchel HG. Evolution of rRNA and origin of mitochondria. Nature. 1981;293:751–5.
39. Galanos C, Freudenberg MA, Joh K, Freudenberg N, Lüderitz O. Bacterial endotoxins: chemical and biological properties. In: Keppler D, Popper H, Bianchi C, Reutter W, editors. Mechanism of hepatocyte injury and death. Lancaster: MTP; 1983:203–13.
40. Lugtenberg B, Van Alphen L. Molecular architecture and functioning of the outer membrane of *Escherichia coli* and other gram-negative bacteria. Biochim Biophys Acta. 1983;737: 51–115.
41. Ramadori G, Hopf U, Galanos C, Freudenberg M, Meyer zum Büschenfelde KH. *In*

vitro and *in vivo* reactivity of lipopolysaccharides and lipid A with parenchymal and nonparenchymal liver cells in mice. In The reticuloendothelial system and pathogenesis of liver disease. H. Lier, Grün M, editors. Elsevier, Amsterdam; 1980:285–95.
42. Freudenberg MA, Freudenberg N, Galanos C. Time course of cellular distribution of endotoxin in liver, lungs and kidney of rats. Br J Exp Pathol. 1982;63:56–64.
43. Amoroso P, Vergani D, Wojcicka BM, McFarlane IG, Eddleston ALWF, Tee DEH, Williams R. Identification of biliary antigens in circulating immune complexes in primary biliary cirrhosis. Clin Exp Immunol. 1980;42:95–8.
44. Penner E, Goldenberg H, Albini B, Weiser MM, Milgrom F. Immune complexes in primary biliary cirrhosis contain mitochondrial antigens. Clin Immunol Immunopathol. 1982;22: 394–9.
45. Stemerowicz R, Möller B, Küther D, Freudenberg M, Galanos C, Hopf U. Are antigenic components of circulating immune complexes (CIC) in primary biliary cirrhosis (PBC) of enterobacterial origin? Eur J Gastroenterol Hepatol. 1990;2:112 (abstract).
46. Hopf U, Möller B, Stemerowicz R, Rodloff A, Lobeck H, Freudenberg M, Galanos C, Huhn D. *Escherichia coli* rough (R) mutants in the gut and lipid A in the liver from patients with primary biliary cirrhosis (PBC). Lancet. 1989;2:1419–22.
47. Burroughs AK, Rosenstein IJ, Epstein O, Hamilton-Miller JMT, Brumfitt W, Sherlock S. Bacteriuria and primary biliary cirrhosis. Gut. 1984;25:133–7.
48. Morreale M, Tsigotis M, Hughes MD, Brumfitt W, McIntyre N, Burroughs AK. Significant bacteriuria has prognostic significance in primary biliary cirrhosis. J Hepatol. 1989;9: 149–58.
49. Burroughs AK, Butler P, Valle F, Baum H, Hamilton-Miller J, Brumfitt W, McIntyre N. M2 antibodies and rough (R) mutants in urine of normal women with recurrent bacteriuria, and women with PBC. J Hepatol. 1990;11:13 (abstract).
50. Butler P, Valle F, Hamilton-Miller JMT, Brumfitt W, Baum H, Burroughs AK. M2 mitochondrial antibodies and urinary rough mutant bacteria in patients with primary biliary cirrhosis and in patients with recurrent bacteriuria. J Hepatol. 1992:in press.
51. Prytz H, Holst-Christensen J, Korner B, Liehr H. Portal venous and systemic endotoxaemia in patients without liver disease and systemic endotoxaemia in patients with cirrhosis. Scand J Gastroenterol. 1976;11:857–63.
52. Jacob AI, Goldberg PK, Bloom N, Degenshein GA, Kozinn PJ. Endotoxin and bacteria in portal blood. Gastroenterology. 1977;72:1268–70.
53. Triger DR, Boyer TD, Levin J. Portal and systemic bacteraemia and endotoxemia in liver disease. Gut. 1978;19:935–9.
54. Hopf U, Ramadori G, Möller B, Galanos C. Hepatocellular clearance function of bacterial lipopolysaccharides and free lipid A in mice with endotoxic shock. Am J Emerg Med. 1984;2:13–19.
55. Matsuura M, Kojima Y, Homma Y. Biological activities of synthetic lipid A analogues. In Bacterial endotoxin: chemical, biological and clinical aspects. Homma Y, Kanegasaki S, Lüderitz O, Shiba T, Westphal O, editors. Westphal Verlag: Chemie Weinheim; 1984:61–72.
56. Johnson AG, Gaines S, Landy M. Studies on the O antigen of *Salmonella typhosa*: V. Enhancement of antibody response to protein antigens by the purified lipopolysaccharide. J Exp Med. 1956;103:225.
57. Anderson T, Möller G, Sjoberg D. Selective induction of DNA synthesis in T and B lymphocytes. Cell Immunol. 1973;4:381–7.
58. Nixdorff KK, Schlecht S, Rüde E, Westphal O. Immunological response to *Salmonella* R antigens. The bacterial cell and the protein edestin as carriers for R oligosaccharide determinants. Immunology. 1975;29:87–102.
59. Galanos C, Rietschel T, Lüderitz O, Westphal O. Interaction of lipopolysaccharides and lipid A with complement. Eur J Biochem. 1971;19:143–52.
60. Möller B, Hopf U, Martin P, Galanos C. Detection and characterization of antibodies against lipopolysaccharides (LPS) from E. coli and free lipid A in healthy subjects and patients with chronic liver diseases. Immunobiology. 1983;165:321 (abstract).
61. Stemerowicz R, Möller B, Martin P, Heesemann J, Wenzel BE, Galanos C, Freudenberg M, Hopf U. Antibody activity against lipopolysaccharides, lipid A and proteins from Enterobacteriaceae in patients with inflammatory liver diseases. Autoimmunity. 1990;7: 305–15.

62. Martini GA, Phear EA, Reuner B. The bacterial content of the small intestine in normal and cirrhotic patients, relation to methionine toxicity. Clin Sci. 1957;16:35–51.
63. Ercilla G, Pares A, Arriaga F, Bruguera M, Castillo R, Rodes J, Vivos J. Primary biliary cirrhosis associated with HLA-DRw3. Tissue Antigens. 1979;14:449–52.
64. Manns MP *et al.* HLA-DRw8 and complement C4 deficiency as risk factors in primary biliary cirrhosis. Gastroenterology. 1991;101:1367–9.
65. Galbraith RM, Smith M, Mackenzie RM, Tee DE, Doniach D, Williams R. High prevalence of seroimmunologic abnormalities in relatives of patients with active chronic hepatitis or primary biliary cirrhosis. N Engl J Med. 1974;290:63–9.
66. Salaspuro MP, Laitinen OJ, Lelitda J, Makkonen H, Räsänen JA, Sipponen P. Immunological parameters, viral antibodies, and biochemical and histological findings in relatives of patients with chronic active hepatitis and primary biliary cirrhosis. Scand J Gastroenterol. 1976;11:3131.

48
Ursodeoxycholic acid alters hepatocyte membrane structure and function: a therapeutic approach?

U. LEUSCHNER, S. GÜLDÜTUNA, T. YOU, S. BHATTI, G. ZIMMER and H. P. DIENES

It has been shown that, in patients with primary biliary cirrhosis (PBC), ursodeoxycholic acid (UDCA) improves liver function tests and symptoms[1-3]. It is still unclear, however, whether UDCA replaces the more apolar, so-called toxic bile acids, chenodeoxycholic acid (CDCA), deoxycholic acid (DCA) and lithocholic acid (LCA) from the hepatocyte or from endothelial cells of the biliary tree, whether this hypothetical replacement is caused by an increased faecal excretion of toxic bile salts[4], a suppression of their synthesis or a shift into different compartments of the circulating bile acid pool[5], or whether UDCA has a direct protective influence on cell structures, without changing kinetics, concentrations or patterns of the toxic bile salts.

The main question is what happens on the molecular level in the hepatocyte, when UDCA is administered. Do bile acids alter cell structures and does a change in the molecular structure mean a change in their functions; is it a permanent or reversible alteration, etc.? Since at present most investigators concentrate on questions of bile acid, phospholipid or cholesterol metabolism, all these questions concerning molecular morphology and function are completely open.

Since in animal experiments CDCA or LCA destroyed basolateral hepatocyte membranes (and to a lesser extent canalicular membranes) when administered orally in dosages of 90–500 mg/kg bodyweight daily over a period of 3 months[6,7], we started our investigations on molecular changes in heptocyte structures with isolated phospholipid membranes. First, we investigated red blood cell membranes; later, basolateral and canalicular hepatocyte membranes. Structure analyses were performed by electron paramagnetic resonance spectroscopy (EPR). Membranes were incubated with CDCA, DCA, UDCA and their conjugates. The results were compared with data from chemical analyses of membrane lipids and with data obtained after incubation of membrane pellets with [^{14}C]tauro-UDCA and ^{86}Rb.

Further, we investigated Na/K-ATPase at basolateral and Mg-ATPase at canalicular hepatocyte membranes and, in patients with primary biliary cirrhosis stages I and II, the expression of HLA class I/II antigens after 9 months therapy with UDCA, 10 mg/kg per day.

RESULTS

The apolar CDCA and DCA increased membrane polarity and fluidity and the incorporation of water. Simultaneously, CDCA dissolved cholesterol and phospholipids from the pellets. UDCA and tauro-ursodeoxycholic acid (TUDCA) were incorporated into phospholipid membranes, decreased polarity, and prevented lipid solubilization. UDCA incorporation was shown by preincubation of membranes with UDCA, several washing procedures with Pi-buffer at pH 7.4, followed by incubation with CDCA. In these experiments incubation with CDCA did not change membrane structure, which means that UDCA must have been fixed to the membrane surface or was incorporated into the membrane texture. Incorporation was also shown by incubation of membranes with labelled TUDCA and ^{86}Rb. ^{86}Rb is not fixed to biomembranes, thus representing the intermembraneous spaces of the pellet. After several washing procedures with buffer, ^{86}Rb has nearly completely disappeared from the pellet; UDCA had not.

Using 16-doxyl-stearic acid and 5-doxyl-stearic acid as different spin labels for the EPR method, we could show that UDCA occupies different sites in the phospholipid membranes than tauro-UDCA, although the two have a similar protective effect.

During CDCA incubation Na/K-ATPase decreased parallel to the increase of membrane polarity and the loss of membrane lipids, while there was no change in Mg-ATPase in canalicular hepatocyte membranes. UDCA decreased the expression of HLA class I/II antigens on hepatocyte membranes.

CONCLUSIONS

UDCA prevents damage of basolateral hepatocyte membranes caused by apolar bile salts. Membrane damage is accompanied by a decrease in Na/K-ATPase, and membrane stabilization by a loss of HLA antigens. Both stabilization of structure and function are probably caused by an incorporation of UDCA into the membrane texture, similar to cholesterol.

A major problem of all investigations on bile acid toxicity is that, to date, no-one has shown that bile acids are really toxic compounds in physiological concentrations, and that no-one knows what a physiological concentration is in which compartment near or inside of living cells. Therefore, we recently started a series of experiments changing bile salt concentrations, incubation times, incubation volumes, temperature and other conditions. These experiments showed that comparable results, as described above, can be obtained with concentrations of 100–300 μmol/l, whereas our investigations presented here had been performed with 2–20 mmol/l concentrations, and other investigators started experiments with even higher concentrations.

References

1. David R, Kurtz W, Strohm WD, Leuschner U. Die Wirkung von Ursodesoxycholsäure bei chronischen Leberkrankheiten. Eine Pilotstudie (abstr.). Z Gastroenterologie. 1985;23:420.
2. Fisher MM, Paradine ME. Influence of ursodeoxycholic acid (UDCA) on biochemical parameters in cholestatic liver disease. Gastroenterology. 1986;90:1725 (abstract).
3. Leuschner U, Fischer H, Kurtz W, Güldütuna S, Hübner K, Hellstern A, Gatzen M, Leuschner M. Ursodeoxycholic acid in primary biliary cirrhosis: Results of a controlled double blind trial. Gastroenterology. 1989;97:1268–74.
4. Stiehl A, Raedsch R, Rudolph G. Acute effects of ursodeoxycholic and chenodeoxycholic acid on the small intestinal absorption of bile acids. Gastroenterology. 1990;98:424–8.
5. Beuers U, Spengler U, Zwiebel FM, Pauletzki J, Fischer S, Paumgartner G. Effect of ursodeoxycholic acid on the kinetics of the major hydrophobic bile acids in health and in chronic cholestatic liver disease. Hepatology. 1992;15:603–8.
6. Miyai K, Price VM, Fisher MM. Bile acid metabolism in mammals. Ultrastructural studies on the intrahepatic cholestasis induced by lithocholic and chenodeoxycholic acids in the rat. Lab Invest. 1971;24:292–302.
7. Leuschner U. Liver tissue injury due to chenodeoxycholic acid: Metabolic pathways and toxicity. In: Paumgartner G, Stiehl A, Gerok W, editors. Biological effects of bile acids. Lancaster: MTP Press; 1978:191–203.

49
Therapeutic strategies which interfere with the immune system

R. POUPON, Y. CALMUS and R. E. POUPON

Primary biliary cirrhosis (PBC) is a good example of a disease in which two distinct processes damage the liver: immunological aggression and injury of hepatocytes by bile acids. Several histopathological and immunochemical features indicate a primary destructive process of intrahepatic bile duct segments and suggest an immunologically mediated mechanism for bile duct loss. In view of this hypothesis of the pathogenesis, most of the drugs evaluated as therapy for PBC during the past 15 years have been chosen for their immunosuppressive and anti-inflammatory properties. Corticosteroids lead to improvement in liver function and in histological features, but their long-term administration causes severe osteopenia[1]. Azathioprine, an immunosuppressive drug evaluated in two double-blind studies, has no beneficial effect on clinical symptoms, biochemical variables or histological progression[2,3]. Further analysis of the second trial, however, indicated that there might be a beneficial effect on survival[4]. In eight controlled trials, D-penicillamine had no beneficial effect on primary biliary cirrhosis[5–12]. Chlorambucil leads to an improvement in biochemical variables, IgM concentrations and some histological features of PBC, but its long-term administration is limited by potentially severe side-effects[13]. Colchicine improves biochemical variables but has no effect on clinical or histological features[14–16]. Recently, promising results have been reported with cyclosporin[17,18]. In both studies there was an improvement in biological variables, and in one there was also an improvement in clinical and histological features. However, there was a very high incidence of side-effects (particularly renal toxicity), showing that prolonged administration requires careful evaluation.

We proposed ursodeoxycholate (UDCA) as a novel therapeutic approach to PBC, on the basis of evidence suggesting that hepatic lesions in chronic cholestatic diseases can result from intracellular accumulation of potentially toxic bile acids. When chronically given to animals, chenodeoxycholate and lithocholate can induce bile duct and ductular proliferation, as well as fibrosis and cirrhosis. In contrast, UDCA is devoid of toxicity both *in vitro* and in humans. We postulated that long-term administration of UDCA, by modifying the concentration and composition of the circulating bile acids, might be beneficial in patients with chronic cholestatic disorders.

To test this hypothesis we conducted an uncontrolled prospective pilot study to investigate the effects of long-term UDC administration on clinical symptoms and biochemical test results in 15 consecutive patients, most of whom had symptomatic stage I–III PBC[19]. The proportion of patients with pruritus requiring cholestyramine was significantly lower at 2 years, as was the proportion of patients with hyperbilirubinaemia. Activities of alkaline phosphatases, γ-glutamyltransferase, alanine aminotransferase and aspartate aminotransferase fell sharply during the first year of treatment, and more slowly thereafter. By contrast, the improvement in bilirubin levels and bromosulphthalein elimination was gradual, with a return to normal values at 2 years. Since bilirubin and BSP elimination truly reflect liver function, this finding strongly suggested that UDCA was beneficial in PBC.

To confirm and extend these data, we designed a randomized, double-blind trial to assess the efficacy and safety of UDCA in patients with PBC[20]. Patients were admitted to the trial regardless of the duration of the symptoms and histological severity. It was a multicentre trial comparing UDCA with a placebo, given the absence of a reference treatment. The end-points chosen to define failure of UDCA treatment were as follows: (a) a doubling of bilirubin concentrations to above 70 μmol/l or a value of more than 200 μmol/l at two consecutive measurements 3 months apart; (b) the occurrence of a serious complication, e.g. gastrointestinal bleeding from oesophageal varices, ascites or encephalopathy; (c) the occurrence of a major adverse effect.

Following randomization, 73 patients with PBC received UDCA (13–15 mg/kg per day) and 73 received the placebo. At entry, the two groups were well matched for age, sex, time since initial diagnosis, and histological severity: in the UDCA group 50% of the patients had stage I–II disease compared to 56% in the placebo group.

The failure rates were significantly different between the two groups ($p < 0.01$, Cox model). One patient in each group withdrew because of adverse effects. After 2 years of treatment the proportion of treated patients with clinically overt disease had fallen significantly ($p < 0.02$); in particular, there was a clear improvement in terms of the severity of pruritus. Patients receiving UDCA showed significant improvements in serum bilirubin, alkaline phosphatase, ALT, AST, GGT, cholesterol and IgM levels ($p < 0.001$), the antimitochondrial antibody titre ($p < 0.01$), and the Mayo risk score ($p < 0.001$). There was a significant improvement in the UDCA group relative to the placebo group in the following histological features: degree of bile-duct paucity, degree of ductular proliferation, degree of portal mononuclear-cell infiltration, degree of piecemeal necrosis, degree of lobular inflammation, degree of parenchymal necrosis and severity of cholestasis. The degree of fibrosis was not different between the two groups. Overall, the UDCA group showed a significant improvement in a multiparametric liver-histology score ($p < 0.002$).

At the end of this controlled trial all the patients received UDCA and were followed up for a further 2 years on the basis of the same criteria. These data will enable us to determine the course of PBC in patients receiving

UDCA, in terms of histological criteria (data not yet available) and the onset of events necessitating liver transplantation. In our opinion the outcome of PBC is no longer a simple question of survival, but must rather be seen in terms of whether patients can be treated medically, or if they develop end-stage disease, by liver transplantation. Forty-eight months after the initial randomization, UDCA has considerably slowed the progression of the disease. Indeed, only two patients in the UDCA group have undergone OLT, compared to 12 patients from the original placebo group ($p < 0.001$, Cox model).

One question which is often posed is whether the therapeutic effect of UDCA depends on the severity of the disease, so we analysed the factors predictive of the response to treatment. The analysis (Cox model) showed that the probability of failure during the first 2 years of treatment with UDCA depended mainly on the extent of liver fibrosis (evaluated by serum markers of fibrosis, such as hyaluronic acid and PIIINP), the severity of portal hypertension (judged by the presence of splenomegaly) and, to a lesser degree, hyperbilirubinaemia.

A case-by-case analysis of the treatment failures indicated that several of the following factors could be involved: non-compliance, abnormal UDCA metabolism, additional hepatic disease (hepatotoxicity due to vitamin A, active autoimmune hepatitis of type 1, chronic active hepatitis due to virus C, and post-biopsy arterioportal fistula).

The mechanisms by which UDCA is beneficial in PBC are only partly known. Nevertheless, one of the main mechanisms is the effect of UDCA on the ileal and hepatic bile acid transport systems. UDCA, or its conjugated form, diminishes the active ileal absorption of cholic and chenodeoxycholic acids (CDCA) explaining the observed lowering of the serum concentration of these two bile acids following treatment with UDCA[21,22]. However, this effect does not explain all the beneficial effects of UDCA: (a) in the perfused isolated liver model, UDCA prevents or reduces the toxicity of cholic, chenodeoxycholic and lithocholic acids[23]; (b) cholestyramine reduces the intestinal absorption of bile acids but does not have a major effect on the progression of the disease; (c) in the short bowel syndrome, treatment with UDCA has a beneficial effect on liver function test results (unpublished data). It has been suggested that UDCA has a cytoprotective effect, directly on hepatocytes. We studied the effects of UDCA and tauro-UDCA alone and in combination on the viability and certain functions of human hepatocytes in primary culture[24]. Tauro-UDCA did not affect intracellular concentrations of CDCA when added concomitantly. CDCA (100–500 μmol/l) induced concentration-dependent increases in LDH leakage and lipid peroxidation and decreases in cellular protein synthesis, albumin secretion and intracellular glutathione levels. Neither tauro-UDCA nor UDCA had similar effects at the same concentrations, nor did they have a protective effect when added concomitantly with CDCA. These results indicate that UDCA has no direct cytoprotective effect when the bile acid concentrations to which hepatocytes are exposed are unchanged. In contrast to hepatocytes in primary culture, hepatocyte couplets have the ability to maintain their polarity and function in short-term culture. In this model the cholestatic potency of certain drugs or substances (such as CDCA or lithocholate) can be demonstrated. It has clearly been shown that UDCA has the ability to prevent bile acid-induced toxicity in this model[25]. In other words, these observations suggest that the cytoprotective effect of UDCA, observed only in a polarized system, is related to its ability to promote canalicular efflux of toxic bile acids. According to these observations, the beneficial effect of UDCA in PBC and other cholestatic diseases could occur in the following way. Initially, UDCA, or one of its conjugates, would directly increase biliary excretion of bile acids; their return to the liver would then be limited by an inhibitory effect of UDCA on their intestinal absorption. Liver cell metabolism and functions would be improved by the sustained reduction in the concentration of endogenous bile acids and the predominant presence of UDCA in the blood perfusing the liver and within the hepatocytes. The mechanisms by which UDCA, a bile acid with very high intrinsic hepatic clearance[26], increases the vectorial transport of bile acids by hepatocytes, are currently under study. Recently, Häussinger and co-workers have provided circumstantial evidence that increased taurocholate intrinsic clearance induced by UDCA is mediated by hepatocellular swelling[27].

Our controlled trial unexpectedly showed that some of the immunological markers of PBC improved with UDCA, suggesting that bile acids and/or UDCA interfere with immune regulation in this disease. HLA molecules, more specifically class I species, are the main targets of the cytotoxic reaction. In normal human liver, HLA expression is limited to sinusoidal and biliary cells; and hepatocytes do not express HLA molecules. In contrast, abnormal expression of class I molecules on hepatocytes is a salient feature of PBC. A study was undertaken to evaluate the effects of UDCA therapy on this expression[28]. Twelve untreated patients with PBC were compared to eight patients treated for at least 1 year with 13–15 mg/kg per day UDCA and to eight control patients without hepatobiliary disease. MHC expression was studied by means of an immunofluorescence technique. No class I molecules were expressed on the hepatocytes of the control subjects. In contrast, there was strong expression on hepatocytes of untreated PBC patients, while UDCA treatment induced a dramatic reduction in HLA class I expression. No class II molecules were expressed in the bile ducts of the controls, whereas there was strong class II expression in the PBC patients, with no significant difference between the treated and untreated patients. These results suggest that cholestasis itself can induce aberrant expression of MHC class I molecules on hepatocytes. The beneficial effect of UDCA at this level could result from an improvement in the cholestasis or a direct effect on hepatocytes. We recently showed that an immune mechanism is not involved in the cholestasis-induced expression of MHC class I molecules, but that cholestasis itself is able to modulate their expression[29]. To further investigate the role of bile acids in HLA expression by hepatocytes, we used human hepatocytes in primary culture. CDCA induced hyperexpression of class I MHC molecules, which was concentration-dependent from 100 to 500 μmol/l. In contrast, UDCA and its tauroconjugate had no significant effect. CDCA, UDCA and tauro-UDCA had no effect on hepatocyte MHC class II expression, which did not exceed 10% of the cells[30]. These results suggest that the reduction in hepatocyte MHC class I antigen expression induced by UDCA could block periportal and lobular cell necrosis by suppressing the cytotoxic T cell target, thereby slowing the progression of PBC.

We also discovered that endogenous bile acids have strong immunosuppressive properties. We assessed the respective effect of cholestasis, CDCA and UDCA using mixed lymphocyte culture as a model of allogenic immune response. CDCA induced a dose-dependent inhibition of the proliferative response (0–150 μmol/l). Mononuclear cells obtained from bile duct-ligated mice had a normal immunostimulatory effect, whereas responder cells obtained from such animals showed a profoundly impaired proliferative response, suggesting that responder T cells are the main target of cholestasis-induced immune defect. In contrast to CDCA, UDCA had no inhibitory effect on the allogenic immune response at concentrations up to 50 μmol/l.

In addition, CDCA, in contrast to UDCA, exhibits strong effects on mononuclear cell activity assessed in terms of cytokine production *in vitro*[31]. Reduced production of various cytokines or expression of their mRNA in the liver has been reported in PBC[32–34] and experimental models of autoimmune disease[35]. This rather unresponsive state may be due, at least in part, to bile acids and may be an important factor in the autoimmune phenomenon. Alleviation of this unresponsive state by UDCA might explain the beneficial effect of the drug on some immune features of PBC.

Until the 1980s, the possible role of bile acids in the initiation of liver injury in humans was only suspected on the basis of the toxicity of whole bile and bile salts, and of studies showing elevations in serum and tissue levels of bile salts in liver diseases. The beneficial effects of UDCA in PBC have provided the first firm evidence that bile acids may in some way be related to liver injury in humans.

These observations raise a series of questions and challenges in clinical research, as well as in cellular and molecular biology: is UDCA capable of modifying the progression and prognosis of other cholestatic diseases of the child and the adult and, more generally, liver diseases in which the enterohepatic bile acid circulation is disturbed? Is it possible and warranted to design UDCA analogues with stronger activities and more specific targets? How might UDCA and these analogues modulate fundamental cell or organelle functions and cell-to-cell interrelationships in the normal and cholestatic liver?

References

1. Mitchison HC, Bassendine MF, Malcolm AJ *et al.* A pilot, double-blind, controlled 1-year trial of prednisolone treatment in primary biliary cirrhosis: hepatic improvement but greater bone loss. Hepatology. 1989;10:420–9.
2. Heathcote J, Ross A, Sherlock S. A prospective controlled trial of azathioprine in primary biliary cirrhosis. Gastroenterology. 1976;70:656–60.
3. Crowe J, Christensen E, Smith M *et al.* Azathioprine in primary biliary cirrhosis: a preliminary report of an international trial. Gastroenterology. 1980;78:1005–10.
4. Christensen E, Neuberger J, Crowe J *et al.* Beneficial effect of azathioprine and prediction of prognosis in primary biliary cirrhosis. Final results of an international trial. Gastroenterology. 1985;89:1084–91.

5. Triger DR, Manifold IH, Cloke P, Underwood JCE. D-Penicillamine in primary biliary cirrhosis: two year results of a single centre, double-blind controlled trial. Gut. 1980;21: 919–20 (abstract).
6. Bassendine MF, Macklon AF, Mulcahy R, James OFW. Controlled trial of high and low dose D-penicillamine in primary biliary cirrhosis: results at three years. Gut. 1982;23:909 (abstract).
7. Epstein O, Jain S, Lee RG *et al.* D-Penicillamine treatment improves survival in primary biliary cirrhosis. Lancet. 1981;1:1275–7.
8. Matloff DS, Alpert E, Resnick RH, Kaplan MM. A prospective trial of D-penicillamine in primary biliary cirrhosis. N Engl J Med. 1982;306:319–26.
9. Taal BG, Schalm SW, Ten Kate FWJ *et al.* Low therapeutic value of D-penicillamine in a short-term prospective trial in primary biliary cirrhosis. Liver. 1983;3:345–52.
10. Neuberger J, Christensen E, Portmann B *et al.* Double blind controlled trial of D-penicillamine in patients with primary biliary cirrhosis. Gut. 1985;26:114–19.
11. Bodenheimer HC, Schaffner F, Sternlieb I *et al.* A prospective clinical trial of D-penicillamine in the treatment of primary biliary cirrhosis. Hepatology. 1985;5:1139–42.
12. Dickson ER, Fleming TR, Wiesner RH *et al.* Trial of penicillamine in advanced primary biliary cirrhosis. N Engl J Med. 1985;312:1011–15.
13. Hoofnagle JH, Davis GL, Schafer DF *et al.* Randomized trial of chlorambucil for primary biliary cirrhosis. Gastroenterology. 1986;91:1327–34.
14. Kaplan MM, Alling DW, Zimmerman HJ *et al.* A prospective trial of colchicine for primary biliary cirrhosis. N Engl J Med. 1986;315:1448–54.
15. Warnes TW, Smith A, Lee FI *et al.* A controlled trial of colchicine in primary biliary cirrhosis. Trial design and preliminary report. J Hepatol. 1987;5:1–7.
16. Bodenheimer H, Schaffner F, Pezzullo J. Evaluation of colchicine therapy in primary biliary cirrhosis. Gastroenterology. 1988;95:124–9.
17. Minuk GY, Bohme CE, Burgess E *et al.* Pilot study of cyclosporin A in patients with symptomatic primary biliary cirrhosis. Gastroenterology. 1988;95:1356–63
18. Wiesner RH, Ludwig J, Lindor KD *et al.* A controlled trial of cyclosporin in the treatment of primary biliary cirrhosis. N Engl J Med. 1990;322:1419–24.
19. Poupon R, Chrétien Y, Poupon RE *et al.* Is ursodeoxycholic acid an effective treatment for primary biliary cirrhosis? Lancet. 1987;1:834–6.
20. Poupon RE, Balkau B, Eschwège E *et al.* A multicenter, controlled trial of ursodiol for the treatment of primary biliary cirrhosis. N Engl J Med. 1991;324:1548–54.
21. Marteau P, Chazouillères O, Myara A *et al.* Effect of chronic administration of ursodeoxycholic acid on the ileal absorption of endogenous bile acids in man. Hepatology. 1990; 12:1206–8.
22. Stiehl A, Raedsch R, Rudolph G. Acute effects of ursodeoxycholic and chenodeoxycholic acid on the small intestinal absorption of bile acids. Gastroenterology. 1990;98:424–8.
23. Kitani K, Kanai S. Interactions between different bile salts in the biliary excretion of the rat. Chem Pathol Pharmacol. 1983;39:139–52.
24. Hillaire S, Ballet F, Franco D, Poupon R. Ursodeoxycholic acid does not protect human hepatocytes in primary culture against bile acid toxicity (Submitted).
25. Thibault N, Ballet F. Tauroursodeoxycholate inhibits actin filament alteration induced by cholestatic agents in isolated rat hepatocyte couplets. Hepatology. 1991;14:263 (abstract).
26. Poupon R, Chrétien Y, Parquet M *et al.* Hepatic transport of bile acids in the isolated perfused rat liver: structure–kinetics relationship. Biochem Pharmacol. 1988;37:209–12.
27. Haüssinger D. The hepatocellular hydratation state: a regulator of liver function cell function. Hepatol Rapid Lit Rev. 1992;6:9–13.
28. Calmus Y, Gane P, Rouger P, Poupon R. Hepatic expression of class I and class II major histocompatibility complex molecules in primary biliary cirrhosis: effect of ursodeoxycholic acid. Hepatology. 1990;11:12–15.
29. Calmus Y, Weill B, Ozier Y *et al.* Immunosuppressive properties of chenodeoxycholic and deoxycholic acids in the mouse. Gastroenterology. 1992;102:1371–7.
30. Hillaire S, Calmus Y, Boucher E *et al.* Bile acids modulate hepatocyte HLA class I expression in human hepatocytes by a transcriptional mechanism. Hepatology. 1991;14:99 (abstract).
31. Calmus Y, Guéchot J, Podevin P *et al.* Differential effects of chenodeoxycholic and ursodeoxycholic acids on interleukin 1, interleukin 6 and TNFα production by human

hepatocytes. Hepatology. 1992;16:719–23.
32. Spengler U, Möller A, Jung MC *et al.* T lymphocytes from patients with primary biliary cirrhosis produce reduced amounts of lymphotoxin, tumor necrosis factor and interferon-γ upon mitogen stimulation. J Hepatol. 1992;15:129–35.
33. Broome U, Eriksson LS, Sundin U, Sundquist K. Decreased in vitro production of tumor necrosis factor in primary biliary cirrhosis. Scand J Gastroenterol. 1992;27:124–8.
34. Shindo M, Mullin GW, Bergasa NV *et al.* Lack of cytokine mRNA expression in the liver of patients with primary biliary cirrhosis. Hepatology. 1992;14:62 (abstract).
35. Satoh J, Seino H, Abo T *et al.* Recombinant tumor necrosis factor α suppresses autoimmune diabetes in NOD mice. J Clin Invest. 1989;84:1345–8.

Index

acetaldehyde 288
acetaminophen 288
acetyltransferase, catalytic function inhibition by autoantisera 162
actin antibodies 210–11
acyclovir 122
Addison's disease 171
  arenal autoantibodies 260
adenine arabinoside 121
  monophosphate 121–2
adenovirus 118
  E1A protein 134–5
    oncogene 119
alcoholic liver disease 187
alcoholic liver injury 208
α-actinin 207
α-antitrypsin deficiency 208
anti-ASPG-R antibodies 185
anti-HBx 24
anti-idiopathic antibodies 167
anti-LC antibodies 185, 215–25
anti-liver cytosol antibodies 215–25
  diagnostic value 220–1
    autoimmune hepatitis 220–1
    hepatic GVHD 221
    viral hepatitis C 221
anti-LKM 1/anti-LC 1 autoantibodies 222, 223 (fig.)
anti-LP antibodies 185
anti-SLA antibodies 185
antigen-presenting cells, antigenic peptide/MHC class II
  complexes in 3–7
antineutrophil cytoplasmic antibodies 324–8
antisense oligonucleotides 123–4
aryl hydrocarbon (dioxin) receptor 264
ASC patients 33
asialoglycoprotein receptor (ASGPR) 227–30
  anti-ASGPR autoantibodies 228–9
  autoreactive T cell response 229–30
  regulation in chronic liver disease/ inflammation 227–8
astrocyte 12
autoantibodies 145–51
  generation hypotheses 161
  Sm antigen 146
  subcellular particles, function inhibition 147–8
autoantigens 145
  molecular biology *see* molecular biology
  subcellular particles associated 146–7
autoimmune (chronic active) hepatitis 102–3, 179–204
  –2, viral hepatitis C relationship 223–5
  age 180
  anti-liver cytosol antibodies 215–25
  autoantibodies 183–4
  autoantibodies for transfer ribonucleic acid 201–4
  biochemical liver tests 183
  causes 251 (table)
  cellular immune reactions 233–8
  complications 253–5
  'definite' 189
  disorders simulating 251 (table)
  family studies 245–6
  gender 180–1
  histology 186
  idiopathic (IACAH) 250–5
    subgroups 250
  immunogenetics 240–7
    HLA system 241–3
  immunoregulatory dysfunction 246–7
  international group recommendations 188–9
  'liver' autoantibodies associated 185 (table)
  natural history 247
  nuclear macromolecules (ANA) 193–6
    immunoblotting 200–1
  onset 180
  overlapping conditions 187
  pathogenic pathways 234 (table)
  population level studies 243–5
  'probable' 189
  signs 182–3
  subtypes 184–6
  symptoms 181–2
  therapy 251–5
  treatment 247

type I 243
type-2, LKM-1 autoantibodies associated, genetics 272–3
autoimmune disease 152
antinuclear antibodies 197–8
to: DNA, single/double/stranded 198
to: nuclear RNP 197–8
to: SS-A/SS-B 197
criteria 169 (table)
primary evidence 169 (table), 170
secondary evidence 169 (table), 172
vs. autoimmunity 169–72
autoimmune disorder 242
autoimmune liver syndromes 152
autoimmune thyroiditis 344
autoimmunity
immunological derangements 166–73
infection associated 172–3
specific therapy 173
autoimmunity vs. autoimmune disease 169–72
autonomous signalling via co-stimulatory molecule 12–13
azathioprine 462

B cells
abortion 166
anergized 166
antigen-specific 4–5
clonal anergy 166
clonal deletion 166
MHC class II with antigenic peptides in 4–5
tolerance 166–7
bacteria, protein expression vector systems 158 (table)
bacteriophage
lambda 153
T-7 158–9
Bacteroides spp. 335
biliary cirrhosis, primary 162, 170, 187, 208, 272, 297, 341–7, 373–80, 423–31
2-oxo acid dehydrogenase complexes 362–3, 373–4, 376 (table), 397
adhesion molecules 437–44
antigen presentation 444
E2 expression 438
MHC expression by biliary epithelial cells 442–4
age 343
animal models 410–20
investigations 411–13
results 413–15
anti-Sp-100 399–400
antibodies to nuclear membrane components 400
anticentromere 398–9
antimitochondrial antibodies (AMA) 343–4, 350–8, 361–2
cross reactivity with M2 antigens 365–6
M2/anti-M2 system 350–1
M4/anti-M4 system 351–3
M8/anti-M8 system 353–5
M9/anti-M9 system 355
associated diseases 344
autoimmunizing B-cell epitopes mapping 366–7
blood group antigens 437
cell surface expression of M2 autoantigens 378–9
cross-reactivity investigations 401–4
affinity separation of anti-PDC-E2/anti-centromere 404
affinity separation of anti-PDC-E2/anti-Sp-100 404
affinity separation of antibody population 403
antibodies analysis by ELISA 401
antibodies analysis by immunoblotting 401
antibodies analysis by immunofluorescence 401
CT scan 344
differential diagnosis 344–5
cholestatic drug reactions 344–5
cholestatic sarcoidosis 345
immune cholangiopathy 345
primary sclerosing cholangitis 345
endoscopic cholangiography 344
enzyme inhibition 375–6
epidemiology 345–7, 379–80
environmental factors 347
genetic factors 346–7
epitopes 376–7
gas transfer studies 344
HLA class I region 383–5, 389 (table)
HLA class II region 385–7, 388, 389
HLA class III region 387
immunogenetic influences 383–94
liver biopsy 341–2
lymphokine production 423–31
MHC antigens 435–7
mitochondria autoantibodies 345–6, 376 (table)
mitochondrial autoantigens, M2 363–5
nuclear autoantibodies 397–401
scleroderma overlap 398–9
serum biochemistry 343
sex 343
symptoms 343
T cells 367–8, 377–8
biliary tract surgery 303

centromere proteins 146 (table), 147
CH-B patients 32–5
IgG anti-HBe detection by E1A 32

chlorambucil 462
cholangiocarcinoma 299–300, 313
cholestatic sarcoidosis 345 (table)
chronic active hepatitis 206–12
  cytoskeleton 206–7
    antibodies 208–10
  smooth muscle antibodies 208
clofibric acid 264–5
co-stimulatory molecule via autonomous signalling 12–13
colchicine 462
collagen disease 193
complement deposition 172
corticosteroids 126, 462
Coxsackivirus B3, myocarditis 172–3
CREST syndrome 344
Crohn's disease 325
CRST (calcinosis–Raynaud phenomena–sclerodactyly–telangiectasia) 398–9
cyclosporine 462
CYP1A 264
CYP4A6 264
cytochrome P 450, naming 261
cytochrome P-450 21-hydroxylase enzymes 387
cytochrome P-450 259–65
  adverse drug reactions against 277–8
    investigations 279–80
    results 280–1
  amino acid sequences 261
  autoantibodies recognizing 262 (table)
  catalytic diversity 260–2
  detoxication of foreign compounds 260
  enzymes shared properties 259–60
  fatty acid sterols catabolism 260–1
  induction by environmental chemicals 263–5
  induction, mechanism 263 (table)
  reactive products, generation 262–3
  subfamilies 261
cytochrome P-450 II D6 269
  autoimmune hepatitis associated 269–74
  cellular immune response 271
  gene regulation 272
  hepatotropic viruses associated 273–4
  LKM-1 autoantibodies effect 270–1
  membrane expression 271
  target antigen of LKM-1 autoantibodies 270
cytochrome P-450 protein autoantibodies 160
cytokines 117, 118
  action on immune response/virus replication 117–19
  cascade 118
  problems mimicing 118–19
  synergism 119
  viral interaction 118–19
cytosol (rat liver), immunodiffusion in 216–18

D-penicillamine 462
deoxyacyclovir 122
dermatomyositis 145, 344
diabetes mellitus
  insulin dependent 171
  P-450 2E elevated 264
diclofenac 289
dideoxyadenine 122
dideoxycytodine 122
dideoxyguanosine 122
dideoxyinosine 122
dideoxynucleosides 122–3
dihydralazine 278
dihydrolipoamide acetyltransferases 362–3
dioxin (aryl hydrocarbon) receptor 264
DNA
  cDNA 156
  replication particles 146 (table)
drug-induced hepatotoxicities 278–9, 284–5
drug-induced immunoallergic hepatitis 278

Eα 131
Epstein–Barr virus 134
erythromycin 264

Factor B (properdin) 387
fibrillarin 146, 148
fluoro-iodo-arabinofurasyl-uracil (FIAU) 123
foscarnet (phosphonoformate) 122

ganciclovir 122
gastritis, atrophic 171
glomerulonephritis 172
  segmental necrotising 324
graft-versus-host disease, anti-liver cytosol antibodies 221
granulocyte-macrophage colony stimulating factor 126
Graves' disease 170

halothane hepatitis 278–9
  protein adducts associated 285–7
heat shock protein genes (hsp 70) 387
hepadnavirus 52 *see also* woodchuck hepatitis virus
hepatitis
  acute, drug induced 160
  autoimmune *see* autoimmune hepatitis
  chronic active *see* chronic active hepatitis
  idiopathic autoimmune 160
  lupoid 206, 208
hepatitis A virus (HAV) 85

histology 85–7
immunopathogenesis 85–8
hepatitis B core antigen, cellular immune reactions 39–46
hepatitis B virus 17, 48
acute infection 61
acute phase antibodies directed against conformational pre-S1 epitopes 21–2
anti-pre-S1 response 19–21
anti-pre-S2 following immunization with pre-S2 containing recombinant particles 22–3
antibodies to, during acute/chronic infection 17–18
antibodies to products of polymerase/X gene 24
antiviral agents 121–4
bone marrow transplantation 126–7
cellular immune reactions to envelope antigens 48–50
chronic carriage 61–2
escape mutants 69
genetic variability 61–76
genome 64–5
genome genetic organization 63 (fig.)
HbcAg 26, 28
HbeAg 26–35
CH-B carriers 32
T cell tolerance 29–32
immunological therapy 124–7
specific 126–7
immunological tolerance in chronic infection 26–35
immunomodulatory agents 124 (table)
infantile infection 27–9
innovative therapies 120–7
intrauterine infection 27–8
lymphocyte/macrophage infection 49
molecular technique 123–4
mutants in HbsAg-negative patients 71–3
mutants in HBsAG-positive patients 65–8
in Pre C sequence 65–8
mutants potential effects 73–5
mutation at nucleotide-126 69
mutations of core gene 68
mutations on Pre S/S genes 68–70
nucleoprotein, CD-4 mediated response specificity 45–6
placental transite 27–8
polymerase chain infection 62
pre C stop codon in acute hepatitis 66 (table)
pre C stop codon in chronic hepatitis 65 (table)
proteins 64–5
semiquantitative assessment of IgM anti-Hbc 23–4
spliced RNA, defective HBV particles 70, 71 (fig.)
terminal protein of polymerase gene 119
women as chronic carriers 27
Hepatitis C virus 90, 105
anti-liver cytosol antibodies 221
autoimmune hepatitis 2 relationship 223–5
autoimmunity 102–3
genetic organization 105–6
histology 96–9
immunology 102–3
immunopathology 96–9
monoclonal antibody production 107, 108 (fig.)
non-structural proteins, monoclonal antibodies 108–10
nucleoprotein, monoclonal specific antibody 110–11
polypeptides, antibody response 106–7
T-lymphocyte response 90–2
hepatobiliary inflammation/injury
experimental 332–7
potential mechanism 331
hepatocellular carcinoma, autoimmune phenomena 148–51
hepatocyte plasma membrane antigen antibodies 185
HLA system 240–3
human immunodeficiency virus (HIV) 49

IgG-class actin antibodies 211
IgG, anti-HBenv 32
IgM, low affinity antibodies 167
immune cholangiopathy 345
immunoabsorption, immunofluorescence with 218–20
immunoglobulin deposition 172
immunoglobulin, Fc portion 167
immunoprotection 139
immunosuppression, virus triggered acquired 141–2
interferon 117–19
α 117, 120, 125, 127
inducible gene activation 131, 132 (fig.)
virus elimination 131–5
α/β 117
antiviral agents 133–5
β 117, 125
gamma 117, 125, 424, 425 (fig.)
immunomodulator action 132–3
inhibitors 134–5
interferon stimulated gene factors (ISGF) 117–18
3α 117
(-1) 117

(−2) 117
(−3) 117–18
gamma 117
interferon-stimulated response element (ISRE) 117–18
interleukin-2 125
iproniazide 278

jejunal villus atrophy 344

kinetochore 146 (table)
Kupffer cells 336

Lac operon 153
Lac Z 153–4
levamisole 124
liver diseases 148
autoimmune, antibodies to recombinant proteins 198–200
liver transplantation 304–5
LKM-1 autoantibodies 184
lymphocytic choriomeningitis (mice) 139–40, 141–2, 143

MHC (HLA complex) 171
MHC-disease association 140
mixed connective tissue disease 145, 344
molecular biology
autoantigen analysis 152–63
clone characterization 156–7
expression cloning 153–6
recombinant protein expression systems 157–60
sera 156
cloned autoantigen applications 160–2
diagnostic antibody detection 160–1
epitope mapping 161–2
protein expression technology 159–60
molecular mimicry 242
multiple sclerosis 170
myasthenia gravis 152, 170

NOMAs (naturally occurring mitochondrial antibodies) 376
nuclear ribonucleoprotein particles, small 146 (table)
nucleolus organizer region-90 (NOR-90) 146, 148
nucleosome 146 (table)

2-oxo acid dehydrogenase complexes 362–3, 373–4, 376 (table), 397

pATH vector system 158
pathogen-derived protein (X) 31
pemphigus vulgaris 170
peptidoglycan–polysaccaride complexes (PG–PS) 335–6
pernicious anaemia 171
peroxisome proliferators 264–5
pET vector system 158–9
pGEX 158 (table), 159
phosphonoformate (foscarnet) 122
Phyllanthus amarus extracts 124–5
polymyositis 145
prednisolone 126
proctocolectomy 303–4
proliferating cell nuclear antigen (PCNA) 146
properdin (factor B) 387
pUC, pBluescript 158 (table)

repertoire renewal process 29
restriction fragment length polymorphism (RFLP) 424–6, 429–30
rheumatoid arthritis 179, 272, 344
ribavirin 123
ribosomes 146 (table)
rifampicin 264

Schistosoma japonicum 159
scleroderma 145, 146, 148, 344, 398–9
sclerosing cholangitis, primary 187, 295–305
ANCA/UC p-ANCA compared 325–7
animal models 331–7
antineutrophil cytoplasmic antibodies 324–8
associated diseases 296 (table)
biochemical abnormalities 296–7
cholangiocarcinoma 299–300, 313
complications 298–9
diagnosis/clinical features 295–6
extracellular matrix 313, 314 (fig.)
histological findings 297
histopathology 307–8
immune mechanisms 310–11, 312 (fig.)
immunogenetics 318–22
immunohistology 309–13
natural history 300–1
pathogenic factors 297–8
prognostic survival model 301
radiological findings 297
staging 308–9
therapy: medical/surgical 302–5
self vs. non-self 166
self-antigen 143
semiquantitative microparticle enzyme immunoassay 23
Shope fibroma virus 119
Sjögren's syndrome 145, 344
subacute sclerosing panencephalitis 272
superantigens 10–11
T cell activation by 10–12
suramin 122
systemic lupus erythematosus 145, 146, 170, 179, 272, 344

antibodies to tRNA 203
nephritis (mouse model) 424
systemic vasculitis 325

T cells
activated 7
activation by superantigens 10–12
antibody synthesis suppression 167
antigen recognition by 9–10
autoreactive response to ASGPR 229–30
CD-4-helper 168
cytotoxic resistant virus variants, viral escape 140–1
cytotoxic response
against HBV nucleocapsid antigens 39–40
molecular analysis of response to HBV nucleocapsid antigens 42–3
HBV tolerance 29
helper function 28–9, 30–3
HLA class II restricted response to HBV nucleocapsid antigens 44–5
immunosuppression, antigen specific 168
lymphokine production 423–31
mediated hepatitis 139–40
non-antigen-specific suppression 168
in primary biliary cirrhosis 367–8, 377–8
response to hepatitis C virus 90–2
tolerance 167 (table), 168–9
tolerance/response to viral antigens (transgenic mice) 142–3
TFA 286–7
anti-TFA antibodies 287–8
3-thiacytidine (3TC) 123
thymosin 125
thymus
cells 28–31
HBeAg access to 28
thyroglobulin 171
thyroiditis, chronic 171
tienilic acid 278
troleandromycin 264
tropomyosin 207
troponin 207
tumour necrosis factor-α (TNF-α) 336, 387, 424, 425 (fig.)
tumour necrosis factor-β (TNF-β) 387, 424, 425 (fig.)

U3 ribonucleoprotein particle 146 (table)
ulcerative colitis 297, 318, 325
antineutrophil cytoplasmic antibodies 324–8
ursodeoxycholic acid 459–61, 462–6
therapeutic strategies 462–6

vector lambda-gt-11 153
vinblastin 207
viral IL-10 118

Wegener's granulomatosis 324–5
Wilson's disease 187, 208, 251 (table)
woodchuck 52
immunobiology 54
woodchuck hepatitis virus (WHV) 52–9
immunomodulation 54–8
chronicity/post-exposure immunosuppression with CsA 56–7
chronicity/post-exposure priming with 55–6
chronicity/tolerance to e-antigen 54–5
late stage modulation of chronic WHV infection 57–8
liver disease 52
neonatal infection 52 (table)